The Clinical Guide to Child Psychiatry

The Clinical Guide
to
Child Psychiatry

EDITED BY
DAVID SHAFFER
ANKE A. EHRHARDT
LAURENCE L. GREENHILL

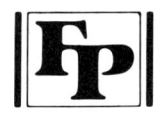

THE FREE PRESS
A Division of Macmillan, Inc.
NEW YORK

Collier Macmillan Publishers
LONDON

Copyright © 1985 by David Shaffer, Anke A. Ehrhardt, and Laurence L. Greenhill

All rights reserved. No part of this book may be reproduced or transmitted in any form or by any means, electronic or mechanical, including photocopying, recording, or by any information storage and retrieval system, without permission in writing from the Publisher.

The Free Press
A Division of Macmillan, Inc.
866 Third Avenue, New York, N. Y. 10022

Collier Macmillan Canada, Inc.

Printed in the United States of America

printing number
1 2 3 4 5 6 7 8 9 10

Library of Congress Cataloging in Publication Data

Main entry under title:

The Clinical guide to child psychiatry.

    Includes index.
    1. Child psychiatry—Handbooks, manuals, etc.
I. Shaffer, David   II. Ehrhardt, Anke A.   III. Greenhill, Laurence L. [DNLM: 1. Mental Disorders—in infancy & childhood. WS 350 C6415]
RJ499.3.C58   1984   618.92′89   84-47887
ISBN 0-02-929020-1

Contents

Introduction		*ix*
Editors and Contributors		*xv*

Part I THE TREATMENT OF SPECIFIC DISORDERS IN CHILDHOOD

DEVELOPMENTAL AND HABIT DISORDERS

1	The Tourette Syndrome and Other Tics *Donald J. Cohen, James F. Leckman, and Bennett A. Shaywitz*	3
2	Nocturnal Enuresis: Its Investigation and Treatment *David Shaffer*	29
3	Infantile Autism *Michael Rutter*	48
4	Childhood Language Disorders *Laura S. McKirdy*	79
5	Stammering and Stuttering *Barry Guitar*	97
6	Psychosocial Management of Short Stature *Heino F. L. Meyer-Bahlburg*	110
7	Abnormal Puberty: Psychological Implications and Treatment Issues *Anke A. Ehrhardt*	145

Affective and emotional disorders

8	Situational Fears and Object Phobias *Suzanne Bennett Johnson*	169
9	Major Depression in Children and Adolescents *Paul J. Ambrosini and Joaquim Puig-Antich*	182
10	Somatoform Disorders *Daniel T. Williams*	192
11	Childhood Obsessive-Compulsive Disorder *Judith L. Rapoport*	208
12	The Diagnosis and Treatment of Anorexia Nervosa *Katherine A. Halmi*	218

Conduct disorders

13	Aggressive Behavior in Middle Childhood *P. Chamberlain and G. R. Patterson*	229
14	The Hyperkinetic Syndrome *Laurence L. Greenhill*	251
15	Juvenile Delinquency *Dorothy Otnow Lewis*	276
16	Disturbance in School *Mark A. Stewart*	293

Special situations

17	Child Abuse and Neglect *Arthur Green*	315
18	Sexual Abuse in Childhood and Adolescence *Judith V. Becker and Linda J. Skinner*	336
19	The Divorcing Family: Its Evaluation and Treatment *Alan M. Levy*	353

Part II EVALUATING PROBLEMS—THE DIAGNOSTIC APPROACH

20	The Initial Clinical Evaluation of the Child *Richard A. Gardner*	371
21	Taking a History *Ian A. Canino*	393
22	The Physical Examination in Child Psychiatry *Laurence L. Greenhill*	409
23	Functional Analysis of Children's Behavior *Richard S. Feldman*	432

24	The Use of Psychological Tests in Clinical Practice with Children *Rachel Gittelman*	447
25	Organization and Use of *DSM-III* *Dennis P. Cantwell*	475

Part III GENERAL NOTES ON TREATMENT APPROACHES

26	Pediatric Psychopharmacology *Laurence L. Greenhill*	493
27	The Behavior Therapies *Tommie G. Cayton and Dennis C. Russo*	519
28	Family Therapy *Virginia Goldner*	539
29	Individual Psychotherapy with Young Children *Hector R. Bird*	554
30	Focused Short-term Treatment in Clinical Social Work *Bobba Jean Moody, Reggie Swenson, Anna Welton, and Penny Goldberg*	566
31	Establishment of Accessible and Relevant Services for Adolescents *Lorraine E. Henricks*	583
	Index	605

Introduction

THE GOAL OF EVERY CLINICIAN who treats a disturbed child is to arrive at an accurate diagnosis and to match this diagnosis with the most appropriate available treatment. In the field of child psychiatry, individual symptoms are rarely pathognomonic, so this process of assessment and treatment is often complex. Most clinicians intuitively adopt a systematic approach—setting a hypothesis, posing questions, making observations, and undertaking investigations to confirm or refute the hypothesis. The clinician with more knowledge of a particular disorder or group of disorders—the specialist or expert—conducts this assessment more efficiently, requiring fewer steps to arrive at a conclusion; he or she also knows of a broader set of treatment alternatives from which to choose the one that is most likely to help the child patient.

The purpose of this book is to have leading specialists explain their approach to the diagnostic procedure and describe what factors they take into account when selecting and providing a treatment. The emphasis is on practice although many of the contributors provide excellent and comprehensive reviews of etiology, epidemiology, and the results of treatment.

Advances in knowledge have made it clear that there is no single therapeutic approach to all child psychiatric problems. We have also learned that although every clinical case may have its idiosyncracies there are important commonalities among patients with similar types of problems and these can be used as a basis for predicting which types of treatment will be most appropriate. In other words, the well-trained child-mental-health professional should be able to decide on which of a variety of treatments is indicated and be in a position to apply that treatment. We expect that many of our readers, while being well versed in one or more therapeutic modalities, will be unfamiliar with others. We therefore include a group of chapters to introduce the reader to various assessment and treatment methods independent of specific diagnostic entities.

Part I deals with specific diagnostic groupings. It is divided into four major sections—developmental and habit disorders, affective and emotional disorders, conduct disorders, and special situations. Each of its 19 chapters formulates a practical approach for the practitioner.

Cohen, Leckman, and Shaywitz, at Yale's Child Study Center, have led the field of research in the biology and treatment of Tourette's Syndrome. In the first chapter, they share their cumulative experience in diagnosing and treating this condition. Shaffer's discussion (chapter 2) of enuresis provides information on the origins and clinical correlates of this common problem and gives a detailed guide to both pharmacological and behavioral treatment and to the factors which might lead a clinician to choose one or the other. Rutter has made a major contribution to knowledge of the epidemiology, cognitive features, and natural history of infantile autism. In chapter 3, he provides a comprehensive guide to the clinical features of this syndrome and explains how he approaches differential diagnosis and management of the pervasive developmental disorders, of which autism constitutes the most important example. McKirdy's chapter on childhood language disorders approaches deviant language development in childhood from a developmental perspective, showing how the disorders present to the practitioner in terms of history and profile, response to audiological and cognitive testing, and the social-emotional behaviors which may be associated with them. Guitar's chapter, which follows, provides a detailed assessment of the chronic stutterer, differentiating his pattern of distinctive misarticulations from the normal phase of dysfluency most children experience temporarily. The chapter closely assesses treatment methods, including fluencey-shaping techniques (metronome-induced rhythmic speech, prolonged speech, controlled respiration, and drug treatments), and attitude/stuttering modification approaches (psychotherapy, desensitization, "easier" stuttering) viewed in terms of the severity of the problem.

Chapter 6, by Meyer-Bahlburg, provides a guide to the assessment of the psychosocial sequalae to short stature, including a comprehensive list of both medical and psychiatric problems and problem-specific recommendations. Few clinicians realize the impact of short stature on the child's relations with family, peers, and other adults, and may, therefore, ignore the need for preventive counseling. Major problems are identified—shyness, withdrawal from peers, avoidance of contact with strangers, inhibition of mobility outside of the home, and harassment. Treatment counseling can take the form of role playing, training in how to "retease" harrassers, enrollment in karate, instruction in grooming and dressing skills, and introduction to self-help organizations. Chapter 7, by Ehrhardt, on abnormal puberty, deals with common behavioral problems experienced by adolescents who undergo normal puberty, as well as the hormonal abnormalities that may occur for some young people, and their impact on behavior. This chapter gives the clinician overview of treatment approaches for adolescents who have to cope with too early or too late puberty, or with gynecomastia, hirsutism, and Turner Syndrome.

The second section addresses the various affective disorders found in children. Johnson (chapter 8) reviews the epidemiology and etiology of object and situational fears and phobias, and the value of different behavior therapy approaches in treating them. A major development in recent years has been interest in the identification of major depressive disorder (MDD) in children. The notion that depression can occur only after adolescence is no longer held. The work of Puig-Antich and other investigators has been very significant in this reappraisal. We are pleased to include chapter 9, written by Ambrosini and Puig-Antich, which outlines the clinical features of MDD and reviews the impact of the disorder on psychosocial relationships, neuroendocrine rhythms, sleep patterns, and hormonal responses, as well as the value of tricyclic antidepressant medication.

The somatoform disorders include conversion phenomena, somatization disorder (Briquet's syndrome), and hypochrondriasis. In chapter 10, Williams provides an excellent guide to the very difficult problem of differentiating these disorders from physical illness and to their treatment with a number of therapies, including hypnosis.

In chapter 11, Rapoport guides the clinician in the diagnosis and treatment of children with obsessive-compulsive disorders. Childhood obsessive illness results in severe impairment which affects the whole family. The chapter includes a section on working with parents and ward staff. Affective disorders involving preoccupations with body weight and food—bulimia and anorexia nervosa—are common psychiatric problems in adolescents. Halmi's chapter (12) highlights methods of assessment and treatment, particularly the use of reinforcement techniques in a hospital setting.

The conduct or behavior disorders comprise the largest number of referrals to child guidance centers and practitioners and are discussed in the third section of Part I. Clinical features frequently include aggressive behavior, and we consider ourselves fortunate to be able to include a contribution by one of the leading experts in this field. Patterson's "coercion theory" of children's aggression has provided a major advance in our understanding of this problem and has also given a rationale for intervention. In chapter 13, Chamberlain and Patterson describe the ways in which social learning principles are applied in treatment and give details of the special assessment procedures required, with a step-by-step guide to the program's implementation.

Although many American practitioners tend to diagnose Attention Deficit Disorder with Hyperactivity (ADDH), this disorder contains heterogeneous subgroups, including the milder conduct disorders, classroom-based problems, aggressivity, and adolescent violence. Family circumstance, social ecology, treatment response, and eventual outcome differ for these subtypes. Greenhill's chapter (14) provides a detailed guide for assessing and treating the child with ADDH or with hyperactivity. Since an accurate diagnosis depends heavily on history taking methods, Greenhill provides a thorough outline for a complete interview, including a history of prior treatments. The chapter concludes with a section on ways to determine a pre-treatment baseline in terms of a mental status examination, psychometric tests, a neurological evaluation, and the use of parent and teacher global rating forms. Methods are outlined for introducing psychostimulants and for explaining this treatment to the parent and child in an appropriate manner.

When the child's conduct disorder reaches severe proportions, he will probably be identified by the legal system and be classified with the administrative term, "delinquent." In chapter 15, Lewis delineates a major public health concern, since the violent adolescent offender creates problems greater than the numbers of individuals involved would suggest. She begins by reviewing the medical, psychiatric, and neurological correlates of delinquency. The assessment section highlights the use of medical and neurological examinations so important in this area, and the mental status and psychological evaluations necessary to uncover psychotic cases, who can then benefit from antipsychotic medications. In chapter 16, Stewart describes the range of conduct problems which are seen in the classroom and how they are best assessed.

The last section of Part I includes three special situations which affect ever-increasing numbers of children and adolescents. Chapter 17, by Green, describes the diagnosis and impact of physical abuse and neglect, provides a list of physical findings, and explains the process of differential diagnosis and intervention strategies. Becker and Skinner (chapter 18) deal with the problem of sexual molestation of children and adolescents, indicating diagnostically relevant behavior symptoms and the ways in which they are elicited. Treatment approaches include individual therapy and group therapy of the affected child, and counseling and family therapy for the parents. In chapter 19, Levy provides an excellent guide to assessment in preparation of an expert opinion on custody and visitation rights for divorcing parents. He discusses the criteria to be considered in making a recommendation and the clinician's therapeutic role in this adversarial situation.

Part II describes common assessment techniques applied in child psychiatry. Gardner (chapter 20) describes the practical techniques used in examining young children. Taking a history for a child patient will include calling on several informants (e.g., parents, teacher, and child) to supplement any account given solely by the child. In chapter 21, Canino provides a systematic history-taking approach which should result in a broad and accurate appraisal of the child's problem. The physical examination of the behaviorally disturbed patient is often overlooked. In chapter 22, Greenhill summarizes a quick but thorough physical approach that gathers most of the data needed to carry out a comprehensive examination of the child. It incorporates many features from the pediatric neurological examination as well as aspects of developmental tests, such as the Denver Developmental. Practitioners should find this section full of practical hints.

The increasing use of behavioral techniques for children requires a somewhat different approach to history taking, one that emphasizes precise examples of the problem behavior, its contingencies and consequences—the so-called "functional analysis." Feldman's chapter (23) provides a guide to the selection of target behaviors, the use of various observational methods, and the systematic rating of the behaviors which will be the focus of the treatment.

Psychological testing of children may be invaluable or misleading. The ability to use the information provided by standard tests critically and appropriately is an essential part of any mental health practice with children. In chapter 24, Gittelman provides an incisive guide to this process, highlighting the strengths of some procedures and the weaknesses of others.

Assessment ends with the assignment of a diagnosis and a prescription for treatment. The organization and use of *DSM-III*, the diagnostic scheme currently in broadest use, is described in detail in chapter 25 by Cantwell, who has played a leading role in both the development and testing of *DSM-III*.

Part III deals with specific treatment approaches. Greenhill (chapter 26) provides a practical overview of management with psychoactive drugs. He addresses pitfalls of the "drug" approach, such as "false medicalization" of child psychiatric disorders, inattention to parental concerns about medications, false beliefs, and negative placebo effects. Placebo trials, drug counseling for the child patient, and management of the difficult adolescent patient are discussed. Controversies affecting the stimulants, such as their alleged diagnostic and age specificity, the so-called dissociation of cognitive and social drug response, and interactions of stimulants with other therapies, are addressed. Practical methods of treatment with other drug classes are provided, including the use of tricyclics, neuroleptics, lithium, propranalol, carbamazepine, and clonodine.

Cayton and Russo have written widely on the application of behavior therapy in child psychiatric disorder. In chapter 27, they review the historical development of behavior therapy and provide an overview of a number of behavioral techniques including desensitization, cognitive, operant, and biofeedback methods. Goldner's chapter (28) reviews the implementation of family therapy as a diagnostic tool, using some of the recent techniques developed by Minuchin and others. In Chapter 29, Bird reviews the priniciples of individual psychotherapy, guiding the reader as to the timing and circumstances in which this type of treatment is indicated. The case examples presented illustrate this approach and can be used as useful teaching models. Chapter 30, by Moody, Swenson, Welton, and Goldberg, discusses the concept of focused short-term social work treatment as a method which gets results. This therapeutic approach is successful because it sets up a workable contract between patient and therapist which targets a reachable goal for the patient.

Henricks (chapter 31), one of the founders of the adolescent outreach program, "The Door," in New York City, introduces the reader to new ways of reaching young people for whom traditional models of psychiatric care have been unsuccessful. Henricks identifies specific principles of service delivery which should be considered in the development of programs for adolescents, such as accessibility, confidentiality, expense, youth participation, and comprehensiveness of services.

The editors hope that this book will be useful to a wide range of professionals at different levels of experience and be a guide to the current knowledge, diagnosis, and treatment of child psychiatric disorders.

The preparation of every book requires the cooperation and hard work of many people. We want to thank all the contributors, as well as Dorothy A. Lewis for her editorial assistance, and our agent, Sandra A. Elkin.

David Shaffer
Anke A. Ehrhardt
Laurence L. Greenhill
New York City, 1984

Editors and Contributors

DAVID SHAFFER, M.D., is Professor of Clinical Psychiatry and Pediatrics at the College of Physicians and Surgeons of Columbia University, and the Director of the Department of Child Psychiatry at the New York State Psychiatric Institute and at Columbia-Presbyterian Medical Center. He has carried out research into the epidemiology of child and adolescent suicide and runaway behavior; the classification and treatment of enuresis; the psychiatric effects of localized head injury; the role of neurological soft signs in the development of psychopathology in children; and the reliability and validity of diagnostic categorization in child psychiatry.

ANKE A. EHRHARDT, Ph.D., is a clinical psychologist with special expertise in the diagnosis and treatment of behavior disturbance in children and adolescents with endocrine abnormalities, and of sex and gender problems. She is currently Professor of Clinical Psychology in the Department of Psychiatry at the College of Physicians and Surgeons of Columbia University and a research scientist at the New York State Psychiatric Institute. She previously co-authored (with John Money) *Man & Woman, Boy & Girl. The Differentiation and Dimorphism of Gender Identity from Conception to Maturity* (1972). Dr. Ehrhardt has done extensive research in developmental psychoendocrinology.

LAURENCE L. GREENHILL, M.D., is a child psychiatrist with special expertise in child psychopharmacology. He is currently Assistant Professor of Clinical Psychiatry at the College of Physicians and Surgeons of Columbia University and serves as Director of the Children's Inpatient Research Unit at the New York State Psychiatric Institute. He previously co-authored (with Baron Shopsin, M.D.) *The Psychobiology of Childhood* (1984). Dr. Greenhill has done research in childhood psychoneuroendocrinology and in the clinical pharmacology of stimulant medication in children.

PAUL J. AMBROSINI, M.D., is Research Fellow in Child Psychiatry at the New York State Psychiatric Institute. His major fields of interest are the psychopharmacology and psychoneuroendocrinology of childhood and major depressive disorders of childhood.

JUDITH V. BECKER, Ph.D., is Director of the Sexual Behavior Clinic at the New York State Psychiatric Institute and Associate Professor of Clinical Psychiatry at the College of Physicians and Surgeons of Columbia University. She has conducted extensive studies in the area of sexual victimization and sexual aggression.

HECTOR R. BIRD, M.D., is Associate Professor of Psychiatry at the University of Puerto Rico School of Medicine and Director of Child Psychiatry at the same institution. He has written on the assessment of children and on transcultural child psychiatry.

IAN A. CANINO, M.D., has held multiple administrative and training positions at Albert Einstein College of Medicine, New York and is presently Deputy Training Director and Associate Clinical Professor in the Department of Child Psychiatry, Columbia University.

DENNIS P. CANTWELL, M.D., is Joseph-Campbell Professor of Child Psychiatry and Director of Residency Training in Child Psychiatry at the Neuropsychiatric Institute, UCLA. He is engaged in research in psychiatric disorders in children with communication problems and has published extensively in this area.

TOMMIE G. CAYTON, Ph.D., is Director of the Behavioral Health Psychology Program at Wilford Hall, USAF Medical Center, San Antonio, Texas. He developed and is Director of the Behavioral Medicine Program for postdoctoral fellows in the Air Force. He has been a school psychologist and has been involved with parent training and classroom management for many years.

PATRICIA CHAMBERLAIN, Ph.D., is Clinic Director of the Oregon Social Learning Center at Eugene, and is currently in charge of the therapy staff there, as well as the Monitor Program. Her current research interest is the measurement and modification of client resistance.

DONALD J. COHEN, M.D., is Director of the Yale Child Study Center and Professor of Pediatrics, Psychiatry, and Psychology at Yale University, as well as Director of the Yale Mental Health Clinical Research Center. He is engaged in research in the Tourette Syndrome and in autism, and has published extensively in these areas.

RICHARD S. FELDMAN, Ph.D., is a research scientist in the Department of Child Psychiatry at the New York State Psychiatric Institute where he teaches and consults in the area of child behavior therapy. He has done basic and applied research in psycholinguistics, verbal conditioning, schizophrenic speech, and behavior modification with children.

RICHARD A. GARDNER, M.D., is Clinical Professor of Psychiatry in the Department of Child Psychiatry at the College of Physicians and Surgeons of Columbia University. He is the author of numerous books and articles in the field, of which the most pertinent to this volume is *Psychotherapeutic Approaches to the Resistant Child* (1975).

RACHEL GITTELMAN, Ph.D., is Professor of Clinical Psychology at the College of Physicians and Surgeons of Columbia University, and the Director of the Department of Psychology at the New York State Psychiatric Institute and at the Columbia-Presbyterian Medical Center. She has conducted research in the diagnosis and treatment of several childhood disorders, including attention deficit, specific developmental, and anxiety disorders.

PENNY GOLDBERG, M.S.W., is Associate Director, Social Work Services, Hospital for Joint Diseases Orthopaedic Institute, New York, N.Y., and is on the faculty of the Mt. Sinai School of Medicine, Department of Community Medicine. Ms. Goldberg has worked extensively with emotionally disturbed and developmentally disabled children and has lectured in the areas of child maltreatment and the impact of a handicapped child on the family system.

VIRGINIA GOLDNER, Ph.D., is Assistant Clinical Professor of Psychiatry at the Albert Einstein College of Medicine, Lecturer in Psychiatry at Columbia University, and Assistant in Psychiatry at the Columbia-Presbyterian Medical Center. She has published widely on family therapy, the psychology of women, and social psychiatry.

ARTHUR GREEN, M.D., is Associate Clinical Professor of Psychiatry at Columbia University College of Physicians and Surgeons, and Director of the Columbia-Presbyterian Family Center. He is also Clinical Director of the Therapeutic Nursery in Babies Hospital, New York City, and is on the faculty of the Columbia Psychoanalytic Center.

BARRY GUITAR, Ph.D., is Associate Professor of Communication Science and Disorders at the University of Vermont, Burlington. His particular area of interest is stuttering in children, about which he has written extensively. His most recent book, cowritten with Theodore Peters, is *Stuttering: An Integration of Contemporary Therapies* (1980).

KATHERINE A. HALMI, M.D., is Associate Professor of Psychiatry at Cornell University Medical College, and Director of Eating Disorders Program at New York Hospital–Westchester Division. She has published extensively on anorexia nervosa and bulimia nervosa.

LORRAINE E. HENRICKS, M.D., is president of the International Institute for Development of Youth Services. She was the founder and for many years administrative director of The Door—A Center of Alternatives, a pioneering program in New York City which identified adolescents in crisis and met their emotional and health needs with a wide variety of activities, rehabilitative services, and outreach programs.

SUZANNE BENNETT JOHNSON, Ph.D., is Associate Professor of Clinical Psychology in Psychiatry at Florida Medical Center, Gainesville. She is also Director of the Diabetes Project Unit, an inpatient treatment program for youngsters in poor diabetic control with emotional and behavioral problems. Her research and clinical activities focus on psychological correlates of children's health with a particular interest in the chronically ill population. Her research on diabetes in children with emotional and behavioral problems has been published widely.

JAMES F. LECKMAN, M.D., is Associate Professor of Psychiatry and Pediatrics at the Child Study Center, Yale University School of Medicine. He is also Associate Director for Neuropsychiatric Research at the Children's Clinical Research Center at the Yale University School of Medicine.

ALAN M. LEVY, M.D., is Associate Clinical Professor of Psychiatry at the College of Physicians and Surgeons of Columbia University, and Chief, Forensic Child Psychiatry Clinic, the Columbia-Presbyterian Medical Center. His published articles have been mainly on child custody.

DOROTHY OTNOW LEWIS, M.D., is Professor of Psychiatry, New York University School of Medicine, and Clinical Professor of Psychiatry, Yale University Child Study Center. She is the author of *Delinquency and Psychopathology* (1976) and editor of *Vulnerabilities to Delinquency* (1981).

LAURA S. MCKIRDY, Ph.D., is Principal of Lake Drive School for Hearing Impaired Children, Mountain Lakes, N.J. She has worked extensively with speech- and language-disordered children in hospital and school settings.

HEINO F. L. MEYER-BAHLBURG, Dr. rer. nat., is a research scientist at the New York State Psychiatric Institute, Associate Professor of Clinical Psychology in the Department of Psychiatry at the College of Physicians and Surgeons of Columbia University, and Pediatric Behavioral Endocrinologist in Psychiatry Service at The Presbyterian Hospital in New York City. His major research is in the area of developmental psychoendocrinology.

BOBBA JEAN MOODY, M.S.W., is Director of the Social Work Department and of Social Work Training at the New York State Psychiatric Institute and Hospital and is Adjunct Associate Professor at the Columbia University School of Social Work and Assistant Clinical Professor in the Department of Psychiatry, College of Physicians and Surgeons of Columbia University. She holds the office of First Vice President in the New York State Society of Clinical Social Work Psychotherapists, is a consultant to Spence-Chapin Services to Families, and maintains a small private practice of psychoanalytic psychotherapy.

G. R. PATTERSON, Ph.D., is conducting full-time research at the Oregon Social Learning Center at Eugene. His last decade's work has been devoted to naturalistic observation techniques, development of assessment instruments, therapy process and maintenance of effects, and especially to evolving and expanding social learning theory. He is currently working on a ten-year longitudinal study of juvenile delinquency and a study of families' coping with post-separation stress.

JOAQUIM PUIG-ANTICH, M.D., is Chief of Child and Adolescent Psychiatry and Visiting Professor of Child Psychiatry at the Western Psychiatric Institute, University of Pittsburgh School of Medicine. He has conducted extensive research and written widely on affective disorders of children.

JUDITH L. RAPOPORT, M.D., is Chief, Child Psychiatry Branch, National Institute of Mental Health. She specializes in the biological aspects of child psychiatry.

DENNIS C. RUSSO, Ph.D., is Director of the Behavioral Medicine Program, Department of Psychiatry, The Children's Hospital, Boston, and Assistant Professor of Psychology, Harvard Medical School. He has published extensively on the psychological management of chronic diseases in children and, with Dr. James Varnie, is co-editor of a recent book, *Behavioral Pediatrics: Research and Practice* (1982).

MICHAEL RUTTER, M.D., is Professor of Child Psychiatry and Honorary Director of the Medical Research Council Child Psychiatry Unit at the Institute of Psychiatry, London. He is Honorary Consultant, The Maudsley Hospital, London. Dr. Rutter has been involved in studying the nature of autistic children's problems and their treatment over the last twenty years.

BENNETT A. SHAYWITZ, M.D., is Director of Pediatric Neurology at Yale New Haven Hospital, Yale University School of Medicine. He is the editor of *Learning Disorders,* the spring 1984 issue of *Pediatric Clinics of North America,* and author of "Diagnosis and management of attention deficit disorders: A pediatric perspective," in that issue.

LINDA J. SKINNER, Ph.D., is Assistant Professor of Psychology at the University of Hartford, Hartford, Connecticut. She works in the area of sexual victimization.

MARK A. STEWART, M.D., is Ida P. Haller Professor of Child Psychiatry at the University of Iowa College of Medicine, Iowa City, Iowa, and head of its Division of Child Psychiatry. His research has focused mainly on the metabolism of peripheral nerve and on aggressiveness in children.

REGGIE SWENSON, M.S.W., is Assistant Director of Social Work for the Children's Service at the New York State Psychiatric Institute, and Instructor in Clinical Social Work, Psychiatry, at Columbia University. He serves as a Field Instructor for both Fordham University and Columbia University Schools of Social Work. In 1982, Mr. Swenson became part-time Co-Director of the North Rockland Family Counseling Center where he utilizes task-focused counseling techniques in his work with children and their parents.

ANNA WELTON, M.S.W., is Assistant Director of Social Work for Adult Clinical Research Services at the New York State Psychiatric Institute and educational coordinator for social work students and staff. She is Adjunct Assistant Professor at the Columbia University School of Social Work and Instructor in Clinical Social Work in Psychiatry at the College of Physicians and Surgeons. Ms. Welton is in private practice in New York City.

DANIEL T. WILLIAMS, M.D., is Associate Clinical Professor of Psychiatry at the College of Physicians and Surgeons of Columbia University, and Director of Pediatric Neuropsychiatry Services at Columbia-Presbyterian Medical Center. He is the author of articles on hypnosis, psychiatric aspects of seizure disorders, and treatment of rage outbursts.

Part I

THE TREATMENT OF SPECIFIC DISORDERS IN CHILDHOOD

DEVELOPMENTAL AND HABIT DISORDERS

1

The Tourette Syndrome and Other Tics

DONALD J. COHEN / JAMES F. LECKMAN / BENNETT A. SHAYWITZ

TICS, OR HABIT SPASMS, are rapid, rhythmic, involuntary movements of individual muscle groups, but they are more easily recognized than precisely defined. Disorders involving tics generally are divided into categories according to age of onset, duration of symptoms, and the presence of vocal, or phonic tics, in addition to motor tics.

Transient tic disorders often begin during the early school years and can occur in up to 15% of all children. Common tics include eye blinking, nose puckering, grimacing, and squinting. Transient vocalizations are less common and include sucking air, coughing, throat clearing, humming, or other distracting noises. Childhood tics may be bizarre, such as licking the palm or poking and pinching the genitals. Transient tics last only weeks or a few months and usually are not associated with specific behavioral or school problems. They are especially noticeable with heightened excitement or fatigue. As with all tic syndromes, boys are three to four times more often afflicted. Familial aggregation of transient tics are also seen. While transient tics by definition do not persist for more than a year, it is not uncommon for a child to have a series of transient tics over the course of several years.

Chronic tic disorders are differentiated from transient ones not only by their duration over many years but by their relatively unchanging character. While transient tics come and go, with sniffing replaced by forehead furrowing or finger snapping, chronic tics such as hemifacial contortion or blinking may persist unchanged for years. Chronic multiple tics (CMT) suggest that an individual has several chronic motor tics. Where to draw the lines between transient tics, chronic tics, and chronic multiple tics is often not an easy task.

Jill Detlor, R.N., Sharon Ort, R.N., and J. Gerald Young, M.D., were essential to the formulation of our approach to assessment and treatment. This chapter reflects the ongoing work of the Yale Child Study Center Tourette Syndrome research group; we appreciate the collaboration with David Pauls, Ph.D., Kenneth Kidd, Ph.D., George Anderson, Ph.D., Diane Harcherik, M.A., Arlen Price, Ph.D., Emanuel Wolff, M.D., Martin Kremenitzer, M.D., Fred Volkmar, M.D., Thomas Lowe, M.D., and others who have shared in the work of this group. The research was supported by the Gateposts Foundation, Mental Health Clinical Research Center grant MH 30929, the Children's Clinical Research Center grant RR 00125, NICHD grant HD-03008, and Mr. Leonard Berger.

The disorder of Gilles de la Tourette, or the Tourette syndrome (TS), can be the most debilitating tic syndrome and is characterized by multiform, frequently changing motor and phonic tics and a range of behavioral symptoms. The prevailing diagnostic criteria include an age of onset between two and fifteen years; recurrent, involuntary, rapid, purposeless motor movements affecting multiple muscle groups; multiple vocal tics; ability to suppress movements voluntarily for minutes to hours; variations in the intensity of the symptoms over weeks to months (waxing and waning); and a duration of more than one year (American Psychiatric Association, 1980, Shapiro et al., 1978; Friedhoff and Chase, 1982). While these criteria appear basically valid, they are not the final word. First, there have been cases of TS that emerged later than age fifteen. Second, the concept of "involuntary" may be hard to define operationally, since some patients experience their tics as having a volitional component—a capitulation to an internal urge for motor discharge accompanied by psychological tension and anxiety. Finally, as will be discussed, the diagnostic criteria do not adequately portray the full range of behavioral difficulties observed in TS patients, such as attentional problems, compulsions, and obsessions.

CLINICAL EXPRESSION OF TS

The polymorphous motor and phonic tics of TS can be characterized by their frequency, complexity, and the degree to which they cause impairment or disrupt the patient's ongoing activities and daily life (see Table 1-1) (Cohen et al., 1982). Extremely frequent tics, occurring twenty to thirty times a minute, such as mouth puckering, nodding, or arm flexion, may be less disruptive than an infrequent tic, occurring several times an hour, such as slamming to the ground or screaming.

Simple motor tics are fast, darting, and meaningless muscular events, but they can be painful (such as jaw snapping) and embarrassing. They are easily distinguished from simple muscular twitches or rapid fasciculations, e.g., of the eyelid or lip. Complex motor tics often are slower, more purposeful in appearance, and more easily described by terms used for deliberate actions (see Table 1-2). They can be virtually any type of movement that the body can produce—gyrating, hopping, clapping, thrusting, tensing arm or neck muscles, fist clenching, and kicking. A patient may hyperextend his thumb or wrist until becoming

TABLE 1-1.
Tourette's Syndrome: Range of Symptoms

Motor
      Simple motor tics: Fast, darting, meaningless
      Complex motor tics: Slow, purposeful

Phonic
      Simple phonic tics: Sounds, noises
      Complex phonic tics: Linguistically meaningful utterances
          Words, phrases, statements
          Coprolalia

Behavioral
      Attention deficit disorder + hyperactivity
      Obsessions and compulsions
      Emotional irritability and lability
      Mirroring and echophenomena

TABLE 1-2.
Motor Symptoms

Simple Motor Tics: Fast, Darting, Meaningless
    Eye blinking, grimacing, nose twitching, lip pouting, shoulder shrugs, arm jerks, head jerks, abdominal tensing, kicks, finger movements, jaw snaps, tooth clicking, frowning, tensing parts of body, rapid jerking of any part of body

Complex Motor Tics: Slower, Purposeful
    Hopping, clapping, touching objects or others or self, throwing, arranging, gyrating and bending, "dystonic" postures, biting mouth or lip or arm, banging head, thrusting arms, striking out, picking scabs, writhing movements, rolling eyes to the ceiling, holding funny expressions, sticking out tongue, kissing, pinching, writing over-and-over the same letter or word, pulling back on a pencil while writing, tearing paper or books, Copropraxia: Giving the finger—cursing through gestures

---

double-jointed, control his diaphragm, cough like a seal, or belch and pass wind; he may kiss people and try to touch them on specific parts of their bodies (usually the breasts or butt, but displaced often to other parts), or punch at the wall. At some point in the continuum of complex motor tics, the term *compulsion* seems appropriate for capturing the organized, ritualistic character of the actions. The need to arrange objects neatly, to do and then redo or undo the same action a certain number of times (e.g., stretching out an arm ten times before writing), or to stand up and push a chair into "just the right position" is compulsive in quality and is accompanied by considerable internal "resistance." These complex motor tics may greatly impair schoolwork, e.g., when a child must tear pages out of textbooks, scribble over a sentence he has just written, stab at his workbook with a pencil, or go over the same letter so many times that the paper is worn thin. Self-destructive behaviors also occur—such as head banging, eye poking, picking at scabs, and sticking oneself with sharp objects.

Phonic tics extend over a similar spectrum of complexity and disruption as motor tics (see Table 1-3). With simple phonic tics, patients emit linguistically meaningless sounds or noises, such as hissing, coughing, spitting, sucking, and sniffing. Complex phonic tics involve linguistically meaningful words, phrases, or sentences, e.g., "Wow!" "Oh, boy, now you've said it," "Yup, that's it," "But, but . . ." Phonic symptoms may interfere with the

TABLE 1-3.
Phonic Symptoms

Simple Phonic Symptoms: Fast, Meaningless Sounds
    Whistling, coughing, sniffling, spitting, screeching, barking, grunting, gurgling, clacking, hawking, hissing, sucking, uh-uh, eeee, ah-uh, ah, and innumerable other sounds

Complex Phonic Symptoms
    Words, Phrases, Statements
        Shut up. Stop that. Oh Ok. I've got to.
        I'm going to get better—right? Right.
        What makes me do this? How about it.
        Now you've seen it, all right, oh boy.
    Rituals
        Counting rituals. Repeating a phrase until it is "just right."
    Speech Atypicalities
        Unusual rhythms, tone, accents, intensity of speech
    Coprolalia: Obscene and aggressive words and statements

smooth flow of speech and resemble a stammer, stutter, or speech clutter. Often, but not always, phonic symptoms occur at points of linguistic transition at the beginning of a sentence, where there may be blocking or difficulties in the initiation of speech, or at phrase transitions. Patients suddenly may alter speech volume, slur a phrase, emphasize a word, or assume an accent.

The most socially distressing complex phonic symptom is coprolalia, the explosive utterance of foul or dirty words or more elaborate sexual and aggressive statements (see Table 1-4). While coprolalia occurs in only a minority of TS patients—from 5 to 40%, depending on the clinical series—it is the most well-known, pathognomonic symptom of TS. Early in the course of coprolalia, a child may mumble the beginnings of words ("fff," "sh, sh") in order to camouflage what he feels impelled to exclaim. Finally, the curses no longer can be contained within; even when he is not particularly excited or angry, he will shout the full explicative. While watching television, playing, sitting at his desk, curse words will pop into his mind and just as quickly be expressed. A child may be very much bothered, as well, by mental coprolalia, incessant or obsessional obscene thoughts or images.

After the emergence of single-word coprolalia, some patients progress to more elaborate forms in which their swearing is embedded in longer statements or takes the form of sexual, hostile, and insulting comments. At first, these comments may be considered by the patient's family as rudeness until their compulsive quality becomes apparent. In its most richly articulated form, coprolalia includes the accurate but socially unacceptable description of another person's appearance, social status, or behavior—"You're the fattest fucking son-of-a-bitch I've ever seen," "What tits," "They should take cripples out and shoot 'em," "Donald Duck . . . Donald . . . bald-headed duck." Needless to say, the response of those to whom such comments are addressed may be socially disastrous and even dangerous for the patient. Yet, this strong social response may be a necessary condition for the patient

TABLE 1-4.
Coprolalia: Obscene and Aggressive Words, Statements, Communications

Sexual and Body Curses
    Shit, fuck, fart, prick, ass, cunt, bastard, asshole, smell my ass, suck my dick, up yours, eat it, piss head, crap, snot

Theological Curses
    Goddamn it. Jesus Christ. Christ.

Combinations
    Fucking Christ shit hole.
    Suck God's dick, asshole, motherfucker.

Racial, Ethnic, and Physical
    Nigger, kike, wop, fatso, cripple, retard, gork, Puerto Ricans eat it!

Complex Aggressive and Sexual Descriptions
    You bald-headed doctor son of a bitch.
    You sickening fat slob. Get your fat ass cut off.
    I'd like to knock your head off, asshole.
    Do you suck your nurse's cunt, Dr. Quinn?

Complex Oppositionals
    I love you, I hate you. You're full of crap—
    I'm sorry. What did I say?

Coproxaxia: Obscene gestures
    Giving the finger. Giving the hand.

to feel the full relief of the inner tension leading up to the tic explosion, as will be described later.

Even for TS patients who recognize themselves to be impulsive or labile, the more complex coprolalic symptoms are felt to be dystonic and to carry with them a greater urgency than their usual ("That's the way I am") conduct. However, at times, the patient and his family may not recognize the symptomatic nature of his short fuse and argumentativeness. This low threshold for arguing and irritability may be dramatically observed in family sessions when there is more than one family member with TS.

Associated Disorders

TS patients often have behavioral difficulties that would justify another psychiatric diagnosis. While there is still uncertainty about whether these difficulties are intrinsic to TS, secondary results, or coincidental, newer genetic and developmental evidence suggests that attentional and compulsive disorders are manifestations of the underlying, genetic TS diathesis or are closely related to it.

The most common behavioral problems associated with TS in childhood involve the regulation of attention and activity. At least 50% (and up to 60% in some series) of children with TS satisfy the diagnostic criteria for attention deficit disorder (poor attention, difficulty concentrating, distractibility, impulsivity) with hyperactivity (fidgety movements, ceaseless activity). The ADD of these patients may originate early in the preschool years and precede the onset of tics, or when tics are so mild they are noticed only in retrospect. Later, ADD tends to worsen with tic severity. This increasing difficulty with attention appears to reflect the underlying psychobiological dysfunctions involving inhibition in TS and may be exacerbated by the strain in attending to the outer world while working hard to remain quiet and still. Attentional problems persist during periods of relative tic remission. While most TS patients do not have primary learning disabilities, and, as a group, their intelligence is normal, attentional problems and hyperactivity profoundly affect school achievement. At least 30 to 40% of TS children have serious school performance handicaps which require special intervention.

In addition to a high frequency of attentional problems, at least 40% of TS patients are burdened with obsessions and compulsions. The family members of TS patients also have an increased frequency of obsessive-compulsive disorder, suggesting a genetic association between these disorders. It is tempting to speculate about the possible adaptive function of compulsive modes of organization in relation to an underlying attentional deficit, but the relationship between these two domains of psychological disturbance remains open for future study.

Phenomenology

The behavioral "inertia" in TS is manifested in many types of symptoms—stereotypic movements, repetitive behavior, obsessions, and compulsions. It is vivid in the tendency of TS patients to imitate what they have just seen (echopraxia), heard (echolalia), or said (palilalia). This mirroring or suggestibility frequently involves behavior that the patient does not admire or actions or speech that the patient considers to be odd, distasteful, or even vulgar. For example, while watching someone forcefully cough, pick at a scab, or scratch himself, a TS patient may think how funny the person looks. The observation will then "take hold" within the patient; he will feel an impulse to repeat what he has seen, to speak with an odd inflection, to accent a syllable just the way he has heard it, or to perform the observed gesture. He will then mimic in order "to clear his head of the impression" or "to see what it feels like." Shortly after this, the patient may then recognize that a new symptom has been added to his repertoire: a caricature has become a tic. A similar need to repeat may initiate a self-mirroring tic. A sniffle that originates during a cold may endure long after the virus has passed. Or an action may become inscribed in the individual's repertoire of tics. A young man in the midst of the breakup of a relationship made an exaggerated, disdainful expression to show his disapproval of his girlfriend and her nastiness. When he recurrently made this sour face in her presence, he thought it was his feelings about her that elicited it. Within a few weeks, however, he knew that his screwed-up grimace had become a new tic and had taken on an autonomous character.

While such modeling or repetition may lead to specific symptoms, patients most often do not know what precipitates or serves as the sensory template for a new tic. A patient will awaken one morning and hop out of bed, and then keep hopping; he will feel an itch and begin poking; while walking, he will start scratching at the ground with his toes or kicking with his heel. A tic appears from out of the blue, an act of unconscious creativity. There may be moments that are most propitious for the emergence of new symptoms, as when patients are particularly anxious, tense, or experiencing a heightened arousal. A touching example of such a new symptom was presented by an affectionate boy who rushed to his mother to greet her with a kiss, only then to be unable to stop kissing. This marked the start of a kissing tic which persisted for many months.

In its most severe forms, patients may have uncountable motor and phonic tics during all their waking hours, with paroxysms of full-body movements, shouting, and self-mutilation. Other patients may have only several tics per minute or fewer. There may be tremendous variability, over short and long periods of time, in symptomatology, frequency, and severity. Children may be able to inhibit, or not feel a great need to emit, their symptoms at school or in the presence of classmates; when they arrive home, tics may erupt with violence and remain distressing throughout the afternoon and evening. It is not unusual for children to "lose" their tics as they enter the doctor's office for "some mysterious reason." Parents may plead with a child to "show the doctor what you do at home," only to be told that he "just doesn't feel like doing them" or that he "can't do it" on command. A child with minimal symptoms may display severe tics with a change in the observational situation —for example, when the clinician is turned away from him and talking with a parent or when the child is allowed to sit alone in the waiting room. The clinician may see a symptom-free patient leave his office and begin hopping, flailing, and barking.

In addition to these moment-to-moment or short-term changes in symptom intensity, many patients have oscillations in severity over the course of weeks and months. This waxing and waning of severity may be triggered by changes in the patient's life; for example, around the time of holidays, children may develop exacerbations which will take weeks to subside. Other patients feel their symptoms show seasonal fluctuations. However, there is no rigorous data on whether life events, stresses, or seasons do, in fact, influence the onset or offset of a period of exacerbation. Once a child enters a phase of waxing symptomatology, a process seems to be triggered which will run its course, usually eight to twelve weeks.

Many TS patients, particularly older adolescents and adults, describe a sensory component to their TS. In the process of emitting a motor or phonic tic, the patient feels a crescendo of bodily tension and anxiety localized to a part of the body, e.g., to the wrist, forehead, arm, or throat. The patient tries to inhibit the movement or sound, but with the passage of seconds or minutes his anxiety mounts to an explosive degree. He then realizes, for the millionth time, that only through a specific, abrupt, forceful movement or sound will he be freed of the unpleasant sensation that is exploding within him. With the emission of the tic, he feels the discharge of internal tension; the sensory experience is muted. However, within seconds to minutes the refractory period passes, and the patient experiences another wave of tension, in the same or another part of the body; as the sensation reaches a nearly irresistible intensity, the patient again is forced into a strong action, movement, or statement to achieve quiescence. At times of stress this sensory-discharge cycle can repeat itself in a wild paroxysm of motor and phonic tics. Patients with this type of coupling between sensory phenomena and tics often experience their tics as having a voluntary aspect: they feel they can control themselves to a degree but then give up control to a force that they cannot bear, a "second will" existing within their psychic world.

However, the relationship between impulse and action in TS is not the same as in healthy individuals. Normally, an impulse or thought becomes engaged in a process of mediation and planning; the impulse carries a motivational valence, and the individual experiences the freedom to choose whether or not to act, whether to fulfill the urge or abstain. In TS an impulse that becomes increasingly powerful is not simply a motive for action of this type. Just as the tickle in the nose is not an urge that is relieved by sneezing but is part of the sneeze, the sensation preceding a tic is closely coordinated with the motor discharge. The need to breathe is felt after we hold our breath for as long as we can and increases just before we take a deep breath, but we do not take in this breath simply because of the felt need. Arguing along this line, one might say that the sensation in TS is a premonition of an action or, somewhat differently, that it represents the biological and psychological process leading to motor discharge, in some way analogous to the aura preceding a seizure or an attack of migraine.

Yet, the phenomenology of TS is more complex than models of breathing, sneezing, or seizing would suggest. While patients feel they capitulate to the internal demands, they also recognize the involvement of their will in shaping tics and in suppressing them for short or long periods of time. Adult patients may hold back their tics in the presence of clients and leave the office when they feel they can no longer abstain. Children will wait until they are home to begin screaming; particularly upsetting tics will be camouflaged. Thus, the sensory component (increasing bodily tension and anxiety) and the motor act which constitute a tic symptom are not bonded as tightly as would be suggested by the term *premonition;* on the other hand, they are more closely coupled than are normal desires and their fulfillment through action. Introspective TS patients have attempted to describe their predicament and the multiple connections between states of feeling and various tics. This effort to introspect and organize experience may be useful therapeutically for these patients, and perhaps for others who find their inner lives confusing.

The range and exotic nature of tics defies any unitary explanation of their biological or psychological meaning. However, the sexual and aggressive nature of many tics, the forceful exertion needed in their execution to bring satisfaction, and the associated attentional difficulties have suggested that TS may represent a dysfunction involving the inhibition of impulses and thoughts that are normally maintained under the control of unconscious mechanisms of censorship. In TS it has appeared that ideation and fantasies which are generally expressed only in sublimated forms or in dreams may come directly into consciousness. And that the step from thought to action may occur too easily and quickly. While the metaphoric nature of such an account is obvious, placing TS symptoms into the perspective of the normal organization of the mental apparatus may be useful for individual patients, who otherwise may feel completely estranged, and for furthering our understanding of phenomenology in TS and elsewhere.

Natural History

In the typical case of TS, behavioral difficulties, such as irritability, frustration, attentional problems, occur during the late preschool years; these problems are prodromal to any tics or accompanied by a few transient tics. Around second or third grade, more persistent tics emerge and then are followed by other motor and phonic symptoms. A rostra-caudal progression of motor tics has been documented in many studies, with eye blinking and other facial tics followed by shoulder shrugging, arm movements, truncal symptoms, and leg movements. Simple tics are followed by complex motor tics. In turn, phonic symptoms usually follow the simple motor tics by months or a year, and then are followed by complex phonic symptoms. The most articulated motor symptoms—compulsions, rituals, and self-destructive acts—and the most complex phonic symptoms—graphic descriptions of sexual acts, rude descriptions, and argumentativeness—usually emerge several years or more after the onset of the simple tics. It has appeared that the most severely afflicted patients tend to have the most severe early behavioral difficulties and relatively early onset of motor tics. However, there are numerous exceptions to this generalization, and there are also cases in which phonic tics have preceded motor tics.

Ultimate social adaptation may be more a function of behavioral and attentional difficulties than of simple motor or phonic tics. Many patients with severe tics achieve adequate social adjustment in adult life, although usually with considerable emotional pain. The factors that appear to be of importance with regard to social adaptation include the seriousness of attentional problems, school achievement, intelligence, degree of family support, and the severity of complex motor and phonic symptoms.

The long-term use of medication often complicates the understanding of natural history and the emergence of social and personality difficulties. Haloperidol, the most commonly prescribed medication, may elicit dysphoria, depression, school and social phobias, and intellectual and attentional dulling, as well as dystonic reactions, akathisia, and Parkinsonian side effects. These side effect may have considerable impact on the child's emerging sense of self-control, autonomy, self-esteem, and cognitive and social competence. In addition to the way in which psychoactive medication may alter how a child's body feels to him and how he experiences the working of his mind, the use of medication may single a child out in school, alter his daily schedule, focus parental and other adult concern on small changes in symptoms and side effects, and tie the child down to the care and attention of many adults.

Today, there is a generation of adults with TS whose childhood development occurred under the influence of changing doses of haloperidol and multiple other standard and experimental medications. These individuals have been preoccupied for many years with symptoms, medications, side effects, with being "victims" of a disease and its treatments. Too often, the developmental tasks of latency and adolescence—individuation, industriousness, autonomy, appreciation of bodily pleasures, coping with confusing motivations—have been derailed; patients have grown up being uncertain about what feelings were really "their own," what feelings were "the Tourette syndrome," what feelings were the result of medication, what feelings were "normal" and what feelings were "sick," what feelings were "private" and what feelings should be shared. Patients with symptoms of self-directed and other-directed aggressiveness and destructiveness are especially burdened during the course of development because of the disastrous consequences of their symptoms and the impossibility of learning about healthy aggression and its channeling.

Because of multiple, interacting forces, some severely afflicted individuals become profoundly maladapted, dependent, isolated, and "chronic" patients. They are burdened by a range of seriously debilitating personality disorders, phobias, and anxiety. Confronted by the clinical problems of such an individual, it is difficult, if not impossible, to sort out the etiological and continuing factors that relate to the severity of the disorder and its natural history, on one hand, and those that relate to social and academic consequences, medication, and medical management, on the other.

Finally, given the socially catastrophic nature of TS, it is not surprising that patients have recurrent minor depressions and occasional major depressions. In adolescence and adulthood, TS patients frequently come to feel that their social isolation, vocational and academic failure, and painful and disfiguring symptoms are more than they can bear; at times, they will consider and attempt suicide.

EPIDEMIOLOGY / GENETICS

It has been estimated that 15% of all schoolchildren have transient tics, and it seems likely that this figure is only somewhat lower for adults. The more carefully one looks, the more tics one finds. The peak incidence of elaborate transient tics seems to coincide with the mean age of onset of TS (seven years) for reasons that are probably connected with biological and psychological maturation at this time. There is no firm epidemiological evidence about the incidence and prevalence of TS. At one time, the disorder was thought to be rare, but with increasing medical recognition and the excellent publicity provided by the national Tourette Syndrome Association, many cases are now being recognized. Based on known cases in Connecticut, we have estimated that the prevalence is at least 1:2,000 (i.e., somewhat higher than autism) for full-blown TS. However, genetic evidence, to be discussed, suggests that TS and multiple tics are on the same spectrum, and this would then increase the prevalence of the TS diathesis at least several fold, perhaps to as common as 1:200 or 1:300.

The question of familial aggregation of TS was first raised in the original nineteenth-century reports, but a genetic basis for TS was not seriously considered until recently. Several genetic studies have been reported and other rigorous studies are far enough along to conclude that there is a strong genetic contribution to TS, with clear familial aggregation of TS and multiple tics (Pauls et al., 1981). Boys are far more often afflicted than girls, and girls may require a stronger genetic predisposition (more afflicted individuals in their family) before they express the disorder. The individuals at highest risk for developing TS appear to be the sons of mothers with TS. For these individuals the chances of developing TS or a related disorder may reach as high as 30%. No specific mode of genetic transmission has been established in TS. Some pedigrees suggest a dominant autosomal gene; however, more data seem explicable on the basis of polygenic models with sex thresholds of expression affecting the trait. As things stand, any number of mathematical models to genetic transmission can be fit to the data. Environmental factors also appear to be important, and there are many sporadic cases of TS that lack a family history of tics or TS.

Perhaps of greater interest than the transmission of the tics, as such, is the increasing evidence of genetic association between TS and other neuropsychiatric disorders, especially ADD and obsessive-compulsive disorder. ADD is commonly found in the prodromal phase of TS and persists with the full expression of the disorder for the majority of children; it appears likely that there are children or adults with ADD and no tics, ADD and motor tics only, or ADD and phonic symptoms, who are suffering from a milder variant of TS. These individuals can be understood as suffering from a *forme fruste* of TS which has not progressed to full expression, perhaps because of biological or environmental protective factors. This hypothesis is especially compelling in relation to children with serious ADD who have siblings or other close relatives with TS or multple tics. However, the TS variant of ADD may not be rare even in nonfamilial cases. Similarly, obsessive-compulsive disorder, without tics or with only a paucity of tic symptoms, is overrepresented in families of patients with TS. Further biological and genetic studies are required to demonstrate the precise nature of the relationship between TS and other disorders. If other disorders are found to be linked genetically with the biological diathesis of TS, these disorders may be distinctive variants, genotypically, from forms of ADD, obsessive-compulsive, or anxiety disorders which are not associated with TS. Genetic heterogeneity is more the rule than the exception in biology.

Etiology

While the genetic factors noted previously appear to be powerful influences in the etiology of TS, they are not found in all cases nor is it known through which mechanisms they operate. Even if the gene(s) underlying the disorder are identified, it will be necessary to explicate their molecular mode of action and to identify specific risk factors that may cause this vulnerability to be expressed. The most intensive research in relation to etiology has focused on neurochemical alterations in the brain (Cohen et al., 1979).

Multiple neurochemical systems have been implicated by pharmacological and metabolic evidence. The most convincing evidence for dopaminergic involvement has come from the dramatic response to haloperidol, exacerbations produced by stimulant medications, and findings of reduced levels of dopamine metabolite in the cerebrospinal fluid (CSF) of patients. Serotonergic mechanisms have been suggested on the basis of reduced CSF serotonin metabolites. The role of the cholinergic system is clouded by contradictory reports; enhancing cholinergic functioning (through use of physostigmine) has been associated both with improvement and worsening of TS. Elevated levels of red-blood-cell choline have been found in TS patients and their relatives, but the relationship of this to brain cholinergic function is unclear. Noradrenergic mechanisms have been most persuasively implicated by observations that clonidine, a drug that inhibits noradrenergic functioning by stimulation of an autoreceptor, may improve motor and phonic symptoms. Noradrenergic involvement has also been suggested by the exacerbation of the syndrome by stress and anxiety and elevated levels of norepinephrine metabolite in the CSF of some severe patients.

It is possible that the expression of TS involves several neurotransmitter systems, operating in a cascading or reinforcing fashion. Various aspects of the disorder may involve different neurotransmitters or the balance between them; e.g., motor tics may express dopaminergic overactivity while severe difficulties with inhibition (e.g., attentional problems) may represent the engagement of noradrenergic mechanisms. There is evidence for interactions between neurochemical systems. For example, clonidine most directly reduces noradrenergic functioning, but downstream it may influence dopaminergic activity. This noradrenergic-dopaminergic interaction appears to require the mediation of the serotonergic system in the raphe. It is likely that other neurotransmitters will be implicated in TS as well. A role for opioid receptors, for example, is suggested by the amelioration of symptoms reported by patients who have used heroin.

A particularly important risk factor in tics and TS is the use of stimulant medication.

Over 25% of all TS patients in some cohorts have had a course of stimulant medication early in the emergence of their behavioral or tic symptoms because they have been diagnosed as having ADD. Over the last several years, series of cases have been reported in which the use of stimulants (methylphenidate, dextroamphetamine, and pemoline) has been correlated with the onset of motor and phonic tics, with pemoline perhaps being the worst offender. It is well recognized that stimulant medications can produce complex stereotypies in animals which disappear when the stimulants are terminated; similarly, several percent of all children treated with stimulant medication will develop simple motor tics (such as eye blinking or nose puckering) which will disappear with reduction or termination of the medication. It is more controversial whether stimulants can actually trigger or produce prolonged chronic multiple tics or TS which will persist following the termination of medication. However, many cases have been reported in which this seems to have occurred (Golden, 1974; Lowe et al., 1982). The most convincing clinical evidence may come from tic-free children who have had two courses of stimulant medication. During the first course, tics have appeared after months of treatment and have stopped with drug termination; during the second course of stimulants, tics have appeared within days and have persisted for months or permanently when stimulants have been withdrawn. These children seem to have had TS kindled by repeated exposure to stimulants. A complication in this story is the fact that some children—but, importantly, not all—who have had TS emerge during the course of stimulant treatment have a family history of TS or tics and perhaps were genetically vulnerable. Further, it is not possible to know whether a subgroup of ADD children who have developed TS with stimulants were already on their way to TS in any case. Detailed neurochemical, genetic, and other studies will be needed to tease out the interacting factors related to stimulant induction and exacerbation of tic syndromes; for instance, we do not know if genetically less vulnerable children require longer treatment or larger amounts of stimulants to precipitate TS or how stimulants affect receptor functioning in children carrying the genetic loading for TS. However, since it is beyond dispute that stimulants cause transient tics, often (but, interestingly, not always) worsen pre-existing tic symptoms, and elicit stereotypies and prolonged alterations in CNS dopaminergic and other systems in animals, it seems likely that for some vulnerable children stimulants precipitate the full expression of TS earlier than it might have appeared or when it might not have developed at all. Available information thus indicates that stimulants should be used cautiously with ADD children who have a close relative with tics, should not be used with ADD children with a first-degree relative with TS, and should be terminated with the onset of tics in children who previously were tic-free.

Several lines of evidence suggest that TS may be heterogeneous biologically: there is variability in the type of symptoms and severity in family history, in response to medication, and in natural history. Extremely severe cases of TS with multiform, ceaseless, and devastating symptoms may be etiologically different from milder forms. While TS cases can be subgrouped on the basis of clinical findings, such as the presence of coprolalia or ADD, further research will be required to determine if these groups are distinctive or represent a spectrum of severity.

DIFFERENTIAL DIAGNOSIS

The differentiation of TS from other tic syndromes may be no more than semantic, especially since recent genetic evidence links TS with multiple tics. Transient tics of childhood are best defined in retrospect. Today, the full-blown case of TS is unlikely to be confused with any other disorder. However, patients who were initially diagnosed before the popularity of TS, received multiple psychiatric diagnoses, including schizophrenia and obsessive-compulsive disorder. The wild thoughts and uncontrolled expression of ideas, in word and action, in TS suggest a psychotic disorder; but TS patients maintain a painful awareness of what they are doing and feeling, and they recognize the "craziness" of their thoughts and actions. While they may feel that thoughts pop into their mind, they do not have the same experience of thought insertion as found in schizophrenia: they recognize the thoughts as their own. Obsessive-compulsive disorder is obviously suggested by the obsessive thoughts and compulsive actions; here, too, the question may be semantic. Patients with TS may satisfy the criteria for obsessive-compulsive disorder; if so, this should be clarified in the diagnostic formulation.

On occasion, it may be difficult to distinguish children with extreme ADD from TS. Restlessness, fidgety movements, impulsive behavior, out-of-context statements, diffuse hyperactivity, fingering and touching objects, and other symptoms in children with severe ADD are also found in TS; many ADD children, on close examination, have a few phonic or motor tics or grimacing and noises that can pass for them. As noted earlier, some ADD children may have variant forms of TS, and only further biological and genetic research will help in making this differentiation for the difficult cases. (There are ongoing clinical studies concerning the treatment of complex ADD patients, with and without tics, using clonidine, an agent of possible value in the treatment of TS.) Where ADD is present in association with TS or multiple tics, this should be noted in the diagnostic formulation.

The differentiation between TS and seizures is made difficult by the presence of abnormal EEGs in up to 40% of patients with TS and the similarity of some complex motor tics to automatisms. In contrast with seizure disorders, TS patients usually can inhibit their movements for a time, do not lose sphincter control, and have a clear consciousness during and following their paroxysms of tics. While they may have trouble falling asleep, may occasionally awake from sleep with movements, and may even have some tics during sleep, TS patients do not have complex or paroxysmal tic activity while sleeping.

The differential diagnosis of TS and epilepsy is complicated by the fact that some patients may have both types of disorders. A teenage boy with a characteristic history of TS also had a grossly abnormal EEG and episodes that started with sensory changes and sometimes a headache; he would lose consciousness and exhibit tonic-clonic movements. The diagnosis of TS in combination with juvenile migraine was made, and treatment for migraine was of use. In contrast, another ten-year-old boy threw himself to the floor, shook uncontrollably, and felt exhausted after his paroxysmal movement; at times, he was wildly and unreasonably aggressive to his sister. Because of this history and the presence of spike-and-wave complexes on his EEG, he was treated with anticonvulsants. This regimen was of no benefit, and he was then diagnosed as having TS, for which treatment was highly successful. A young man was considered to have TS because of his complex motor symptoms, starting late in adolescence, in which he would throw himself forward and curse or shout, lift up a telephone receiver and talk in short, incoherent sentences, or pull himself into a fetal position. He had an aura before these spells and some memory for them. The unusual natural history, minimum of simple tics, and presence of a temporal lobe spike focus suggested that this was not TS; depth electrode recordings confirmed the presence of an epileptogenic focus, which was removed surgically. When in doubt, a therapeutic trial of anticonvulsants may make sense. Subtle tics may simulate EEG abnormalities, so repeat and sleep EEGs may be useful.

Autistic and retarded children may display the entire gamut of TS symptoms, including simple and complex motor and phonic tics, echolalia, palilalia, and coprolalia. The autistic child's need to preserve sameness in his environment and routines, stereotypic hand flapping and other movements, and bizarre posturing also are reminiscent of TS. Some autistic children have elaborate compulsions. Whether an autistic individual requires the additional diagnosis of TS may remain an open question until there is a biological or other diagnostic test. On the side of diagnosing TS would be a positive family history, characteristic age of onset and progression of tics, severity of simple motor and phonic tics, in addition to the more typical autistic complex stereotypies and compulsions, and presence of coprolalia. We have seen TS in association with a number of other developmental, neurological, and medical disorders, and it is possible that CNS trauma or deviations may predispose a child to the expression of the disorder, particularly if there is a genetic history.

A broad range of neurological diseases are associated with motor symptoms, including disorders of the basal ganglia and various degenerative conditions. Wilson's disease, subacute sclerosing panencephalitis (SSPE), Sydenham's chorea, and other such conditions can be noted in a grand rounds presentation, along with various dystonias. These syndromes are differentiated from TS by their range of persistent neurological findings, such as spasticity, chorea, seizures, or deterioration, as well as by various laboratory tests. Children with esophageal reflux may develop habitual neck torsion and head bobbing—Sandifer's syndrome—but this is unlikely to be confused with TS.

Although prevailing diagnostic criteria would require that all children who for at least one year have suppressible multiple motor and phonic tics, however minimal, should be diagnosed as having TS, in practice we deviate from this rigorous research approach. In talking with families, and thinking about the disorder as clinicians, we tend to consider severity and associated features (particularly complex motor and phonic symptoms, as well as attentional problems and general disinhibition) in the diagnosis of TS. For the meticulous, hard-working boy, we are willing to use the term "nervous habits," quaint as it may sound, to cover his throat clearing, facial grimacing, and occasional shrugging. Universities, corporate headquarters, and Congress are filled with such men. Although their symptoms may meet formal criteria for the diagnosis of TS, it would seem to be stretching the diagnosis beyond the best interests of the patients. However, since there are genetic implications, and some families and patients will want to have full disclosure of the physician's thoughts, the clinician may want to raise the possible relationship betweeen the patient's symptoms and TS. The problem is, while not everyone who twitches has TS, in the absence of diagnostic tests it may be hard to draw the line. For research purposes it is necessary to maintain clear diagnostic criteria with appropriate specification of severity and compensatory assets.

ASSESSMENT

Investigation of the child with tics requires the usual medical and psychiatric history, with particular emphasis on attentional and behavioral difficulties.

The nature, severity, frequency, and degree of disruption produced by the motor and phonic tics needs to be carefully assessed from the time of their emergence until the present. It is important to determine their onset, progression, waxing and waning, and factors that have worsened or ameliorated their status. A critical question concerns the degree to which they have interfered with the child's social, familial, and school experiences or have upset the family. In usual clinical practice it is very useful to monitor symptoms over a few months in order to assess their severity and fluctuation, impact on the family, and nature of the child's and family's adaptation. This monitoring can be facilitated if the family keeps records or uses standard rating forms (e.g., a list of tic symptoms and a behavioral checklist, such as the Conner's parent-teacher questionnaire). (See Appendix).

Child psychiatric clinicians are not likely to focus exclusive attention on the tic symptoms, but other physicians may be more likely to emphasize the tics and lose sight of the child. During the evaluation of a child with TS, the clinician must assess the child's other areas of functioning and difficulties, particularly school performance, the presence of attentional and learning difficulties, and relationships with family and peers. Before receiving a diagnosis, the child and family may think the child is going "crazy." By the time of his evaluation, the child may be extremely distressed by his own experiences and by the kind of criticism he has received from parents who have scolded, cajoled, bribed, threatened, and perhaps beaten him to stop his "weird" and embarrassing behavior. During evaluation, therefore, family issues, including parental guilt, need to be addressed. Relevant factors elicited through careful diagnostic evaluation can then be approached through clarification, education, and therapeutic discussion with the child and family.

Careful assessment of cognitive functioning and school achievement are indicated for children having school problems. The nature of this assessment is similar to that for other children with school-performance problems. TS children with school-performance difficulties often do not have clearly delineated learning disorders, and the average IQ of TS patients is normal; rather, their problems tend to lie in the area of attentional deployment, perseverance, and ability to keep themselves and their work organized. Many have difficulties with penmanship (graphomotor skills) and compulsions which interfere with writing. Determining specific problem areas will help in the recommendation of alternatives (e.g., use of a typewriter or more emphasis on oral reports).

Neurological examination should include documentation of neuromaturational difficulties and other neurological findings. About half of TS patients have nonlocalizing, so-called soft neurological findings suggesting disturbances in the body schema and integration of motor control. While these findings have no specific therapeutic implications, they are worth noting, probably strengthen the diagnosis of TS, and may define a clinical subgroup. Neurological findings also are important as baseline data, since the use of medications, such as haloperidol, may cloud the neurological picture.

As noted previously, the EEG is often abnormal in TS, but EEG findings are usually nonspecific. Children with paroxysmally abnormal tracings sometimes have been treated as epileptic, but anticonvulsants are of no consistent value in TS. Computed tomography of the brain generally produces normal results, and the EEG and computed tomography are not necessary for the diagnosis or treatment of TS. Yet, clinicians who tend to worry are likely to feel comforted by a normal EEG and computed tomograms; at the least, other disorders affecting movement (such as a seizure or basal ganglia disorder) are more or less ruled out. Additional chemical studies which can be considered in the biological work-up include electrolytes, calcium, phosphorous, ceruloplasmin, liver-function tests—all related to movement difficulties of various types. In practice, TS is rarely confused with these disorders today, since the history and findings in TS are distinctive.

Previous medications must be reviewed in detail during assessments. If a child has received stimulant medications, it is important to determine what the indications for the medications were, whether there were any preexisting tics or compulsions, and the temporal relationship between the stimulants and new symptoms. Catecholaminergic agonists are contained in other drugs, such as in antihistamine combinations used in treating allergies and in medications used for asthma. If a patient with TS is on a stimulant or a drug containing an ephedrinelike agent, discontinuation should be strongly considered. If such drugs were used in the past, it is important to know their effects. Children who developed tics on stimulants may have shown improved attention and learning with the use of these medications.

It is quite common that children will have been tried on other medications—such as haloperidol—before being seen for assessment by the current clinician. The child's response to these medications needs to be assessed. What dosages were used, what were the initial positive and negative responses to the drug, why was the medication discontinued? A family may report that haloperidol was not useful for a child or that he had unacceptable side effects. A careful history may reveal that he improved on haloperidol but then developed akathisia which was not recognized, or that the side effects were dose related and probably controllable. Was the medication used at the correct dosage, with good enough monitoring, for a long enough time? Patients also may not recognize important side effects of a drug. Thus, families may not appreciate that their child's fearfulness or school phobia may be related to haloperidol and not primarily to psychological issues.

When a child is currently on a medication but is still having serious tic or behavioral difficulties, hard clinical judgment is called upon. In practice, TS patients today will frequently be on haloperidol, clonidine, a phenothiazine, or some combination when they are evaluated. The clinician will have to decide whether to increase the medication and see if the child improves or discontinue the medication and observe the child's response. Discontinuation from haloperidol may lead to severe withdrawal-emergent exacerbation wwith worsening of symptoms—far beyond what they ever were—for as long as two to three months. Thus, if haloperidol is withdrawn, it cannot be expected that the child's "real" status will be visible for quite a while. Some children may improve for a few weeks after haloperidol is stopped and then exacerbate after a further week or so, remain worse for a while, and then gradually improve. With discontinuation of haloperidol, cognitive blunting, feeling dull, poor motivation, school and social phobias, excessive appetite, and sedation may lift rather quickly, over days to several weeks, while emergent tic symptoms remain or become worse. Thus, the decision to discontinue haloperidol may be harder than the one to initiate it; withdrawal must be planned so as to disrupt the child's life as little as possible. Often, families and children will have great difficulty in tolerating the discontinuation and will need a good deal of support from the physician, including the possibility of hospitalization.

If a child is on clonidine and is not benefiting, a tapering of the medication over one or two weeks may lead to a short period of exacerbation lasting several days and up to a few weeks. This exacerbation typically is milder than with haloperidol and children only rarely seem to get worse during withdrawal than they were before the initiation of treatment. Less is known about withdrawal from phenothiazines, but withdrawal-emergent dyskinesias and exacerbations occur as with haloperidol.

A clinician will have to decide whether to try to "clean out" a child's system by discontinuation of all medication or to change dosage when symptoms are poorly controlled. The presence of serious side effects would probably lead us to attempt detoxification, but only careful assessment of the child's and family's coping and response to intervention can guide the clinician in proceeding down either path.

The assessment of a child with TS usually requires a number of hours spent with the child and family. During the course of this assessment, the clinician will be in a good position to learn about the fluctuations of symptoms; as the child becomes more comfortable, he will show his symptoms with less suppression or inhibition. Also, the identification of symptoms by the clinician and family will be important in determining the baseline against which treatment can be assessed. Only when there is confidence in the doctor is a child or adult likely to acknowledge the most frightening and bizarre symptoms—e.g., obsessive thoughts, rituals, and "disgusting" habits. A teenage boy after many hours admitted, with great shame, that he soiled his underwear during his complex motor tic which involved straining down; this symptom responded well to medication and could be monitored only because he was comfortable enough to admit its presence. Families may recognize a particular behavior as a tic only after they have been educated about possible symptoms.

It is useful to have a detailed behavioral history of the extended family, including tics, compulsions, attentional problems, learning disorders, and the like. A grandfather's TS may have been diagnosed Sydenham's chorea, an uncle may have been thought simply to be odd or weird. Parents, like their children, may be embarrassed in acknowledging their own symptoms. When a father is asked about his obvious lip-puckering and throat-clearing tics, he may at first deny that he has ever had any tics or that he ever "noticed" them. Only when the mother says, "Well, dear, you do sometimes clear your throat when you're nervous," will he be able to "remember" his childhood and current symptoms. There is no substitute for the clinician's observational abilities, patience, and tact.

Patients with long-standing TS, like other patients with chronic disorders, have complex medical, school, and social histories. The process of assessment includes the reconstruction of these histories. The various types of treatments, their results, and what they have meant to the child and family are pieced together. Unless the clinician knows what has been tried before, why it was tried, and why it did not work, he is likely to repeat unsuccessful approaches. An important aspect of this type of assessment is the understanding of what the family contributed to earlier therapeutic difficulties and successes and what the family's previous pleasant and, more often, unsatisfying, experiences with the medical and educational communities have been. A well-conducted assessment allows the family to feel that their full story has been heard—sometimes for the first time after having seen many physicians. This assessment process of clarification and integration can be therapeutically important and lead to an easing of the immediate crisis. In addition, nothing is more important for developing confidence than the family's and child's belief that the clinician has understood (a) where they have been, and (b) how they are coping (in their own best ways) with the tragedy they have experienced or are now experiencing.

Families often will ask during the course of an evaluation if TS is a "medical" or "emotional" disorder. These terms carry with them ideological and psychological weight. A well-conducted assessment, in which all sectors of the child's development and current functioning are discussed, is an important step in undoing an epistemologically mischievous disjunction between an isolated body and detached mind. While it is clear that TS arises on the basis of neurophysiological dysfunction, and thus is "biological," it is equally apparent that its manifestations affect the child in many areas of his life. Thus, the treatment of TS must address the child in many areas of his life. Thus, the treatment of TS must address the child as a whole person and not just as a collection of physical symptoms. This orientation to TS and its treatment can be conveyed implicitly during the assessment—as the clinician analyzes medical, psychosocial, and psychological issues—but usually requires explicit discussion at the end of the evaluation.

A complication encountered during the assessment of a child with TS is that parents may themselves have TS or disorders associated with it. There are several implications of this multigenerational sharing of symptoms and underlying troubles. A clinician may feel inhibited in fully sharing his impressions of the child's social and personality problems because he may observe similar difficulties in the parents, or fear that he may hurt their feelings. At times, the relationship between the clinician and family may be strained because of attentional problems, impulsivity, or obsessional features in the parents which are similar to the problems of the child. Also, parents may feel an additional burden of guilt if they recognize that they have contributed genetically to their child's disorder. On the other side, parents with tics or TS are likely to be more sympathetic to their child's dilemmas and to appreciate how life can proceed in spite of them. And they may be interested in receiving treatment for themselves, or other family members, if there is success in the treatment of the child.

TREATMENT

The decision about whether to treat, and with what form of treatment, will depend not only on the primary diagnosis but on the degree to which TS or the tics are intefering with the child's normal development. The primary emphasis in management of TS must be on helping the child to navigate the normal developmental tasks—for the school-age child: to feel competent in school, develop friendships, experience trust in his parents, and enjoy life's adventures. Many children with multiple tics and TS do well in moving onward with development; for them, treatment to ameliorate the tics generally is not indicated. Natural parental upset about the tics requires lengthy, calm discussion and education about available treatments. If treatment is decided upon by the child, family, and physician, developmental issues must constantly be reassessed.

Monitoring

Unless there is a state of emergency, the clinician usually can follow a patient for several months before a specific treatment plan is organized. The goals of this first stage of treatment are to establish a baseline of symptoms; define associated difficulties in school, family, and peer relationships; obtain necessary medical tests; and monitor, through checklists and interviews, the range and fluctuations in symptoms and the specific contexts of greatest difficulty; and establish a relationship.

Reassurance

It may become apparent that the child's tics are of minimal functional significance. Even if a child satisfies the criteria for TS, he may have good peer relationships, school achievement, and sense of himself, and no treatement may be needed. If parents have read about TS, they may be worried about the child's future. In general, the severity of TS announces itself within a short period following its appearance; by the time a child has had TS for two to three years, one can guess with reasonable accuracy how severe the disorder ultimately will be. Thus, for a thirteen-year-old boy with mild TS which first appeared at age seven, one can reassure the family that it will become no worse than what they have already seen. For these cases, we tend to tell families that while their child can be diagnosed as having TS, it is not the same severity or type of disorder as what they might hear about in regard to TS, and that "in the old times" their child probably would have simply been called "a nervous child." For transient single tics, such reassurance is fully appropriate. Because of the clear genetic factors involved in TS, families deserve to know about the emerging knowledge in this area even if they are reassured about the nature of their child's disorder.

Chemotherapy

The only effective treatments for the simple and complex motor and phonic symptoms of TS are pharmacological. Psychotherapy may be useful for children with TS as it relates to personality and adjustment difficulties, peer relationships, etc., just as for any child with a medical problem, but as a rule tics are not responsive to psychotherapy. Behavior modification, hypnotherapy, and relaxation methods have been tried with TS with little success; perhaps they may be synergistic with pharmacotherapy, but there is no firm evidence supporting this. Some patients are able to learn methods of self-control, particularly as they grow older.

Several classes of medication are used in the treatment of TS today.

HALOPERIDOL. Since the 1960s, haloperidol has been the mainstay of treatment of TS. During the first years of its use, dosage was rapidly increased to very high levels (up to 200 mg/day), followed by gradual reduction. However, it is now accepted that haloperidol is most effective at quite low doses, and patients generally are started at 0.5 mg/day and slowly increased up to 3-4 mg/day, usually in twice daily dosage. Impressive benefits are seen at these low doses—patients may have almost complete remissions with few side effects (Shapiro and Shapiro, 1982). Those who do not respond to low doses of haloperidol may sustain a reduction of symptoms at higher doses (10-15 mg), but results are never as satisfying and side effects intervene to limit the drug's usefulness. While there has been a suggestion that patients with a family history of TS may respond better to haloperidol than those without, other studies, including our own, do not indicate that family history or EEG abnormalities are specifically associated with good response.

Up to 80% of patients with TS initially benefit from haloperidol, sometimes dramatically. However, long-term follow-up suggests that only a smaller number, perhaps 20-30%, continue haloperidol for an extended period of time. Patients discontinue the drug because of the emergence of side effects, including excessive fatigue, weight gain, dysphoria, Parkinsonian symptoms, intellectual dulling, personality changes, feeling like a "zombie," and akathisia. Parkinsonian and acute dystonic reactions can be controlled with anti-Parkinsonian agents (1-2 mg/day of Cogentin). The akathisia is somewhat less responsive to anticholinergic agents. School phobias generally appear during the first weeks of treatment with low doses of haloperidol and while the tic symptoms are improving; social phobias in adults may involve acute anxiety about going to work or performing at work and, like school phobia, can be extremely disabling. When these phobias are not recognized as drug side effects, they can continue for months; they remit within weeks of haloperidol discontinuation. Intellectual dulling leads to marked worsening of school and work performance. Children who are "A" students and have friends may be started on haloperidol because of their tic symptoms, only to become "C" students, dysphoric, and isolated. To counter the attentional difficulties produced by the drug, some clinicians have prescribed methylphenidate in combination with haloperidol, with apparently good results. However, the association between stimulant medications and tics suggests that adding a stimulant to haloperidol should be considered experimental and performed only with informed consent and careful monitoring until long-term effects can be assessed.

Haloperidol has been incriminated in the onset of tardive dyskinesia (TD). In patients with TS, the appearance of new facial or hand movements may be hard to assess. Are these tics? Is TD appearing? We have seen orofacial movements consistent with a suspicion of TD disappear after a number of weeks following the discontinuation of haloperidol. Because of animal studies suggesting an increased likelihood of TS with multiple discontinuations and reintroductions of neuroleptics, it is probably wise not to use haloperidol intermittently or with frequent drug holidays. Withdrawal exacerbations also make this usually not feasible.

Anti-Parkinsonian agents generally are not prescribed until they are required for the remediation of specific side effects—Parkinsonian tremor or rigidity, dystonia, oculogyric crisis, or akathisia. However, some clinicians prefer to start low doses of these agents once the haloperidol is above a certain threshold, perhaps 2 mg/day, because of the fear of the occurrence of these side effects in school and the great anxiety they cause. Since anti-Parkinsonian agents have their own side effects, prophylactic use may be unwise. However, patients should be instructed about haloperidol's potential side effects and should have an anti-Parkinsonian drug at home and with them on trips in the event that they do develop Parkinsonian symptoms. Also, patients and families should be told to watch for unusual new symptoms which may be mistaken for TS but which may represent a side effect of the haloperidol. For example, a teenager began to have repeated episodes, lasting many minutes, of thrusting his tongue and deviating his jaw. After a while, these episodes lengthened, and he would hold his tongue and jaw in a rigid position for hours. He became frightened of going to school or being with friends. This dystonic reaction was not diagnosed until haloperidol was discontinued for other side effects.

CLONIDINE. The first report in 1979 of the value of clonidine in treating TS has been followed by other case reports and open and closed trials suggesting that from 40–70% of TS patients benefit from its use (Cohen et al., 1980). Clonidine has been approved by the FDA only for use in hypertension, but clinicians can prescribe it without special government approval for TS as long as they understand its indications and share the basis for their decision with the family and child. Formal FDA acceptance of clonidine's value in TS is likely. Clonidine's mode of action appears to be different from that of haloperidol; clonidine primarily inhibits noradrenergic functioning while haloperidol alters dopaminergic functioning. As noted earlier, however, some interactions between the central dopaminergic and noradrenergic systems may be involved in the pathophysiology of TS, and there is some evidence that clonidine may indirectly affect central dopaminergic neurons. In addition to reducing the simple motor and phonic symptoms in TS, clonidine seems especially useful in improving attentional problems and ameliorating complex motor and phonic symptoms.

In general, clonidine is started at low doses of 0.05 mg/day and slowly titrated over several weeks to 0.15–0.30 mg/day (3 μg/kg/day). Doses of 0.4 mg are not infrequent, but doses above 0.5 mg/day are more likely to lead to side effects. Patients may experience the need for their next dose, when the medication is working effectively, by sensing an increasing anxiety, frequency of symptoms, or irritability. Unlike haloperidol, which may lead to clear improvement within a few days, clonidine tends to have a slower onset of action. When larger doses are used earlier, improvement may occur sooner, but there may be more sedation. With slower titration to therapeutic levels, clonidine may take three weeks or longer to show a beneficial effect. Even before tics are reduced, the patient may experience a reduction in tension, a feeling of being calm, or a sense of having a "longer fuse". A gradual decrease in complex motor tics and compulsions also may precede clear improvement in simple tics. In the most successful cases, attentional, behavioral, and complex phenomena seem more responsive than the simplest tics. Evaluation of the medication's effectiveness may not be possible before three to four months. When there is a positive response, improvement may progressively appear even many months and up to a year or more later. Patients gain confidence in themselves, adjust better to school, feel less irritable, and have fewer tic symptoms. These therapeutic benefits reinforce each other. Since clonidine has only recently been used in TS, the longest individual treatment has lasted for about four years. Children with extremely severe TS have benefited from this length of time, and only very slight increases in medication have been required.

The major side effect of clonidine is sedation, which appears early in the course of treatment and especially if the dose is increased quickly, but which tends to abate after several weeks. A few patients have dry mouth, but children seem to have this less often than adults. We have documented that clonidine continues to decrease salivary flow even after years of treatment. Rarely, patients will feel that things are "too bright," perhaps because of impairment of pupillary constriction. At higher doses there may be hypotension and dizziness, and this is more likely if clonidine is given at high doses quite early or if it is increased to over 0.4 or 0.5 mg/day. At lower doses blood pressure is not clinically affected, although a fall of several mm mercury in diastolic and systolic pressure can be detected. Slight prolongation of the P-R interval in the electrocardiogram has been noted, but this has not been considered of significance. No other medical or clinical side effects have so far emerged.

Before clonidine is prescribed, it is wise to obtain an EKG and routine blood studies. However, no alterations in standard blood-chemistry measures or hemogram have been found.

Haloperidol and clonidine have been used in combination, but there is only anecdotal information about this approach. The combination has been used in two clinical situations: (1) for patients whose symptoms are not fully controlled on haloperidol, or who are having serious side effects when medication is increased, yet who cannot have their haloperidol fully discontinued because of the severity of symptoms or the emergence of an exacerbation with tapering; and (2) for patients who are on clonidine but still having motor and phonic symptoms. It has appeared that patients can be managed with smaller doses of haloperidol if clonidine is added to the regimen and, on the other hand, that haloperidol may improve the tic control for some patients on clonidine. In general, quite small doses of both medications have been used when the drugs are combined, and no serious side effects have been reported in addition to what is seen with the drugs used individually.

PIMOZIDE. Pimozide is a potent neuroleptic widely used in Europe in the treatment of psychosis; several open and blind clinical studies have shown pimozide to be at least as effective as haloperidol in the treatment of TS and probably less sedating. Clinical experience with children is limited because the drug is not yet available in the United States. Pimozide is a diphenylbutylpiperidine derivative, chemically distinctive from haloperidol, clonidine, or the phenothiazines. Its mode of action appears to be preferential inhibition of postsynaptic dopamine receptors.

Treatment with pimozide is initiated at 1 mg/day, and dosage is gradually increased, on clinical indications, to a maximum of 6-10 mg/day (0.2 mg/kg) for children and 20 mg/day for adults. Because of its long half-life (55 hours), one daily dosage may be feasible. Major side effects are similar to haloperidol, including: Parkinsonism, akathisia, drowsiness, insomnia, and dizziness, as well as depression, nervousness, and other adverse behavioral effects. Anti-Parkinson agents are useful. Pimozide causes EKG changes in up to 25% of patients, including T-wave inversion, U waves, Q-T prolongation, and bradycardia. EKG changes are observable within one week and at doses as low as 3 mg/day. The manufacturer recommends discontinuation of pimozide with the occurrence of T-wave inversion or U waves, seen in up to 20% of patients; dosage should not be increased if there is prolongation of the Q-T interval (corrected). At least three cardiac deaths have occurred in healthy young men. As with haloperidol, tardive dyskinesia must be considered a long-term possibility. In addition to the usual clinical and laboratory monitoring, patients receiving pimozide should receive an EKG before treatment, every several months, and at points of dosage increase.

PHENOTHIAZINES AND OTHER MEDICATIONS. While haloperidol has often been thought to be specifically useful in TS, it now appears that some patients respond as well to phenothiazines when doses and side effects are equivalent (Friedhoff and Chase, 1982). On the other hand, phenothiazines have no greater value than haloperidol. For the patient who cannot tolerate haloperidol, a trial with a phenothiazine may be indicated; dosages are similar to those used in the treatment of schizophrenia and with the same side effects.

Agents that affect cholinergic functioning have not found a place in the treatment of TS. Physostigmine given intravenously has been used to study cholinergic mechanisms; even those investigators who have found a reduction in TS symptoms have found no way of using agents like physostigmine clinically. Lecithin has been tried with little benefit. Agents affecting serotonergic functioning also have been found not to be useful, but rigorous studies are quite limited. It is very likely that other medications with more specific modes of action will be utilized with TS during the next several years.

CHOICE OF MEDICATION. The clinician's choice of a first drug is a difficult decision. Haloperidol has the longest "track record," and its therapeutic benefits and side effects are well defined; the only other major contender as a first drug today is clonidine, which is less well defined and less likely to be dramatically effective. Those clinicians who lean toward clonidine as a first drug do so because of its limited side effects and positive effect on attention; however, where a rapid response is needed, haloperidol may be more effective. Until more evidence accumulates, or other drugs become available, it will be hard to decide if a patient should have a several-month course of clonidine before starting haloperidol or the other way around. If a patient is started on haloperidol, it may be difficult to discontinue because of withdrawal symptoms, which are not attenuated by clonidine at usual doses. Some clinicians have added low-dose clonidine to low-dose haloperidol with good results, but no controlled studies have been reported. Whether pimozide will become an alternative to haloperidol will depend on the seriousness and frequency of side effects when it is more widely used.

When used alone, antidepressant medications either worsen or are not useful in the treatment of TS. However, TS patients may develop serious depressions, and then the use of antidepressant medication should be considered. In these situations, antidepressants have been added to other, ongoing TS treatment (haloperidol, clonidine) with good results. Complicating the assessment of depression in TS is the fact that both haloperidol and clonidine may elicit lowered spirits or dysphoria. Therefore, a trial of no medication might be considered before the addition of an antidepressant, especially if the depression emerges soon after the use of another medication and with no apparent psychosocial precipitant. Various minor tranquilizers have been used in the treatment of TS with no apparent benefit on the tic symptomatology; however, individual patients seem to have benefited from these medications when used to help alleviate anxiety or improve sleep. As such, their use for TS patients should follow usual guidelines.

Academic Intervention

Children with attentional and learning problems require educational intervention similar to the approaches used in the treatment of other forms of ADD and learning disabilities. TS patients may require special tutoring, a learning laboratory, a self-contained classroom, a special or residential school, depending on the severity of school and associated behavioral problems. It may be difficult to convince a school district of the need for special-school provisions for a bright TS patient who does not have specific learning disabilities but whose attentional problems limit his optimal functioning. Since TS is an uncommon disorder, schools need to be informed about the nature of TS and the ways it affects attention and learning; sometimes the physician must actively serve as a child's advocate.

Children with TS sometimes are kept as homebound students because their symptoms are thought to be too disruptive for the classroom. Most difficult for teachers are phonic symptoms. If a child is homebound, he is being deprived of his legal rights for the least restrictive educational environment and an adequate education. We consider this an emergency situation, demanding intensive medical and legal intervention. When children stay at home, their TS symptoms are likely to exacerbate, as they exert less control and are exposed to the tedium of no outside diversions and the intense, often negative or ambivalent interactions with parents. A chain reaction may be set up in which bad symptoms lead to worse symptoms and increasing isolation from normal forces of socialization. Even more than tics, school difficulties and appropriate school placement require prompt clinical intervention, and we place our first emphasis in this area.

Genetic Counseling

Parents and older TS patients want to know about genetic risk for siblings and offspring. Since the precise mode of inheritance is still not known, only generalizations are possible. Parents considering having another child should be told that having a first-degree relative (parent or sibling) with TS increases the risk of having the disorder from 1 in many hundreds or thousands to 1 in 4 or 5. The risk is higher by far for male offspring. For a young adult with TS who is thinking about having a child, genetic counseling must be done cautiously and with sensitivity about the meaning of the information. As previously noted, the offspring of a mother with TS are at quite high risk. At present, there is no method for prenatal diagnosis. In providing genetic counseling, it is important to emphasize the uncertainties, as well as the increasing knowledge about treatment. A high-risk family might consider abortion if the fetus is male, to reduce the likelihood of the expression of TS; however, such a decision is highly charged with feelings, and the definition of the clinician's role in such a situation is beyond the scope of this discussion.

Multiply Handicapped TS Patients

The most difficult treatment problems arise for the adolescent or adult with long-standing, severe TS and multiple associated social and academic difficulties. It is not uncommon for these most severely afflicted individuals to have few personal or social resources and to be locked into intensely ambivalent relationships with their exhausted families. Disentangling what is "Tourette's" and what are the manifold consequences of chronicity, disorganization, and various medications may be a major, long-term therapeutic task. Patients may no longer know what is under their control, in any sense of this term, and what is primarily a manifestaion of their TS. Reconstructing their experience and trying to understand what they are doing is a goal of the therapeutic work. Medication withdrawal and side effects confuse matters and make it difficult to assess any intervention. Most pathetic are the young adults who exhibit self-mutilation, such as poking their eyes or banging their heads, during TS crises; perhaps equally painful are those patients who have become chronically dependent and unable to function on their own but who have nobody to whom to turn.

For the young adult who has had serious interferences with school achievement, socialization, and personality development, a thorough rehabilitation program is required. The patient may need vocational guidance, a half-way-house program, psychotherapy, family counseling, and advocacy, in addition to judicious use of medication. Even in desperate situations, therapeutic commitment combined with the patient's determination and courage may lead to satisfying therapeutic results. The treatment is facilitated if there is a therapeutic team which can be mutually supportive and can work together to find social and financial resources during the many months when the patient may be dependent and demanding.

Clinicians and the patient must recognize that episodes of exacerbation are to be expected. At such times, months of hard-won progress may seem to dissipate in days without a trace. During such exacerbations, when a patient may start to hurt himself again and "fall apart," it is natural for the physician to become disappointed and angry, for the patient to sense this, and for the treatment relationship to end; the patient may feel enraged and utterly discouraged. Clinicians, like parents, may cajole, bribe, and threaten. It may be difficult for the physician to know how to set limits that can be used by the patient to regain a sense of inner control, and to know when such behavioral approaches are an expression of anger. However, if a therapeutic alliance can be maintained, it is possible to weather the storm and for this shared experience to strengthen the treatment relationship as the patient re-stabilizes.

Short-term hospitalization may be of use during crises. However, TS patients may be unwelcome on an inpatient neurology or psychiatry service because of their disruptive and often bizarre behavior. Phonic symptoms are as difficult to tolerate in a hospital as in school. When patients are hospitalized, there is a tendency to use medication for sedation, not only because of the patient's needs but because of the anxiety of the clinical staff and other patients. Yet, the availability of an inpatient service willing to accept a TS patient in crisis can be reassuring for both the patient and the physician.

CONCLUSION

TS is a chronic and usually lifelong disorder in which the simple motor and phonic tics may interfere less with development than complex tics (compulsions), complex phonic symptoms, and associated attentional and behavioral problems. Evaluation must include careful attention to personality development and school achievement; intervention includes reassurance and support, medication if needed, and guidance and advocacy in relation to appropriate school placement. Throughout the assessment and treatment, target symptoms should include not only motor and phonic symptoms but an individual's full range of functioning. The major goal of treatment is to help the child succeed in moving along the various lines of development. The use of medication that interferes with these achievements runs the risk of creating patients who are socially more disadvantaged than had they been left undiagnosed. Being maintained on psychoactive medications for many years poses many medical and behavioral toxicological risks that require careful scrutiny.

Family therapy, psychotherapy, and behavior-modification approaches have limited value in regard to the motor and phonic tics, but they should be considered for the behavioral and psychological problems that may compound TS or be elicited in a family because of the stress of a chronic neuropsychiatric disorder. As with any chronic disorder, periods of exacerbation are likely to lead to anxiety and stress which may further exacerbate the condition. The clinician's availability and a long-standing relationship are especially important at such times. One reassuring fact for families and patients with TS is that TS has become an area of active clinical-research interest and more has been learned in the past few years than in the preceding century (Friedhoff and Chase, 1982; Leckman and Cohen, 1983).

REFERENCES

American Psychiatric Association. 1980. *Diagnostic and statistical manual of mental disorders (DSM-III)*. Washington, D.C.: APA.

Cohen, D. J., Detlor, J., Shaywitz, B. A., and Leckman, J. F. 1982. Interaction of biological and psychological factors in the natural history of Tourette syndrome: A paradigm for childhood neuropsychiatric disorders. In *Gilles de la Tourette syndrome: Advances in neurology,* vol. 35, ed. A. J. Friedhoff, and T. N. Chase, pp. 31-40. New York: Raven Press.

Cohen, D. J., Detlor, J., Young, J. G., and Shaywitz, B. A. 1980. Clonidine ameliorates Gilles de la Tourette syndrome. *Arch. Gen. Psych.*, 37:1350-1357.

Cohen, D. J., Shaywitz, B. A., Young, J. G., Carbonari, C. M., Nathanson, J. A., Lieberman, D., Bowers, M. B., Jr., and Maas, J. W. 1979. Central biogenic amine metabolism in children with the syndrome of chronic multiple tics of Gilles de la Tourette: Norepinephrine, serotonin, and dopamine. *J. Am. Acad. Child Psych.*, 18:320-341.

Friedhoff, A. J., and Chase, T. N., eds. 1982. *Gilles de la Tourette syndrome: Advances in neurology*. vol. 35. New York: Raven Press.

Golden, G. S. 1974. Gilles de la Tourette's syndrome following methylphenidate administration. *Dev. Med. Child Neurol.*, 16:76-78.

Leckman, J. F., and Cohen, D. J. 1983. Recent advances in Gilles de la Tourette syndrome: Implications for clinical practice and future research. *Psychiat. Dev.* 3:301-316.

Lowe, T. L., Cohen, D. J., Detlor, J., Kremenitzer, M. W., and Shaywitz, B. A. 1982. Stimulant medications precipitate Tourette's syndrome. *J. Am. Med. Assoc.*, 247:1729-1731.

Pauls, D. L., Cohen, D. J., Heimbuch, R., Detlor, J., and Kidd, K. K. 1981. Familial pattern and transmission of Gilles de la Tourette syndrome and multiple tics. *Arch. Gen. Psych.*, 38:1085-1090.

Shapiro, A. K., and Shapiro, E. 1982. Clinical efficacy of haloperidol, pimozide, penfluridol, and clonidine in the treatment of Tourette syndrome. In *Gilles de la Tourette syndrome: Advances in neurology,* vol. 35, ed. A. J. Friedhoff, and T. N. Chase, pp. 383-386. New York: Raven Press.

Shapiro, A. K., Shapiro, E., Brunn, R. D., and Sweet, R. D. 1978. *Gilles de la Tourette's syndrome*. New York: Raven Press.

APPENDIX. Yale Tourette Syndrome Symptom List (Revised)

Patient _____ I.D.# _____ Date ___/___/___

Rate Each Symptom by Putting the Appropriate Number in the Box Each Day. (Use the reverse side for any detailed comments.)

Rater __ 1. Patient
       __ 2. Mother
       __ 3. Father
       __ 4. Other

0 = Not at all or symptom free
1 = Just a little
2 = Pretty much
3 = Very much
4 = Extreme
5 = Almost always

Date	Mon	Tue	Wed	Thur	Fri	Sat	Sun

Simple Motor

	Mon	Tue	Wed	Thur	Fri	Sat	Sun
Eyeblinking							
Other facial tics							
Head jerks							
Shoulder jerks							
Arm movements							
Finger or hand movements							
Stomach jerks							
Kicking leg movements							
Tense parts of body							
Other							
Other							

Sum of Simple Motor Symptoms _____

Complex Motor

	Mon	Tue	Wed	Thur	Fri	Sat	Sun
Touching part of body							
Touching other people							
Touching objects							
Can't start actions							
Hurts self							
Finger or hand tapping							
Hopping							
Picks at things (clothing, etc.)							
Copropraxia							
Other							
Other							

Sum of Complex Motor Symptoms _____

(continued)

APPENDIX. Yale Tourette Syndrome Symptom List (Revised) (continued)

Date	Mon	Tue	Wed	Thur	Fri	Sat	Sun
Simple Phonic							
Noises							
Grunting							
Throat clearing							
Coughing							
Other							
Other							

Sum of Simple Phonic Symptoms _____

Complex Phonic							
Words							
Repeats own words/sentences							
Repeats others speech							
Coprolalia (obscene words)							
Insults (lack of inhibition)							
Other							
Other							

Sum of Complex Phonic Symptoms _____

Behavior							
Argumentative							
Poor frustration tolerance							
Anger, temper fits							
Provocative							
Other							
Other							

Sum of Behavior Symptoms _____

# of Days _____

2

Nocturnal Enuresis: Its Investigation and Treatment

DAVID SHAFFER

CLINICAL FEATURES

Nocturnal enuresis is a chronic condition characterized by the involuntary passage of urine during sleep in children age four or older. An enuretic child or adolescent will usually wet once or several times during night sleep but may also do so during brief daytime naps. Most children who present for treatment will be wet several times a week and most will have been wet all of their lives.

Enuretic incidents are most likely to occur between midnight and 3:00 A.M. (Rapoport et al., 1980). A minority of enuretics will awaken after micturition, and the occurrence of this phenomenon has no known significance for diagnosis, treatment, or prognosis.

About one in six of younger enuretics (i.e., those aged between four and seven years) will also have occasional or regular daytime incontinence (Bloomfield and Douglas, 1956). Many enuretic children will experience urinary frequency and urgency during the day, the significance of which is discussed later.

Some enuretic children will be dry when sleeping away from home, although this pattern is rarely sustained if the vacation, hospital admission, etc., is a prolonged one. This is probably a consequence of disturbed sleep and has no particular significance for etiology or prognosis. It may anger parents who often feel that the child who is only wet at home is being incontinent on purpose.

EPIDEMIOLOGY AND NATURAL HISTORY

At age three, approximately 25% of children wet their beds at least once a week. Of these, 20% will have become completely dry by their fourth birthday (Shaffer, 1980). However, of the children who are still wet at age four, only 6% will go on to become dry by their fifth birthday. The rate at which children spontaneously become dry will persist at this low level throughout childhood and adolescence. Approximately 1% of eighteen-year-old males will still be regularly wet (Shaffer, 1980). Practitioners should, therefore, be cautious in predicting spontaneous recovery for any enuretic child over the age of four.

Most enuretics have never been dry. However, a small proportion of children, more often boys than girls, will only start to wet in middle childhood, usually between the ages of five and seven. This condition is called *secondary,* or *onset,* enuresis. Secondary enuresis rarely starts before the age of five (Miller, 1973). Although secondary enuresis may often appear to have been precipitated by a stressful event such as starting school, the birth of a sibling, or a separation experience (Werry and Cohrssen, 1965), the rate of psychiatric disturbance is no higher in this group than among primary enuretics, and by no means all secondary enuretics have emotional or behavior problems (Novick, 1966; Rutter et al., 1973). A single longitudinal study has indicated that secondary enuretics are less likely to remit spontaneously than primary enuretics of the same age (Miller et al., 1960).

In younger children enuresis is as common among boys as among girls (Rutter et al., 1973). However, enuresis is more common in boys than girls after age seven. In part, this is because boys show slower rates of spontaneous remission than girls, and in part, because they are more likely to develop secondary enuresis than girls (Oppel et al., 1968; Miller et al., 1960).

Enuresis rarely stops suddenly. The usual pattern of acquiring continence is that the child wets with diminishing frequency until enuresis only occurs sporadically, often in association with an intercurrent infection or at the time of acute stress (Miller et al., 1960).

Associated Conditions

Psychiatric Symptoms

Psychiatric symptoms are found in about one-fifth of all enuretic children (Rutter et al., 1973). The proportion of bed wetters with associated psychiatric problems will of course be higher among those referred for treatment to a psychiatric clinic and lower among those referred to a pediatrician or urologist. Enuretic girls are more likely to have an associated psychiatric disturbance than enuretic boys, and disturbance is also more common in children who are wet during both day and night. Psychiatric problems are as common in older enuretics as in younger ones. Disturbed enuretic children show a full range of psychiatric problems, but they are somewhat more likely to have anxiety symptoms and a degree of social withdrawal than other psychiatric patients. Despite reports in the clinical literature, studies on more representative populations reveal no particular association between enuresis and other habit disorders such as motor tics and nail biting (Rutter et al., 1973).

Although the psychodynamic literature indicates that enuretic children are especially likely to be passive and/or passive aggressive and to show dependent personality characteristics, there is no convincing evidence of any characteristic dynamic or personality structure in the large and very heterogenous population of children who wet the bed (Achenbach and Lewis, 1971).

It should be emphasized that although the majority of enuretic children show no signs of any psychiatric disturbance, most are significantly distressed by their condition, and many otherwise well-adjusted enuretic children will show an increase in social confidence and independent behavior after successful treatment (Hedge and Shaffer, in preparation).

Developmental Disorders

A proportion of enuretic children, and in particular boys, have a history of mild to moderate developmental speech lag, and some have persistent articulation difficulties lasting into middle childhood (Hallgren, 1957; Kolvin et al., 1972). Like all children with speech delay, these enuretics are at greater risk for learning difficulties.

Urinary Tract Abnormalities and Infections

Associated urinary tract infections are found about five times more often in enuretic than in nonenuretic girls (Meadow et al., 1969). The urinary tract infections found in enuretic children most commonly have no obvious anatomic cause. It is not clear whether the processes that underlie the urinary infection lead to the enuresis or whether enuresis itself might predispose to urinary infection. Urination in a recumbent posture may facilitate ascending infection. There is some suggestion that this may be the case because the excess of urinary infection in enuretics is confined to girls, who are more prone to ascending infection than boys, and also because there is some evidence that recurrence of urinary infection is more likely in enuretics than in non-enuretics (Dodge et al., 1970).

DIFFERENTIAL DIAGNOSIS

Enuresis needs to be distinguished from other causes of nocturnal incontinence, such as any cause of *polyuria* (e.g., diabetes, renal disease, diabetes insipidus, etc.). The differentiation is not usually difficult. The undiagnosed polyuric child will usually be ill and show other symptoms, will wake before being incontinent, and their symptoms will be of recent and acute onset.

Nocturnal epilepsy may result in incontinence without waking. However, the frequency of incontinence is likely to be considerably less than in the usual enuretic, and there may be other clinical features to suggest the diagnosis. In practice very few cases of nocturnal epilepsy present as cases of enuresis.

ETIOLOGY

Enuresis is probably determined by both biological and experiential factors acting separately or in conjunction. Many theories have been put forward to explain the condition. These include a basic disturbance of sleep rhythm; subacute urethral obstruction with detrusor muscle hypertrophy and bladder hypertonicity; a need to display aggression in an indirect fashion, etc. However, only three convincing factors have been found in reported studies (for a review, see Shaffer, 1984).

Genetics

Enuresis is clearly genetically determined—75% of all enuretics will have a first-degree relative who wet the bed after the age of five, and the concordance rate for enuresis is significantly higher in monozygous than in dizygous twins (Bakwin, 1961).

Bladder Disturbances

A significant proportion of enuretics appear to show a functional bladder disturbance, both symptomatically and on testing (Starfield, 1967; Shaffer et al., 1984). In the normal person an increase in urinary volume is accommodated by a concomitant reduction in bladder tone, which maintains the bladder pressure at a more or less constant level up until the occurrence of the micturition contraction. However, in a substantial proportion of enuretics relatively small increases in urinary volume will be accompanied by increased intravesical pressure. This presumably follows from a failure of the bladder to accommodate to the regular inflow of urine and is mediated by the autonomic nervous system under midbrain control. Bladder relaxation during filling—at least in animals—is facilitated by the tricyclic antidepressants (Shaffer et al., 1979), and this may be one mode of their action in this condition. High bladder tone may also be responsible for urinary symptoms such as urgency and frequency which occur in many enuretics.

Social-Learning Factors

There is some evidence that enuresis is more common among children who are not toilet trained at all or who were late in being toilet trained (Kaffman and Elizur, 1977). Furthermore, enuresis occurs more often among children who are living in institutions (Stein and Susser, 1965) and in children reared under unfavorable social and family circumstances. These factors may each be associated with inadequate social-learning opportunities. The efficiency of social learning may also be reduced if the parents of the enuretic child are extremely tolerant toward the symptom. This could be because the parents themselves were enuretic as children and may, therefore, either be more sensitive to the distress experienced by their own enuretic child; because they wish to deny the importance of a condition that they may feel they have passed on to their child; or, if they were not adequately treated themselves, because they have a feeling of helplessness about the condition. Thus it is not uncommon to find that no one in the family will talk about the problem, which becomes a well-known but unspoken secret within the family. Similarly, enuresis is often well tolerated in children's institutions, bed-wetting being regarded as symptomatic of some underlying distress rather than as a habit disorder in its own right. It is likely that this otherwise praiseworthy tact and consideration leads to a diminution of negative contingencies for the enuresis and may serve to perpetuate the condition.

Whether or not enuresis can ever be regarded as symptomatic of an underlying psychiatric disturbance is unclear. As mentioned earlier, only a minority of enuretics have associated psychiatric symptomatology, and disturbed enuretics appear to respond as well to purely symptomatic treatments as those who are not disturbed (Shaffer, 1984). Furthermore, controlled studies indicate that psychotherapy alone will not cure enuresis. These findings all suggest that associated psychopathology should not be regarded as a cause of enuresis. Given the heritability of the condition and the fact that there are enuretics who will wet less frequently during school vacations, others who relapse at times of stress, and others who only start to wet after a traumatic episode, it is probably most sensible to regard enuresis as a biological condition which may be influenced by stress or inadequate social learning at a critical period of development, rather than as a symptom of some underlying psychopathological process.

Assessment of the Enuretic Child

History: To Make the Diagnosis

Ascertain the frequency, periodicity, and duration of symptoms to exclude causes of sporadic incontinence such as a seizure disorder. Determine whether there is associated daytime incontinence and/or polyuria. If there is daytime incontinence, this will require a specific treatment program of its own. Daytime symptoms that are suggestive of polyuria will need full medical investigation.

Determine whether there is a positive family history of enuresis. If so, it will make the diagnosis of functional enuresis more likely. If that affected relative is the accompanying parent, the knowledge may be helpful in dealing with such processes as projective identification between parent and child which may interfere in the therapeutic process.

If the enuresis is secondary, i.e., had its onset after a period of prolonged dryness, determine whether it followed a traumatic event or was associated with other physical symptoms suggesting an underlying physical illness. It seems likely that quite often a "precipitating" stress event represents an attempt by the parent or child to assign meaning to the problem and is not causally related to the onset of secondary enuresis. Nevertheless, the psychological weight of the stress will need to be acknowledged and then taken into account in the clinical management of the case.

History: To Ascertain the Presence of Associated Features

Inquire about the presence of behavioral and emotional symptoms. Ask about language milestones and ascertain whether there are any persistent articulation or speech difficulties. If there are abnormalities, make special inquiries about school progress and any possible associated learning difficulties.

Determine the quality of social relationships and behaviors indicative of poor self-confidence. Inquire about symptoms that could indicate associated intercurrent urinary tract infection such as episodic pyrexia, gastro-intestinal symptoms (e.g., nausea and vomiting), or genito-urinary symptoms (e.g., dysuria and urgency).

History: To Plan Treatment

As with any chronic condition, find out why the parent has decided to seek help now rather than at some previous time. A common reason is preparation for a forthcoming vacation away from home. If this is the case, the practitioner will be unwise to suggest lengthy baseline observations and a slowly effective treatment. Other reasons for seeking referral may include unrelated family or child crises which may need attention quite independently of the enuresis.

Inquire about the previous use of common home managements, e.g., fluid restriction, rewards and punishments, and waking the child at night before the parent goes to sleep. Most parents have used one or the other of these methods before seeking professional help. The rewards and punishments will usually have been of a material nature, such as cash or gifts or withholding of an allowance, or inconsistent social punishments, such as scolding or shouting followed by apologetic or reparative behaviors. The reward will often have been given after some delay (e.g., "If you are dry for a week, then you can have . . .") and provided inconsistently. These approaches will have been predictably ineffective but may well have contributed to a feeling of hopelessness in the parent ("I have tried everything").

There is no evidence that fluid restriction is an effective management technique, but wetting in some children is controlled with night waking. If this procedure has never been used, it should be included as a preliminary management approach.

Inquire about unusual parental managements, e.g., the use of physical punishment, or the opposite, e.g., an excessively solicitous or sympathetic approach. The punitive parent will rarely comply with the demands of complex conditioning techniques. Their child is also likely to have associated psychiatric problems that will require separate interventions.

A different problem occurs among parents who identify strongly with the distress of their enuretic child. Some parents will insist that enuresis is a symptom of underlying unhappiness and maladjustment, and they may find it especially difficult to comply with a behaviorally oriented treatment that focuses on the wetting behavior. They may insist on less focused therapy. In such cases the unhappiness and maladjustment should be regarded as associated and not underlying conditions, and both merit and should receive their own specific treatments. This should be explained to the parent.

There is also a group of parents who feel certain that children can control wetting if they choose to. They may cite episodes of dryness when the child is away from home as evidence for their belief. In some this may be a cloak for hostility to the child, although they may stop short of physical punishment. In others the parent feels overwhelmed by the problem, and their assertion that the symptom can be controlled may relieve them from facing an unmanageable situation. In either case the parents may state that they do not wish to become personally involved in the treatment. It is sometimes alleged that this will only interfere with the child's development of independence. Special attention will have to be given to working with such parents to allow them to take the active role in the treatment that may be required.

Inquire about previous special treatments. Conditioning treatment will often have been used without expert instruction or guidance. An apparatus may have been purchased by mail order or prescribed by a professional who is unfamiliar with the many practical problems that arise during treatment. Before accepting that conditioning treatment has failed in a previous trial, inquire about its duration and which, if any, problems were encountered. More often than not, the treatment will have been abandoned prematurely by parents or child because of difficulties that could have been overcome with more adequate explanation and supervision (see later discussion). Similarly, an initial cure may have been achieved with conditioning treatment and have been followed by a relapse. Under these circumstances some parents may be reluctant to provide the child with a further course of treatment even though this is the correct procedure to follow.

If medication has been used, inquire about its nature, dose, duration, and efficacy, and whether or not (or which) side effects were encountered. Ascertain what the parents' attitude is toward medical treatment.

Obtain information that will help you plan the treatment that is probably going to be most effective, e.g., conditioning treatment. Inquire whether the child sleeps alone or with siblings, what is the disposition of the parents' and the child's bedrooms, where the parent normally spends the later part of the evening after the child goes to bed, and the relative times of going to bed of the parent and the child. Effective management of conditioning treatment may require direct interventions from the parent both in the early and in the later parts of the evening.

INVESTIGATIONS

Physical Examination

All children should have a routine physical examination with special note being made of any apparent congenital malformations. Because congenital malformations are often multiple, the presence of one in any system may call for a more extensive uro-genital examination.

All children should also have a clean catch specimen of urine examined for bacteriuria. This examination should be repeated on at least two separate occasions for girls.

A more detailed uroradiological or full medical investigation is only called for if there is (1) bacteriuria or symptoms suggestive of recurrent urinary tract infections, (2) a history of episodic enuresis associated with dysuria, urgency, and frequency, (3) a clear history of polyuria.

Psychometric Evaluation

If in examining the child there is an apparent articulation or speech disorder and/or if there is any history suggestive of current learning difficulties or problems at school, IQ or reading ability should be assessed with the appropriate psychometric tests.

Mental-Status Evaluation

Determine what the child has been told about the causes, prevalence, treatment, and prognosis of enuresis. In particular, explore whether the child feels the bed-wetting to be his or her own fault, and how common the child understands the condition to be among other children. Many children are sure that they are unique in being enuretic. Others anticipate that treatment will involve injections or surgical operations on their genitalia.

Determine whether to be cured of enuresis figures in a "three-wishes" probe (i.e., "If you could have three wishes which could come true, what would they be?"). Many parents misinterpret embarrassment or denial by their child as a sign of indifference, and this may affect attitudes to the problem and treatment.

Ascertain from the child who else in the family or in the child's peer group knows about the condition and what the child's attitude is to this. Both secrecy in the family and teasing by siblings or peers may need to be addressed in the final treatment plan. Inquire about the nature of the child's social relations with other family members. If the condition is episodic, attempt to ascertain whether the child has had features of depression during the periods of incontinence.

AVAILABLE TREATMENTS

General Reassurance and Record Keeping

About 10% of enuretic children will show a significant diminution in their wetting frequency after an initial visit to a practitioner who has provided nothing more than reassurance and requested systematic recording of each dry and wet night over a two-week period (Shaffer et al., 1968).

Reassurance is addressed to both the child and the parent. It should be made clear that enuresis is a biologically based condition that may be made worse by stress and that it will often cause adverse psychological consequences or be associated in a non-causal way with other psychiatric problems. It should be stated very explicitly that enuresis is not a willful behavior under the child's conscious control. Younger children should be told that they are not alone in suffering from the condition and that it is common in their age group. Reassurance is also provided by discussing the excellent prognosis that can be expected from satisfactory treatment.

The record keeping is usually done by maintaining a "star chart," i.e., a chart on which a star or other sticker is placed if the child was dry on the previous night. Many parents will say that their child is too old to use stars or stickers, but even youngsters in their early teens appear to obtain satisfaction and social reinforcement from a graphic display of their progress.

It is important to stress that children should keep and complete the star chart themselves but that they should show it to the parent each day. The parent should then offer appropriate social reinforcement if there has been a dry night. If the parent decides to keep the chart ("in the interest of accuracy"), then the child will have a reduced sense of participation. If the child keeps the chart and does not show it on a daily basis to the parent, the opportunity for social reinforcement for success is reduced.

Very little is known about which children respond to these measures, which may be assumed to reduce anxiety and optimize social reinforcement for success. Their subsequent relapse rate is unknown, and their clinical and personality characteristics have not been studied.

Night Waking and Fluid Restriction Before Bed

Waking a child during the night and restricting fluids before bedtime are commonsense measures frequently adopted by the parents of younger children who are still wet at night. Roberts and Schoellkopf (1951) investigated these practices intensively in a community study and concluded that they did little to increase the chances of a dry night. The only controlled study into night lifting and fluid restriction in older children was that carried out by Hagglund (1965) on a group of psychiatric inpatients. He found that although there was an initial reduction in the frequency of wetting, the response was short-lived, and after three months the group treated was wet as often as a no-treatment control group.

However, it may be that these practices are more effective in the majority of bed wetters who are never referred for specialist treatment. A good response to waking the child before the parent retires and ensuring that he or she passes urine at that time may be one of the factors that deters some parents from seeking professional help. If a parent has never used night lifting, it is probably worthwhile suggesting that systematic observations be made for one week during which waking is carried out, and for one week when the child is allowed to sleep through the night as usual. If these observations indicate more dry nights during the period of waking, the procedure should be given a more extensive trial.

Surgery Treatment

A rationale for the surgical treatment of enuresis—usually urethral dilatation, meatotomy, or bladder-neck repair—has been suggested by Mahony (1971). The reasoning is that many enuretics have a sub-critical obstructive lesion of the urinary outflow tract, most commonly anterior urethral valves or meatal stenosis alone or in combination with bladder-neck obstruction. The purported pathological entities have come under critical review (Manley and French, 1970; Cendron and Lewpinard, 1972) and their relevance to common enuresis has been questioned. The interventions listed do not appear to alter the urodynamic properties of the bladder. Attempts to modify the neurological control of the bladder by division of the sacral nerves (Torrens and Haldt, 1979) or the detrusor by bladder transection have also been disappointing (Jankneget et al., 1979). There have been no controlled surgical treatment studies. The hazards of surgical intervention are well documented (Smith, 1969) and include urinary incontinence, recurrent epididymitis, and aspermia.

Psychotherapy

Controlled studies have shown that psychotherapy alone does not cure or reduce the frequency of enuresis (Werry and Cohrssen, 1965; DeLeon and Mandell, 1966). This is not, of course, to say that psychotherapeutic principles and sensitivity is not required in the clinical management of this problem, just as they may be in any doctor-patient interaction.

Hypnosis

Two studies have suggested that hypnotherapy may be effective in reducing wetting frequency (Bauman and Hinman, 1974; Olness, 1975). However, these studies have been inadequately designed, without control groups, and the duration of improvement has not been documented. Furthermore, it is not clear whether only hypnotizable children will respond favorably to this form of management.

Pharmacotherapy

Of the many drugs that have been used to treat enuresis (for a historical review of this subject, see Blackwell and Currah, 1973), most studies have involved three main drug groups: the amphetamines, the anti-cholinergics, and the tricyclic anti-depressants.

AMPHETAMINES. The rationale for using amphetamines is that they reduce the depth of sleep. However, there is no evidence that enuretics sleep either more heavily or any differently than nonenuretic children (Rapoport et al., 1980). A double-blind study (McConaghy, 1969) found amphetamines to be no more effective than placebo and to be markedly inferior to either conditioning treatment or imipramine. There is, however, some suggestion that amphetamines may shorten the duration of conditioning treatment (Young and Turner, 1965), although this is thought to be an effect on learning behavior rather than on the enuresis itself.

ANTICHOLINERGIC DRUGS. Drugs such as belladonna, propantheline, and methscopolamine have been used extensively to treat bed-wetting. The rationale for their use is that they inhibit detrusor contraction and that in non-enuretics their use is associated with urinary retention. However, a number of double-blind controlled studies have now been carried out and none have shown them to have a significant antienuretic effect (Wallace and Forsyth, 1969; Rapoport et al., 1980).

TRICYCLIC ANTIDEPRESSANTS. The efficacy of imipramine in suppressing bed-wetting was first reported by MacLean in 1960. Since then, careful studies (Shaffer et al., 1968; Rapoport et al., 1980) have been carried out which confirm their effectiveness. The newer, related class of drugs, the tetracyclics, such as maprotiline, also appear to be effective antienuretics (Simeon et al., 1981).

Studies comparing tricyclics such as imipramine, amitriptyline, nortryptyline, and desmethylimipramine show that all have a similar antienuretic effect (Blackwell and Currah, 1973; Rapoport et al., 1980). With imipramine this is closely related to the total plasma concentration of imipramine (IMI) and its principal metabolite desipramine (DMI). The optimum effect appears to be reached with a combined IMI-DMI plasma level at or above 60 mg/ml, which may require a nighttime dose of between 1 and 2.5 mg/kg (Jorgensen et al., 1980). Providing that dosage is adequate, the effect is usually noted within one week of starting treatment. Because children receiving the same oral doses of imipramine may show very different plasma levels (Rapoport et al., 1980) standard dosage schedules will not always provide a good guide to adequate doses. Careful studies (Rapoport et al., 1980; Jorgensen et al., 1980) have noted that the clinical effect wears off in a substantial proportion of patients still receiving medication. This tolerance becomes apparent between two and six weeks after treatment has begun. There is no evidence that children ever show a delayed response.

Imipramine will reduce wetting frequency in about 85% of bed wetters and will suppress wetting completely in about 30%. Relapse after withdrawal of medication may be immediate or delayed, but within three months of stopping treatment nearly all children treated with imipramine will be wetting again at or near their previous wetting frequency (Shaffer et al., 1968). The technique of stopping the drug—gradual or abrupt withdrawal—does not seem to influence the relapse rate. The effect of very prolonged treatment has not been studied. However, variations in duration with periods of less than six months do not influence outcome.

A number of studies have shown that imipramine produces a hypertensive effect in children. The magnitude of this effect is directly related to serum levels of IMI and DMI (Lake et al., 1979). Side effects from the tricyclic compounds used in therapeutic doses are uncommon if the serum level of combined IMI-DMI is below 50 mg/ml. They are invariably present if it is above 100 mg/ml. The most frequent unwanted effects are dry mouth, dizziness, headache, and constipation. Some hyperactive children may show a worsening of their restlessness and distractibility. The tricyclic drugs should not be prescribed for children under the age of four years. Goel and Shanks (1974) have reported a number of cases of acute tricyclic poisoning in this age group, although poisoning was most common in the untreated younger siblings of the enuretic children, who had taken the drug accidentally.

Most authors advise against a dose exceeding 5 mg/kg (Rohner and Sanford, 1975) and it has been suggested that if doses higher than 3.5 mg/kg are given, EKG monitoring should be used to detect signs of conduction delay (Saraf et al., 1978). Manifestations of toxicity include cardiac irregularities, convulsions, hallucinations, retention of urine, and ataxia. Death, when it occurs, is usually due to a cardiac arrhythmia.

Retention-Control training

In 1948 Smith suggested that enuresis could be treated by training children to defer micturition during the day. Paschalis et al. (1972), Stedman (1972), and Miller (1973) have described a treatment procedure whereby enuretic children are instructed to delay micturition in increments of 2 to 3 minutes each day after feeling the urge to void. Tokens were provided each time this was done, just *before* use of the toilet (the token after micturition might have the effect of reinforcing rather than deferring micturition). This continues for twenty days, by which time the children should be deferring micturition for forty-five minutes on each occasion. In a controlled treatment study, half the children adopting this procedure and none of the controls became dry at night (Paschalis et al., 1972).

However, these positive findings have not been confirmed by others (Harris and Purohit, 1977; Fielding, 1980). In Fielding's study comparisons were made between treatment with the bell and pad only (see later) and four weeks of retention-control training *followed by* the bell and pad. Bell and pad was far superior to retention control in reducing night wetting in both nocturnally and diurnally enuretic children. Functional bladder capacity was measured before and after treatment and no significant increase was noted among the night wetters regardless of cure. Given that retention control is a time-consuming and questionably effective treatment, there is at present no clear indication for its use alone or in combination with other procedures.

Conditioning

HISTORY AND DESCRIPTION. Pfaundler (1904) devised an alarm system to alert nurses after their patients had wet the bed. He noted that when this was done many children stopping wetting. Despite this early report of a successful treatment for enuresis, the method was not generally applied for another thirty years when Mowrer and Mowrer (1938) described a similar device. The Mowrer apparatus (known as bell and pad), with some technical refinements, has continued in use and constitutes the most effective form of therapy now available. The device usually consists of an auditory signal linked to two electrodes, either in the form of perforated metal or foil sheets separated by an ordinary cotton sheet, or electrode strips placed on a single plastic sheet running parallel in a spiral pattern. The presence of urine effects contact between the two electrodes and triggers the alarm.

THEORETICAL BASIS. A number of theories have been advanced to explain the efficacy of the alarm system. In the classical-conditioning paradigm, bladder distension or the micturition contraction is assumed to be the indifferent stimulus (IS). Treatment introduces the auditory signal which becomes the unconditioned stimulus (US) in proximity to the IS, which then acquires the properties of a conditioned stimulus (CS) leading to the conditioned response (CR) (waking). Support for a conditioning model is provided by the findings that: (a) when the introduction of the US is delayed treatment is ineffective; and (b) extinction of the CR after initial cure can be inhibited by intermittent reinforcement (Finley et al., 1973) and by overlearning (Young and Morgan, 1972). These are features that would be expected from a classical-conditioning model.

However, it seems likely that other learning processes are also involved. The "gadget effect" in which the child becomes dry when the apparatus is placed on the bed but not switched on (DeLeon and Mandell, 1966) suggests that avoidance learning, a form of operant conditioning, may also be important. The effectiveness of a twin-signal apparatus designed by Lovibond (1964) and Hansen (1979) lends support to this. The apparatus emits a moderate-volume auditory signal when micturition is first detected and a second much louder aversive noise several seconds later. Hansen has demonstrated its efficacy in enuretic children who did not respond to conventional bell-and-pad treatment and postulates that avoidance learning (to avoid the second loud, aversive noise) may be being coupled with classic conditioning to result in cure. Crosby (1950) put forward the view that the apparatus worked primarily through punishment training. He devised an instrument that applied an electric shock to the legs of the child after micturition. In fact, this instrument has proved no more effective than the Mowrer device and is understandably less acceptable to both parents and children (Lovibond, 1964). Turner (1973) has pointed out that the use of the bell and pad focuses the family's attention on the wetting habits of the child and that dry nights are more liable to be noted and rewarded by praise. He suggests that social learning is an important component in the efficacy of the treatment program.

CURE RATES. Cure rates vary in different studies from 60 to 90%. Acceptable success rates have been reported among the retarded (Sloop and Kennedy, 1973; Smith, 1981) and non-retarded institutionalized children. "Cure," defined as fourteen nights of continuous dryness, is usually reached during the second month of treatment (Kolvin et al., 1972). In retarded individuals it has been found that the initial treatment may profitably be increased to as many as six months (Smith, 1981) or the simultaneous use of stimulant drug such as methylamphetamine (Young and Turner, 1965) can be employed, but this also increases the likelihood of relapse. Young and Morgan (1973) and Dische et al. (1983) have examined the characteristics associated with a delayed response to treatment. Significant factors are maternal anxiety, disturbed home background, and a failure of the child to waken with the alarm. Age of the child and initial wetting frequency was not significantly related to delay. Response may also be hastened by increasing the intensity of the auditory stimulus (Finley and Wansley, 1977).

TREATMENT DROPOUT. Treatment dropout is a major problem. A high proportion of families discontinue treatment before the child is dry. The elements in treatment that are most likely to lead to dropout are: (1) failure to understand or to follow the instructions; (2) failure of the apparatus to waken the child; and (3) irritation at false alarms (Turner, 1973). These are all more likely when the treatment is self-administered, e.g., when the bell is purchased by mail order, or when the treatment is not fully understood by the prescribing therapist, or when the time taken to provide instructions is inadequate.

RELAPSE. Relapse after initial cure is another major problem with this form of treatment. Turner, summarizing results from studies in which follow-up was maintained for at least a year, determined that the average relapse rate within a year of completing treatment was 35%. Young and Morgan (1973) found that relapses were more likely in older children but failed to find other factors associated with the phenomenon.

Two techniques appear to reduce the relapse rate. The first, *intermittent reinforcement,* may involve the use of special apparatus designed to waken the patient contingently (i.e., shortly after wetting) in only a proportion of enuretic events (Finley et al., 1973). Such apparatus is not readily available and the treatment requires a great deal of parental cooperation. Lovibond (1964) has suggested that by using conventional apparatus on only three or five days each week similar results may be obtained. It should be noted that if that approach is used, the time taken to reach initial cure may be lengthened.

Overlearning is the second technique. Young and Morgan (1972) found that if children who have reached criterion, i.e., who have been dry for fourteen consecutive nights, are *then* given a fluid load of two pints before retiring (designed to reinduce wetting and with it the triggering of the bell), the relapse rate is reduced from 35 to 11%. This approach has the advantage of not delaying the initial "cure."

Despite these problems, the bell and pad offer an opportunity of a cure to the great majority of bed wetters. However, its successful use requires that the therapist be acquainted with practical problems that are likely to arise during treatment and that he or she be available for a fairly intensive level of support and guidance during the early stages of treatment.

"Dry-Bed" Procedure. Azrin, Sneed, and Foxx (1974) reported that treatment time with the bell and pad could be shortened by a number of other procedures grouped under the name of the "dry bed" program. These include (a) retention-control training (see earlier section), (b) training the child to waken rapidly, (c) reinforcement for correct micturition during the day, etc. Although Ballard and Woodroofe (1977) and Azrin and Thienes (1978) have proposed that these procedures could be modified to make the use of the bell and pad unnecessary, other reports (Nettelbeck and Langeluddecke, 1979) indicate that without the simultaneous use of an alarm apparatus the so-called dry bed training produces substantially the same results as no treatment at all.

The dry-bed procedure (Azrin and Thienes, 1978) is complicated. On the first afternoon a variation of *retention training* is carried out. The child is encouraged to drink large quantities of a favorite beverage to increase the frequency of micturition and with it the number of opportunities for learning. If the child feels the need to urinate, he or she is asked to hold for increasingly longer periods of time; when urination is necessary, the child is asked to lie on the bed as if asleep and then go to the bathroom, role playing what they will have to do at night. This is rewarded with praise and another drink.

Just before bedtime, the child is asked to role play a self-correction procedure that will have to be carried out in the middle of the night, i.e., taking off pajamas, removing sheets, and putting them back on. Fluids continue to be given until the child falls asleep. There is a discussion about the rewards for being dry, and once having fallen asleep, the child is awoken hourly until 1:00 A.M. Additional fluids are given on each awakening until 11:00 P.M. If dry, the child is asked to rehearse yet again what will have to be done if he or she feels the need to pass urine, and if the child urinates, he or she is praised for correct toileting. If incontinent, these children are wakened by the parent, reprimanded for wetting, directed to the bathroom to finish urination, and asked to go through the self-correction procedure. If dry the next morning, they are allowed to stay up for an extra hour the next night and other social reinforcement is offered. If wet the next morning, they are once again required to change their bed and pajamas and to do a large number of positive practices in correct toileting, both in the morning and one-half hour before bed the following night.

Mattsson and Ollendick (1977) have reported adverse affects from this very intensive approach, stating that preschool children may react to such methods with temper tantrums or withdrawing behavior, and the parents may also become upset and need a good deal of support. Given the suggestions that the simultaneous use of the bell and pad is essential to achieve cure, it is questionable whether its use can be justified.

PRACTICAL GUIDE TO TREATMENT

Advice to the Parent

Point out to parents and child that enuresis is a common problem. Aim to reduce punitive behavior if it is present and provide the parents with an explanation that educates them away from feeling that the child "can help it if he wants to." Present an optimistic view of your ability to treat the condition, but anticipate the difficulties of treatment at the time of the first contact. In particular, inform parents that the modal time taken for cure is around three months and that many children may not wake up to the noise of the bell but that this can usually be dealt with. Set a maximum duration of treatment, e.g., six months. If continence has not been achieved at that time, then state in advance that treatment will be discontinued for a year before being recommenced.

Point out that relapses after an initial cure occur quite frequently, but these can usually be treated effectively with the same treatment method.

Initial Observation

Initial observation should be carried out for two weeks after the first visit. During this period it may be found that the child is only wet infrequently, or the child may, in fact, stop altogether. As noted earlier, observations are recorded on a simple star chart, the child sticking in a star whenever he or she has a dry night. If this is displayed for the rest of the family to see, the social rewards for being dry may themselves have a therapeutic effect. During this period of baseline observation, various simple interventions, such as night lifting can be systematically assessed.

Choice of Nonpharmocological Treatment

There is no good evidence to suggest that daytime training has any advantage over a night-waking treatment. Every effort, therefore, should be made to treat the child by a night-conditioning method. This safe, although tedious, form of treatment is more likely to result in a permanent cure than any other known method.

Ideally, a demonstration of how to fit the bell and pad on the patient's bed should be given on a clinic couch with both parents and child present. The first follow-up, which can be by telephone, should take place a few days after the apparatus has been provided to deal with any difficulties that the patient or parents might experience.

Many children are not woken by the alarm and parents should be warned of this possibility before treatment is started. Sleeping arrangements may need to be altered, so that if the parents hear the bell, they can waken the child after it has sounded. The volume of the alarm may be increased by placing it on a resonating surface, rather than on solid furniture or the floor. Booster alarms of differing volumes and tones are available and are often helpful. Some children will turn the bell off before going to bed, and parents should be advised to place the apparatus as far from the child's bed as possible, so that it is out of easy reach. The parent should check that the switch is on before retiring to bed. Once the alarm has sounded, the child should rise, turn off the alarm, and pass urine in a convenient toilet or urinal. He or she should then be encouraged to assist the parents in removing the wet sheets. The child will in almost all cases return to sleep without delay. There is no evidence that resetting the alarm in the middle of the night shortens treatment time, and it may result in fatigue and premature conclusion of the treatment.

False alarms cause irritation to the family. They may be due to contact betwen the metal clips or sheets through movement or else through worn intervening sheet. Both the top and intervening sheet should be sufficiently large to be able to be tucked in under the mattress, thus securing the metal sheets in position. Dische (1973) has pointed out that another cause of false alarms may be inadequate laundering of the intervening sheet. Urinary electrolytes deposited in the soiled sheet may facilitate conduction by perspiration. A checklist for problems arising during treatment is provided in Table 2-1.

Overlearning

After the child has been dry for two continuous weeks, the parents should be told that the chances of relapse can be reduced by continuing with the bell and pad for a further two weeks, during which time the child is encouraged to drink up to two pints of fluid at night before retiring. In a very few cases this will result in a complete breakdown of continence and the procedure should then be abandoned, however, in most cases continence at night is maintained despite this stress. Instructions for overlearning are provided in Table 2-2.

Drug Treatment: Indications

The bell-and-pad method results in cure in a high proportion of cases and is therefore the treatment of choice. Nevertheless, there are a number of situations in which treatment with imipramine or other tricyclic drugs is appropriate. Examples are: (a) when it is important to obtain an immediate short-term effect, as when a child is first seen just before going away on vacation; (b) in a situation in which the wetting has become the focus of aggressive and hostile behavior on the part of parents or siblings—a rapidly effective treatment may serve

TABLE 2-1.
Problem Checklist for Conditioning Treatment

Problem	Solutions
1. "The bell doesn't work."	a. Check batteries and apparatus. b. Check that porous separating sheets are being used. c. Make sure that child is not turning off alarm before going to sleep or immediately after sounding. Get parent to check if alarm is on after child is asleep and place alarm out of easy reach.
2. "The bell goes off but does not wake the child."	a. Increase the volume of the alarm by placing it on an empty can or other resonating surface. b. Rearrange sleeping arrangement so that parent can wake the child.
3. "The bell goes off and the child wakes, but no cure."	a. Check on consistency of treatment. b. Check for possible reinforcing factors in night waking, e.g., mother doing all the work, with no tasks left for the child. c. Check on delay between alarm sounding and child rising. Should not exceed 30 minutes. d. Prescribe d-amphetamine 5 mg at night.
4. "False alarms."	a. Check that separating sheets are: 　1. not threadbare. 　2. rinsed through each day. 　3. big enough to prevent slippage.
5. "The child is cured but relapses."	a. Repeat treatment.

TABLE 2-2.
Overlearning Instructions for Patients Who Have Completed Initial Course of Behavior Therapy

1. Approximately 30 minutes before you plan to be asleep drink 1½ pints of fluid over a period of 10-15 minutes.
2. Go to bed with the alarm set up and on.
3. Don't worry if you wet—that is the idea.
4. If the bell goes off, carry out the usual procedure, i.e., get up, turn bell off, and empty bladder.
5. Carry on for 14 nights, *unless:* You have more than 3 wet nights in the space of 7 nights. If you have that many wets, stop extra fluids, and carry on with the bell until the next appointment.

to reduce the stresses in the family until a time when the bell and pad can be used; (c) when the bell and pad is impractical (this should be a conclusion based on actual experience rather than anticipation, for some apparently disorganized and inadquate families seem able to use the bell and pad successfully under the most difficult circumstances, even for example when the enuretic child is sharing the bed with a sibling); and (d) after failure of conditioning treatment.

Imipramine is probably the drug of choice. Dosage should start at a level of 1 mg/kg in a single undivided dose taken before bedtime. The average seven year old weighs approximately 25 kilograms and a starting dose of 25 mg/night is convenient for this age group.

Dosage should be increased until there are either significant side effects or until a maximum level of 3 mg/kg is reached.

Conclusion

Enuresis is a common but extremely distressing condition for most children. Its treatment requires skills in psychotherapeutic management, behavior therapy, and psychopharmacology. Despite the difficulties involved, the successful treatment of an enuretic child is a truly satisfying experience that makes a significant impact on the child's life and further development.

References

Achenbach, T. and Lewis M. 1971. A proposed model for clinical research and its application to encorpresis and enuresis. *J. Am. Acad. Child Psych.,* 10:535-54.

Azrin, N. H., Sneed T. J., and Foxx, R. M. 1974. Dry bed: A rapid method of eliminating bed-wetting (enuresis) of the retarded. *Behav. Res. Ther.,* 11:427-434.

Azrin, N. H., and Thienes, P. M. 1978. Rapid elimination of enuresis by intensive learning without a conditioning apparatus. *Beh. Res. Ther.,* 9:342-54.

Bakwin, H. 1961. Enuresis in children. *J. Ped.,* 58:806-819.

Ballard, R. J., and Woodroofe, P. 1977. The effect of parent-administered dry-bed training on nocturnal enuresis in children. *Beh. Res. Ther.,* 15:159-165.

Bauman, F. W., and Hinman, F. 1974. Treatment of incontinent boy with non-obstructive disease. *J. Urol.,* 3:114-116.

Blackwell, B., and Currah, J. 1973. The psychopharmacology of nocturnal enuresis. In *Bladder con-*

trol and enuresis, ed. I. Kolvin, R. MacKeith and S. R. Meadow, pp. 231-257. Clin. in Dev. Med., no. 48/49. London: Heinemann/SIMP.

Bloomfield, J. M., and Douglas, J. W. B. 1956. Bedwetting—prevalence among children aged 4-7 years. *Lacet i,* 850-852.

Cendron, J., and Lepinard, V. 1972. Maladie du Col Vesical chez l'enfant. *Urol. Int.,* 27:355-360.

Crosby, N. D. 1950. Essential enuresis: Treatment based on physiological concepts. *Med. J. Aust.,* 2:533-543.

DeLeon, G., and Mandell, W. 1966. A comparison of conditioning and psychotherapy in the treatment of enuresis. *J. Clin. Psychol.,* 22:326-330.

Dische, S. 1973. Treatment of enuresis with an enuresis alarm. In *Bladder control and enuresis,* ed. I. Kolvin, R. MacKeithy, and S. R. Meadow. Clin. in Dev. Med., no. 48/49. London: Heinemann/SIMP.

Dische, S., Yule, W., Corbett, J., and Hand, D. 1983. Childhood nocturnal enuresis: Factors associated with outcome of treatment with an enuresis alarm. *Dev. Med. Child Neurol.,* 25:67-81.

Dodge, W. F., West, E. F., Bridgforth, M. S., and Travis, L. B. 1970. Nocturnal enuresis in 6-10-year old children. *Am. J. Dis. Child.,* 120:32-35.

Fielding, D. 1980. The response of day and night wetting children and children who wet only at night to retention control training and the enuresis alarm. *Beh. Res. Ther.,* 18:305-317.

Finley, W. W., Besserman, R. L., Clapp, R. K., and Finley, P. 1973. The effect of continuous, intermittent and placebo reinforcement on the effectiveness of the conditioning treatment for enuresis nocturna. *Beh. Res. Ther.,* 11:289-297.

Finley, W. W., and Wansley, R. A. 1977. Auditory intensity as a variable in the conditioning treatment of enuresis nocturna. *Beh. Res. Ther.,* 15:181-185.

Goel, K. M., and Shanks, R. A. 1974. Amitryptyline and imipramine poisoning in children. *Brit. Med. J.,* 1:261-263.

Hagglund, T. B. 1965. Enuretic children treated on fluid restriction or forced drinks. A clinical and cystometric study. *Ann. Paediat. Fenn.,* 11:84-90.

Hallgren, B. 1957. Enuresis: A clinical and genetic study. *Acta. Psychiat. Neuro. Scand.,* 32(suppl. 114).

Hansen, G. D. 1979. Enuresis control through fading, escape, and avoidance training. *J. of Applied Behav. Anal.,* 12:303-307.

Harris, L. and Purohit, A. 1977. Bladder training and enuresis: A controlled trial. *Beh. Res. Ther.,* 15:485-490.

Hedge, B., and Shaffer, D. Behavior changes in children during treatment of enuresis. (in preparation).

Jankneget, R. A., Moonen, W. A., and Schrienemechars, L. M. H. 1979. Transection of the bladder as a method of treatment in adult enuresis nocturna. *Brit. J. Urol.,* 51:275-277.

Jorgensen, O. S., Lober, M., Christiansen, J., and Gram, L. F. 1980. *Clin. Pharmokin.,* 5:386-393.

Kaffman, M., and Elizur, E. 1977. Infants who become enuretics: A longitudinal study of 161 kibbutz children. *Monogr. Soc. Res. in Child. Dev.,* Vol. 42(2):170.

Kolvin, I., Taunch, J., Currah, J., Garside, M. F., Nolan, J., and Shaw, W. B. 1972. Enuresis: A descriptive analysis and a controlled trial. *Dev. Med. Child. Neurol.,* 14:715-726.

Lake, C. R., Mikkelsen, E. J., Rapoport, J. L., Zavadil, A. P., and Kopin, I. J. 1979. Effect of imipramine on norepinephrine and blood pressure in enuretic boys. *Clin. Pharm. Ther.,* 26:647-653.

Lovibond, S. H. 1964. *Conditioning and enuresis.* Oxford: Pergamon Press.

Mahoney, D. T. 1971. Studies of enuresis. I. Incidence of obstructive lesions and pathophysiology and enuresis. *J. Urol.,* 106:951-958.

Manley, C. B., and French, R. S. 1970. Urinary tract infection in girls: Prevalence of spina bifida occulta. *J. Urol.,* 103:348-351.

McConaghy, N. 1969. A controlled trial of imipramine, amphetamine, pad and bell, conditioning and random awakening in the treatment of nocturnal enuresis. *Med. J. Aust.,* 2:237-239.

Mattsson, J. L. and Ollendick, T. H. 1977. Issues in training normal children. *Beh. Ther.,* 8:549-553.

Meadow, S. R., White, R. H. R., and Johnston, N. M. 1969. Prevalence of symptomless urinary tract disease in Birmingham school children. *Brit. Med. J.,* 3:81.

Miller, F. J. W., Court, S. D. M., Walton, W. S., and Knox, E. G. 1960. *Growing up in Newcastle-upon-Tyne.* London: Oxford University Press.

Miller, P.M. 1973. An experimental analysis in retention control training in the treatment of nocturnal enuresis in two institutionalized adolescents. *Beh. Ther.,* 4:288-294.

Mowrer, O. H., and Mowrer, W. M. 1938. Enuresis: A method for its study and treatment. *Am. J. Orthopsych.,* 8:436-59.

Nettelbeck, T., and Langeluddecke, P. 1979. Dry-bed training without an enuresis machine. *Beh. Res. Ther.,* 17:403-404.

Novick, J. 1966. Symptomatic treatment of acquired and persistent enuresis. *J. Abnorm. Psychol.,* 71:363-368.

Olness, K. 1975. The use of self-hypnosis in the treatment of childhood nocturnal enuresis. *Clin. Ped.,* 14:273-279.

Oppel, W. C., Harper, P. A., and Rider, R. V. 1968. Social, psychological and neurological factors associated with enuresis. *Ped.,* 42:627-641.

Paschalis, A. P., Kimmel, H. D., and Kimmel, E. 1972. Further study of diurnal instrumental conditioning in the treatment of enuresis nocturna. *J. Beh. Res. Exp. Psych.,* 3:253-56.

Pfaundler, M. 1904. Demonstration eines Apparetes zur selbstatig Signalisierung stattgehabter Bettnassung. *Verhandlungen der hesellschuft Kinde. heilkd.,* 21:219-20.

Rapoport, J. L., Mikkelsen, E. J., Zavardil, A., Nee, L., Gruenau, C., Mendelson, W., and Gillin, C. 1980. Childhood enuresis. II. Psychopathology, tricyclic concentration in plasma, and antienuretic effect. *Arch. Gen. Psych.,* 37:1146-52.

Roberts, K. E., and Schoellkopf, J. A. 1951. Eating, sleeping, and elimination practices in a group of 2½ year olds. *Am. J. Dis. Child,* 82:144-152.

Rohner, T., and Sanford, E. 1975. Imipramine toxicity. *J. Urol.,* 114:402.

Rutter, M. L., Yule, W., and Craham, P. J. 1973. Enuresis and behavioural deviance: Some epidemiological considerations. In *Bladder control and enuresis,* ed. I. Kolvin, R. MacKeith, and S. R. Meadow, pp. 137-147. Clin. in Dev. Med., no 48/49. London: Heinemann/SIMP.

Saraf, K., Klein, D., Gittlelman-Klein, R., Gootman, N., and Greenhill, P. 1978. EKG effects of imipramine treatment in children. *J. Am. Acad. Child Psych.,* 17:60-69.

Shaffer, D. 1980. The development of bladder control. In *The scientific foundations of developmental psychiatry.* ed. M. Rutter, pp. 129-137. London: Heinemann.

Shaffer, D. 1984 (in press). Enuresis. *In Modern approaches, second edition,* ed. M. Rutter and L. Hersov. Oxford: Blackwell Scientific.

Shaffer, D., Costello, A. J., and Hill, J. D. 1968. Control of enuresis with imipramine. *Arch. Dis. Child.,* 43:665-671.

Shaffer, D., Gardner, A., and Hedge, B. 1984 (in press). Behavior and bladder disturbance in enuretics: The rational classification of a common disorder. *Dev. Med. Child Neurol.*

Shaffer, D., Stephenson, J. D., and Thomas, D. V. 1979. Some effects of imipramine on micturition and their relevance to their anti-enuretic activity. *Neuropharm.,* 18:33-37.

Simeon, J., Maguire, J., and Lawrence, S. 1981. Maprotiline effects in children with eneuresis and behavioral disorders. *Progress in Neuropsychopharm.,* 5:495-498.

Sloop, E. W., and Kennedy, W. A. 1973. Institutionalized retarded nocturnal enuretics treated by a conditioning technique. *Am. J. Ment. Def.,* 77:717-721.

Smith, D. R. 1969. Critique of the concept of vesical neck obstruction in children. *J. Am. Med. Assoc.,* 207:1686–1692.

Smith, L. J. 1981. Training severely and profoundly mentally handicapped nocturnal enuretics. *Beh. Res. Ther.,* 19:67–74.

Starfield, S. B. 1967. Functional bladder capacity in enuretic and non-enuretic children. *J. Paediat.,* 70:777–781.

Stedman, J. M. 1972. The extension of the Kimmel treatment method for enuresis to an adolescent: a case report. *J. Beh. Ther. Exp. Psych.,* 3:307–309.

Stein, Z. A., and Susser, M. W., 1965. Socio-medical study of enuresis among delinquent boys. *Brit. J. Prev. Soc. Med.,* 19:174–181.

Torrens, M., and Haldt, L. 1979. Bladder denevation procedures. *Urol. Clin. North Am.,* 6:283–293.

Turner, R. K. 1973. Conditioning treatment of nocturnal enuresis: Present studies. In *Bladder control and enuresis,* ed. I. Kolvin, R. MacKeith, and S. R. Meadow, pp. 195–210. Clin. in Dev. Med., no. 48/49. London: Heinemann/ SIMP.

Wallace, I. R., and Forsyth, W. I. 1969. The treatment of enuresis: A controlled clinical trial of propantheline, propantheline and phenobarbitone, and placebo. *Brit. J. Clin. Pract.,* 23:207–210.

Werry, J. S., and Cohrssen, J. 1965. Enuresis: An etiologic and therapeutic study. *J. Ped.,* 67:423–431.

Young, G. C., and Morgan, R. T. T. 1972. Overlearning in the conditioning treatment of enuresis. *Beh. Res. Ther.,* 10:147–151.

Young, G. C., and Morgan, R. T. T. 1973. Rapidity of response to the treatment of enuresis. *Dev. Med. Child Neurol.,* 15:488–496.

Young, G. C., and Turner, R. K. 1965. C.N.S. stimulant drugs and conditioning treatment of nocturnal enuresis. *Beh. Res. Ther.,* 3:93–101.

3

Infantile Autism

MICHAEL RUTTER

THE SYNDROME OF INFANTILE AUTISM was first delineated by Kanner (1943) as an "inborn autistic disturbance of affective contact." The term specified that the most striking feature comprised an abnormality of social development, and emphasized that the disorder was constitutionally determined and present from the earliest stages of development. Nevertheless, because autistic children were so grossly abnormal in their behavior and because they lacked adequate reality testing, at first the condition came to be grouped with the psychoses of childhood. This classification was unfortunate in its misleading implication that autism constituted some form of disease state that had affected a previously normal child. The general recognition that this was not the case and that, instead, it involved a serious and widespread distortion of the developmental process has led to the recent adoption of the term *pervasive developmental disorders* to describe the general class of conditions of which autism constitutes the most important example (American Psychiatric Association, 1980).

CLINICAL CHARACTERISTICS

The diagnostic criteria for autism are five: (1) an onset before thirty months of age; (2) a particular form of deviant social development; (3) a particular form of deviant language development; (4) stereotyped behaviors and routines; and (5) the absence of delusions, hallucinations, and schizophrenic-type thought disorder (Rutter, 1978; American Psychiatric Association, 1980; Rutter and Garmezy, 1983).

The most characteristic elements of the deviant social development are a lack of social reciprocity and emotional responsiveness, usually combined with a relative failure in specific bonding. Thus, during the first year, autistic infants may not take up an anticipatory posture or put up their arms to be picked up in the way that normal infants do. Similarly, during the toddler phase, most autistic children do not follow their parents about the house or run to greet them when the parents return after having been out; they tend not to go to their parents for comfort when they are hurt or upset; and frequently they do not develop the bedtime kiss-and-cuddle routine followed by so many normal children. They may or may not approach adults and they may or may not be distressed by separation, but in any case, they are inclined *not* to use a specific relationship as a source of security, comfort, and anxiety relief. It used to be said that autistic children lacked eye-to-eye gaze, but it is not the amount of gaze that is characteristic of autism; rather it is its abnormal quality. Ordinarily, eye-to-eye contact serves to modulate social interactions and it is this quality that is lacking in autism. That is, autistic children tend not to look at people's faces when they want something or when they are being spoken to, and they fail to use the engagement and aversion of eye contact to regulate the reciprocal to and fro that characterizes normal social interchange. Often autistic children have a rather unexpressive face, so that it may be difficult to gauge their emotions, but most typical of all is their lack of modulation of their emotional expression according to the emotions of others. In addition, there is a lack of cooperative group play with other children, a failure to make personal friendships, and an apparent lack of empathy, with an impaired ability to perceive other people's feelings and social responses.

Most autistic children are markedly delayed in their acquisition of speech, but it is the *deviant* qualities of their language development that are most characteristic of the syndrome. Before speech develops, there is a deficit in the understanding of spoken language and, when this is severe, often there is a lack of response to being called or spoken to—so that at first the child may appear deaf. Babble tends to be both reduced in amount and abnormal in quality, without the speechlike cadences or the varied vocal "play" with different combinations of sounds typical of normal babble. Moreover, autistic children's babble lacks the qualities of social communication; and there is a lack of other forms of communication, such as pointing with the index finger, or gesture and mime, to indicate need or to make social responses to other people's overtures. When speech develops, perhaps the most striking feature is its limited usage for social purposes. The speech of the normal toddler is intensely social, with much to and fro "chat," much following the parents around the house to talk about this and that, and many attempts to sustain a conversation with reciprocity and responsiveness to the communications of the other person. In contrast, young autistic children tend to speak little, much of what they say lacks these social qualities, and there is a lack of reciprocity so that sustained conversations are few and, if present at all, are confined to topics relevant to the children's particular preoccupations of the moment. Young autistic children are rarely able to describe their activities at other times or in other places. In addition, their spoken language tends to be stereotyped in form, with delayed and inappropriate echoing of what they or others have said previously; there is abnormal egocentric language usage and, often, I-you pronominal reversal. Occasionally, neologisms may be used and, more often, there is idiosyncratic word usage.

Stereotyped behaviors and routines constitute the third set of features that characterize autism. Play tends to be repetitive, with little imagination or variety; often autistic children spend hours endlessly lining up objects, making patterns, or whirling things. Frequently this is accompanied by stereotyped repetitive movements—especially rapid hand and finger mannerisms near the eyes but toward the limits of their field of vision. Young autistic children rarely engage in make-believe games and their use of toys is both diminished and lacking in symbolic or creative qualities. Pretend play with dolls or teddy bears is uncommon. There is little unelicited imitation of others and little spontaneous participation in imitative games such as pat-a-cake or social gestures such as waving good-bye. Often there is an apparent preoccupation with the smell or feel of objects, instead of an interest in their appropriate functional usage. Some autistic children develop intense attachments to unusual objects such as stones, tin cans, or bottle openers. Often in middle childhood (and sometimes when younger), there is a preoccupation with routes, timetables, numbers, dates, or patterns—interests that tend to be pursued to the exclusion of other activities. Rigid routines in play, eating habits, or daily activities are common, and sometimes there is a resistance to any changes in the environment. Food fads are common; often they take an atypical form in their favoring of extremely strong savory tastes (such as pickles, yeast extract, or mustard) that most young children dislike.

Associated Features

About three-quarters of autistic children show some degree of mental retardation, but the condition does occur in children of normal intelligence. Usually the intellectual deficit is most marked for verbal skills and least evident for visuospatial abilities, but this pattern is not invariable. However, it is very characteristic for autistic children to perform much better on tasks requiring mechanical or rote-memory skills than on those that necessitate abstraction, conceptualization, sequencing, or the extraction of meaning.

Most autistic children have a normal physiognomy and their serious expression may convey a (usually) misleading impression of high intelligence. Nevertheless, although their facies is normal in structure, it lacks the emotional expressiveness and responsiveness of the normal child. Minor congenital anomalies are somewhat more frequently present than in the general population, but these have no diagnostic importance (as they are present in a wide range of conditions as well as in many entirely normal children), and serious physical stigmata are unusual. In a minority of cases, autism is associated with some neurological disorder, of which infantile spasms, tuberous sclerosis, and congenital rubella are among the more common. Somewhat more frequently, however, there is some form of neurodevelopmental impairment as evident in such signs as poor coordination or the abnormal persistence of mirror movements or choreiform activity.

Epidemiology and Course

The general-population prevalence of autism as defined in the foregoing is about 2 to 4 cases per 10,000 (Lotter, 1966), but the rate varies according to the strictness of the diagnostic criteria employed. Many mentally retarded children show some, but not all, features of the syndrome, and if these autistic-like conditions are included, the prevalence figure rises to some 21 per 10,000 in the general population and about half of all children with an IQ below 50 (Wing and Gould, 1979). Autism is less frequent among the most profoundly retarded (IQ below 20) but otherwise the rate of autism goes up as the IQ goes down. Autism is more frequent in boys than in girls, in a ratio of about 3 to 1, but there is some suggestion that autistic girls tend to be more seriously affected and also more likely to have a family history of cognitive problems (Tsai et al., 1981; Lord et al., 1982). About 2% of the siblings of autistic children suffer from the same condition—a rate fifty times that in the general population (Rutter, 1967). Although a family history of autism is rare, one of speech delay is more common. August, Steward, and Tsai (1981) found that some 15% of the siblings of autistic children compared with 3% of the siblings of Down's syndrome individuals have language disorders, learning disabilities, or mental retardation. Folstein and Rutter's (1977) twin study showed a 36% pair-wise concordance rate for autism in monozygotic twins compared with 0% in dizygotic twins; the concordance rates for cognitive abnormalities were 82% and 10%, respectively.

The data suggest an important genetic component that probably applies to a predisposition to language and cognitive abnormalities of which autism constitutes a part, rather than to the inheritance of autism per se. Earlier studies found that autism was somewhat more common in children born to middle-class parents, but more recent investigations have shown no appreciable variation by social class and it may well be that the earlier association was an artifact of referral or diagnostic practices (Rutter and Garmezy, 1983).

By the time they reach adulthood, some two-thirds of autistic individuals are still severely handicapped and unable to look after themselves, yet about 5 to 17% are working, leading some kind of social life, and holding their own in the community (Lotter, 1978). The prognosis is strongly influenced by the children's IQ and language skills. If the IQ is below about 50 on performance tests, it is almost certain that the autistic child will remain severely handicapped throughout life; if there is gross language impairment still evident at five years of age in spite of an IQ above 50, the child may make a fair adjustment but a good outcome is unlikely; if nonverbal intelligence is within the normal range *and* if there is a useful level of spoken language by age five with no more than a mild comprehension defect, there is a 50-50 chance of good social adjustment in adult life (Rutter, 1970). Nevertheless, even among the most mildly afflicted autistic children, very few achieve complete normality.

Epileptic seizures develop during adolescence in about a quarter of all cases, but the likelihood of seizures is much greater in autistic children with severe mental retardation (Rutter, 1970; 1983a). The age pattern of onset of seizures in autism differs from that in nonautistic individuals who are most likely to have their first seizures in early childhood (Deykin and MacMahon, 1979). A small proportion of autistic individuals show a deterioration in adolescence with a loss of language skills associated with inertia, decreasing activity, and sometimes an intellectual decline (Gillberg and Schaumann, 1981; LeCouteur, 1983).

About half of autistic children gain useful speech; usually this occurs by age five years but it can occur much later. Even among the autistic individuals who achieve a normal, or near-normal, level of language competence, there are often continuing abnormalities in language usage and speech delivery (Rutter, 1970). In some cases there is a monotonous flat delivery; in others speech is staccato. Frequently language appears formal and pedantic and often among adolescents it is mainly made up of obsessive questions related to their preoccupations of the moment. Difficulties in using concepts of emotions usually persist. Many autistic children show some improvement in their social relationships as they grow older; however, continuing abnormalities of some degree are almost invariable. Often there is a growing interest in people and a wish to have friendships, but in the great majority of cases, a lack of social reciprocity and a relative unawareness of other people's feelings make deep friendships unlikely.

DIAGNOSTIC ASSESSMENT

History-taking

Before proceeding to more systematic questioning, it is important to allow parents to express their own concerns and worries about their child. This is necessary if the clinician is to be able to deal adequately with the parents' reasons for seeking referral, as the question of what is the matter with their child may not be the issue foremost in their mind (Cox and Rutter, 1983). Moreover, parents will likely know their child better than anyone else and it is always helpful to pay attention to the features that have aroused their concern. Also, of course, it is usually appropriate to make the first focus of treatment those aspects of the child's behavior that are causing the most distress or disturbance in the family at the time of clinic attendance (Howlin et al., 1973; Hemsley et al., 1978).

It is both good sense and a matter of courtesy to start systematic questioning with the problems presented by the parents. As with any psychiatric disorder, it is crucial to ask for detailed descriptions of actual behavior; general summary statements are not sufficient. Thus, if the parent says "Johnny never seems happy," it would be necessary to ask such questions as: "How does he show that he is not happy?" "What does he do (say) when he is miserable?" "How can you tell what he is feeling?" "When was he last like that?" "Are there times when he is different from that?" etc., etc. The object is to build up a coherent picture of the child's feelings, behavior, and relationships with respect to each of the key symptoms, with information on such items as severity, frequency, circumstances when shown, precipitating or ameliorating factors, time of onset, duration, and how dealt with by the parents (Rutter, 1975; Cox and Rutter, 1983). Of course, the clinician must decide on the likely relevance of the behavior in question in order to decide how thoroughly to pursue the issue. But, in this connection, the "relevance" may concern either matters of diagnosis or treatment. Thus, if the main complaint is "temper tantrums," the symptom may be of little importance with respect to differential diagnosis. On the other hand, if that is the prime concern of the parents, it will be important in planning treatment to work out effective and adaptive responses that are likely to reduce the frequency and severity of tantrums and to make them more readily manageable. That requires a systematic functional analysis of the child's behavior (Mash and Terdal, 1981; Berger, 1983; Yule, 1983)—meaning an identification of the environmental circumstances associated with the occurrence or nonoccurrence of the behavior, predisposing situations, precipitating factors, responses that appear to perpetuate the behavior, and responses that seem to cut it short. Almost always the clinician will have to guide the parents to consider specific aspects that might be important, with questions such as, "Does it matter where he is?" "Is it affected by who is with him?" "Do they occur more often at some times of day than others?" "What was he doing just before the last tantrum began?"

DEVELOPMENTAL SEQUENCE. Having obtained an adequate account of the presenting complaints, it will be necessary next to obtain further information on those aspects of development and of current behavior that are crucial either to differential diagnosis or to treatment. As autism is a developmental disorder, usually it is most convenient to begin with a chronological account of development. Rather than go immediately to questions of pregnancy and delivery, however, it may be preferable to start by asking the parents *when* they first became concerned that something might be not quite right with the child's development, and *what* it was that aroused their concern at that time. Particularly with a first child, the parents' concern may have been aroused long after the child first showed delays or distortions in development. Accordingly, it is helpful to inquire whether, with hindsight, the parents think that all was well before they first became concerned (and, if not, what it was that might have been abnormal). Having established the time and nature of those first indications of concern, it is generally easiest to go back to the time of pregnancy and work forward systematically up to the present time. All the usual questions on development are applicable. Thus, it is necessary to ask about illnesses and drugs during pregnancy, the course of the delivery, the duration of gestation, birth weight, whether there were any difficulties immediately after birth, whether there were any problems with feeding or sleeping, whether the infant received any form of special care in the neonatal period (such as incubators), and so forth.

Information should be sought on the usual developmental milestones. Most parents do not remember at all accurately when milestones occurred if they were within the normal range, but they are more likely to recall if they were delayed. Accordingly, it is important to focus on that aspect first before going on to tie down the time more exactly. When seeking to date milestones, reference should be made to *familiar* landmarks rather than to ages as such. Thus, for example, it might be appropriate to ask whether the child was walking on his first birthday, or when they moved to a new house, or at the time of his first Christmas, or when the second child was born.

Particular attention needs to be paid to the developmental aspects of play, socialization, and language. With respect to the milestones of language it is crucial to be quite specific on what is being asked about. Parents are very inclined to interpret all manner of sounds as speech, and especially as "mama" and "dada." Consequently, it may be wise to ask very focused questions such as, "When did he first use simple words with meaning—that is words other than mama and dada?" "What were his first words?" "How did he show that he knew their meaning?" In addition to the first use of single words, it is important to ask about babble, the use of two- or three-word phrases, the use of pointing or gesture or mime, the following of instructions, and immediate or delayed echoing. Again, it is generally most profitable to concentrate on key age periods that are easily remembered by parents (because they coincide with some memorable event or occasion), rather than to ask for exact dating. It is helpful to identify some occasions that the parents obviously remember reasonably clearly and then to focus on what the child was like at that time. In doing so, an attempt should be made to determine what the child was like at about two years, thirty months, three years, and four years.

Few parents think of socialization in terms of milestones or indeed in terms of specific behaviors. As a result, although the topic may be introduced by some general question such as "how affectionate was he as a toddler?" it will always be necessary to proceed with a series of focused questions directed at eliciting information on key aspects of social relationships and social responsiveness at particular ages. Thus, for the six- to twelve-month age period it would be necessary to ask whether the child turned to look the parents directly in the face when they spoke to him, whether he put up his arms to be lifted, whether he nestled close when held, whether he protested when left, whether he laughed and chortled in response to parental overtures, whether he was comforted by being picked up and cuddled, and whether he was wary of strangers. Similarly, with toddlers, questions should be asked about whether the child greeted the parents when they came back from being out (by going to the door on hearing it being opened, on running to be picked up, or by smiling and saying "mama," "dada," etc.); whether he sought to be cuddled when upset or hurt (did he come to you or did you have to go to him?); whether he differentiated between the parents and others to whom he went for comfort; whether he showed separation anxiety; and whether he could be "playful," entering into the spirit of to and fro in a teasing or make-believe game.

Similarly, precise questions are required to elicit an adequate account of the child's play at particular ages. Thus, for example, to determine whether play was normal at age two years, the clinician should ask about the child's use of toys and other objects. Did he recognize the appropriate use of miniature toys, as by pushing toy cars along the floor making car noises, or rather did he tend to spin the wheels, feel the texture of the paint, or listen to the sound of a wind-up car? Was there any pretend play—as with the use of toy tea sets, dolls, etc? Would the pretend play vary from day to day and would the pretend element be used to create any sort of sequence or story (with the toy cars racing each other or being parked in the garage or being used to go to grandma's home)?

Having obtained a history of the development of play, social interaction, and language —with special reference to the first five years—it is necessary to obtain a comparably specific account of the child's current behavior in these areas of functioning. Before proceeding to direct questioning on particular features, it is helpful to get an overall picture of the child's activities by asking how he spends his time on return from school or on a weekend. Such a description usually provides a lifelike portrayal of the bleakness or richness of the child's inner and outer worlds and focuses attention on the activities and experiences to be asked about in greater detail. For adequate evaluation to be possible, it is essential that the specific questioning be based on some sort of systematic scheme that ensures that each of the crucial facets is covered.

LANGUAGE. Thus, with language and language-related functions (as shown in table 3-1), the questioning should deal in turn with imitation, so-called inner language, comprehension of language, vocalization and babble, language production, word-sound qualities, phonation, and speech rhythm (Rutter, 1974). Imitation in a toddler will be evident by waving good-bye or by baby games such as peekaboo or pat-a-cake. A slightly older child might be expected to copy his parents' vacuuming or mowing the lawn or, indeed, their idiosyncratic social mannerisms. Inner language refers to a child's ability to use a symbolic code in his thought processes, as reflected, for example, in his meaningful use of miniature objects or in pretend play or drawing.

There are several different aspects of language comprehension. Thus, "hearing behavior" includes hearing as such (as shown by the child looking up when an airplane flies overhead, going to the door when the bell rings, or looking up in response to a noise outside); listening and attention (by alerting when called, looking at the person who is speaking to him, watching faces); and understanding of spoken language (as shown by the child's ability to follow instructions given without visual, contextual, or gestural cues). Especially with a young nonspeaking child, most parents naturally adopt the habit of using pointing, gesture, and demonstration when speaking and, often, are unaware that they do so. Accordingly, once again, questions need to be specific with regard, for example, to whether the child would follow an instruction to fetch something from another room. Would he do so if it was something unfamiliar? Would he follow a two- or three-part instruction (such as go to the hall and fetch my gloves out of the bottom drawer)?

Current vocalization and babble, of course, is relevant only if the child is not yet speaking. But with a nonspeaking child it is important to inquire about the amount, range, type, and rhythm of the child's sounds. Does the child "talk" to himself or to you? Are a wide variety of sounds strung together with complex inflections and speech cadences so that sometimes, from the other side of the room, it almost sounds as if the child *is* speaking? Does he babble back when you speak to him (i.e., does it have a reciprocal, social quality)?

When the child is communicating at all, it is important to assess the mode of communication, its complexity, its quality, its amount, and its social usage. The clinician will want to know whether the child uses speech or gesture and, if speech, whether this is accompanied by normal gestural accompaniments (pointing, arm movements, etc.). The parent should always be asked how the child indicates that he wants something. If he takes the

TABLE 3-1.
Scheme for Speech and Language

1. *Imitation*
2. *Inner Language*
3. *Comprehension of Spoken Language*
    Hearing
    Listening and Attention
    Understanding
4. *Vocalization and Babble*
    Amount
    Complexity
    Quality
    Social Usage
5. *Language Production*
    Mode (gesture, speech, etc.)
    Complexity: syntactical and semantic
    Qualities (echoing, stereotyped features, etc.)
    Amount
    Use of social communication
6. *Word–Sound Production*
7. *Phonation*
8. *Rhythm*

parent by the arm, does he grasp the hand or the wrist, does he look at the parent to engage their attention, does he point with a finger or just an outstreched arm, etc.?

An estimate of the mode of complexity of the speech used may be obtained by asking about the average length of utterances, whether the small connecting words (such as prepositions and conjunctions) are included, the range of vocabulary, the use of tenses other than the present, and the flexibility of grammatical constructions. The qualities to be asked about include pronominal reversal (with particular reference to I-you confusion), immediate and delayed echoing, stereotyped phrases, made-up words (neologisms), and odd or idiosyncratic use of words or language. Parents should be asked about the amount that the child talks and the circumstances in which he does so. Particular attention should be paid to the social qualities of the child's communications—whether he "chats" in a to-and-fro fashion, whether he can sustain a conversation with reciprocal interchange (i.e., whether the child's communications show a response to what has been said to him, beyond an answer to a direct question), whether what he says shows an interest in the other person, whether he can give an account of what he did at another time (such as at school or when visiting grandma's), and whether his speech is accompanied by appropriate variations in emotional expression and use of eye-to-eye gaze. Last, there should be questioning on the child's articulation of speech —that is, his pronunciation; and the phonation and rhythm of speech. Often the autistic child's speech is curiously flat or staccato, without the normal ebb and flow of ordinary language usage.

SOCIAL INTERACTIONS. A scheme for questioning about social interactions is even more necessary than with language because (a) most loving parents tend to perceive some affection in even the most autistic children, (b) parents who feel negative toward their child may wrongly describe him as generally unresponsive because he is so with them, and (c) there is no generally accepted set of constructs about the development of social relationships. A possible scheme of questioning is outlined in table 3-2; however, the particular structure used in assessment matters less than that there is some structure to ensure systematic coverage. The most basic question is whether the child differentiates between people; is his response to his parents reliably different from his response to family friends or to strangers—and how is that differentiation manifest?

The next issue is whether the child shows selective attachments or bonds. It should be appreciated that although in a normal child the phase of clinging, separation anxiety, and wariness of strangers usually lasts only to age three or four or five years, the phenomenon of social bonding is a life-long human characteristic (Rutter, 1980). Questions should be asked after the features specific to early childhood, but the main focus should be on the quality of specific attachments to provide security and reduce anxiety. Does the child stay close to his parents in a strange situation, does he go to them for comfort when upset, does he become clingy when anxious or frightened, does his manner of greeting show pleasure when he sees his parents, does their holding him relieve his distress?

With respect to the child's social overtures, the important question is not whether he approaches other people (many autistic children will do that), but rather *how* social overtures are made and in what circumstances. In the normal child most social approaches involve a friendly facial expression, some show of positive emotion, the appropriate engagement of mutual gaze, and some expression of interest in the other person or his activities. It is necessary, therefore, to obtain a detailed description of just what the child does when he seeks to engage the attention of someone else to determine whether these characteristics apply.

Much the same applies to the style of the child's response to other people's overtures to him. Does he look directly at them, does he smile, and does he show pleasure? The feature of reciprocity is also crucial: does the child show an appropriate response to what the other person says or does; is there a sequence of social dialogue with a to and fro; and do the child's

TABLE 3-2.
Scheme for Social Interaction

1. *Differentiation Between People*
2. *Selective Attachment*
    Source of security or comfort
    Greeting
    Separation anxiety
3. *Social Overtures*
    Frequency and circumstances
    Quality: visual gaze, facial expression, and emotions
4. *Social Responses*
    Frequency and circumstances
    Quality: eye-to-eye gaze, facial expression, and emotions
    Reciprocity
5. *Social Play*
    Spontaneous imitation
    Cooperation and reciprocity
    Pleasure in the other person
    Humor
    Excitement

emotions and facial expressions vary according to those of the other person? Finally, in what ways, if any, does the child play *with* someone else? Does he *seek* play with other people or does he have to be *brought* in to social play? Will he do something together with his parents, sharing, cooperating, and taking turns (as in building with blocks or playing a board game, ball, musical games, or chasing games)? If so, does he show pleasure or humor in relation to *other* people's activities in a shared game? Can he follow rules? Does he show social excitement (i.e., joining in the spirit of the occasion)? In short, not only will he go through the mechanics of a shared game but is this accompanied by a range of emotions appropriate to the social elements in the interaction? Is there a playful quality to the social interactions?

PLAY. There is a similar need for some kind of structure to questioning about play (see table 3-3). Together with social interactions, these tend to constitute the two aspects least well dealt with in history-taking by trainees. The social aspects of play have been considered already in terms of interest, playfulness, reciprocity, and emotional expression. Play also constitutes a good guide to the child's cognitive level. Curiosity in the environment is an important quality: does the child explore new toys and show an interest in the world about him; does he seem interested in finding out how things work (toys, tools, household gadgets, etc.) and how successful is he in doing so? What is the complexity of the child's play—can he do puzzles on his own (how many pieces?), can he build things with blocks or cope with other constructional toys; what does he draw; how good is he in understanding and following the rules of games; how inventive is he in his play? One particular feature that usually is impaired in autism concerns imaginative play. Accordingly, questions need to be asked about make-believe play, dressing up, and pretend games (tea parties, playing school, cops and robbers, etc., etc.) with special reference to the extent to which this is spontaneous, creative, and varying.

Third, attention should be paid to the content, type, and quality of the child's play.

TABLE 3-3.
Scheme for Play

1. *Social Aspects*
    Interest
    Playfulness
    Reciprocity
    Interest
    Emotional expression
2. *Cognitive Level*
    Curiosity
    Understanding of how things work
    Complexity: puzzles, drawing, rule following, inventiveness
    Imagination: pretend elements, creativity, spontaneity
3. *Content, Type, and Quality*
    Initiation
    Variability or stereotypy
    Unusual preoccupations
    Unusual object attachments
    Rituals and routines
    Resistance to change
    Stereotyped movements
    Interest in unusual aspects of people or objects

Many autistic children seem to lack the ability to initiate and organize their own play. It is helpful to ask what the child does if left to his own devices—will he play in an appropriate fashion or does he tend to engage in repetitive activities or motor stereotypies? What toys or games will he choose if that is left up to him, or does he not use toys or games? Also, in most cases play tends to be lacking in variability and creativity, so that questions should be asked on these features. Of course, too, attention needs to be paid to the abnormal qualities of play that tend to be characteristic of autism: routines and rituals (are there things that he insists have to be done in a special way or in a special order—what about with mealtime or bedtime or dressing or going places?); resistance to change (does he mind if you change the ornaments or rearrange the furniture or vary your household routine?); unusual preoccupations (has he got any special interests that tend to preoccupy him to the exclusion of other activities, such as with numbers, dates, routes, or things like that?); unusual object attachments (does he have any things that he likes to carry around with him all the time or that he collects?); and interests in unusual aspects of people or objects (does he tend to smell or feel things inappropriately—either with toys or with people?).

OTHER BEHAVIORS. In addition to coverage of the features most characteristic of autism, it is necessary in all cases to question systematically about other aspects of the child's emotions, behavior, and relationships that might exhibit abnormal features. Table 3-4 provides a possible list of headings for this purpose.

Observation/Interview of Child

So far as possible, all the issues covered in the history-taking should be assessed by direct observation of the child. For that purpose, it is highly desirable to see the child in situations that vary greatly in their social context and demands, as each is likely to tap rather different dimensions of the child's functioning. Psychological testing provides the opportunity of observing the child in a structured setting with the context explicitly task oriented. Often this

TABLE 3-4.
Scheme for Systematic Questioning on Other Symptoms

1. *Emotions*
   Misery/depression
   Worrying/anxiety
   Fears/phobias
   Anger/tantrums
	4. *Conduct Difficulties*
	   Lying
	   Stealing
	   Truanting
	   Violence

2. *Aggression/Destructiveness*
   To others
   To self
   To objects
	5. *Somatic Aspects*
	   Headaches, stomach aches, etc.
	   Hypochondriasis

3. *Social Relationships*
   Parents
   Siblings
   Peers
   Other adults
	6. *Routine Activities*
	   Sleeping
	   Eating
	   Micturition and defecation

	7. *Habits, Etc.*
	   Tics and mannerisms
	   Thumb sucking, nail biting, etc.
	   Obsessions and compulsions

situation shows the child at his best. The school provides another task-oriented environment, but one that differs in the crucial respect of its being a group setting rather than a one-to-one interaction, and in terms of the less close supervision that that entails. In all cases it will be essential to obtain a detailed report from teachers of the child's behavior at school. However, in addition, it may be valuable to make a school visit for a direct observation of the child in the classroom and playground, and for a discussion of treatment goals and plans with the teachers in the context of the child's behavior and attainments at school.

At the clinic the opportunity should be taken of seeing the child with his family—both in order to observe the quality of his interactions with them and in order to assess behavior in that more familiar social milieu. This may be done in the waiting room but also it may be helpful to have part of the interview time with the family as a whole. As well as providing information on the child's behavior, it should be informative on the nature of the parents' interactions with the child and on their style of coping with his difficult behavior. If the parental account of the child's behavior at home is discrepant from that seen at the clinic, a home visit will be essential in order to determine whether there is indeed such situation variability (and, if so, what seems to regulate it), or whether the parents are misinterpreting or misperceiving what the child does.

Finally, the child should be seen by the clinician in a less structured setting than that provided by psychological testing, and with a social rather than a task orientation. The room should be uncluttered, with a few well-chosen toys appropriate to the child's interests and developmental level on view. These should be selected to provide the opportunity for some form of social interaction and joint play and for the use of imagination and make-believe (a doll's house with family figures may be most suitable for young children). Some additional toys may be kept in reserve on a side table. Initially, after an appropriate social greeting, it may be useful to take a somewhat passive role in order to see how the child uses both the toys and the social situation. Then, according to circumstances, the clinician may take a somewhat more active role—socially, verbally, and with respect to task structure—in order to see how the child responds. However the session is organized and whatever the order followed, it is important to provide a varying social and emotional "stimulus" to the child so that his reciprocity and responsivity may be evaluated. Although, obviously, it is necessary to tailor the session to the needs, interests, and capabilities of the individual child, there are also great advantages in ensuring that there is broad comparability between the diagnostic interviews with different children. Unless the interview conditions are comparable, it will not be possible to know whether variability in the children's behavior is a function of changes in the interview or differences in the children.

Table 3-5 summarizes the key elements to be taken note of in observations of the child. Ordinarily, a visit to a clinic and an interview with a doctor whom he has not met before will create a degree of initial social inhibition in a normal child, but with a lessening as the child becomes more at ease and "gets to know" the doctor. This may not occur with a socially unresponsive autistic child—either in terms of the initial inhibition or the change as the interview proceeds. The quality of the child's social interaction with the clinician and of his play should be assessed in terms of the features discussed earlier. The range, quality, and social appropriateness of the child's emotions should be noted, together with the extent to which emotional expressiveness accompanies social overtures and responses. The child's use and understanding of language should be observed systematically according to the language scheme given in table 3-1, with whatever systematic attempts to elicit language as are necessary. Of course, too, all abnormal behaviors shown should be noted, with attention to smelling or feeling objects, response to parts of the clinician rather than to him or her as a

TABLE 3–5.
Observation of Child

    (i) Unstructured with family (clinic and home)
    (ii) Structured and task oriented (psychological testing)
    (iii) Socially oriented, with less structure (psychiatric interview)
    (iv) Group setting with task orientation (school)

1. *Social Inhibition/Disinhibition*
2. *Social Interaction*
3. *Play*
4. *Emotions*
5. *Language*
6. *Abnormal Behaviors*

person (e.g., feeling the clinician's hair), motor stereotypies, self-destructive behavior (such as wrist biting or head banging), routines or rituals, and stereotyped play or speech.

Cognitive Assessment

Because of its importance in diagnostic evaluation, prognosis, and planning of treatment, an accurate assessment of the child's current level of cognitive performance is crucial (see table 3–6). Psychological testing is an essential element in such an assessment, but the testing should never be considered in isolation (Berger, 1984). In all cases the history from the parents and from the teachers of the child's behavior at home and at school should be used to provide an estimate of cognitive level; this should also be made on the basis of what has been observed of the child's behavior in different settings. Whenever the estimates from history and from observation do not agree with test findings, this must be regarded as a matter for further investigation. It is *never* permissible to conclude that the test findings provide the "true" picture. It is not uncommon for autistic children to have specific skills (often in rote memory, visuospatial skills, mental arithmetic, or music) that are substantially above those evident on routine psychological testing. In such instances, it is necessary to observe the reported skills in the setting in which they occur and, if necessary, to undertake specific testing to assess their validity. Also, sometimes autistic children perform very much better in some settings than others. But some parents overestimate their children's skills either because they do not appreciate the cues that are being provided inadvertently, or because they misinterpret the meaning of the child's behavior in terms of the cognitive skills required. In such circumstances, it is necessary both to provide a valid estimate of the child's level of cognitive functioning at home and to help the parents appreciate the meaning of that level in terms of the child's needs.

Social maturity may be assessed by asking the parents specific questions about the child's performance in the areas of self-help (e.g., whether he can dress himself without help, manage buttons and shoelaces, get his clothes right way round, etc.); household activities (in terms of his helping with washing up, clearing the table, etc., and his ability to run errands or go shopping); and use of objects (whether he can use scissors, the radio, record player, etc.). The Vineland Social Maturity Scale (Doll, 1953) provides systematic coverage that gives rise to a score representing an overall social age or social quotient. The Mecham (1958) scale does much the same for language development.

As already discussed, the cognitive level of the child's play may be determined from

TABLE 3-6.
Cognitive Assessment

(i) History of child's behavior at home and at school
(ii) Observation in different settings
(iii) Psychological testing

1. *Social Maturity*
    Self-help: feeding, toileting, dressing, etc.
    Household activities: washing up, shopping, errands, etc.
    Use of objects: tools, scissors, etc.
    Vineland Social Maturity Scale
2. *Play*
    History
    Observation
    Lowe and Costello
3. *Intelligence*
    Curiosity in environment
    Finding out how things work
    Style of problem solving
    Social maturity
    Play
    Merrill-Palmer Scale/WISC-R
4. *Language*
    History
    Observation
    Reynell Developmental Language Scales
    Peabody Picture Vocabulary Test
5. *Scholastic Attainment*

both history and observation. If a more detailed and accurate evaluation is required, the Lowe and Costello (1976) scale may be employed, although this need not be included as routine.

The child's general intelligence should be assessed from his curiosity in the environment, the extent to which such curiosity is systematically applied to new situations, his ability to find out how things work, his style of problem solving (does he work things out or try responses at random?), his social maturity, and his play. In addition, of course, it will always be necessary to apply standardized tests (see Berger and Yule, 1972). For young children, or for seriously retarded older children, the Merrill-Palmer scale (Stutsman, 1948) tends to be the most useful because most children find it interesting, verbal items can be omitted in the case of children with substantial language impairment, and the scoring provides a means of dealing with items refused. For school-age children who are not severely retarded, the Wechsler Intelligence Scale for Children—Revised (Wechsler, 1974) is the most satisfactory test in terms of the range of cognitive skills covered, the quality of its standardization, and its provision of both a performance IQ score and a verbal IQ score. However, the test has a floor of an IQ just below 50, so that other tests will be required to differentiate within the range of moderate or severe retardation. The Wechsler Intelligence Scale for Preschool Children (Wechsler, 1967) is occasionally suitable for younger, more able, autistic children but, on the whole, it is not well accepted by very disturbed or mentally retarded autistic children in the preschool age range. The colored version of Raven's Progressive Matrices (Raven, 1960) provides an alternative test of visuospatial problem-solving skills and sometimes there may be an advantage in using a board form of the test (Clark and Rutter, 1979). For very young children, the Bayley (Bayley, 1969) scales may be needed.

It is sometimes wrongly asserted that many autistic children are "untestable"; however, this should not be the case if the testing is skillfully undertaken by a psychologist experienced in the assessment of autistic children. Certainly, it is true that many autistic children are difficult to test and that patience, ingenuity, and persistence may be required. However, if the situation is appropriately structured, if a test at a suitable level is employed, and if care is taken to interest the child in the test items, testing should be possible in almost all cases. Nevertheless, it is crucial to start with easy items, as some autistic children tend to adopt a stereotyped response following repeated failure (Clark and Rutter, 1979). Also, it is important to ensure that the child attends to and understands the instructions. Some variations from the standard procedure laid down in the manual may be necessary for this purpose (although such variations should be kept to a minimum as they make scores noncomparable with those used in standardization). With most young autistic children, items that require complex verbal instructions or a verbal response are best avoided. In scoring the child's responses, items refused or not attempted should be disregarded. As with any other form of psychological testing, it is important to evaluate the validity of the IQ estimate in terms of the consistency and logical coherence of the pattern of responses. There should be considerable reservations about findings if there is not a systematic trend for a higher proportion of easier items than difficult items to be passed, or if the subtest scores fail to fall into a meaningful pattern. When the scores are inconsistent in a way that throws doubt on the validity of the scores, the only safe procedure is to repeat the testing on another occasion.

The child's language skills, in addition to being assessed from the history and from observation, should be evaluated in quantitative terms by means of standardized testing. A range of tests is available for this purpose (see Mittler, 1972), but the most generally useful are the Reynell (1969) developmental language scales as they provide measures of both the comprehension and expression of spoken language. The Peabody Picture Vocabulary Test (Dunn, 1965) may also be useful as a simple measure of vocabulary recognition.

Finally, with school-age children it will be important to assess their scholastic attainments. Because autistic children's understanding so often lags behind their rote learning, it is important to use tests that measure both. The Neale Analysis of Reading Ability (Neale, 1958) does this satisfactorily with its separate scores for reading accuracy, comprehension, and rate.

In individual cases further psychological testing may be required in order to provide systematic information on other skills, but the tests mentioned constitute those needed for routine use in relation to the assessment of cognitive skills.

Medical Examination

As with any child referred for developmental problems, an adequate screening for medical conditions is essential. This requires appropriate questioning in the history-taking with regard to pregnancy and perinatal complications, to illnesses with a possible neurological component (such as meningitis or encephalitis), and to epileptic seizures (or other attacks involving impairment of consciousness). Obviously, too, there must be inquiries regarding any kind of developmental disorder or delay (including specific language disorders, reading difficulties, and mental retardation), or mental illness, in family members. A general physical examination is needed to alert the physician to the need to investigate further with respect to any possible medical conditions that may be suspected. The skin should be examined for adenoma sebaceum—the rash associated with tuberous sclerosis—and systematic attention should be paid to the possible presence of minor and major congenital physical anomalies. In all cases, there should be a systematic neurodevelopmental assessment, using one of the various schemes that have been tested and found satisfactory (e.g., see chapter 22). The findings should serve to identify areas of particular difficulty (such as poor motor coordination) that may need to be studied in more detail, or taken into account in planning treatment.

Also, because language delay (a common presenting complaint) may be secondary to deafness, systematic audiometric examination by someone experienced in the testing of handicapped children is essential in all cases. In addition there should be a careful auriscopic examination of the ears. The testing of hearing in a young, behaviorally disturbed, non-speaking, unresponsive child can sometimes be a matter of extreme difficulty and it is common for repeat testing to be necessary. In cases of doubt, there may be a need for further, more specialized testing by an audiologist with expertise in this area. Clinical testing of visual acuity should also be a matter of routine as should funduscopy. Again, when there is any doubt about the child's vision, there should be referral to an ophthalmologist with experience in the testing of young handicapped children.

Medical Investigations

In terms of the need for routine medical investigations, the child suspected of having autism should be treated in the same way as any other child with a disorder of development. In the absence of specific indications, the yield in terms of positive findings indicating treatable medical conditions (or even those of relevance for genetic counseling) is quite low. Accordingly, although opinions differ on the matter, probably the number of investigations should be kept to the minimum needed for safety (Kirman, 1984). However, blood and urine should be taken for metabolic screening, including amino acid chromatography, and for serological evidence of intrauterine infection (as by toxoplasmosis or cytomegalic disease). In addition, there should be tests for phenylketonuria, maple syrup urine disease, histidinemia, and homocystinuria; together with an assessment of blood lead levels. Probably chromosome studies, including examination for the "fragile X," should now be done as a matter of routine if facilities are available. Protein-bound iodine should be determined if there is any suggestion of hypothyroidism, and serum copper and ceruloplasmin should be determined if there is any indication of Wilson's disease or if there has been a significant regression in development. A skull Xray is justified for the occasional identification of relevant intracerebral calcification. An EEG is rarely contributory in the absence of seizures, and, particularly in view of the difficulty of EEG examination with disturbed, unresponsive children, there is no need to make it a routine procedure. A CAT scan may be very helpful if there is any question of a localized cerebral lesion but it, too, is not warranted as routine.

DIFFERENTIAL DIAGNOSIS

Multiaxial Procedure

Because it is usual for autistic children to have multiple problems, it is essential to approach the question of differential diagnosis in a stepwise fashion if one is not to get lost in a thicket of overlapping possibilities. It is in just such a situation that multiaxial systems of diagnosis come into their own. Undoubtedly, the adoption of such an approach in *DSM-III* (American Psychiatric Association, 1980) was a step forward; unfortunately, the particular scheme adopted has many disadvantages, the most serious of which is the placement of intellectual level on the same axis as psychiatric disorder (Rutter and Shaffer, 1980). The multiaxial scheme based on *ICD-9* (World Health Organization, 1978) is better suited for the purpose, with its five axes of intellectual level, specific developmental disorders, psychiatric syndromes, medical conditions, and abnormal psychosocial situations (Rutter et al., 1975) (see table 3-7).

The first step requires determination of the child's current intellectual level. For most practical purposes a simple subdivision according to the child's nonlanguage cognitive skills is adequate: normal (i.e., an IQ of 70 or more), mildly retarded (50-69), moderately retarded (35-49), severely retarded (20-34), and profoundly retarded (below 20). However, in order to assess the meaning of the child's behavior, it is necessary to derive some estimate of the child's overall mental age (MA).

The second step involves a parallel exercise with respect to language development, except that there must be the additional question of whether the level of language is discrepant with the child's mental age. Of course, general intelligence and language do not develop precisely in parallel and it is common for mentally retarded children's language to lag somewhat behind their mental age. Accordingly, it would not be appropriate to diagnose a *specific* delay in language unless the language level is at least a year or so below the mental age (although, obviously, the difference that is clinically significant will vary with age and a lesser difference may be significant if the MA is very low).

The third step is a consideration of whether the child's behavior is appropriate for his chronological, mental, or language age. The essence of autism lies in the *deviance* of development, and the diagnosis cannot be made if the child's behavior is in keeping with the rest of his development (i.e., if socialization and language are delayed but not otherwise abnormal). Of course, no exact parallels between socialization, language, and general cognition should be expected; the question is whether there is deviance in relation to all concepts of developmental level. Whereas, it is helpful to consider deviance in relation to the child's own developmental level, often it may be appropriate to go straight to the basic question of whether the child's language, social interactions, and behavior would be considered normal or near normal for *any* phase of development. If the answer is that they cannot, the fourth

TABLE 3-7.
Procedure for Differential Diagnosis on a Multi-axial System

1. Determine Intellectual Level
2. Determine Level of Language Development
3. Consider Whether Child's Behavior Is Appropriate for
    (i) Chronological age
    (ii) Mental age
    (iii) Language age
4. If Not Appropriate, Consider Differential Diagnosis of Psychiatric Disorder According to
    (i) Pattern of social interaction
    (ii) Pattern of language
    (iii) Pattern of play
    (iv) Other behaviors
5. Identify Any Relevant Medical Conditions
6. Consider Whether There Are Any Relevant Psychosocial Factors

step is to consider the differential diagnosis of psychiatric conditions that might be responsible for the deviant patterns of behavior. The fifth and sixth steps then, respectively, concern the presence of any relevant medical conditions, and of relevant psychosocial factors.

Psychiatric Conditions

The differential diagnosis of psychiatric conditions leading to abnormalities of language, socialization, and play is also easier if taken according to a series of steps. The first question is whether there was ever a period of normal development. The issue here is *not* whether obviously autistic behavior was evident from the outset (usually it has not been so), but rather whether the development of language, cognition, social interactions, and play was proceeding entirely normally during the early years of infancy and childhood. In practice, in most cases this is almost impossible to determine with respect to development before eighteen months or even two years. However, by the age of two years, sufficient skills are to be expected for a reasonable estimate to be made of the normality or abnormality of development, provided the appropriate specific questions have been asked. Autism usually occurs without any clear-cut period of prior normal development, but in about a fifth of cases development seems to have been quite normal up to the age of two or two and a half years. The usually accepted diagnostic criteria demand an onset at or before thirty months. However, there do seem to be occasional cases with a clinical picture indistinguishable from autism with an onset shortly after that (see Lotter, 1966; Rutter et al., 1967; Folstein and Rutter, 1977).

If there has been a period of normal development up to the age of two or two and a half years, the possibilities of elective mutism, disintegrative psychosis, and schizophrenia have to be considered in addition to autism. Electively mute children may be rather socially withdrawn and unresponsive (see Rutter and Garmezy, 1983), but they differ from autistic children in (a) speaking normally in some situations, (b) not showing abnormalities in spoken language (other than delay in some cases), (c) showing appropriate social attachments and social reciprocity with at least some people, and (d) not showing the autistic abnormalities in play.

Disintegrative psychosis is a rare condition in which a period of normal development is followed, usually at about age two to four years, by a profound regression and behavioral disintegration (Heller, 1930). The clinical picture after the phase of regression is often somewhat similar to autism and the differentiation may be difficult, if not impossible, in cases with an onset before thirty months. However, the profound loss of interest in objects and of cognitive skills generally—often with loss of bowel and bladder control—in disintegrative psychosis is rather different from the usual onset with autism. *DSM-III* classifies the condition as an organic dementia but this seems an unjustified inference. It is true that in many cases the onset follows some clear-cut brain disease such as encephalitis (Corbett et al., 1977), but that is far from always the case. There are well-reported series of patients with the clinical picture of disintegrative psychosis but without any clear-cut evidence of brain disease or damage (Evans-Jones and Rosenbloom, 1978). At present, its etiology remains unknown and it is uncertain whether or not it is linked in any way with autism.

The rare syndrome of acquired aphasia with convulsions (Landau and Kleffner, 1957; Cooper and Ferry, 1978; Bishop, 1984) may occasionally be difficult to differentiate from autism or disintegrative psychosis. In this condition social and language development proceeds normally for some years but then over a period of weeks or months both receptive and expressive language is lost. In most cases there are a few seizures and generalized EEG abnormalities at the time of onset but usually neither persist. The children show a profound disorder of language comprehension characterized by a deviance of pattern as well as impairment (Bishop, 1982). In some cases there is recovery but usually substantial language impairment remains. The lack of general intellectual deterioration and the presence of normal social reciprocity differentiate acquired aphasia from the pervasive developmental disorders, but differential diagnosis may be difficult at first if the frightening experience of loss of the ability to understand what people are saying leads to social withdrawal and behavioral disturbance.

Ordinarily there is no difficulty differentiating autism from schizophrenia, in that the latter condition arises much later in childhood with a quite different set of symptoms (Kolvin, 1971; Eggers, 1978; Rutter, 1972; Kydd and Werry, 1982). However, there are a few reported cases of children in whom there has been a serious disorder of development from early childhood, in some instances from before thirty months, but in which the pattern of symptomatology suggests an unusually early onset of schizophrenia (Cantor et al., 1982). Such cases are said to differ from autism in terms of (a) relatively good social relationships with normal use of eye-to-eye gaze; (b) the presence of thought disorder; (c) sometimes the presence of delusions and hallucinations (although these are exceedingly difficult to determine in a young child); (d) marked hypotonicity; and (e) often a family history of schizophrenia. The nosological validity of schizophrenia beginning in infancy has not been established but certainly it may be accepted that there are serious nonautistic disorders of development manifest at that age.

But it would be unwarranted to assume that all such nonautistic conditions are schizophrenic in origin. *DSM-III* has a category of "childhood onset pervasive developmental disorders" for conditions with an onset after thirty months of age in which there is a gross and sustained impairment in social relationships but no delusions, hallucinations, or thought disorder. Such disorders vary in the extent to which they resemble autism, but the differentiation lies in terms of the later age of onset according to current diagnostic practice. Although the existence of such conditions is in no doubt, the *DSM-III* decision to provide specific diagnostic criteria is much more questionable. At present, little is known about these disorders or the extent to which they constitute a homogeneous group, and their nosological validity remains untested. In recognition of this lack of knowledge it seems preferable to keep to some diagnostic term that emphasizes our current ignorance, such as "*other* childhood onset pervasive developmental disorders" or, in the less satisfactory *ICD-9* terminology, "*other* childhood psychosis."

If the child's development has been abnormal from the outset, elective mutism, disintegrative psychosis, and these various onset disorders can all be ruled out. However, the fourth possibility of an abnormal pattern of bonding secondary to parental neglect or abuse, or to an institutional upbringing has to be considered. In these cases there may be language delay, deviant social interactions, and various abnormalities of behavior (including motor stereotypies). However, the picture differs from autism in terms of (a) normal social reciprocity; (b) the seeking of attachments; (c) the use of language for social communication; and (d) an absence of the specific autistic abnormalities of language. Also, it would be unusual for there to be any gross impairment of language comprehension.

The differential diagnosis of language delay as a presenting complaint involves consideration of a rather wider range of conditions (Rutter, 1974). Usually these can be distinguished from autism in terms of their pattern of language but, as most also differ in not showing deviance in social interactions or in patterns of play, they will not be considered further here. However, occasional difficulty may be experienced in cases of a severe developmental disorder of receptive language associated with social and behavioral problems. In such cases there may well be echolalia in association with the language delay, but there will not be delayed echoing, stereotyped utterances, and a failure to use language for social communication. Also, although the children may show social shyness and withdrawal, they will not show the lack of social attachments and reciprocity characteristic of autism, nor will they exhibit the abnormalities of play.

In practice, differential diagnosis presents most difficulties in two rather different situations. First, as the Camberwell general-population survey (Wing and Gould, 1979) clearly indicated, many children with moderate or severe mental retardation show some, but not all, of the features of autism. The differentiation from autism is most problematical with children who are very seriously retarded (say those with an MA below two years), because their level of skills is so low that it is very difficult to determine whether or not development is deviant as well as delayed. With very young children the question may have to be deferred until they are older. However, if the IQ is below 35 or so, the question is of little or no moment in that the presence of severe mental retardation is likely to be the main determinant of both the prognosis and pattern of treatment. The matter is of somewhat greater importance in the case of children with mild or moderate mental retardation. Nevertheless, it has to be accepted that we lack the knowledge to decide precisely where to draw the diagnostic distinctions, or indeed whether they should be drawn at all. For the moment at least, it seems best to restrict the diagnosis of autism to disorders that fully meet the criteria outlined here and to classify the others as *atypical autism, atypical pervasive developmental disorder,* or some such category of that kind.

The second area of difficulty concerns the differential diagnosis of autistic-like disorders in individuals of normal intelligence, but without the marked language deviance or delay usually considered essential for the diagnosis of autism. Some investigators have argued that these represent a condition separate from, but possibly related to, autism—so-called Asperger's syndrome (Wing, 1981) or "schizoid personality" * (Chick et al., 1979; Wolff and Barlow, 1979; Wolff and Chick, 1980). The lack of empathy and feeling for people, the deviant styles of communication, the unusual and constricted intellectual interests, and the idiosyncratic attachments to objects all suggest that the disorders constitute a milder variant of autism. However, whether that is true of all disorders within the rather broad concept of schizoid personality is less certain. It is evident that we lack the knowledge for a valid differentiation and classification of these serious disorders of social development. In the absence of that knowledge there is little profit in arguing over the niceties of these diagnostic distinctions at the periphery of the concept of autism. What *is* important for both prognosis and treatment is a careful delineation of the nature of the child's assets and deficits. Thus, in this group of autistic-like disorders in children of normal intelligence, the clinician should seek to determine whether there is a social and emotional *incapacity* (as well as poor performance), together with the specifics of the abnormalities in social functioning.

Finally, of course, diagnosis needs to be made with respect to the further axes of medical conditions and of abnormal psychosocial situations. The issues here are similar to those that arise in children with any form of psychiatric disorder. However, as already noted, it is not enough to note the presence of "abnormal" psychosocial situations. The

---

* This term applied by Wolff and her colleagues is unfortunate in that it is quite uncertain whether this constitutes the same condition as the personality disorder of the same name as diagnosed in adults. The *DSM-III* category "schizoid disorder of childhood or adolescence" also does not appear synonymous with the disorder discussed here.

clinician must also consider the overall style of family functioning in relation to the autistic child, the ways in which the family react to and deal with the child and with his particular problems of behavior, the impact of the autistic child on the rest of the family, the feelings and attitudes aroused in parents and siblings by having an autistic child, and the specific family concerns in relation to the child.

Obviously, too, it is necessary to determine the parents' own ideas on what is the matter with their child, what they have been told by previous advisers, and what treatments the child has had previously and is having now.

PLANNING TREATMENT

Goals, Strategies, and Principles

In deciding on an appropriate plan of treatment, it is necessary to start with a consideration of the goals (see table 3-8). As with any developmental disorder the first aim must be to foster normal development. In deciding how this should be done, we need to take account of what is known about the *normal* developmental process and about the factors that facilitate optimum development, as well as what is known on the *abnormal* features that interfere with development in autistic children (Rutter and Sussenwein, 1971; Rutter, 1984). In other words, there has to be a focus on the mechanisms that underlie normal growth and maturation in order to provide what is needed to promote these mechanisms, but it is also necessary to know which autistic features cause interference so that steps can be devised to reduce or circumvent that interference.

Table 3-9 outlines the approach with respect to language development. Normal children acquire their language skills through conversational interchange in a social context. Autistic children need the same but, because of their handicaps, it is necessary to provide planned periods of structured reciprocal interaction. Parents may be asked to set aside some thirty minutes per day for an uninterrupted period of play and conversation with their autistic children. The time should be kept relatively short both because such structured interactions with an unresponsive child are quite hard work for parents and because it is important for parents to lead their own lives and spend time with their nonautistic children. The main need is not to give the child "words" (although, of course, these are useful) but rather to facilitate social communication. The problem is that autistic children tend not to use language for social purposes. Moreover, unlike deaf children, if they lack speech they tend not to use gesture or mime in its place. The solutions lie in a focus on communication (encouraging any and all forms of communication and not just speech per se), on the differential use

TABLE 3-8.
Goals of Treatment

1. *To Foster Normal Development*
    a) Cognitive
    b) Language
    c) Social
2. *To Promote Learning*
3. *To Reduce Rigidity and Stereotypy*
4. *To Eliminate Nonspecific Maladaptive Behaviors*
5. *To Alleviate Family Distress*

TABLE 3-9.
Aim: Promotion of Language Development

Need	Problem	Solution
1. Social/conversational interchange	Social isolation	Planned periods of interaction / Promotion of social development
	Lack of reciprocity	Structured reciprocal interchange
2. Social communication	Failure to use language socially	Teaching to do so / Differential reinforcement / Focus on communication (rather than speech per se)
3. Linguistic capacity	Incapacity	Direct teaching at appropriate level / Use of alternative mode (signing)

of praise to encourage communication, and on teaching that is deliberately structured to provide an emphasis on social usage of language (Hemsley et al., 1978; Howlin, 1980, 1981). There is value in providing specific training in the use and understanding of spoken language, but treatment has a greater effect on the *usage* of language than on basic language *capacities*.

Inevitably, children's progress in language is limited by the severity and extensiveness of the biological incapacities. Some autistic children will never learn to speak regardless of what is done, whereas others will acquire extensive spoken language even in the absence of any form of specific treatment. All studies have demonstrated huge individual differences in outcome and in response to language training (Howlin, 1980; Rutter, 1980). By and large, language training is most effective when there is evidence of some limited language skills before treatment commences—as shown by some understanding of language; by speechlike cadences in babble, by the presence of imitation and of pretend play, and by some echoed speech. Speech training has little to offer the mute child without any of these linguistic and prelinguistic skills. Direct teaching (using operant and other techniques) needs to be geared to the child's developmental level. But also, if there is little or no progress with speech in spite of the presence of some understanding of language, it may be worthwhile introducing sign language (Carr, 1979; Bonvillian et al., 1981; Kiernan, 1983).

Similar considerations apply with respect to socialization (see table 3-10). In the normal child it seems that attachment and social relationships are promoted by intense personal interaction that is pleasurable to the child, that is responsive to the child's needs, and that provides comfort and security at times of stress and distress (Bowlby, 1969; Rutter, 1981). The sheer duration of interaction is less important than these personal qualities. The problem for autistic children lies both in their lack of social approaches and in their lack of responsiveness to *other* people's overtures to them. The solution lies in the parents' (or therapist's) deliberate *intrusion* into the children's solitary activities, so that the children need to interact with other people in order to engage in their preferred activities (Rutter and Sussenwein, 1971). This must be done in a way that makes the social interaction pleasurable to the child but, still, the interactions must be structured so that they are reciprocal and social, rather than solitary. Another consideration is that caretaking should be personalized;

TABLE 3-10.
Aim: Promotion of Social Development

NEED	PROBLEM	SOLUTION
1. Intensive personal interaction that is pleasurable, responsive, comforting	Lack of social approach / Lack of reciprocity	Structured interaction with social intrusion
2. Personalized caretaking	Institutional upbringing	Avoidance of residential care in early childhood
3. Social cognitive capacity	Incapacity	Direct teaching (social-skills training)

hence prolonged institutional care should be avoided, especially in early childhood. It is necessary, too, to recognize the importance of autistic children's social incapacities. So far, we lack knowledge as how to remedy these deficits but presumably direct teaching may be helpful and social-skills training has a place in treatment.

As well as fostering normal development, there has to be a concern to promote autistic children's learning more generally (see table 3–11). It has been shown that autistic children can and do profit from schooling and that systematic teaching in an ordered environment is more effective than freer permissive approaches (Bartak, 1978; Schopler et al., 1982). Autistic children lack self-direction and there is a need to structure the learning situation appropriately, providing guidance and supervision, not just at the beginning, but throughout task performance. The learning tasks should be broken down into a series of manageable small

TABLE 3-11.
Aim: Promotion of Learning

NEED	PROBLEM	SOLUTION
1. Attention to cues	Lack of self-direction	Structured learning situation / Breakdown of learning task into small steps
	Interference from deviant behaviors	Reduce deviant behaviors
	Overselectivity	Avoidance of extra prompts
2. Ability to apply skills in new situations	Context specificity	Focus on natural environment (home and school) / Limited use of residential treatment / Structure for generalization
3. Understanding of meaning	Comprehension defect	Monitoring of learning / Focus on meaning
4. Persistence to cope with difficulties	Adverse response to failure	Error-free learning

steps. Also, they should be programmed (through "chaining" elements, "prompt fading," and other techniques) to encourage the autistic child to be able to work on his own (Rincover and Koegel, 1977). In common with other mentally retarded children, many autistic children tend to focus on one cue to the exclusion of others (Lovaas et al., 1979). One consequence is that learning tends to be *worse* if autistic children are given extra prompts or cues that are not inherent in the discrimination required for the learning task (Schreibman, 1975; Koegel and Rincover, 1976; Nelson et al., 1980). Because autistic children's learning tends to show a handicapping context specificity, therapeutic efforts need to be focused on the child's natural environment at home and at school. Residential treatments have not proved satisfactory as a general solution. But, in addition, it is necessary to organize training in such a way as to encourage generalization of learning (Holman and Baer, 1978; Wahler et al., 1979; Handleman and Harris, 1980). Throughout all teaching there is a need to focus explicitly on meaning and on understanding, as autistic children otherwise tend to learn by rote without attention to the concepts involved. This problem also means that the autistic child's learning needs to be carefully monitored to assess whether he is understanding what he is learning mechanically. Because autistic children tend to respond to failure by retreating into a stereotyped style of response (Clark and Rutter, 1979; Koegel and Egel, 1979; Volkmar and Cohen, 1982), it is important to organize their learning tasks to put a premium on success with the minimum opportunity for error.

The third major goal of treatment is the reduction of the rigidity and stereotypy that pervades so many aspects of autistic children's functioning. The techniques to be employed include that of "graded change" (Marchant et al., 1974). In essence, this involves the bringing about of major changes through a series of very tiny steps, each of which is so small that it is accepted by the child as not amounting to any noticeable alteration in pattern. Such changes may involve physical structure (as the gradual cutting down of inconveniently large attachment objects), timing, routine, or indeed any aspect of behavior. Another approach is provided by attention to the environmental features that seem to elicit stereotyped behaviors or which increase the frequency of their occurrence. Often stereotypies tend to be at a maximum in barren, bleak, unstimulating environments (Baumeister, 1978); hence, so far as possible, it is desirable that autistic children are kept actively engaged in play or work, with ample provision of toys and activities, and with structured opportunities for personal interactions. Autistic children tend to be at their worst in unstructured situations (Clark and Rutter, 1981) and, sometimes, the experimental provision of extra sensory stimulation may reduce stereotypies in severely retarded *autistic* children (Goodall and Corbett, 1982; Murphy, 1982). Stereotyped behaviors may also be reduced by the introduction of alternative behaviors or activities that are incompatible with, and hence compete with them.

The fourth goal of treatment involves the elimination of nonspecific maladaptive behaviors, such as tantrums, aggression, fears, and bed-wetting. For the most part, behavioral approaches provide the most suitable form of intervention (Howlin et al., 1973; Hemsley et al., 1978). These require a functional analysis of behavior and an application of the various principles of learning. Since the principles are the same as those that apply to the use of behavioral methods with other psychiatric conditions, they will not be considered further here.

Pharmacological interventions have a place, albeit a rather limited place, in treatment. There are no drugs that are specific to autism but drugs may be useful for the control of specific behaviors. For example, the major tranquilizers may serve to reduce agitation, tension, and overactivity (Corbett, 1976; Campbell, 1978), although care is needed in their usage because of the possibility of adverse effects on learning (Taylor, 1983). Phenothiazines have the limitations of sedation as a side effect, but, on the whole, they are safer than the butyrophenones (such as haloperidol). The latter have been found to have more powerful effects in some studies (DeMyer et al., 1981), but the side effects of dystonic reactions make them troublesome drugs. Stimulants are *contra*indicated as a treatment of hyperactivity in mentally retarded autistic children, not only because they are ineffective but also because they may increase stereotyped behavior (Aman, 1982). Hypnotics have an occasional place in the treatment of sleep disturbance but habituation develops rapidly, as it does in normal children. Accordingly, they are of use mainly at times of crisis or as an adjunct in the early stages of introduction of a behavioral program. Claims have been made that megavitamin therapy benefits some autistic children (Rimland et al., 1978), but the limited available evidence suggests that it is unlikely that vitamins constitute a generally effective form of treatment in most cases. A recent report (Geller et al., 1982), based on just three children, suggested that there may be some behavioral improvement following the pharmacological reduction of raised serotonin levels but, so far, this remains an experimental approach.

The fifth major goal of treatment is the alleviation of family distress. The parents and siblings of handicapped children face many difficulties and carry many burdens; this is especially the case with autistic children, many of whom are unresponsive and unrewarding to be with, difficult to play and talk with, and demanding in their need for supervision, structuring, and control. Often, the family are very puzzled by their child's abnormal behavior and hence worried and uncertain about what they should do. It is important to help them gain an understanding of their child's behavior. Families should have full feedback on the results of the diagnostic appraisal. This may take more than one session and the feedback should include an understanding of the nature and patterning of the child's problems; his developmental level with respect to the key areas of functioning, educational and other needs, and as much information as it is possible to give on the probabilities of the child's later development and outcome in later childhood and in adult life.

But, also, it is necessary that parents learn *what* to do. They should be helped to gain effective problem-solving skills by, in effect, engaging them as cotherapists (Schopler and Reichler, 1971; Hemsley et al., 1978; Holmes et al., 1982). Most parents find that the acquisition of practical means of coping with their child's difficulties is in itself helpful in reducing their worries and anxieties. Nevertheless, the treatment focus on the autistic child is likely to have implications for the balance of relationships and for the pattern of life in the family as a whole. It is important to be sensitive to the needs of each parent as an individual and with respect to their marital relationship, and to the needs of other children in the family. *What* parents are expected to do for their autistic child and *how* they are expected to do it must be adapted to the personal situation and characteristics of each family. But, also, the therapist must be alert to the irrational guilt felt by many parents, to despair and depression when their child seems to make so little progress, to anger and frustration aroused by the parents' difficulty in dealing with resistant problems, to disappointment or hostility at the child's lack of affection and social response, and to resentment over having a handicapped child. These are normal and understandable reactions experienced at some time by most parents of seriously handicapped children, but counseling and casework are needed to help parents realize that they are not alone in these feelings, that love and anger can coexist, and that there are ways of coming to terms with these troubling feelings and of channeling them in positive directions. Of course, too, direct advice and guidance may enable parents to deal with these family matters in a more constructive and adaptive fashion. Genetic counseling should be given, to provide both information and the opportunity to discuss the implications that follow from it.

Last, families require practical help with such matters as baby-sitting arrangements, holiday provisions for handicapped children, financial allowances for which they may be eligible, dental care, and special educational provision.

Overall Treatment Program

So far, treatment has been discussed in terms of the multitude of separate elements that are required. In conclusion, these need to be brought together to constuct an overall treatment program with at least three key features: (1) appropriate medical care; (2) special educational provision; and (3) a home-based program for the family (see table 3-12). Medical care needs to be planned on the basis of the diagnostic assessment. However, it should be recognized that there can never be a "once-and-for-all-time" diagnostic appraisal. Not only may circumstances change (with the onset of seizures or the occurrence of new behavioral problems), but also the earlier assessment may have been in error. This is particularly the case with hearing deficits, and if there is any reason for doubt, the appraisal should be repeated.

A careful analysis of educational requirements should form the basis of selection of a suitable class, unit, or school. In many cases a unit specially designed for autistic children may be best, but it should not be assumed that this is necessarily preferable. In some cases facilities for mentally retarded or for language-impaired children may be equally (or more) appropriate, especially if there can be flexibility in the provision of special help of one kind or another. A few of the more intellectually able, and more mildly handicapped, may even be most suitably placed in a regular school if means can be found to adapt the school situation to cater to any special individual needs of the autistic child. In most circumstances, day schooling is preferable for younger autistic children, but it is necessary that residential schooling be available for those who require it, for reasons associated with their own handicaps, family needs, or geography. Whatever the schooling decided upon, there should be consideration of whether any extra facilities (such as speech therapy) are needed. It will always be necessary to let the school have a report of findings and recommendations, and in

TABLE 3-12.
Overall Treatment Program

1. *Appropriate Medical Care*
    a) Treatment of medical conditions (when present)
    b) Correction of hearing/vision defects
    c) Dental care
    d) Genetic counseling
    e) Discussion with parents of diagnosis, prognosis, and treatment
2. *Special Educational Provision*
    a) Suitable class, unit, or school
    b) Extra facilities as required
3. *Home-Based Program for Family*
    a) Use of behavioral/developmental methods
    b) Drugs (when appropriate)
    c) Counseling
    d) Practical Help
    e) Inpatient care (when needed)
    f) Self-Help groups
    g) Books

most cases it is desirable to pay a visit to the school to discuss how the child's needs may be met most satisfactorily.

Finally, there must be a therapeutic program for the family. It should be home based in the sense that it is planned to tackle problems as, and how, they arise in the home environment. Almost always this means that there should be at least one prolonged home visit to observe the child, to appraise parent-child interaction, and to note any particular features of the house or neighborhood that have implications for treatment. There are advantages in undertaking much of the treatment in the home itself, but practical considerations may impose limits on how far that is possible. The elements that should be included in such a home-based approach have, for the most part, been discussed previously; they include the use of behavioral/developmental methods of treatment, drugs where appropriate, counseling, practical help, the availability of inpatient care for the very few occasions when it is necessary as an adjunct to deal with specific problems, putting the family in touch with parent self-help groups, and suggesting books that they might find helpful.

In the great majority of cases there is no need to admit the child to hospital,* as all investigations can be undertaken as an outpatient, and treatment is best provided at home and at school. However, occasionally, short-term admission may be needed when there is severely disturbed behavior that is resistant to treatment and, rarely, long-term hospital care may be required. The National Society for Autistic Children, open to both parents and professionals, provides both information and a source of mutual self-help that most parents find beneficial; accordingly, families should be asked if they wish to be put in touch with the society (or with other self-help groups). Also, some parents find it useful to read further on autism. Lorna Wing's book for parents (Wing, 1980) is a good example of what is available, as is Janet Carr's (1980) book for the parents of mentally handicapped children.

The intensity of treatment and the frequency with which the family needs to be seen vary greatly. In most cases it is desirable to start by seeing the parents every week or so, making visits less frequent as problems diminish and as the family learns how to manage those that remain (Hemsley et al., 1978; Holmes et al., 1982). Intermittent outpatient attendance is not usually adequate. Autistic children's needs and problems change as they grow older and it seems that, even after parents have learned effective coping strategies, most need to be seen every few months to deal with new issues and to reconsider the use of behavioral approaches.

Systematic evaluations have shown that the benefits of treatment in both the short term and long term are real and worthwhile, albeit modest. This applies to both special schooling (Bartak, 1978) and to work with parents (Hemsley et al., 1978). Nevertheless, it is also apparent that there is immense variation in outcome, with some autistic children remaining very severely handicapped in spite of all therapeutic endeavors.

References

Aman, M. C. 1982. Stimulant drug effects in developmental disorders and hyperactivity: Toward a resolution of disparate findings. *J. Aut. Dev. Disor.*, 12:385-398.

American Psychiatric Association. 1980. *Diagnostic and statistical manual of mental disorders (DSM-III)*. Washington, D. C.: APA.

---

* The proportion of autistic individuals requiring hospital care is somewhat greater in adolescence than in early childhood but still it is a small minority.

August, G. J., Stewart, M. A., and Tsai, L. 1981. The incidence of cognitive disabilities in the siblings of autistic children. *Br. J. Psych.,* 138:416–422.

Bartak, L. 1978. Educational approaches. In *Autism: A reappraisal of concepts and treatment,* ed. M. Rutter, and E. Schopler. New York: Plenum Press.

Baumeister, A. A. 1978. Origins and control of stereotyped movements. In *Quality of life for severely and profoundly retarded people,* ed. C. E. Meyers, pp. 353–384. American Association on Mental Deficiency, series 3. Washington, D.C.: Research Foundation for Improvement.

Bayley, N. 1969. *Manual for the Bayley scales of infant development.* New York: Psychological Corp.

Berger, M. 1984 (in press). Psychological assessment and testing. In *Child and adolescent psychiatry: Modern approaches,* 2nd. ed., ed. M. Rutter, and L. Hersov. Oxford: Blackwell Scientific.

Berger, M., and Yule, W. 1972. Cognitive assessment in young children with language delay. In *The child with delayed speech,* ed. M. Rutter, and J. A. M. Martin. Clin. in Dev. Med. no. 43. London: Heinemann/SIMP.

Bishop, D. V. M. 1982. Comprehension of spoken, written, and signed sentences in childhood language disorders. *J. Child Psychol. Psych.* 23:1–20.

Bishop, D. V. M. 1984 (in press). Classification of childhood language disorders. In *Language development and communication problems,* ed. W. Yule, M. Rutter, and M. Bax. Clin. in Dev. Med. London: Blackwell Scientific/SIMP.

Bonvillian, J. D., Nelson, K. E., and Rhyne, J. M. 1981. Sign language and autism. *J. Aut. Dev. Disor.,* 11:125–138.

Bowlby, J. 1969. *Attachment and loss. I. Attachment.* London: Hogarth Press.

Campbell, M. 1978. Pharmacotherapy. In *Autism: A reappraisal of concepts and treatment,* ed. M. Rutter, and E. Schopler. New York: Plenum Press.

Cantor, S., Evans, J., Pearce, J. and Pezzot-Pearce, T. 1982. Childhood schizophrenia: Present but not accounted for. *Am. J. Psych.,* 139:758–762.

Carr, E. G. 1979. Teaching autistic children to use sign language: Some research issues. *J. Aut. Dev. Disor.,* 9:345–360.

Carr, J. 1980. *Helping your handicapped child: A step-by-step guide to everday problems.* Harmondsworth, Middx.: Penguin, 1980.

Chick, J., Waterhouse, L., and Wolff, S. 1979. Psychological construing in schizoid children grown up. *Brit. J. Psych.,* 135:425–430.

Clark, P., and Rutter, M. 1979. Task difficulty and task performance in autistic children. *J. Child Psychol. Psych.,* 20:271–285.

Clark, P., and Rutter, M. 1981. Autistic children's responses to structure and to interpersonal demands. *J. Aut. Dev. Disor.,* 11:201–217.

Cooper, J. A., and Ferry, P. C. 1978. Acquired auditory verbal agnosia and seizures in childhood. *J. Speech Hear. Disor.,* 43:176–184.

Corbett, J. 1976. Medical management. In *Early childhood autism,* 2nd ed., ed. L. Wing. Oxford: Pergamon Press.

Corbett, J., Harris, R., Taylor, E., and Trimble, M. 1977. Progressive disintegrative psychosis of childhood. *J. Child Psychol. Psych.,* 18:211–219.

Cox, A., and Rutter, M. 1984 (in press). Diagnostic appraisal and interviewing. In *Child and adolescent psychiatry: Modern approaches,* 2nd ed., ed. M. Rutter and L. Hersov. Oxford: Blackwell Scientific.

DeMyer, M. K., Hingtgen, J. N., and Jackson, R. K. 1981. Infantile autism reviewed: A decade of research. *Schiz. Bull.,* 7:388–451.

Deykin, E. Y., and MacMahon, B. 1979. The incidence of seizures among children with autistic symptoms. *Am. J. Psych.,* 136:1310–1312.

Doll, E. A., 1953. *The measurement of social competence: A manual for the Vineland social maturity scale.* Minneapolis: American Guidance Service.

Eggers, C. 1978. Course and prognosis of childhood schizophrenia. *J. Aut. Child. Schiz.,* 8:21–36.

Evans-Jones, L. G., and Rosenbloom, L. 1978. Disintegrative psychosis in childhood. *Dev. Med. Child Neurol.,* 20:462–470.

Folstein, S., and Rutter, M. 1977. Infantile autism: A genetic study of 21 twin pairs. *J. Child Psychol. Psych.,* 18:297–321.

Geller, E., Ritvo, E. R., Freeman, B. J., and Yuwiler, A. 1982. Preliminary observations of the effect of fenfluramine on blood serotonin and symptoms in three autistic boys. *N. Eng. J. Med.,* 307:165–169.

Gillberg, C., and Schaumann, H. 1981. Infantile autism and puberty. *J. Aut. Dev. Disor.,* 11:365–372.

Goodall, E., and Corbett, J. A. 1982. Relationships between sensory stimulation and stereotyped behaviour in severely mentally handicapped children. *J. Men. Def. Res.,* 26:163–175.

Handleman, J. S., and Harris, S. L. 1980. Generalization from school to home with autistic children. *J. Aut. Dev. Dis.,* 10:323–324.

Heller, T. 1969. Pub. in German, 1930. About dementia infantilis. Translation in *Modern perspectives in international child psychiatry,* ed. J. G. Howells. Edinburgh: Oliver and Boyd.

Hemsley, R., Howlin, P., Berger, M., Hersov, L., Holbrook, D., Rutter, M., and Yule, W. 1978. Training autistic children in a family context. In *Autism: A reappraisal of concepts and treatments,* ed. M. Rutter, and E. Schopler. New York: Plenum Press.

Holman, J., and Baer, D. M. 1979. Facilitating generalization of on-task behavior through self-monitoring of academic tasks. *J. Aut. Dev. Disor.,* 9:429–446.

Holmes, N., Hemsley, R., Rickett, J., and Likierman, H. 1982. Parents as co-therapists: Their perceptions of a home-based behavioral treatment for autistic children. *J. Aut. Dev. Disor.,* 12:331–342.

Howlin, P. 1980. The home treatment of autistic children. In *Language and language disorders in childhood,* ed. L. A. Hersov, M. Berger, and R. Nicol. Oxford: Pergamon Press.

Howlin, P. 1981. The effectiveness of operant language training with autistic children. *J. Aut. Dev. Disor.,* 11:89–106.

Howlin, P., Marchant, R., Rutter, M., Berger, M., Hersov, L., and Yule, W. 1973. A home-based approach to the treatment of autistic children. *J. Aut. Child. Schiz.,* 3:308–336.

Kanner, L. 1943. Autistic disturbances of affective contact. *Nerv. child,* 2:217–250.

Kiernan, C. 1983. The use of non-social communication techniques with autistic individuals. *J. Child Psychol. Psych.* 24:339–376.

Kirman, B. 1984 (in press). Mental retardation: medical aspects. In *Child and adolescent psychiatry: Modern approaches,* 2nd ed., ed. M. Rutter and L. Hersov. Oxford: Blackwell Scienctific.

Koegel, R. L., and Egel, A. L. 1979. Motivating autistic children. *J. Abnorm. Psych.,* 85:418–426.

Koegell, R. L., and Rincover, A. 1976. Some detrimental effects of using extra stimuli to guide learning in normal and autistic children. *J. Abnorm. Child Psych.,* 4:59–61.

Kolvin, I. 1971. Psychosis in childhood—a comparative study. In *Infantile autism: Concepts, characteristics, and treatment,* ed. M. Rutter. Edinburgh: Churchill Livingstone.

Kydd, R. R., and Werry, J. S. 1982. Schizophrenia in children under 16 years. *J. Aut. Dev. Disor.,* 12:343–358.

Landau, W., and Kleffner, F. 1957. Syndrome of acquired aphasia with convulsive disorders in children. *Neurol.,* 7:523–530.

Le Couteur, A. Unpublished data, 1983.

Lord, C., Schopler, E., and Revick, D. 1982. Sex differences in autism. *J. Aut. Dev. Disor.,* 12:317–330.

Lotter, V. 1966. Epidemiology of autistic conditions in young children. I. Prevalence. *Soc. Psych.,* 1:124–137.

Lotter, V. 1978. Follow-up studies. In *Autism: A reappraisal of concepts and treatment,* ed. M. Rutter, and E. Schopler. New York: Plenum Press.

Lovaas, O. I., Koegel, R. L., and Schreibman, L. 1979. Stimulus overselectivity in autism: A review of research. *Psychol. Bull.,* 86:1236–1254.

Lowe, M., and Costello, A. J. 1976. *The symbolic play test.* Windsor: National Foundation for Educational Research.

Marchant, R., Howlin, P., Yule, W., and Rutter, M. 1974. Graded change in the treatment of the behaviour of autistic children. *J. Child Psychol. Psych.,* 15:221–227.

Mash, E. J., and Terdal, L. G., eds. 1981. *Behavioral assessment of childhood disorders.* New York: Guilford Press.

Mecham, M. 1958. *Verbal language development scale.* Minneapolis: Educational Test Bureau.

Mittler, P. 1972. Psychological assessment of language abilities. In *The child with delayed speech,* ed. M. Rutter, and J. A. M. Martin. Clin. in Dev. Med., no. 43. London: Heinemann/SIMP.

Murphy, G. 1982. Sensory reinforcement in the mentally handicapped and autistic child: A review. *J. Aut. Dev. Disor.,* 12:265–278.

Neale, M. D., 1958. *Analysis of reading ability.* London: Macmillan.

Nelson, D. L., Gergenti, E., and Hollander, A. C. 1980. Extra prompts versus no extra prompts in self-care training of autistic children and adolescents. *J. Aut. Dev. Disor.,* 10:311–322.

Raven, J. C. 1960. *Guide to using the coloured progressive matrices.* London: H. K. Lewis.

Reynell, J. 1969. *Reynell developmental language scales.* Slough: NFER.

Rimland, B., Callaway, E., and Dreyfus, P. 1978. The effects of high doses of vitamin B_6 on autistic children: A double-blind crossover study. *Am. J. Psych.* 135:472–475.

Rincover, A., and Koegel, R. L. 1977. Classroom treatment of autistic children. II. Individualized instruction in a group. *J. Abnorm. Child Psychol.,* 5:113–126.

Rutter, M. 1967. Psychotic disorders in early childhood. In *Recent developments in schizophrenia,* ed. A. J. Coppen, and D. Walk. Ashford, Kent: Headley Bros.

Rutter, M. 1970. Autistic children: Infancy to adulthood. *Sem. Psych.* 2:435–450.

Rutter, M. 1972. Childhood schizophrenia reconsidered. *J. Aut. Childhood Schiz.,* 2:315–337.

Rutter, M. 1974. The child who is slow to talk. *Update* (March), pp. 777–786.

Rutter, M. 1976. *Helping troubled children.* New York: Plenum Press.

Rutter, M. 1978. Diagnosis and definition. In *Autism: A reappraisal of concepts and treatment,* ed. M. Rutter, and E. Schopler. New York: Plenum Press.

Rutter, M. 1980. Attachment and the development of social relationships. In *Scientific foundations of developmental psychiatry,* ed. M. Rutter. London: Heinemann Medical.

Rutter, M. 1981. *Maternal deprivation reassessed.* 2nd ed. Harmondsworth, Middx.: Penguin.

Rutter, M. 1983. Cognitive deficits in the pathogenesis of autism. (The Kenneth Cameron Memorial Lecture.) *J. Child Psychol. Psych.,* 24:513–531.

Rutter, M. 1984. The treatment of autistic children. *J. Child Psychol. Psych.* (in press).

Rutter, M., and Garmezy, N. 1983. Developmental psychopathology. In *Social and personality development. Carmichael's manual of child psychology,* vol. 4, ed. E. M. Hetherington. New York: Wiley.

Rutter, M., Greenfield, D., and Lockyer, L. 1967. A five to fifteen year follow-up study of infantile psychosis. II. Social and behavioural outcome. *Brit. J. Psych.,* 113:1183–1199.

Rutter, M., and Shaffer, D. 1980. *DSM-III:* A step forward or back in terms of the classification of child psychiatric disorders? *J. Am. Acad. Child Psych.,* 19:371–394.

Rutter, M., Shaffer, D., and Sturge, C. 1975. *A guide to a multi-axial classification scheme for psychiatric disorders in childhood and adolescence.* London: Institute of Psychiatry.

Rutter, M., and Sussenwein, F. 1971. A developmental and behavioral approach to the treatment of pre-school autistic children. *J. Aut. Child. Schiz.,* 1:376-397.

Schopler, E., Mesibov, G., and Baker, A. 1982. Evaluation of treatment for autistic children and their parents. *J. Am. Acad. Child Psych.,* 21:262-267.

Schopler, E., and Reichler, R. J. 1971. Parents as co-therapists in the treatment of psychotic children. *J. Aut. Child. Schiz.,* 1:87-102.

Schreibman, L. 1975. Effects of within-stimulus and extra-stimulus prompting on discrimination learning in autistic children. *J. Appl. Beh. Anal.,* 8:91-112.

Stutsman, R. 1948. *Guide for administering the Merrill-Palmer scale of mental tests.* New York: Harcourt Brace and World.

Taylor, E. 1984 (in press). In *Child and adolescent psychiatry: Modern approaches,* 2nd ed., ed. M. Rutter and L. Hersov. Oxford: Blackwell Scientific.

Tsai, L., Steward, M. A., and August, G. 1981. Implication of sex differences in the familial transmission of infantile autism. *J. Aut. Dev. Disor.,* 11:165-173.

Volkmar, F. R., and Cohen, D. J. 1982. A hierarchical analysis of patterns of noncompliance in autistic and behavior-disturbed children. *J. Aut. Dev. Disor.,* 12:35-42.

Wahler, R. G., Berland, R. M., and Coe, T. D. 1979. Generalization processes in child behavior change. In *Advances in clinical child psychology,* vol. 2, ed. B. B. Lahey, and A. E. Kazdin. New York: Plenum Press.

Wechsler, D. 1967. *Wechsler preschool and primary scale of intelligence.* New York: Psychological Corporation.

Wechsler, D. 1974. *Wechsler intelligence scale for children (revised).* New York: Psychological Corporation.

Wing, L., 1980. *Autistic children: A guide for parents.* London: Constable.

Wing, L. 1981. Asperger's syndrome: A clinical account. *Psychol. Med.* 11:115-130.

Wing, L., and Gould, J. 1979. Severe impairments of social interaction and associated abnormalities in children: Epidemiology and classification. *J. Aut. Dev. Disor.,* 9:11-30.

Wolff, S., and Barlow, A. 1979. Schizoid personality in childhood: A comparative study of schizoid, autistic, and normal children. *J. Child Psychol. Psychiat.* 20:29-46.

Wolff, S., and Chick, J. 1980. Schizoid personality in childhood: A controlled follow-up study. *Psychol. Med.,* 10:85-100.

World Health Organization. 1978. *International classification of diseases.* Geneva: World Health Organization.

Yule, W. 1984. Behavioral approaches. In *Child and adolescent psychiatry: modern approaches,* ed. M. Rutter and L. Hersov. Oxford: Blackwell Scientific, in press.

4

Childhood Language Disorders

LAURA S. MCKIRDY

ONE OF THE MOST SIGNIFICANT social and cognitive developmental milestones in the first year is the emergence of the first word and the child's subsequent rapid establishment of a wide variety of verbally based communication skills. For the majority of children, the basic language acquisition process is completed by age four, and children of this age are fluent speakers of their native language. The language learning process is usually so smooth that it is taken for granted. However, normal speech and language development requires a complex neurophysiological and psychological foundation. Abnormalities in any portion of this substructure frequently present, as their most obvious symptom, deviant speech and language. The major portion of this chapter will deal with childhood language problems, but a brief survey of speech disorders will also be presented.

SPEECH AND SPEECH PROBLEMS

Speech and language will therefore be discussed as if they were entirely separate functions, but in reality there is considerable overlapping between the two. Within the current context, speech will refer to the vocal-motor aspect of communication involving one or a combination of the processes of: (1) articulation, (2) voice, and (3) fluency. Speech is dependent on effective motor planning and control of the airstream and orofacial musculature. Structural or functional abnormalities such as a cleft lip and/or palate, velar weakness or paralysis, dental malocclusions, etc., all lead to speech defects but spare language function. For example, a child with a cleft palate may have considerable difficulty making himself understood because of impaired pronounciation and severe hypernasality, but might have no difficulty understanding the speech of others or formulating his ideas for verbal expression. As further illustration of the separation between speech and language, Lenneberg (1962) and Fourcin (1975) both report on patients who are so severely dysarthric that they have no intelligible vocal speech, yet show normal language comprehension. In the case of Fourcin's patient (a quadriplegic athetoid), the dissociation between language and speech was dramatically illustrated when at age thirty he was given access to a special foot-controlled typewriter, which enabled him to communicate with others for the first time. He demonstrated a high level of written language and functional competence in mathematics, skills he achieved largely through self-education.

There are a diversity of problems that cause speech defects. Only a brief listing will follow to familiarize the reader with the usual classification system and to clarify the distinction between speech problems and language problems (although speech and language disorders do often coexist).

Voice disorders are abnormalities of voice production, commonly due to disease of the larynx, such as vocal nodules, vocal fold paresis (Ingram, 1975), or to difficulty in controlling and directing the air stream through the vocal tract resulting in problems with volume, sustaining vocalization, or resonance. *Rhythm disorders* involve problems in fluency, including stuttering and cluttering. *Articulation disorders*, impaired pronunciation of the sounds of speech, are caused by problems such as:

a. *structural abnormalities*—cleft palate; absent or underdeveloped tongue; abnormalities of the lips or teeth; disproportions of mandible or maxilla; velopharyngeal disproportion or malfunction; inadequate nasal airway due to grossly enlarged adenoids or congenital nasal defects.
b. *dysarthrias*—defects of innervations of the lips, tongue, palate, or related organs resulting in paresis, poor coordination, involuntary movements (e.g., cerebral palsy).
c. *verbal apraxias*—difficulty with motor planning for speech resulting in poor ability to control the articulators voluntarily and consistently in the presence of good use of the oral mechanism for vegetative functions such as chewing and swallowing.
d. *articulation problems secondary to other disorders* such as overall delayed development (e.g., mental retardation), hearing impairment, auditory perceptual problems, and faulty learning.

The reader is referred to Ingram (1975) or Travis (1971) for more information about speech disorders. Each type of speech disability has been studied extensively, and there is a separate literature devoted to theory and treatment of each of the various speech problems.

Childhood Language Problems

The remaining portions of this chapter will deal with childhood language problems, an area that has come under study in only the last fifteen to twenty years coinciding with the rapidly expanding interest in language in general. This interest in language was particularly stimulated by the work of Chomsky (1957), who posited a human innate "language acquisition device." Later, this idea was expanded by psycholinguists who were interested in language acquisition (e.g., Bloom, 1970; Brown, 1973) and the interrelationships between language and thought (e.g., Vygotsky, 1962; Sinclair-de-Zwart, 1969).

Language: A Definition

Within the current context, language will be described as a complex process that (a) places into words our perceptions and concepts about the world (words being simply "a conventional system of arbitrary signals," [Bloom and Lahey, 1978]); (b) subserves central portions of reflective thought; and (c) permits us to communicate with others who use the same conventional code. The predominant language of human communities is an auditory-oral system and in many cultures this oral system has a written counterpart.

Just as speech problems can occur without language problems, the opposite can occur as well. A familiar adult clinical disruption of language which may spare speech is seen in some forms of adult aphasia following a cerebral vascular accident where pronunciation remains clear but where there is obvious difficulty comprehending and using language. For example, the dysnomic patient may grope in search of a particular word, but when it is ultimately found it is frequently clearly articulated.

The child with a language disorder does not necessarily have the same problems as the adult aphasic. He has not lost language, he has instead failed to develop it. To have some feel for the child's difficulty, it is useful to imagine being a stranger in a foreign country, where an unfamiliar and unusual language is spoken. The language lacks the accustomed melody, rhythm, and word boundaries. (For English-speaking people, Chinese is a good example.) When faced with such an exotic language, one attempts to communicate through gestures, pantomine, tone of voice, and facial expression. These nonverbal means, however, may not be effective as even body language varies from culture to culture. One's difficulties in communication in this foreign country are compounded by a series of problems: vocabulary limitations, differences in the suprasegmental code (melody, volume), and differences in the nonverbal codes (body language). The language-disordered child experiences all or some of the difficulties of the stranger in his attempts to learn to use language. He has difficulty not only with vocabulary, but with decoding all symbols including gestures, pantomime, and facial expressions. To further complicate his problem, the auditory input that the language-disordered child receives may be distorted, seeming to come through static; or it may seem to occur too quickly for him to discriminate individual words or the sounds of speech.

Imagine the confusion and frustration of being in such communicative isolation and the adverse effects this isolation would have on social, emotional, and intellectual growth. While such severe and pervasive impairment of language is unusual, even mild difficulty can have enormous impact.

Learning Disorders and Language Problems

With this background in mind, it is not surprising that there is increasing recognition of the relationship between many forms of learning disabilities and difficulty with language. Our educational system assumes that children will enter school with well-developed language and that they will continue to acquire new language skills to meet curricular demands (ASHA, 1980). A large vocabulary, ability to follow directions, and ability to express oneself all are important prerequisites for being able to learn. Poor language skill can cause severe interference in academic endeavors, disrupting listening, speaking, reading, and writing. Even subtle impairment of language can have profound adverse impact on school success (Wiig and Semel, 1980). The development of thought and the development of language reciprocate and each feeds upon the other in the growth process. For example, in order to learn about the history of a country, the child must be able to think about (mentally represent) events that occurred in the past, not the immediate perceptual present, and be able to gather this new information verbally either through reading or listening to a teacher. During this process both new vocabulary and new concepts will be acquired laying a foundation for further learning. For a comprehensive discussion of the interdependence of language and learning see Blank et al., (1978).

Developmental Problems

A problem in the development of speech and/or language therefore has impact beyond what is immediately apparent, resulting in problems in almost all spheres of development. Distortions and disruptions in communication between the child and his family, teachers, and peers can result in problems in emotional and social adjustment. These adjustment problems may themselves become the focus of clinical attention when in fact the speech and/or language difficulty is at the root and in need of treatment.

Finally, poor language skill affects the development of thought processes themselves, depriving the child of vital tools for mental organization, memory, representing and thinking about the world to himself, and for gaining information about the past and future.

INCIDENCE OF SPEECH AND LANGUAGE DISORDERS

There are a large number of children who suffer from speech, language, and language-related learning disorders, but exact numbers are difficult to obtain. The most comprehensive information available is from the White House Mid-Century Conference reported in 1952, indicating that about 5% of the total population between ages five and twenty-one demonstrate some form of communication problem (Healey et al., 1981). Without defining exactly what is meant by a language disability, a 1976 report of the Department of Health, Education, and Welfare estimates that approximately 3.5 million children ages four to seventeen years had some degree of language disability (cited in Healey et al., 1981).

NATURE OF CHILDHOOD LANGUAGE DISORDERS

Psycholinguistic Orientation

A major difficulty in discussing childhood language disorders is that there is confusion among professionals regarding the nature of the problem. Reflecting this confusion is the variety of names that have been used as labels. Bloom and Lahey (1978) use the broad term *language disorder* to refer to "any disruption in the learning of a native language" (p. 290) irrespective of the etiology, arguing for the importance of describing the behavior rather than trying to identify a specific diagnostic entity with the limited knowledge we have at this time. Theirs is a psycholinguistic approach to the study of language disorders, focusing on three aspects of language: (1) its form (syntax—the grammar, word order, and tense, for example); (2) its content (semantics—the ideas that are formulated and the words chosen to represent the ideas); and (3) its use (pragmatics—the way language is used, including the rules governing what is "proper" to say and in what circumstances). Deviant language is described as variations from age-expected behavior in any or all the categories of form, content, or use.

Neurological Orientation

Others view the problem of deviant language development from a neurological perspective and focus their diagnostic attention on the underlying processes that may be impaired and therefore interfere with normal language acquisition. Terms such as *childhood aphasia* or *dysphasia* (Myklebust, 1954, McGinnis, 1963) and *developmental aphasia* (Eisenson, 1972) are used to emphasize the similarity between the language acquisition problems of the child and the language problems of the adult aphasic and serve to focus on the overall difficulty with symbolization found in both populations. As knowledge about childhood language problems increases, the use of the term *aphasia* has diminished and is generally reserved to describe loss of language after a period of normal development. Acquired aphasias in children, as in adults, result from left hemisphere lesions (trauma, tumors, cerebral vascular accidents). Lenneberg (1967) reports that acquired aphasias occurring during childhood, up to the early teens, are transient; but the same lesions occurring after age seventeen are irreversible 50% of the time.

The terms *specific language deficit* (Benton, 1965; Stark and Tallal, 1981), *language processing disorder* (Butler, 1981), and *central auditory processing disorder* (Keith, 1981) also stem from the neurological orientation. The focus here is on underlying central auditory processing skills which are thought to be essential for the successful acquisition of language, such as the ability to perceive rapid acoustic transitions in speech (Tallal and Stark, 1980). There is evidence that some children with language disorders do have difficulty with certain auditory tasks which are measured by two types of sophisticated audiological tests. These tests are described in detail by Jerger (1981) and Keith (1981) and include:

1. auditory brainstem evoked response audiometry where click sounds are presented to one ear and the corresponding electric activity is picked up by surface electrodes on the vertex and mastoid and then averaged by computer. Patients with brain stem abnormalities tend to show delayed peak latencies or the absence of certain peak responses.
2. special diagnostic speech audiometry, whereby words and sentences are made difficult to understand by a variety of methods including filtering, time compression, and presence of competing messages. Two test paradigms are currently used. In one, the target message is presented to one ear and the competing message to the opposite ear. This type of test is thought to be sensitive to auditory disorders at the level of the temporal lobe. In the other, the target message is presented to one ear and degraded by either filtering, temporal alterations, or a competing message to the same ear. The degraded message must be transmitted and processed at higher auditory centers. These tests are thought to be particularly sensitive to brain stem lesions.

The clinical value of tests of central auditory processing at this time is questionable; not only do language-disordered and/or learning-disordered children perform poorly on many of the tests, but so too do children with normal language and no learning disabilities (Rees, 1981). Rees summarizes the issue well, stating that "... no one has developed an intelligible account of how these central auditory processing skills, or the lack of them, relate to language acquisition or academic learning.... This area is as yet in a state of experimental exploration" (p. 118).

Medical Advances

More precise information about the nature of language disorders may come from technical advances in the neurological sciences. It is now possible to detect abnormalities in the brain through CAT and PET (position-emission tomography) scans. Regional blood-flow changes and local glucose utilization have been studied and are yielding information about the functional organization of the central nervous system (Ferry, 1981). These diagnostic advances may provide answers regarding the underlying abnormalities in brain function that result in problems of language acquisition.

IDENTIFYING THE LANGUAGE-DISORDERED CHILD

Primary vs. Secondary Language Disorders

While researchers must follow a direction dictated by their hypotheses about the nature of language disorders and thus focus on a particular aspect of the problem (e.g., central auditory processing abilities), the clinician must approach the problem practically, drawing upon available information from a variety of sources to direct his diagnostic procedure. For purposes of planning effective intervention, it is useful to separate those language disorders that occur secondary to some other overriding problem (such as mental retardation) from those that exist primarily independent of other problems. Usually this diagnosis is made by the process of elimination.

Language may fail to develop normally for a number of reasons, the most common of which are (1) hearing impairment, (2) mental retardation, (3) severe emotional disturbance, and (4) severe social deprivation. Any of these problems is serious enough in and of itself to cause difficulty in learning to understand and use language. However, the presence of one of these problems does not preclude the possibility of a coexisting language disorder. Evaluation by an interdisciplinary team is, therefore, necessary to isolate the etiologic and maintaining causes for the speech and language problem and to implement the treatment regimen.

Table 4-1, adapted from Myklebust (1954), summarizes key features of each of the common disorders that result in significant interference with language development.

Diagnosis

The diagnostic process has three primary components: the case history; the examination and observation of the child; and recommendations either for further testing or for treatment.

CASE HISTORY. It is usually best to take the case history without the child present because: (1) the child may be very active, or otherwise demanding of his parents' attention, making conversation difficult; and (2) it is easy for adults to assume that the child who does not communicate normally also does not understand, and there is a tendency to talk about him as if he were not present. It is not possible to evaluate exactly what a child might interpret from a parent interview, but it is likely that he will realize that he is the source of concern and he may greatly misinterpret what he hears.

The history itself should focus on any factors that may have led to central nervous system damage or to impaired hearing sensitivity. Ferry (1981) stresses the importance of

TABLE 4-1.
Language Disorders: History and Findings on Examination

Type of Disorder	History	Audition	Cognition	Social-Emotional	Language
Primary Language Disorder	Delayed language development. May be slow development in other areas as well. May be learning problems. Suggestion of prenatal or perinatal problem causing CNS insult. Any of a variety of prenatal or neonatal high-risk factors.	Normal peripheral sensitivity. Central auditory test battery may show deficits. May be poor auditory perceptual skills. May use hearing inconsistently.	Inconsistent, scattered profile. Performance IQ at or approaching normal. Wide verbal performance gap. May demonstrate visual-perception problems also. Little symbolic play.	Tries to relate, not oblivious or bizarre. May be easily frustrated; dependent on caregivers. Emotional range may be restricted.	Problem in comprehending and/or using language. May be little or no speech. May be little or no ability to follow directions. May use unusual words or phrases. May be grammatical errors which interfere with communication. May be echolalia. Inconsistent ability to say words. Little or no gesture language.
Hearing Impairment	Parents report inconsistent or no response to sound. May hear certain sounds and not others. Exposure to high-risk factors during pregnancy (rubella). Frequent upper respiratory infections. Ototoxic drug exposure. Meningitis.	Audiologic testing shows conductive or sensorineural hearing loss.	Nonverbal intelligence normal (unless other accompanying problems). Scans environment visually; explores using other intact senses. Plays symbolically.	Responsive and alert to others through vision.	May use elaborate gesture system and pantomime depending on age. Watches faces closely for cues. May understand and use some oral language depending on severity of loss. Pronunciation may be very poor, volume unregulated, voice quality poor.

(*continued*)

TABLE 4-1. (continued)

Type of Disorder	History	Audition	Cognition	Social-Emotional	Language
Mental Retardation	General slow development in all areas: motor, social, speech, self-help.	Hearing normal on audiologic testing.	Marked retardation in both verbal and performance IQ.	Commensurate with mental age.	Commensurate with mental age.
Severe Emotional Disturbance (e.g., childhood schizophrenia, autism)	Withdrawn and in own world. Does not make eye contact. Stereotyped, repetitive motor behavior. May have begun to speak and then stopped. Many anxieties.	Hearing normal on audiologic evaluation. Central auditory test battery may show processing problems.	Difficult to test. May perform well on manipulative tasks. Suggestion of good mental ability in some areas of behavior.	Unresponsive to others. May show stereotyped or bizarre, unpredictable behavior.	May be mute. May be echolalic. Language rarely used for communication.

Source: Adapted from Myklebust (1954).
Note: Although these disorders are presented as discrete entities, in clinical experience there is considerable overlapping, and a child may have more than one problem simultaneously.

reviewing: the prenatal period including maternal nutrition, infections, use of drugs; labor, delivery, and perinatal records; problems that would predispose the child to a language disorder such as asphyxia; and postnatal medical problems such as recurrent otitis media or meningitis. A family history of learning or speech problems should also be investigated.

Since hearing loss can easily be mistaken for a language disorder, additional factors suggestive of hearing impairment should be reviewed. Relevant information includes: maternal ingestion of ototoxic drugs, maternal rubella or cytomegalic inclusion disease, RH incompatibility; history of frequent upper respiratory infections, high fevers; failure to wake to noises, or lack of response to some sounds (e.g., the mother's voice, the phone ringing) and good response to other sounds (e.g., the father's voice or a car horn) suggestive of an uneven hearing loss impairing high frequencies more than low frequencies; use of a rich pantomime system by the child for communication (Northern and Downs, 1978; Alexander Graham Bell Association, 1978).

Developmental milestones should be reviewed. Tables 4-2 and 4-3 summarize major milestones in the development of hearing, speech, and language and can be used as a guide to establishing whether the child's behavior in these areas falls within normal limits or is significantly delayed. There are commercially available checklists which can be completed based on the case history, e.g., the Receptive-Expressive Emergent Language Scale (Bzoch and League, 1978) and the Verbal Language Development Scale (Mecham, 1959). Because deficits in speech, hearing, and language are so potentially damaging to social, emotional, and intellectual development, it is best to refer early when there is a delay in development. *Any suspicion at any age* of hearing loss is sufficient cause for immediate referral. A delay of six months or more in meeting speech or language milestones is significant. In either case the starting point should be a referral for an audiological evaluation. If there is no indication of impaired hearing, a referral to a speech and language pathologist is indicated.

In addition to reviewing milestones, it is helpful to ask about the way in which the child and family communicate. Families frequently unconsciously compensate for their child's deficits in language and report for example, that although the child's speech is poor he "understands everything." It is a good idea to observe the child interacting with the family. In the latter instance this observation usually reveals that the family spontaneously use rich body language, maintain visual contact with the child, point and gesture without realizing they are doing so to assist the child in understanding. Conversely, one may observe a situation where no such supports are being offered and there is very little interaction of any kind.

EXAMINATION OF THE CHILD. Having completed a history and observation of parent-child interaction, the next step is to "interview" the child himself. When one is accustomed to establishing rapport by speaking with a child, the nonverbal child presents a unique challenge and formal examination procedures may not be possible. The goal of the evaluation is to obtain a picture of the child's typical speech and language and the conditions under which it varies. In order to do this, it is best to set up a relaxed, play situation with low demands for speech. Although it is tempting to ask the child questions, this generally is ineffective and counterproductive. A play activity with toys that can be manipulated such as a dollhouse and furniture or a garage and cars with accompanying play figures captures the interest of most children. Using these materials, one can begin to assess the child's comprehension of spoken language and his compensatory use of other supporting environmental cues.

For example, the examiner may, after playing quietly for a minute or so, say, "I want to put the daddy in the car. Can you find the car?" The child can respond nonverbally if he has understood the question; if he has not, the examiner can point to the object so that the child can successfully comply with the request. The more successes that can be arranged, the more

TABLE 4-2.
Early Signs of Normal Hearing

Birth-3 months
   Startled by loud sounds
   Soothed by mother's voice

3-6 months
   Localizes source of sounds by turning
   Enjoys sound-making toys
   Imitates own babbling sounds

6-10 months
   Responds to own name
   Demonstrates comprehension of common words (no, bye-bye)

10-15 months
   Points to familiar objects on command
   First word emerges

SOURCE: Alexander Graham Bell Association (1978).

communication the child will offer. The examiner must watch and listen closely to the verbalizations, gestures, direction of visual regard, and facial expressions of the child. All the child's communication attempts may be distorted and difficult to understand, but may still be discernible to the careful observer.

Observations of how the child uses his hearing are important. Are his responses consistent and timely or does there seem to be an unusual delay in response? Does he respond once to a sound and not again? Is he easily distracted auditorially by sounds in the environment? Does he understand speech or are visual supports required? Does he confuse similar-sounding words? *Any* suspicious auditory behavior merits audiological evaluation by a competent pediatric audiologist.

The pattern of the child's communication should also be noted. Does he use his voice to get attention? Is the volume and pitch of voice monitored and appropriate to the situation? Does he use language to communicate? Is his pronunciation intelligible, consistent, and age appropriate? Is his speech fluent or are there unusual pauses? Does he appear to grope for words? If he cannot speak, does he try to communicate by pointing, gesturing, shifting eye gaze? Is he frustrated when you do not understand? If so, how does he behave? Does he withdraw or begin to act out?

With a child who has subtle language problems it is sometimes possible to have the youngster explain what his communication difficulties are. It is worth asking if he has trouble understanding or speaking, and suggesting that he describe the problem to you.

In addition to eliciting information about hearing, speech, and language, the child's behavior in the play situation provides additional information about his nonverbal development. For example, the child may organize the toys into a symbolic, recognizable unit; or he may line them up, perseverating until each toy is perfectly aligned; or he may pick up and mouth the materials. Each form of response must be assessed according to appropriateness for the child's age. For example, mouthing of toys is appropriate in a twelve month old but highly inappropriate for a four year old.

USE OF AN INTERDISCIPLINARY TEAM. Based upon the information obtained from the history and examination, a determination is made of what further testing and treatment are required. A interdisciplinary team may be called upon to complete the assessment. This team

TABLE 4-3.
Speech and Language Milestones

	0–6 Months	6–12 Months
Development of Comprehension	Understands gestures such as outreached arms to be picked up.	Shares direction of gaze with mother. Understands familiar words and short commands.
Development of Speech Sound Production	Babbles repetitively varying speech sounds, pitch, volume.	Imitates sounds of others. "Talks" to self in mirror. First-word approximations ("dada" for daddy). Uses sound playfully.
Development of Vocabulary		5–6 words.
Development of Syntax		Single words only.
Development of Semantics		At preverbal stage may point, gesture, nod. When use of words begins, expresses various meanings through single words (Greenfield and Smith, 1976).

	12–18 Months	18–24 Months
Development of Comprehension	Continues development of ability to understand but comprehension linked closely to the here and now. Points to objects named. Follows a one-step command.	Comprehends about 300 words. Understands most linguistic units but as holophrases not separate words (Berry, 1969). Comprehension continues to be tied to the here and now.
Development of Speech Sound Production	Front consonants beginning to be used with consistency (p, m, w); vowels ah, ee, oo.	Continued growth in ability to approximate words. Simplification processes applied in articulation, giving speech characteristic "baby accent." Pronunciation refinements continue until about age 8 (Ingram, 1976).
Development of Vocabulary	Variable rate of development 6+ words.	50–75 words.

(continued)

89

TABLE 4-3. (continued)

	12–18 Months	18–24 Months
Development of Syntax	Continuation of holophrases; or sequential use of single words.	Begins to combine 2 words to express numerous relationships understood from context such as: 1) existence—e.g., This daddy (meaning, This is a daddy). 2) agent-object—e.g., Daddy car (meaning, Daddy is driving the car). 3) agent-action—e.g., Daddy push (Daddy is pushing my carriage). 4) location—e.g., Daddy chair (Daddy is sitting on the chair). 5) possession—e.g.., My Daddy (This is my Daddy). 6) recurrence—e.g., More Daddy (I want Daddy to come home). 7) negation—e.g., No Daddy (This is not Daddy, it is Uncle Bob). (Bloom and Lahey, 1978)
Development of Semantics	Meaning inferred from contextual cues by the listener from the child's use of single words in a variety of situation.	

	24–36 Months	36–48 Months
Development of Comprehension	Understands 500–900 words. Begins to listen to stories for up to 20 minutes and to enjoy familiar ones. Can identify action in pictures. Identifies familiar objects by use.	Comprehends 1,500–2,000 words.
Development of Speech Sound Production		Consonants *p, m, h, n, w, b* used consistently in words by 90% of all children.
Development of Vocabulary	Uses about 250–450 words.	Rapid growth of vocabulary. Uses 1,000–1,500 words. Can respond to wide range of questions.

	24–36 Months	36–48 Months
Development of Syntax	3–4 word utterances which begin to coordinate earlier relationships into more complex structures. Begins to use inflections such as plural s.	4–6+ word utterances. Grammar becomes increasingly accurate.
Development of Semantics	Can count to 3.	Greater ability to reason using language. Language not as tightly bound to reality. Asks many questions. Can recite nursery rhymes. Names primary colors. Ables to relate a past experience.

	48–60 Months	60–72 Months
Development of Comprehension	Understands about 2,500 words. Can follow 3 commands.	Understands 13,000 words. Can begin to predict. Understands language related to time.
Development of Speech Sound Production	b, k, g, d, t, ng used consistently in words by 90% of all children; f begins to be used.	Speech sounds appearances and initial stabilization of s, sh, ch, y, ng, d used by 90% of all children. The following sounds may develop late and be used by 90% of all children between ages 6 and 8: l, r, sh, ch, v, th, j, s, z, and blends.
Development of Vocabulary	1,500–1,800 words.	2,300 words.
Development of Syntax	Increasing use of compound and complex sentences.	Corrects own grammar. Develops use of relative clauses.
Development of Semantics	Developing ability to use language socially. Can define words. Much pretend play. Tries new words.	Able to retell stories. Concepts of time, number, space, and speed developing. Can categorize likeness and difference. Becomes able to relate past and present.

may include: (1) medical specialists as indicated, such as an otologist, pediatric neurologist, child psychiatrist, etc.; (2) a speech and language pathologist; (3) an audiologist; (4) educational specialists, such as a learning-disabilities specialist, teacher; and (5) a social worker. Each team member makes a unique contribution to the overall picture, but it is extremely important that a team consensus regarding diagnosis and treatment be presented to the family so that they have a cohesive understanding of their child's problems and needs.

AUDIOLOGIST. As has been previously stated, the single most important diagnostic consideration for the child with a speech and/or language problem is to determine if his hearing is normal. A clinical audiologist, preferably an individual with special training in pediatric audiology, is best equipped to make this determination. (The American Speech, Language, and Hearing Association [ASHA] maintains a directory of audiologists and speech and language pathologists who meet their requirements for membership and certification. ASHA certification provides some assurance of the competency of the practitioner particularly in states where there is no licensure.)

There is no need to wait until a child reaches a particular minimum age to make an audiological referral. It is possible to test the hearing of even young infants reliably using a combination of observational and conditioned-response audiological measurements, and tests that do not require active cooperation from the child, such as impedance testing and auditory-evoked responses. (See Northern and Downs, 1978, for a discussion of audiological assessment techniques with children.) Several testing sessions will probably be needed to make an accurate determination of hearing level especially if a hearing loss is suspected. Testing will provide information about the degree and type of hearing loss (e.g., sensorineural, conductive, mixed), and the site of lesion (if any). It will establish etiology and need for medical follow-up, as well as provide recommendations for amplification and any necessary training.

SPEECH AND LANGUAGE PATHOLOGIST. The speech and language pathologist is often the first person contacted by the physician or family of the child with a speech and language problem. The speech and language pathologist (who should be ASHA certified) is trained to identify possible etiologic and maintaining causes for the speech and language problems and to provide an in-depth assessment of the child's current level of language functioning using a combination of behavioral observations and formal tests. Based on this diagnostic assessment, recommendations for further testing (e.g., audiological evaluation) and suggestions for a course of action to remediate the problem (e.g., participation in individual speech and language therapy) will be made. The speech/language pathologist is prepared to devise and implement a treatment program to improve the child's problems in speech and language. Open communication between the referring physician and the pathologist is important. Sometimes physically based problems, such as brief sporadic lapses of consciousness, which are in need of medical management may be observed during the ongoing course of therapy.

The speech and language pathologist also has expertise in identifying *subtle* disorders in language that can interfere with learning. These include word-finding problems, difficulty in understanding and using specific syntactic structures, poor comprehension of lengthy narratives, inability to draw conclusions from verbally presented data, etc. The speech and language pathologist therefore plays a central role in elucidating and treating the problems of the language-disordered child.

MEDICAL SPECIALISTS. Depending upon the presenting symptoms, judicious selection of appropriate medical specialists is indicated. For example, if an underlying hearing impairment is identified through audiological evaluation, an otological consultation is warranted. Similarly the pediatric neurologist can be helpful in evaluating the language-disabled child by: helping to identify etiology; locating areas of the brain involved and degree of involvement; evaluating if the disorder is static or progressive; selecting additional diagnostic tests; prescribing medication when appropriate; and interpreting findings to families (Rapin and Wilson, 1978). However, it may not be possible or practical for all language-disordered children to be seen by a pediatric neurologist. Ferry(1981) suggests the following criteria for referral to a pediatric neurologist:

1. Any acquired language disorder in a previously normal child.
2. The presence of language disorder associated with seizures.
3. Any progressive neurological disorder with associated language impairment.
4. Language disorder with an associated hemiparesis.

PSYCHOLOGIST. The psychologist will identify strengths and weaknesses in the child's intellectual functioning through the administration of a battery of nonverbal and verbal tests. In addition, the psychologist will observe and assess social and emotional development. In interpreting results of psychological testing, it is important to consider verbal and nonverbal (performance) protocols separately. There is usually a disparity between the two when there is a language disorder, and the total IQ score is thereby suppressed and misleading. The information gathered in psychological testing and analysis of the component subtests is of great importance in planning an effective and complete remedial program and is useful in identifying any coexisting factors (e.g., perceptual problems) that could interfere with learning.

EDUCATIONAL SPECIALISTS. With the advent of the Education for All Handicapped Children Act (P.L. 94-142), public schools have become increasingly involved in the diagnosis and planning for children with speech and language problems even during the preschool years. The law specifies an evaluation process for the identification and subsequent classification of handicapped children by a child-study team. Once the child is "classified," an individual educational plan is developed for him through the joint effort of the child-study team, parents, teacher, and if appropriate, the child himself. Unfortunately, the local child-study team may not include an audiologist, speech and language pathologist, or medical specialists (ASHA 1980). It is, therefore, necessary to review classification reports carefully to be sure that complete and accurate information has been gathered. Conversely, useful diagnostic information gathered in assessments occurring outside of the school setting may never reach the people who are directly responsible for helping the child. It is suggested that when an interdisciplinary approach has been used, those educators who will be working directly with the language-disordered child should participate in team discussions. They can offer firsthand information about the various options available to the child within the school (e.g., individual tutoring, special-class placement, resource rooms, etc.), so that a realistic and coordinated treatment and follow-up plan can be developed.

SOCIAL WORKER. The social worker will aid in implementing the treatment plans through management of such problems as transportation difficulties and meeting the cost of the various therapies. Since many language-disordered children have concomitant emotional problems, the social worker will conduct patient and family counseling.

Intervention for Language Disorders

Preschool Years

It is generally agreed that intervention for a language disorder should be begun as early as possible, not only to take advantage of the early plasticity of the central nervous system but also to prevent the development of additional problems which result from the communication difficulty. The optimal starting time is during the period of normal speech and language acquisition—the first three to four years of life.

Enrollment in a program of speech and language therapy is the primary treatment of choice for the child with a language disorder. The age of the child and the severity of the problem will determine the frequency and type of therapy.

PARENT-INFANT PROGRAM. The parent (or other primary caregiver) and infant are seen together on a regular schedule (e.g., once a week for one hour). The therapist demonstrates language-stimulation techniques and serves as a model for the parent who then uses the strategies on a day-to-day basis at home. A structured monitoring process is important to ensure that progress is being made.

INDIVIDUAL SPEECH AND LANGUAGE THERAPY. The child is seen for therapy several times a week in a carefully devised treatment program directed at improving speech and language. The parent is also instructed in methods of reinforcing therapy objectives at home.

GROUP LANGUAGE THERAPY. Several children, usually three to five, who share similar difficulty in language are grouped for training and experience in using language appropriately in a social setting. It is the author's strong clinical bias that group therapy can be used to supplement individual therapy but cannot be substituted for it with preschoolers.

HANDICAPPED CHILDREN. Since the advent of P.L. 94-142, preschool programs for handicapped children have become widely available. It is important to inquire about the qualifications of the staff and the composition of a class before referring a language-disordered child. There may be a variety of disabled children grouped together (including children with severe emotional disturbance, orthopedic handicaps, serious mental retardation, etc.). The staff may not include the regular services of a speech and language pathologist knowledgeable about language disorders. Such an environment is not appropriate for a child with a primary language disorder and may in fact further confuse him. Appropriate preschool programs do exist, but they must be chosen carefully. If possible, a firsthand observation of the setting is suggested.

BALANCING TREATMENT. While great stress has been put on the importance of speech and language therapy for the preschooler, the intervention program must address not only his language needs but must attend to his needs in other areas of development as well (motor, social, emotional, and intellectual). Several therapies may be needed simultaneously and have to be juggled to provide for a balanced overall program. A child may, for example, flourish with individual speech and language therapy alone; or he may need additional therapies for perceptual problems, or a structured introduction to learn how to behave in a group. Regular reassessment is required to ensure that optimal progress is attained.

School-Age Child

When the child reaches school age, it is important to coordinate the efforts of school personnel with those specialists who have been working with him prior to his entry into school. As stated previously, children with problems in language acquisition do subsequently seem to be at risk for other learning problems (Ingram, 1975) and require long-term monitoring and treatment.

A continuum of special services is available within most public schools and it is important to select the most appropriate alternative for language-disordered children. The continuum ranges from placement in a special school to placement in a regular classroom with no special, direct help to the child. Intervening possibilities include: (1) enrollment in a class for children with language disorders or learning disorders; (2) partial enrollment in a special class and partial mainstreaming; (3) enrollment in a regular class with resource room assistance; and (4) enrollment in a regular class with individual or group speech and language therapy. The selection of the most appropriate alternative must be made on an individual basis, and the decision reviewed regularly and altered as the child improves and changes.

The outlook for the language-disordered child is optimistic. Those children who have the benefit of proper treatment beginning as early as possible can make remarkable progress and bring great satisfaction to all who are involved.

REFERENCES

Alexander Graham Bell Association. 1978. Hearing alert.
ASHA. 1980. Language and learning disabilites. Position statement (draft), Ad Hoc Committee on Language Disabilties A.S.H.A., 22:628–636.
Benton, A. L. 1965. Developmental aphasia and brain damage. *Cortex,* 1:40–52.
Berry, M. F. 1969. *Language disorders of children. The bases and diagnoses.* New York: Appleton-Century Crofts.
Blank, M., Rose, S., and Berlin, L. 1978. *The language of learning: The preschool years.* New York: Grune and Stratton.
Bloom, L. 1970. *Language development: Form and function in emerging grammars.* Cambridge, Mass.: MIT Press.
Bloom, L., and Lahey, M. 1978. *Language development and language disorders.* New York: Wiley.
Brown, R. 1973. *A first language: The early stages.* Cambridge, Mass.: Harvard University Press.
Butler, K. G. 1981. Language processing disorders: Factors in diagnosis and remediation. In *Central auditory and language disorders in children,* ed. R. W. Keith. Houston: College-Hill Press.
Bzoch, K. R., and League, R. 1978. *Assessing language skills in infancy.* Baltimore: University Park Press.
Chomsky, N. 1957. *Syntactic structures.* The Hague: Mouton.
Eisenson, J. 1972. *Aphasia in children.* New York: Harper and Row.
Ferry, P. C. 1981. Neurological considerations in children with learning disabilities. In *Central auditory and language disorders in children,* ed. R. W. Keith. Houston: College-Hill Press.
Fourcin, A. J. 1975. Language development in the absence of expressive speech. In *Foundations of language development,* vol. 2, ed. E. H. Lenneberg and E. Lenneberg, pp. 263–268. New York: Academic Press.
Greenfield, P., and Smith, J. 1976. *Communication and the beginnings of semantic structure in one-word speech and beyond.* New York: Academic Press.

Healey, W., Ackerman, B., Chappell, C., Perrin, K., and Stormer, J. 1981. The prevalence of communicative disorders: A review of the literature. Final report 1981 of American Speech-Language-Hearing Association.

Ingram, D. 1976. *Phonological disability in children.* London: Edward Arnold.

Ingram, T. T. S. 1975. Speech disorders in childhood. In *Foundations of language development,* vol. 2, ed. E. H. Lenneberg and E. Lenneberg, pp. 195-261. New York: Academic Press.

Jerger, S. 1981. Evaluation of central auditory function in children. In *Central auditory and language disorders in children,* ed. R. W. Keith. Houston: College-Hill Press.

Keith, R. W., ed. 1981. *Central auditory and language disorders in children.* Houston: College-Hill Press.

Lenneberg, E. H. 1962. Understanding language without ability to speak: a case report. *J. Abnorm. Soc. Psychol.* 65:419-425.

Lenneberg, E. 1967. *Biological foundations of language.* New York: Wiley.

McGinnis, M. 1963. *Aphasic children.* Washington, D.C.: Alexander Graham Bell Association.

Mecham, M. 1959. *Verbal language development scale.* Philadelphia: Educational Publishers.

Myklebust, H. 1954. *Auditory disorders in children: A manual for differential diagnosis.* New York: Grune and Stratton.

Northern, J. L. and Downs, M. P. 1979. *Hearing in children.* Baltimore: Williams and Wilkins.

Rapin, I., and Wilson, B. C. 1978. Children with developmental language disability: Neurologic aspects and assessment. I. In *Developmental dysphasia,* ed. M. A. Wyke. New York: Academic Press.

Rees, N. S. 1981. Saying more than we know: Is auditory processing disorder a meaningful concept? In *Central auditory and language disorders in children,* ed. R. W. Keith. Houston: College-Hill Press.

Sinclair-de-Zwart, H. 1969. Developmental psycholinguistics. In *Studies in cognitive development: Essays in honor of Jean Piaget,* ed. D. Elkind and J. Flavell, pp. 315-336. New York: Oxford University.

Stark, R. E., and Tallal, P. 1981. Selection of children with specific language deficits. *J. Speech Hear. Disor.* 46:114-123.

Tallal, P., and Stark, R. E. 1980. Speech perception of language delayed children. In *Child phonology: Perception,* vol. 2, ed. G. Yenikomshian, C. Ferguson, and J. Kavanaugh. New York: Academic Press.

Travis, L. E., ed. 1971. *Handbook of speech pathology and audiology.* New York: Appleton-Century-Crofts.

Vygotsky, L. 1962. *Thought and language.* Cambridge, Mass.: MIT.

Wiig, E., and Semel, E. 1980. *Language assessment and intervention for the learning disabled.* Columbus, Ohio: Charles E. Merrill.

5

Stammering and Stuttering

BARRY GUITAR

STUTTERING IS A DISORDER OF SPEECH that may appear in a child soon after he or she begins to speak in two- and three-word phrases. The age of onset is generally three years. Symptoms usually begin as repetitions of sounds, words, and/or phrases, and then progress to tense blockages of speech, often accompanied by visible tremors of the lip, tongue, or jaw. In the advanced state, stuttering may be accompanied by fear of speaking and avoidance of social situations. The term *stammering* is used by British authors to designate tense blockages, in contrast to the repetitive form of the symptom which is termed *stuttering*. Conforming with American practice, I will use the term stuttering in referring to all forms of this disorder.

NORMAL CHILDHOOD DYSFLUENCY

In its earliest form, stuttering is not clearly distinguishable from normal childhood dysfluency, although some differences may be discerned. Most normal children go through periods of dysfluency as they learn to speak. When they begin to put words together into phrases, at about two years of age, dysfluencies are common. Word and part-word repetitions are often heard. Interjections such as "uh" and silent pauses are also evident (Bloodstein, 1981). As the normal child reaches his or her fourth, fifth, and sixth years, the dysfluencies diminish in frequency. Moreover, repetitions of syllables and words are not heard as often as repetitions of phrases and sentences (Johnson, 1955). In normally speaking children these dysfluencies occur on less than 3% of the syllables spoken (Floyd and Perkins, 1974).

The author would like to express his appreciation for many helpful editorial suggestions by Dr. Barry Nurcombe, professor and director of child psychiatry, College of Medicine, University of Vermont; Dr. Oliver Bloodstein, professor, Department of Speech Pathology and Audiology, Brooklyn College; and Suzanne Crane, Department of Communication Science and Disorders, University of Vermont.

In addition, normal children are characteristically unaware of their dysfluencies and do not react to them with fear, frustration, or tension.

Developmental Stuttering

Like their normal peers, children who become chronic stutterers show speech dysfluencies as they are learning to speak in phrases and sentences. Some of the dysfluencies of stuttering children, however, may be distinctive. Evidence from retrospective studies suggests there are four major differences between stuttering children and their normal peers:

1. Stuttering children show more frequent dysfluencies. More than 7% of the syllables spoken by stuttering children are dysfluent, compared to less than 3% for normal children (Floyd and Perkins, 1974).
2. Stuttering children often abruptly stop voicing in a repeated syllable, such as in "Mu(stop)-Mu(stop)-Mu(stop) Mommy" (Stromsta, 1965).
3. Stuttering children's dysfluencies tend to be more sound, syllable, and word repetitions rather than the phrase repetitions, pauses, and interjections shown by their normal peers (Johnson, 1959).
4. When stuttering children repeat a sound, syllable, or word, they have more units of repetition than their normal-speaking peers. They may say "Ca-Ca-Ca-Ca-Can I go?" rather than "Ca-Can I go?" (Johnson, 1959).

In general, stuttering children will appear to be more impeded in their speech than normal children. As a result, they soon begin to react to their difficulty by overtensing their speech musculature as if trying to squeeze words out. Vocal tension can be heard, along with pitch rises during both repetitions and prolongations of sounds. At the same time, they may verbalize their frustration and respond with anger or withdrawal to a severe experience of stuttering.

The development of stuttering at this early stage is marked by recurrence and remission. The stuttering child may be struggling severely for months and then go through a period of weeks with mild stuttering or none at all. For most stuttering children, this period of development occurs between two and six years. Approximately 4% of all children go through this stage of real stuttering and about three-fourths of them outgrow it by the time they reach puberty. The 1% who continue to stutter, usually show an increased severity in both behavioral and emotional symptoms as time goes on. The symptoms may worsen gradually or, in some cases, become severe almost overnight. When the stuttering child experiences frustration or disapproval for his stuttering, he responds with increasing effort to speak fluently. This effort leads to frozen articulatory postures, increased facial contortions, associated body movements, and longer and more consistent periods of stuttering. These increases in severity are memorable, punishing experiences. They teach the child to become afraid of talking when dysfluency might occur. Fear of stuttering is added to frustration. Extraneous sounds, pauses, and retrials become evident in the child's speech as he tries to avoid becoming blocked. He commonly uses word substitutions, increasingly avoids particular people, and becomes more and more wary of speaking situations. On top of it all, negative reactions from his listeners convince the stuttering child that his speech is shameful and that he is inadequate as a speaker.

Associated Conditions

Language and Articulation Disorders

Possibly one-quarter of those children who become chronic stutterers are slow in their development of language and articulation (Van Riper, 1971). These children may improperly pronounce sounds, particularly fricatives (*s, z,* etc.) and glides (*r,l*). Their syntax and vocabulary may be immature. These deficits may be a reflection of generally slow development of neural substructures responsible for fluency in speech and language production. Over the years, maturation of the child's nervous system may allow him to catch up in language and articulation. Whether or not the child develops normal fluency may depend on how he reacts to his speech and language problems. If he becomes frustrated with being misunderstood because of his articulation problem, he may hesitate when he speaks. If he has difficulty finding the proper linguistic forms to express his thoughts, he may fill his speech with even more dysfluency than before. If significant adults respond to this extra hesitation with punishment, the child may grow afraid of talking. These emotional reactions to childhood language and articulation disorders may exacerbate any tendency toward dysfluency.

Cluttering

Cluttering is characterized by rapid, often unintelligible speech which seems disorganized. A multitude of fillers (parts of words, repeated syllables, verbalized hesitations, such as "uh" or "um") are thrown into the speech; moreover, the speaker often begins one sentence only to stop it in midstream and begin another. The child who clutters is usually unaware of the problem and is not bothered by it. Clinical researchers such as Van Riper (1971) suggest that the subgroup of stutterers (perhaps 25% of all stutterers) who have language and articulation problems are sometimes clutterers as well. These children begin talking late, demonstrate poor articulation and delayed language, and become stutterers only after a period of fluent, but cluttered speech. At some point, their dysfluencies increase and they become aware of them.

Emotional Problems

Children who stutter will show a range of emotional reactions to the trauma of being unable to speak fluently. Frustration, fear, and shame are common. A few children will respond to the frustration with aggression, hostility, hyperactivity, and overtalkativeness. Some will respond to the fear and shame by avoiding social situations. Most children who stutter, however, will have mild emotional responses to it and will not need special treatment beyond speech therapy.

There are a small number of stuttering children who have serious emotional problems. Somewhat less than 10% of child stutterers have an unusual stuttering pattern that is accompanied by a controlling exploitive personality (Van Riper, 1971). These children might, for example, throw temper tantrums whenever their parents try to leave them with a baby-sitter. Often they become skilled at finding their parents' vulnerabilities and, using these vulnerabilities, they have taught their parents to cater to their immediate needs rather than deal with underlying emotional problems. These children usually begin their stuttering late, after four years of age. They have a consistent monosymptomatic pattern that may be accompanied by symbolic gestures such as biting or sucking. They make little attempt to hide their stuttering and, in fact, show little avoidance of speaking in social situations.

One case we worked with was a four-year-old boy whose father was extremely busy in his business and whose mother was occupied with a new baby. This child's early symptoms included severe facial squeezing in his stuttered moments. Frequently the child would hit himself in the face during a block. Another case we know is an adult stutterer who has repeatedly failed to profit from some of the best stuttering therapy in the country. When he stutters, he glares at his listener as he purses his lips into a sucking gesture and raises his head high, as if to trumpet his affliction.

Etiology

Inheritance

There is evidence that inheritance plays a part in stuttering. The distribution of stuttering universally favors males by a 3.5:1 ratio. Studies of stutterers' families suggest a sex-limited inheritance pattern that may pass on a predisposition to stuttering either via a single gene or the combined effect of several genes (Andrews and Harris, 1964; Kidd and Records, 1979). At least one twin study has shown a significantly higher concordance for stuttering in monozygotic as opposed to dizygotic twins (Howie, 1975).

Interaction with Environment

The environment also plays a significant part in stuttering. The twin study by Howie (1975) disclosed many instances of nonconcordance in identical twins. One might presume, therefore, that the environment was acting differentially on or was experienced differentially by the two members of the twin pair. Moreover, it is not uncommon to find that the children of severe stutterers go through a period of abnormally severe dysfluency while learning to speak. With thoughtful nurturing on the part of the parents, these children often outgrow the dysfluency and have no trace of it as adults (Speech Foundation of America participants, personal communication, 1981).

Etiological Subgroups

Various genetic, congenital, behavioral, and emotional forces may combine in unique ways to produce subgroupings of stutterers with different etiologies, different developmental patterns, and, to a lesser extent, different symptoms. Clinical observations by Van Riper (1971) and empirical investigations (factor analytic, in some cases) by Berlin (1955), Riley and Riley (1980), Liebetrau and Daly (1981), and others suggest that four subtypes of stutterers might be distinguishable: (a) those with motor coordination problems, (b) those for whom an emotional trauma was a precipitating factor and emotional maladjustment is a maintaining factor; (c) those who have difficulty with articulation and language development; (d) those for whom auditory perception and auditory processing are distinctly different from normal.

It has not been established how these various etiological factors could bring about the repetitions, prolongations, and tense articulatory blockages seen in stuttering. One may speculate, however, that for each of these subgroups, the moment of beginning to speak is an event fraught with ambivalence and conflict, a time when sensory-motor processes are difficult to control. As Bloodstein (1981) suggests, this anticipation of difficulty can easily be imagined to lead to breakdown of the smooth processes of speech.

ASSESSMENT

The major aims of assessment are to: (a) determine whether or not the child has a stuttering problem; (b) ascertain the severity of behavioral and emotional concomitants; (c) devise a remediation approach suited to the severity of the stuttering and to the resources of the child and his family. Diagnosis and treatment are carried out in public schools, as well as in hospitals, universities, and private clinics. A major difference between the school setting and the other settings is that parents are consulted initially in the latter but in schools are called in after the child is identified as having a problem by the speech-language pathologist or the teacher. A limitation of the school setting is that parents are not optimally involved in the diagnosis and therapy. The diagnostic procedures I will describe involve the parents fully and are more typically followed in a clinic setting.

Observation of Parent-Child Interaction

Observation can be done informally by noting the interaction of the parent and child in the waiting room. It is preferable, however, to arrange a more formal observation in which the parents and child can be audiotaped and videotaped (with their consent) while they interact. It is important to determine whether the parents' speech is rapid in relation to the expected comprehension level of the child, and whether the child is stressed by the parents' style of interaction (see the section on parent-child interaction treatment).

Interview with Parents

The interview with the parents is conducted with the child out of the room. Care should be taken to allow the parents to express their view of the child's disorder. When they have fully expressed their perspectives on the problem, questions may be asked about the present stuttering symptoms, onset and development of the stuttering, the child's reaction to his or her stuttering, the family's reactions to the stuttering, their assumptions about the cause, and what situations make the stuttering increase and decrease.

In this initial conference the clinician should try to sense whether the parents blame themselves for the stuttering. In this regard, it can be helpful to inform the parents that stuttering is usually the result of multiple, often unknown, factors and that their greatest contribution will be to help muster the forces that promote the growth of fluency. If the clinician is fairly sure at this point that the child's problem is stuttering, he or she should assess the willingness and ability of the parents to change the family environment so that it may increase their child's fluency. This probing of the potential for change is a continuing process that will extend throughout the diagnosis and beyond.

Interview with Child

A complete assessment of a child's stuttering problem may take several sessions and include trial therapy. Initial considerations are to determine whether stuttering really exists and to assess its severity. Observation of the child with the parents plus the parents' description of the stuttering will give the clinician a headstart on this decision. In these two sources and in his or her own interaction with the child, the clinician looks for indications that the child is having excess dysfluency and is aware of it. The clinician also tries to determine if the child is showing signs of struggle, shown either by vocal tension or facial grimacing. Some children may suppress their symptoms and replace them with extraneous sounds and gestures to get difficult words started. More serious problems are characterized by more struggle, more tension, and more avoidance behavior. If it is possible, the initial interview with the child is tape-recorded so that the clinician can later measure the frequency of stuttering and the speech rate (Guitar and Peters, 1980).

A second consideration is assessment of the child's emotional involvement. Again, the parents' description is added to information gathered through observation of the parent-child interaction and in the clinician's own interaction with the child. Evidence of *frustration* may be seen in pitch rises, struggle behavior, and accessory body movements to break free of a moment of stuttering. Excessive talkativeness, inability to sit still, and aggressiveness also denote frustration. Evidence of *fear* may be seen in these speech characteristics: avoidance of words, retrials, pauses, extraneous sounds as starters, and jerky or choppy breathing during speech. A rigid, guarded style of interaction and reluctance to talk and to enter speaking situations may be general behavioral indicators of the fear of stuttering. Evidence of *shame* associated with stuttering may be seen in poor eye contact, especially during and immediately after a stutter, as well as an extreme unwillingness to discuss stuttering or imitate it in trial treatment.

During interaction with the child, the clinician should be alert to accompanying speech and language problems. Typically, voice and articulation problems can be heard in the spontaneous speech of the child. Articulation problems detected in this way should be formally assessed with the Goldman-Fristoe (Goldman and Fristoe, 1969) or another articulation test battery, since a stuttering child may deliberately reduce his or her linguistic output to avoid stuttering. Language ability should be screened via a test such as the Northwestern syntax screening test (Lee, 1969). Hearing should be tested as a matter of course, even though hearing problems are not routinely associated with stuttering. In addition, reading, learning, and intelligence deficits may be detected through discussion with parents and teachers.

If the parent-child interaction is characterized by extreme controlling behavior on the part of the child and the stuttering symtoms fit the pattern of psychogenic stuttering described earlier, further probing of the stuttering symptom is warranted.

Differential diagnosis of psychogenic stuttering can often be made via trial treatment. If psychogenic stuttering is suspected, the slow speech and metronome remediation approaches described in a later section should be tried. If these do not change the symptom, the child should be asked to sing a familiar song along with the clinician. If singing also does not produce fluency, the stuttering is more likely to be psychogenic, particularly when general behavior suggests this. Stuttering of this nature will not yield to typical remediation strategies; referral to a child-guidance clinic is indicated.

Interpretation of Results

The possibility that the child is *normally dysfluent* should first be ruled out. If the child is younger than six, has only occasional repetitions of whole words and phrases, and is not bothered by them, chances are good that he or she is a normally dysfluent child. If the parents are concerned, especially if there is a history of stuttering in the family, the clinician may reassure the parents of the probable normalcy, but suggest that the child be reevaluated in six months or if the dysfluency worsens.

If the problem turns out to be a speech, language, or hearing disorder other than or in addition to stuttering, ensure that appropriate treatment is begun. Results from formal articulation, language, and hearing tests can give a clear indication of a problem. Voice disorders can be detected via careful listening to the quality of the child's voice in spontaneous speech. Often the treatment for stuttering will eliminate an accompanying voice problem.

Interpreting information about the child's stuttering is, in part, a matter of determining where the child is on a severity continuum. The disorder progresses from easy repetitions to repetitions with tension and/or prolongations, and then becomes distinctly more severe when complete blockages appear. As blockages progress, they increase in severity going from very brief silent pauses to longer pauses with evident signs of struggle and tremor. Then, as habits of escape and avoidance are learned, the moments of stuttering become suffused with extraneous sounds and accompanying body movements. Treatment of more severe stuttering may take longer and result in less complete recovery.

Emotional aspects of stuttering—moderate or great amounts of frustration, fear, and/or shame—may not be as likely to benefit from treatments that focus only on behavior. These children may benefit more from approaches that modify emotional responses as well as the stuttering behavior.

The possibility that the stuttering symptom is psychogenic must be considered. If all signs point to this etiology, regular stuttering therapy is not likely to alleviate the problem. Treatment of stuttering may accompany psychotherapy or may be used after psychotherapy, if stuttering remains.

A major consideration in the treatment of children is the influence of the child's home environment. Factors that make speaking more difficult for the child should be identified and eliminated.

If the child's parents are insightful and cooperative, they will be the most important source of help. It is extremely beneficial if the parents can, in the initial interview, suggest sources of speaking pressure on the child. It is even better if they also can, with the clinician's guidance, formulate some tentative plans to reduce these pressures. Parents who can do this much at the beginning will usually work diligently with the clinician over the course of therapy to improve the child's speaking environment. Other parents may be less able or less willing to participate in a program of environmental change. Because of feelings of guilt, helplessness, or other concerns, they may be reluctant to participate in a program of remediation. If the parents show resistance, the clinician should try to determine its source. Negative experiences in the past with counselors or misconceptions about their role may be amenable to change. In many cases parents who are initially resistant will become deeply involved in searching out pressures on the child and finding ways to relieve them. In other cases treatment of the child in the clinic will have to counteract unchanging speaking pressures at home.

TREATMENT

This section will review evidence on the effectiveness of a variety of therapies for stuttering and will make some specific recommendations for practical treatment.

Fluency-Shaping Approaches

Most modern versions of fluency-shaping therapies use programmed learning to instate fluent speech and shape it to take the place of stuttering in the child's everyday environment.

RHYTHMIC SPEECH. There have been few careful studies of rhythmic speech with children. Brady and Brady (1972) used metronome-induced rhythmic speech with young stutterers and reported immediate improvement in their clients, with some relapse over a follow-up period of almost two years. In an analysis of a large number of studies of various stuttering therapies for both children and adults, Andrews, Guitar, and Howie (1980) found twenty-seven studies of rhythmic speech. While the studies generally showed considerable change during treatment, relapse rate was high. Andrews and Ingham (1972) suggest rhythmic speech often results in relapse because the fluency produced by this treatment is so unlike normal speech. This effect may not be so pronounced for younger children. At least one eminent speech pathologist husband-and-wife team used rhythmic speech very successfully with their own severely stuttering daughter (Van Riper and Van Riper, personal communication).

SLOW SPEECH. Studies by Adamczyk (1959) and Ryan and Van Kirk (1974) suggest that teaching the stutterer to become fluent by first using a slow form of speech with prolonged vowels and consonants (prolonged speech) can be effective. These studies of children did not present results of follow-up measures on their subjects. However, the Andrews et al. (1980) metaanalysis of stuttering treatments, referred to earlier, examined forty-seven reports of prolonged speech with children and adults, many of whom did have follow-up, and concluded that this was a particularly effective way to treat stuttering.

CONTROLLED RESPIRATION, AIRFLOW, AND/OR GENTLE ONSET OF PHONATION. This approach is probably effective insofar as it inhibits habitual avoidance and escape responses which block the flow of air and the onset of phonation at the initiation of speech. Although data are not available on the effects of these treatments on children alone, several experimenters have included children in their subject populations. Among these are Azrin and Nunn (1974) who reported on the effectiveness of taking a breath before speaking and Webster (1974, 1975) who reported on the effectiveness of beginning speech with breathy phonation and prolonged syllables. Both reports suggest good immediate effect; Webster's reports noted that 70% retained fluency up to two years after treatment.

DRUG TREATMENTS. The major drug to be used for stuttering children has been haloperidol. The earliest study of haloperidol was conducted by Gattuso and Leocata (1962) on fifty children. They reported complete recovery in 80% after a month's treatment. Other studies, which have included adults as well as children, have shown that haloperidol shows marked improvement in some patients (Tapia, 1969; Prins, Mandelkorn, and Cerf, 1974; Rantala and Petri-Larmi, 1976). Although other drugs have been tried for stuttering, none have been found as powerful in reducing the severity of the symptom as haloperidol. Unfortunately, there are such strong negative side effects from this drug that it appears to be an inappropriate treatment for adults (Andrews and Dozsa, 1977). Whether it is useful for children is not clear.

Attitude/Stuttering Modification Approaches

Attitude/stuttering modification approaches are not easily categorized nor have they been carefully assessed. Their major aims are to reduce environmental (especially communicative) pressures on the child and to build up the child's tolerance for these pressures on his or her speech. These approaches also use techniques that teach the child not to be afraid of a stutter, but instead to relax and utter the word with a minimum of struggle.

PSYCHOTHERAPY. The parents of the stuttering child may receive counseling from the clinician. In this context the parents can learn to ease the environmental pressures on the child. If this results in an accepting home environment, the child's dysfluencies are expected to diminish gradually rather than being compounded by avoidance and escape behaviors.

Play therapy with the child may be used alone or may be accompanied by counseling with the parents. The aim of play therapy is to help the child express emotions freely. This is expected to diminish dysfluency as the child's self-acceptance and security increase. Carryover to the home usually involves gradual participation by the parents in play therapy. Using this approach involving both mother and child, Wyatt and Herzan (1962) reported "marked improvement" with 83% of children two to six years and 63% of children seven to fifteen years. Egolf et al. (1972) reported that parents trained to display acceptance in interactions with their children were able to bring about reductions in frequency and severity of stuttering. These changes were maintained several months after treatment. Guitar et al. (1981) reported in a single case study that an effective and long-lasting treatment of stuttering could be achieved by having parents study videotapes of their interactions with their child over the course of several months. In this case, decreases in the mother's speech rate were correlated with decreases in the child's easy, repetitive stuttering; decreases in the mother's directive, nonaccepting comments were correlated with decreases in the child's tense, struggled stuttering.

DESENSITIZATION. Desensitization begins by creating an environment in which the child is naturally fluent. Into this undemanding environment the therapist gradually introduces more and more pressure, but ensures that the child stays fluent. Through repeated reintroduction and withdrawal of the supposedly disruptive stimuli, the therapist hopes to toughen the child to the sorts of pressures experienced outside the clinic. There do not appear to be reports of systematic evaluation of this approach. Van Riper (1973, chap. 14), however, gives an excellent description of desensitization procedures.

EASIER STUTTERING. This approach is based upon the idea that stuttering is maintained by escape and avoidance behaviors. Treatment focuses on helping the stutterer to unlearn maladaptive behaviors and to learn new ways of speaking that, while they are not stutter-free, are smoother, less struggled, and approximate normal speech in most instances. This less punishing way of stuttering will supposedly reduce the expectation of difficulty. This in turn will provide fewer stimuli for maladaptive ways of talking. Three studies of this approach used with children (Prins, 1970; Prins and Nichols, 1974; Prins, 1976) reported that a little more than half of the children rated themselves much or completely improved six months after the end of treatment. One of the best descriptions of procedures for this approach is by Dell (1979).

Recommended Treatment Plans

The possible courses of treatment derive from information gathered in the diagnostic procedure (see figs. 5-1a and 5-1b).

PSYCHOGENIC STUTTERING. In this case referral is made to a child-guidance or child-psychiatry unit. If stuttering persists after psychotherapy, a prolonged speech program is instituted.

NORMAL DYSFLUENCY. Parents are counseled about normal dysfluency and encouraged to slow their speech rate. Child is rechecked in six months.

BEGINNING OR MILD STUTTERING. In many cases where children show some emotional involvement with their mild stuttering, such as evidence of frustration, fear, and/or shame, parents will want to become involved in the treatment program. For these parents, parent-child interaction therapy as described in Egolf et al. (1972) and Guitar et al. (1981) will be appropriate. Where the parents are not able to be involved in treatment, a program of desensitization (Van Riper, 1973) will be helpful. Desensitization should be designed to build tolerance to the individual child's most devastating internal and external pressures. If either

1. DIAGNOSIS

```
      ┌─────────────────────────────────────┐
      │ a) Observe Parent-Child Interaction │
      │ b) Confer with Parents              │
      │ c) Interact with Child              │
      └─────────────────────────────────────┘
                       │
              Is Problem                              ┌──────────────────────┐
              Normal Dysfluency? ──── Yes ──────────▶ │ Parents Advised      │
                       │                              │ of Normal Dysfluency;│
                       No                             │ Recheck in 6 Mos.    │
                       │                              └──────────────────────┘
              Is Stuttering                           ┌──────────────────────┐
              Purely Psychogenic? ──── Yes ─────────▶ │ Refer to             │
                       │                              │ Psychotherapist      │
                       No                             └──────────────────────┘
                       │
      ┌─────────────────────────────────────────────┐
      │ Make Tentative Assessment of Severity       │
      │ of Behavioral and Emotional                 │
      │ Symptoms. Assess Potential                  │
      │ for Parent Involvement in Treatment.        │
      │ Determine Appropriate Stuttering Therapy.   │
      └─────────────────────────────────────────────┘
```

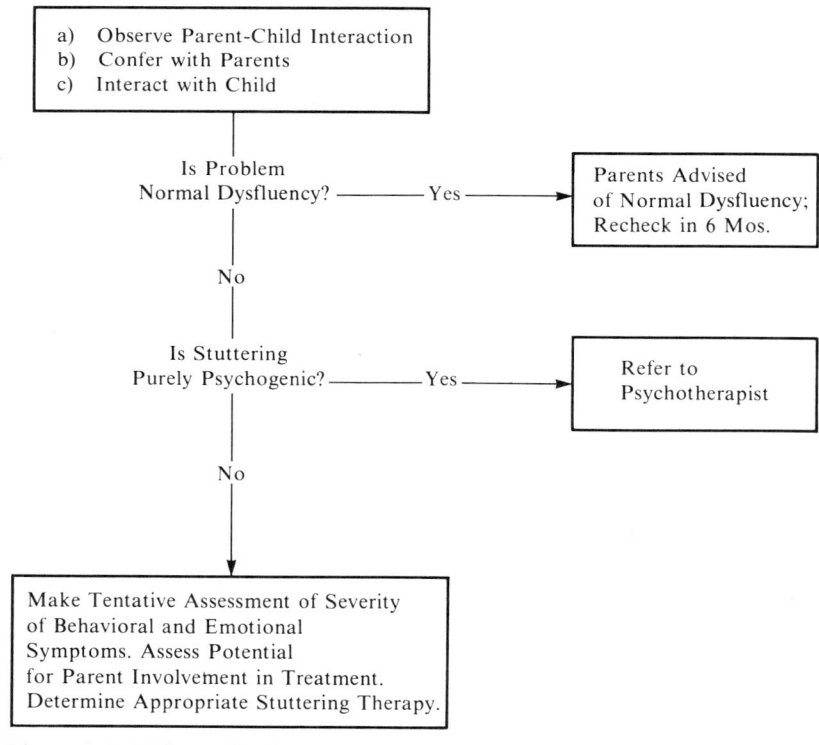

Figure 5.1a Diagnosis of stuttering in child. (*adapted from Dr. Gavin Andrews et al., School of Psychiatry, University of New South Wales, Australia*).

II. TREATMENT

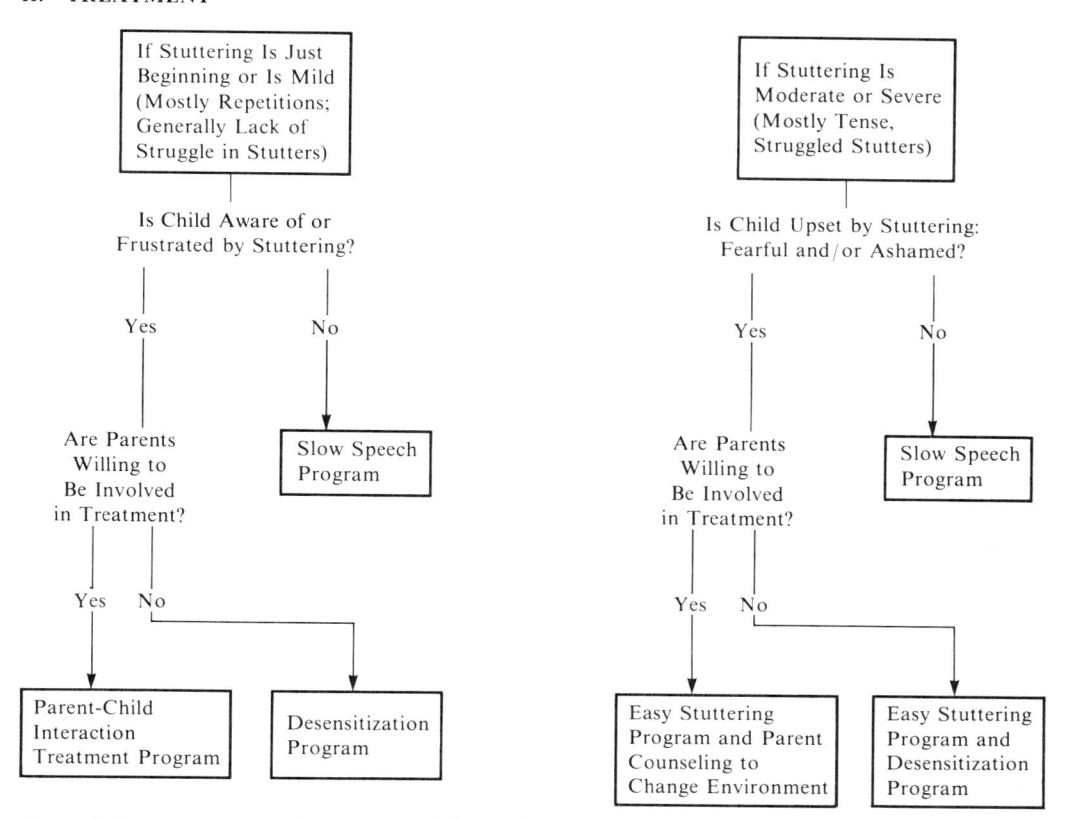

Figure 5.1b. Treatment of stutterng in child. *(adapted from Dr. Gavin Andrews et al., School of Psychiatry, University of New South Wales, Australia).*

the parent-child interaction or the desensitization program does not change the stuttering into normal dysfluency, the therapy should be supplemented by a prolonged speech program (Ryan, 1974; Guitar and Peters, 1980).

If the child shows little or no evidence of frustration, fear, and/or shame the stuttering will often be resolved by a program of prolonged speech. Parents should be involved in the therapy by having them slow their rates of speech at home and by entering fully into transfer and maintenance stages.*

MODERATE TO SEVERE STUTTERING. If there is evidence of more severe symptoms and emotional invovement, the child will need to be desensitized to the stuttering itself. A program of counterconditioning to the moment of stuttering and to the stigma of stuttering will be appropriate. This should be followed by training the child to stutter in an easier, more normally dysfluent fashion. Both components are featured in the approaches of Van Riper (1973, chap. 15) and Dell (1979). Once these treatments are underway, parents should be

---

*Transfer refers to the process of carrying the child's fluency from the clinic into the home setting. Maintenance involves all strategies used to keep fluency levels high in the real word setting.

involved in making the home environment accepting of the easier forms of stuttering. Residual stuttering may be handled by a program of prolonged speech if the stuttering does not become essentially like normal dysfluency.

A few children do not appear to be greatly upset by their moderately severe stuttering. They can be started in a program of prolonged speech which will involve their parents in transfer maintenance. Even the most severe stutterers will lose their symptom immediately if the program is run properly. If this procedure fails to produce results, a more careful analysis of emotional components should be carried out and treatment to remedy these (see earlier) may be needed.

REFERENCES

Adamczyk, B. 1959. [Use of instruments for the production of artificial feedback in the treatment of stuttering]. *Folia Phoniat.,* 11:216–218.

Andrews, G., and Dozsa, M. 1977. Haloperidol and the treatment of stuttering. *J. Fluency Dis.,* 2:217–224.

Andrews, G., Guitar, B., and Howie, P. 1980. Meta-analysis of the effects of stuttering treatment. *J. Speech Hear. Disor.,* 45 (3):287–307.

Andrews, G., and Harris, M. 1964. *The syndrome of stuttering.* Clin. in Dev. Med., no. 17. London: Heineman Spastic Society Medical Education and Information Unit.

Andrews, G., and Ingham, R. 1972. Stuttering: An evaluation of follow-up procedures for syllable-timed speech/token system therapy. *J. Commun. Disor.,* 5:307–319.

Azrin, N. H., and Nunn, R. G. 1974. A rapid method of eliminating stuttering by a regulated breathing approach. *Beh. Res. Ther.,* 12:279–286.

Berlin, A. J. 1955. An exploratory attempt to isolate types of stuttering. *Speech Monogr.,* 22:196–197.

Bloodstein, O. 1981. *A handbook on stuttering.* Chicago: National Easter Seal Society.

Brady, J. P., and Brady, C. N. 1972. Behavior therapy of stuttering. *Folia Phoniat.,* 24:355–359.

Dell, C. 1979. *Treating the school age stutterer: A guide for clinicians.* Memphis: Speech Foundation of America.

Egolf, D., Shames, G., Johnson, P., and Kasprisin-Burelli, A. 1972. The use of parent-child interaction patterns in therapy for young stutterers. *J. Speech Hear. Disor.,* 37:222–232.

Floyd, S., and Perkins, W. H. 1974. Early syllable dysfluency in stutterers and nonstutterers: A preliminary report. *J. Commun. Disor.,* 7:279–282.

Gattuso, R., and Leocata, A. 1962. L'Haloperidol nella terapia della balbuzie. *Clin. ORL,* 14:227–234.

Goldman, R., and Fristoe, M. 1969. *Goldman-Fristoe test of articulation.* Circle Pines, Minn.: American Guidance Service.

Guitar, B., Kopff, H., Kilburg, G., and Conway, P. Nov., 1981. Parent verbal interactions and speech rate: A case study in stuttering. Paper presented at American Speech, Hearing, and Language Association Convention, Los Angeles, Calif.

Guitar, B., and Peters, T. Nov. 1980. *Stuttering: An integration of contemporary therapies.* Memphis: Speech Foundation of America.

Howie, P. 1975. The role of genetic factors in stuttering: A twin study. Doctoral thesis. University of New South Wales, Australia.

Johnson, W. 1955. A study of the onset and development of stuttering. In *Stuttering in children and adults,* ed. W. Johnson, and R. R. Leutenegger. Minneapolis: University of Minn. Press.

Johnson, W. and Associates, *The onset of stuttering.* Minneapolis: University of Minn. Press.

Kidd, K., and Records, M. 1979. Genetic methodologies for the study of speech. In *Neurogenetics,* ed. X. O. Breakfield. New York: Elsevier.

Lee, L. 1969. *Northwestern syntax screening test.* Evanston, Ill.: Northwestern University Press.

Liebetrau, R., and Daly, D. 1981. Auditory processing and perceptual abilities of organic and functional stutterers. *J. Fluency Dis.,* 6:219-231.

Prins, D. 1970. Improvement and regression in stutterers following intensive therapy. *J. Speech Hear. Disor.,* 35:123-135.

Prins, D. 1976. Stutterers' perceptions of therapy improvement and of posttherapy regression: Effects of certain program modifications. *J. Speech Hear. Res.,* 41:452-463.

Prins, D., Mandelkorn, T., and Cerf, A. 1974. Effects of haloperidol upon stuttering. *A.S.H.A.,* 16:508.

Prins, D., and Nichols, A. 1974. Client impressions of the effectiveness of stuttering therapy: A comparison of two programs. *Brit. J. Disor. Commun.,* 9:123-133.

Rantala, S.-L., and Petri-Larmi, M. 1976. Haloperidol (Gerenase) in the treatment of stuttering. *Folia Phoniat.,* 28:354-361.

Riley, G., and Riley, J. 1980. Motoric and linguistic variables among children who stutter: A factor analysis. *J. Speech Hear. Disor.,* 45:504-514.

Ryan, B. P. 1974. *Programmed therapy for stuttering in children and adults.* Springfield, Ill.: C. C. Thomas.

Ryan, B. P., and Van Kirk, B. 1974. The establishment, transfer, and maintenance of fluent speech in 50 stutterers using delayed auditory feedback and operant procedures. *J. Speech Hear. Disor.,* 39:3-10.

Stromsta, C. 1965. A spectrographic study of dysfluencies labelled as stuttering by parents. *De therapia vocis et loquelae,* vol. 1, 13 Congr., Int. Soc. Logoped. Phoniat.

Tapia, F. 1969. Haldol in the treatment of children with tics and stutters—and an incidental finding. *Psychiat. Quart.,* 43:647-649.

Van Riper, C. 1971. *The nature of stuttering.* Englewood Cliffs, N.J.: Prentice-Hall.

Van Riper, C. 1973. *The treatment of stuttering.* Englewood Cliffs, N.J.: Prentice-Hall.

Webster, R. L. 1974. A behavioral analysis of stuttering: Treatment and theory. In *Innovative treatment methods in psychopathology,* ed. K. S. Calhoun, H. E. Adams, and K. M. Mitchell. New York: Wiley.

Webster, R. L. 1975. An operant response shaping program for the establishment of fluency in stutterers. *DSH Abstracts,* 15:136.

Wyatt, G. L., and Herzan, H. M. 1962. Therapy with stuttering children and their mothers. *Am. J. Orthopsych.,* 23:645-659.

6

Psychosocial Management of Short Stature

HEINO F. L. MEYER-BAHLBURG

PATIENTS WITH SHORT STATURE commonly experience chronic stress in relation to three aspects of everyday life: (1) the role of stature in social interactions, (2) stigmatization by deviant appearance, and (3) the physical environment. Infants already react differently to people of various sizes (Brooks and Lewis, 1976; Weinraub and Putney, 1978). Among children and adolescents, height is not only taken as an indicator of chronological age but also of social and cognitive developmental status. In adults height correlates with perceived levels of authority or academic status (Wilson, 1968) and with such success indicators as initial salary after training (Deck, 1968) or attainment of higher positions, even when the influence of social background and formal education has been controlled (Schumacher, 1982). Ethological studies have shown that physical size markedly affects interpersonal spacing, with relatively shorter persons being accorded less personal space than others (Hartnett et al., 1974; Caplan and Goldman, 1981).

Stigmatization by deviant appearance, be it in terms of size, obesity, or somatic deformities, may evoke ambivalence and avoidance in nonstigmatized persons (Richardson, 1976). For short stature in particular, Feldman (1975) has noted the many negative connotations in our language that are associated with the word *short,* for instance, "shortsighted," getting the "short end of the stick," being "short of money," etc. With regard to the physical environment, every severely short individual experiences major physical inconveniences in everyday life: tables and chairs, shelves and appliances, staircases, buses, store counters—all are typically designed for average-sized people and present physical obstacles for the short person.

This chapter is dedicated to William Shields, businessman and community organizer, and to Thomas Aceto, Jr., M.D., pediatric endocrinologist, who together—in developing the Buffalo chapter of the Human Growth Foundation and the Department of Pediatric Endocrinology of the Children's Hospital of Buffalo, New York—set up an exemplary cooperation between a regional tertiary care center and the community at large.

CLASSIFICATION

"Short stature"* is a relative concept. There are no systematic data available regarding at what height relative to the norm people tend to see themselves as "short" or are perceived as such by others. In the pediatric literature, a height of two standard deviations below the mean of the reference population is often taken as an indication for medical screening for a growth disorder. Some adolescents may be worried about short stature although their height falls in the average range; in these cases, it is often the comparison to other tall family members that raises the issue.

A stature of two standard deviations or more below the age norm corresponds to about 2.5% of all children and adults at each age group. This represents approximately six million short-statured persons in the total population of the United States. Most of these constitute normal variations of growth. The number of short-statured people with significant underlying medical disorders is considerably smaller. There is currently no universally accepted classification system for growth disorders. Any current textbook of pediatrics, endocrinology, and particularly pediatric endocrinology will provide overviews of the major forms (e.g., Underwood and Van Wyk, 1981). Some of the more widely used terms are given in table 6.1; the list presented there is not exhaustive nor are all categories mutually exclusive.

Familial short stature is a term traditionally used for short-statured children and adults who come from similarly short-statured families. Some authors (Underwood and Van Wyk, 1981) reject the term as misleading, since "familial" short stature is increasingly found to result from specific nutritional, endocrine, or other conditions. Constitutional growth delay probably represents the largest group of short-statured children. These are basically slow growers that, belatedly, will reach normal height; the condition is often accompanied by delayed puberty. The usefulness of this term is also under debate because a number of such individuals have been identified as having borderline hormonal (or other) abnormalities. In skeletal dysplasias, skeletal proportions and the shape and size of the limbs, trunk, and skull tend to be abnormal—in many cases severely so. More than fifty different forms have been identified. The categories of endocrine disorders, growth disorders related to systemic diseases, and growth disorders associated with chromosome anomalies are self-explanatory. Dysmorphic short stature (nearly identical to such older terms as "primordial dwarfism" and overlapping with "intrauterine dwarfism") consists of numerous syndromes of short stature in association with a variety of associated physical abnormalities; the etiology is poorly understood. Finally, psychosocial short stature (see chap. 17) refers to growth impairment that is induced by an adverse home environment and is often associated with a reversible growth-hormone deficiency and other medical as well as behavioral abnormalities. The mechanism of growth failure in these patients is not yet understood; many seem to belong to the spectrum of child abuse and neglect (Money et al., 1972; Green et al., 1984).

Apart from variations in the severity of the growth deficit, the different categories of growth disorder are associated with specific variations in appearance and somatic functions which may constitute syndrome-specific stressors, both physical and psychosocial. Some syndromes are also accompanied by cognitive and/or behavioral impairments.

---

*The prescientific terms *dwarf* for disproportionate forms and *midget* for proportionate forms of severe short stature should not be used because of their diagnostic ambiguity and their misleading connotations which may be harmful to such patients.

TABLE 6-1.
Diagnostic Categories of Short Stature (Selected)

Familial short stature (hereditary, nutritional)
Constitutional growth delay
Skeletal dysplasias
    achondroplasia
    hypochondroplasia
Growth disorders resulting from endocrine abnormalities
    growth-hormone deficiency — hereditary
                              — secondary to brain tumor or trauma
                              — idiopathic
    growth-hormone resistance
    thyroid-hormone deficiency (cretinism)
    cortisol excess (Cushing's syndrome)
    premature sex-hormone excess (e.g., congenital adrenal hyperplasia; precocious puberty)
Growth disorders related to systemic diseases
    pulmonary disease (asthma, cystic fibrosis)
    congenital heart disease
    malabsorption syndrome
    renal disease
    chronic anemias
Growth disorders associated with chromosome anomalies
    Turner's syndrome (46,XO and related mosaics)
    Down's syndrome
Dysmorphic short stature
    Noonan's syndrome
    Russell-Silver syndrome
Psychosocial short stature

BEHAVIORAL DEVELOPMENT

Physical and Sensory Functions

Short-statured individuals tend to be at a physical disadvantage in body-contact sports and other activities requiring body mass and/or height. Many of the medical syndromes are associated with more specific impairments. For instance, the spine and limb deformities of the skeletal dysplasias may make walking difficult and painful. Pubertal development and the response to sex hormones is impaired in many hypopituitary patients, so that muscle development and physical strength may remain below expectations even if the growth deficit is taken into consideration. Systemic diseases associated with short stature are usually accompanied by impairment of general energy level. Vision is often compromised in patients with pituitary tumors, especially craniopharyngioma; patients with certain skeletal dysplasias are at risk for auditory problems.

Intelligence and Learning

In contrast to common prejudices, intelligence-test studies of the major syndromes show little difference from control samples of norm populations—that is, the vast majority of short-statured patients have no impairment of intellectual function. There are some exceptions, however. Constitutional delay of growth is found with markedly increased frequency in lower socioeconomic strata and particularly in socially disadvantaged families (Lacey and Parkin, 1974; Christiansen et al., 1975; Vimpani et al., 1981). As expected under these circumstances, these children as a group do less well on tests of mental ability and educational attainment than control groups, although one has to stress that the group differences are modest and that the vast majority of these children also have normal intelligence. In children with psychosocial short stature as in other children who suffer from neglect and abuse, intellectual and educational functioning are often drastically impaired; change of the social environment tends to result in marked improvement of mental abilities (Campbell et al., 1982).

Due to their particular body morphology, early motor development is typically delayed in achondroplastic children which in the past has sometimes given rise to the suspicion of mental retardation. However, in the psychometric tests of mental abilities as used in later childhood and adulthood, achondroplastic patients, as well as most of the other forms of skeletal dysplasia, do not differ from controls (Rogers et al., 1979; Todorov et al., 1981). Where the development of brain and/or spinal cord is affected by skeletal deformities, a variety of neurological abnormalities can be found (Yamada et al., 1981), sometimes including impairment of intelligence as in the small minority of achondroplastic patients with hydrocephalus.

Most growth-hormone-deficient patients have normal intellectual functioning (Money et al., 1967; Meyer-Bahlburg et al., 1978), and growth-hormone treatment does not seem to affect intelligence. In hypopituitarism with extensive brain damage due to tumor or other trauma, intellectual functioning may be impaired to varying degrees, although the majority of such children have general IQ scores within the normal range (Clopper et al., 1977; Galatzer et al., 1981). Congenital hypothyroidism, if not treated from early infancy on, is associated with marked intellectual impairment; yet such cases have become rare in the industrialized societies.

In the older medical literature, Turner's syndrome was often described as being associated with mental retardation. This erroneous conclusion was probably based on the initial identification of several Turner's patients in institutions for the mentally retarded. Many Turner's patients have marked but relatively isolated cognitive weaknesses. This is particularly pronounced in the area of spatial perception, which is associated with impairment of spatial orientation in everyday life and with difficulties in geometry and related school subjects. However, overall intelligence is normal (Shaffer, 1962; Money, 1964; Garron, 1977).

A number of rare growth disorders are associated with various degrees of mental retardation, for instance, the so-called cerebral dwarfism (Castells et al., 1974), which may account, at least in part, for the statistical overrepresentation of short-statured children among populations of educationally subnormal or retarded (Vimpani et al., 1981). Note, however, that even in short-stature syndromes associated with a high risk of mental retardation—e.g., Down's syndrome—one sometimes finds individual patients with normal or even superior intellectual functioning. Thus, prognostic counseling must be done with extreme caution in order to prevent self-fulfilling prophecies.

Psychiatric Sequelae

Short stature in childhood and adolescence has predictable effects on everyday interactions with other people which lead to typical forms of long-term adjustment. In interactions with adults, short children tend to evoke behavior that is more appropriate for the level of children of their height age than of their chronological age. Adults tend to baby or infantilize and to overprotect; they are likely to expect and demand less from short children than from their age mates, and these children may learn to evade pressures and demands by acting younger than their chronological age. The overall long-term result may be socialization according to height age rather than chronological age, i.e., social retardation, age-inappropriate dependency on the parents, and lack of age-appropriate assertiveness.

In interaction with peers, especially of the same sex, socialization according to height age also may take place. The probably more important psychopathogenic factor for the short-statured child comes from being at the lowest end of the dominance hierarchy, under constant competitive pressure with little hope for relief. Behaviorally, the most common consequence is withdrawal, either into total isolation from peers (with or without increased interaction with adults) or in the form of preferential interaction with younger children; in the case of boys, one may also see an avoidance of male peers coupled with a (nonromantic) association with girls. These withdrawal syndromes are typically accompanied by a lack of assertiveness and intense inferiority feelings. A number of short-statured persons manage to establish "joking relationships" (Money, 1975) with their peers which in the extreme may propel them into the role of class clown or mascot. A small additional minority develops hyperassertiveness bordering on aggression, probably a form of overcompensation.

Short stature is a highly conspicuous characteristic and presents a stigma of its own. Additional stigmatization may be brought about by other features of individual syndromes such as head and limb deformities in skeletal dysplasias, truncal obesity in hypopituitary dwarfism, or webbed neck in Turner's syndrome. Such features may engender avoidance or outright rejection by both peers and adults. In some cases the physical stigmata may lead to rejection, neglect, and even abuse by the parents themselves, with the typical long-term sequelae not specific to short stature.

Whereas the often associated "cuteness" of the short-statured appearance may lead to a degree of popularity during childhood, avoidance and rejection are much more common peer reactions in adolescence. Severe degrees of isolation, loneliness, depression, coupled with an unusual degree of dependence on the parents are frequent. Both the short stature itself and the often associated delay or lack of pubertal maturation seriously compromise the participation in the heterosocial dating scene which further aggravates the alienation from the peer group. Age-appropriate development of general social, heterosocial, and educational-vocational skills is usually at risk and often impaired; dropping out of school, or later, avoiding employement altogether may be the outcome. This picture tends to be exacerbated when the patient lacks the socioeconomic and/or intellectual capacities that will allow him or her to compensate for some of the immediate effects of being short. Of course, the outcome depends to a large extent on parental attitudes and behavior. It may be quite dismal if the parents have not been able to accept the short-statured child from infancy on, or if they develop marked resentment and rejection at a later age. On the other hand, there is a substantial number of short-statured children, even with severe degrees of growth disorder, who develop quite well and apparently without major psychiatric scars. Parental supportiveness and general stability of the environment (rare, if any, relocations) enhance the chance for a favorable outcome.

This sketch of risks and potential outcomes of the development of short-statured children is based on our own experience with hundreds of such patients and on clinical reports by others, especially Money and his coworkers (e.g., Money, 1975). There are as yet no epidemiologic psychiatric studies of short stature, due to the great variability of short-stature syndromes and the difficulty of finding relatively homogeneous samples in sufficient number.

In spite of the psychosocial difficulties noted, the majority of short patients, even if severely stunted, are employed as adults, in a great variety of careers (Stace and Danks, 1981b,c; Folstein et al., 1981). A significant minority of even the most severely short-statured individuals get married (Money et al., 1980; Stace and Danks, 1981c; Folstein et al., 1981).

To what extent temperament and personality (Money, 1975) or psychosocial and psychiatric status (Holmes et al., 1982) vary between syndromes has not been sufficiently studied. One might expect that psychosocial disadvantages increase with the severity of the growth disorder and its associated stigmata and physical impairment. Yet the medical heterogeneity within a given syndrome, the small sample sizes, the assessment methods chosen, and the lack of comparative studies of adult samples do not permit any general statements at this time.

Direct treatment of their growth disorder is possible for a minority of patients. The psychiatric effects of such treatment, especially of growth-hormone treatment in hypopituitarism, are variable: initial jubilation may be followed by frustration and disappointment with exacerbation of depressive or irritable features (Rotnem et al., 1979), since in most cases the noticeable effects of growth-hormone treatment develop only very gradually, and the end result is highly variable (Burns et al., 1981). Some patients experience a "readjustment syndrome" (Money and Pollitt, 1966), i.e., an ambivalent or frankly negative reaction to catch-up growth that may threaten the special social niche they have become accustomed to. Others enjoy lasting benefits. Where sex-hormone treatment is indicated, especially for the induction of puberty, such treatment seems to be beneficial psychologically (Ehrhardt and Meyer-Bahlburg, 1975; Taipale, 1979). However, when postponed to late adolescence or young adulthood, growth-hormone treatment and/or sex-hormone treatment may come too late to help the patient catch up in social maturation. Also, the endocrinologist may encounter marked reluctance and refusal of treatment by the patient, a variation of the readjustment syndrome.

ASSESSMENT

Because of the chronic effects of short stature on the interaction of the patients with their social environment, every child with a growth disorder should undergo screening for developmental and psychosocial risk factors as well as for psychological problems existing at the time of initial identification. One should not wait until marked maladjustment has developed. Ideally, this type of systematic screening is made a standard component of every growth-disorder clinic.

In this section we will mainly limit the discussion to specific problems of growth disorder; an assessment of these should always be accompanied by general psychiatric screening procedures.

Physical Examination

In the majority of cases, the patients will have had an appropriate medical work-up when they are referred for psychosocial evaluation and management. A number of cases will be sent from schools, other agencies, and sometimes practicing physicians without a thorough medical work-up. It is mandatory that all such cases be referred to growth specialists. Usually, this will be a pediatric endocrinologist, and sometimes other pediatric subspecialists with a particular focus on growth disorders. Since medical knowledge in this area is rapidly advancing, private practitioners who are not working in direct association with a growth-disorder clinic may not be able to render a proper diagnostic examination. As a rule, the growth specialist will refer the patient to additional pediatric specialists, e.g., neurologists, orthopedists, geneticists, etc., as needed. It is mandatory that the mental-health specialist obtain a total overview of all results of the various medical examinations that have bearing on behavioral development and future medical treatments. This will vary from syndrome to syndrome. For instance, in hypopituitarism secondary to pituitary tumors, neurological and ophthalmological examinations will be very important. In skeletal dysplasias, the degree of functional impairment of limbs and joints with its implications for mobility will be of particular interest. In Turner's syndrome, there is a question of additional physical abnormalities, such as webbed neck, that may have important psychosocial consequences. In short stature due to congenital cardiac abnormalities, cardiac function may limit the children's physical activity level and put them at an additional disadvantage with their peers.

Functioning in the Physical Environment

For moderately to severely short-statured patients from preschool age on, a systematic review of the physical home environment should be performed. The patient's functioning in the physical environment should be compared to that of normal-sized children of the same age. Any physical object that does not allow the development of age-appropriate independence should be noted. In most cases this review can easily be performed by the parents or, if old enough, by the patients themselves, especially when provided with an item checklist (see the Physical Environment Checklist, PECL-H, in the Appendix).

A similar review should be performed in school, usually by the teacher, guidance counselor, or school nurse (see the checklist, PECL-S, in the Appendix). Other places where the patient spends much time, such as relatives' homes, clubs, or—for the older adolescent and young adult—the workplace, should be similarly reviewed. Either of the physical environment checklists in the Appendix can be used for those purposes. In addition, it is important to look into problems arising in the use of public and other transportation that might interfere with the age-appropriate development of independent geographical mobility.

Psychiatric Sequelae

Once a patient is known to have a growth disorder, there is a set of predictable problem areas: the discrepancy of apparent and chronological age with the ensuing problems of social perceptions/interactions and self-image; the patient's conspicuousness in the peer group; and the physical/functional impairments associated with certain syndromes. The assessment will aim to identify the severity of these problems and to evaluate the coping by patient and family.

A note on apparent age: apparent age does not only vary with relative height deficit, but also with other features, especially the appearance of the face. For instance, growth-hormone-deficient children and adolescents tend to have younger-looking faces than children with skeletal dysplasias. For two adolescents with equal height deficits, the one with late or no pubertal development tends to look younger than the one who entered puberty at the average age. Clothing and hairstyles of short-statured patients need to be compared to those of their peers. Since it is often difficult to get age-appropriate clothing for small persons, many short-statured children wear the clothes of those who are a number of years younger, which additionally influences the response of the social environment. Parents and patients should be questioned independently about this issue; often, the parents are not aware of what an important and sensitive topic the clothing issue is for their child, especially in teenage years.

Misunderstandings of the medical condition and related misconceptions may have a major influence on both the patient and the parents as well as on their mutual interaction; this area needs to be explored. Physical treatment, where available, presents its own group of psychological issues.

Even if the child is referred because of acute behavioral problems, the assessment usually includes a preventive component, since there are a number of routinely predictable crisis points, such as a change of schools (i.e., facing a new peer group) or medical treatment decisions (e.g., onset of growth-hormone treatment, or continuation of growth-hormone vs. initiation of sex-hormone administration). These crisis points need to be mapped out for future planning of psychosocial intervention.

The psychiatric assessment should include the following major sections:

Medical Aspects
History of the growth problem as experienced by parents and child.
Understanding of the medical condition and associated misconceptions, worries, and fears.
Child's and parents' coping with medical treatment.

Social Aspects
Apparent age of the child.
Everyday skills and independence.
Child-family interaction.
Child-teacher interaction.
Child's interaction with adults outside the home.
Child-peer interactions in neighborhood and school.
Psychosexual development.

Self-Image
A detailed assessment guide is included in the Appendix.

Educational-Vocational Development and Goals

School records should be reviewed at the primary evaluation and periodically thereafter. If there are discrepancies between academic performance and ability level in terms of test results, the situation should be carefully reviewed with patient, parents, and teachers. Apart from the variety of specific learning deficits and emotional problems that may affect short-statured children, emotionally caused performance problems may result from specific short-stature-related harassment and teasing from peers, self-image problems, and the like. In addition, one should always screen for special skills, strengths, and interests that may be fostered to help self-image problems.

In the older child, and especially in the adolescent, the assessment should include a review of educational-vocational goals and interests of both parents and the patient, including what limitations are expected because of short stature. Many of these may be quite exaggerated. Also, the examiner should find out whether the adolescent patient has started having age-appropriate experiences in part-time paid work so that he or she starts acquiring work- and income-related skills, habits, and attitudes.

Psychometric Examination

Unless recent test records are available, we prefer to have a basic intelligence test such as the Wechsler administered as part of our baseline evaluation. This is mandatory for syndromes where specific cognitive weaknesses are likely to occur, as in Turner's syndrome or in children with growth-hormone deficiency due to pituitary tumors. Whenever there are academic performance problems, the standard work-up for such problems, usually involving a battery of achievement tests, should be done.

Summary of Evaluation

Whatever the standard format of evaluation reports may be in a given office or clinic, we recommend that the results of the initial broad-band evaluation be summarized in terms of a very detailed and concrete list of both medical and psychiatric problems followed by problem-specific recommendations. Not only a short-term treatment plan should be developed, but also a tentative long-term plan through late adolescence, listing the most likely crisis and decision points that may involve preventive or therapeutic intervention from pediatric psychiatry, such as predictable changes of school, or probable timing for surgery and hormone treatment where applicable. Both the basic problem list as well as the long-term plan will facilitate the evaluation of the effectiveness of therapeutic work as well as the long-term psychosocial management of these patients especially when there are fluctuations in staff.

PSYCHOSOCIAL MANAGEMENT

The overall goal of the psychosocial management of short-statured patients is an adult individual who is financially self-supportive, is able to pursue a career commensurate with his or her intellectual capacity, functions well socially, and is reasonably happy. Psychosocial management must be geared toward preventing maldevelopments for which short-statured patients are at risk and toward correcting them where they are present. This requires, from early childhood until at least late adolescence, intermittent monitoring—at least annually—of the patient's functioning in all major spheres of everyday life, followed by counseling and therapeutic intervention as necessary. The degree of professional involvement required will vary from family to family, depending on parental skills and children's temperamental makeup. While short-stature conditions call for a specific focus of assessment and intervention, most of the management techniques, in addition to the specific issues dealt with in counseling, are not unique to short-statured patients but are used with many clinical populations. To date, the application and adaptation of such techniques for short-statured patients is justified only by "clinical experience." Because of the great variability of disorders and their associated physical conditions, and because of the chronicity of the risk that short stature presents, it is very difficult to conduct systematic psychiatric treatment studies; none has yet been published.

Physical Examinations and Medical Treatment

The physician should make a conscious effort to interact with the child in an age-appropriate manner, even if the child regresses to an age-inappropriate style, which is particularly likely under the stress of medical examinations. In this fashion, the physician can be a very useful behavioral model for the parents. Nurses, receptionists, and other office and clinic personnel should be instructed and supervised accordingly.

In offices or clinics with relatively large numbers of short-statured patients, the presence of a short-statured staff member can be a bonus for child patients and can provide a useful model of adult functioning. In our experience, paid professionals as well as volunteers can assume this function. However, if the staff member or volunteer has a severe form of short stature, the parents and some adolescents with less severe disorders may need some reassurance as to what they can expect for their own physical development.

Note that most short-statured patients are highly sensitive to seemingly innocuous or harmless jokes and remarks. Physicians and other staff should avoid indications of curiosity and surprise concerning the medical condition and its implications—a problem for which medical students, residents, and new auxiliary staff members especially should be prepared —and should guard against tease words, jokes, and poorly informed remarks about physical characteristics or expectations for the future. For adolescents and adults with severe short stature who have difficulties getting on the examination table, offer a stool or your assistance but do not lift them onto the table except with mutual agreement (Bailey, 1973).

Many patients will need hospitalization for medical work-ups, the initiation of growth-hormone treatment protocols, or surgery. As recommended for pediatric hospitalizations in general, the patient should have adequate preparation for hospital routine and procedures to be performed; arrangements for mother's moving in should be made, especially for younger children and for older children with marked regressive tendencies and separation anxiety. For children with medical-related phobias, for example needle phobias, desensitization procedures should be tried.

Patients in need of long-term medication (especially hormone injections), and their parents, need careful monitoring of compliance, and the help of visiting nurses or school nurses may be required. Early changeover to (supervised) self-treatment by the children themselves —which in some cases may commence well before the teenage years—should be encouraged. Some physicians or nurses will need a reminder that usual drug prescriptions may have to be lowered because of the often dramatically lower weight of short-statured patients.

Particular attention should be given to weight control, especially in patients with skeletal dysplasias where excess weight may aggravate bone deformities and where restrictions of physical mobility decrease energy expenditure. Also, quite a few parents of short-statured children tend to overfeed their children in the vain hope of achieving improved growth.

The physician should be aware of the potential financial pressures the parents of short-statured children may be under and involve the appropriate social worker and/or charitable organization if available.

Medical Education

DIAGNOSIS DURING PREGNANCY. The proliferation of diagnostic methods such as amniocentesis, Xrays, sonograms, etc., leads with increasing frequency to the detection of growth disorders before birth with the implicit option of termination of pregnancy if the diagnostic procedure was done early enough. We are urgently in need of data on parents' reactions and resulting management guidelines. According to the data collected by Stace and Danks (1981a, p. 169), it is likely that such a prenatal diagnosis will cause great distress with need for intense counseling, particularly if it is too late for pregnancy termination.

DIAGNOSIS IN INFANCY. As Stace and Danks (1981a) have found in their extremely useful survey of the reactions and questions of parents of seventy-four children with skeletal dysplasias, there is no single time and mode of counseling to suit all. The majority of parents want to know early or at least as soon as the physician has made the diagnosis of the growth disorder. The diagnosis should include an explanation of the name of the syndrome and of alternate terms, as well as of such outdated terms as *dwarf* or *midget* since the parents are likely to hear or read about them. It is particularly important that the diagnosis be combined with prognostic information. Since this information may have profound and lasting, sometimes very adverse, effects on the parent-child relationship, it is mandatory that the physician carefully plan such diagnostic sessions ahead of time, schedule enough time to allow for parents' questions and discussion, and provide follow-up appointments within a few days. The optimal arrangement is probably an initial joint session with the physician and a well-informed mental-health specialist such as a psychiatric social worker or nurse, child psychologist, or psychiatrist, and subsequent appointments set up with the latter. The accent here has to be on "well-informed." Mental-health workers who do not have the necessary medical and prognostic information about the condition at hand are of only very limited value and may be counterproductive. We recommend separate sessions that give the parents an opportunity to voice their personal fears and worries as well as joint sessions to establish openness and prevent misunderstandings. Additional key family members ought to be involved in counseling.

Detailed prognostic counseling should include: expected growth pattern and adult height; associated medical conditions; etiology (with particular attention to parental guilt feelings and blaming); physical mobility; treatment options (including operations and appliances where appropriate, and the prevention of folk cures such as forced feeding); expected general health and life expectancy; intelligence and educational/vocational future; social and psychosexual development; and the implications for family planning on the part of the parents as well as the child. Prognostic counseling will typically extend over several sessions and parts of it will have to be repeated at future office or clinic visits and be taken up with the child at appropriate stages in his or her development. Pictorial material and simple diagrams should be used as much as possible—e.g., diagrams showing normal and abnormal bone growth, the pituitary as a source of growth hormone, egg and sperm formation, and the occurrence of mutations. We find it beneficial to have the parents and the child repeat to us what we tell them so that we can immediately correct misunderstandings. We also let them report to us what they have learned from other sources such as relatives, friends, books, etc., and counter any misinformation and misconceptions they have acquired elsewhere.

LATER DIAGNOSIS. Many growth disorders do not become apparent before the later preschool years and some only in late childhood or early adolescence. Typically, in such cases the child and his or her family have already developed a habitual way of dealing with the short stature by the time they come to pediatric attention, and the medical work-up needs to be accompanied by a thorough psychologic/psychiatric evaluation as discussed in the assessment section. Both prognostic counseling and psychosocial intervention, if necessary, need to go hand in hand.

Where growth-hormone treatment is possible as in hypopituitarism or where treatment with weak androgens such as oxandrolone is beneficial as for instance in Turner's syndrome, the physician should try to keep the expectations of parent and child on a realistic level.

Physical Environment

The goal in terms of physical environment is to assure that the short-statured child develop age-appropriate autonomy, avoid an undue restriction of physical activities and geographical range, and be prepared from early on to develop self-help tactics in coping with a physically inadequate environment inside and outside the home. On the basis of the earlier review of the physical environment, concrete suggestions can be made on how to improve the situation. In the home, sturdy boxes, stools, and stepladders may be placed in various locations. Cords may be attached to switches, or switches may be relocated. There are attachments to closet rods; or lower rods can be built in.

The school has to provide a desk and chair arrangement so that the child's legs get support and do not dangle, which may cause fatigue and pain. Frequently, special arrangements have to be made for a severely short child to use certain water fountains and toilets, which usually are not accessible to his or her classmates. If climbing stairs is a big problem, the exceptional use of an elevator or the assignment to a classroom on the first floor may be indicated. If a severely short-statured child is being enrolled in a new school, we recommend taking care of this environmental planning ahead of time. We like the child to visit the school beforehand. The school personnel can then conduct a review of the physical environment with the child to make the necessary arrangements and to familiarize the child with them. By doing so the child and the school staff will know how to handle the physical problems and can concentrate on the social ones when the child meets the other students. In particularly severe cases of skeletal dysplasia, it may be advisable to select a school that is (1) small enough to minimize walking, and (2) has most, if not all, classes on the ground floor. Special efforts may have to be made to assist the child in carrying books between classes (Bailey, 1973).

Quite a few parents want to spare their son or daughter the discomfort of using school buses or other public transportation and resort to driving the child to school and other places, or otherwise keeping them around the home. Unfortunately, such arrangements may train the child in undue dependence. Since keeping up with other children's geographical ranges may be a problem for severely short-statured children, especially with skeletal dysplasias, the use of adequately sized (or adjusted) bikes is recommended. With proper training in traffic rules, the bike may provide sufficient access to a wide range of locations. The use of school buses and other public transportation, especially on routes that the child or adolescent is going to use regularly, may take some extra practice and sometimes a talk with the bus driver, etc. After age sixteen, driving a car becomes an issue. A number of models can now be equipped with orthopedic appliances in such a way that they can be driven by most severely short-statured people.

There are many physical features of the environment that cannot be changed or accommodated, especially counters in shops and restaurants, shelves in supermarkets, and the like. To prevent the development of a habit of avoidance, the child should be encouraged to use persistence and assertiveness in finding solutions and/or get the staff to assist if necessary. Also, telescoping metal devices are available to enable one to do such things as reach items on high shelves, insert money into and dial pay phones, and press buttons in elevators (Bailey, 1973).

Psychiatric Sequelae

APPARENT AGE. Along with a thorough instruction about the psychosocial risks of short stature and the goals of the intervention, the parents need to be made aware of any discrepancies of their child's apparent age from his or her chronological age, especially with regard to characteristics that can be changed, such as clothing. To deal with the clothing problems of short-statured children, there is always the temptation to stick with clothes and shoes designed for much younger children. Because of the social consequences, we strongly recommend that the parents make all attempts to provide age-appropriate attire. This may require tailor-made clothing or self-tailoring. In some big cities there are stores available that specifically cater to moderately short-statured people. Occasionally, tailor-made apparel can be directly ordered from factories in other countries such as Hong Kong or Taiwan. Concerning the special effort or increased expenses required, parents should keep in mind that it is better to have somewhat fewer but age-appropriate pieces of clothing available than plenty of age-inappropriate outfits. Age-appropriate clothing, hairstyle, and facial makeup are particularly important to adolescents with short stature, and they might find it useful to learn how to make their own clothes. Girls with delay or failure of puberty may consider the use of padded bras.

Parents of severely short children should be made conscious of the fact that the wear of clothing is increased because of the need to slide in and out of normal-sized chairs, etc. In patients with deformed feet, shoe wear will be excessive. Special shoes may be necessary to provide comfort and increase the weight-bearing surface of the feet (Bailey, 1973).

EVERYDAY SKILLS AND INDEPENDENCE. A detailed discussion of items on the Vineland Social Maturity Scale (or a similar instrument) that show the child has fallen behind his or her age group will allow those areas where the delay is directly due to the physical condition (for instance, the difficulty many young children with skeletal dysplasias have in buttoning their clothes) to be separated from those that are due to inadequate training or unnecessary restrictions. Instructive and supportive counseling in association with itemized diaries for monitoring and/or straightforward behavior-modification programs may be appropriate.

Many children with skeletal dysplasias will have problems with the early milestones, for instance with head control (especially in achondroplasia), with locomotion because of disproportionate limbs and/or hypotonia, and with object manipulation because of short fingers (Stace and Danks, 1981b). Parents need to be instructed that these delays are unrelated to the development of intelligence. They need to learn that toilet training with these kinds of handicaps will be more difficult than usual and that they need to be more tolerant of accidents. Teaching children to wipe their bottoms by reaching a hand between their legs (front to back for the girls) will be helpful (Stace and Danks, 1981b). To facilitate dressing, the parents should choose garments that open right through at the front, with buckles (clips) or zippers with large rings, rather than buttons. A shoulder opening may help getting clothes over the head. Shoes that are buckled or elasticized rather than laced also help these children to manage earlier on their own (Stace and Danks, 1981b).

CHILD-FAMILY INTERACTIONS. Many parents and other caretakers are not aware to what extent they contribute to the social retardation of their short-statured child. They should be guided into comparing their own style of verbal and nonverbal communication with their child, their expectations and demands, to what is typical of average-sized children in their environment—be it relatives, neighbors, or schoolchildren. Sometimes, seeing themselves in interaction with their child on videotape is very instructive. The parents should set as their own goal to have their short-statured child undergo the normal experiences and pressures of childhood and adolescence as much as possible. Parents and patients may need help with many other items listed in the assessment guide. Techniques will involve instructive and supportive counseling, family-therapy sessions, behavior-modification programs, as well as individual therapy for parents (especially those with major problems in accepting their child) and for the patients themselves.

In the case of children with the initial psychosocial evaluation performed at the toddler stage or later, we recommend giving the parents an appropriately modified problem list with management recommendations that they can make use of at home. This is particularly important in parents with limited access to professional counseling.

Where parental rejection leads to child neglect and abuse, placement of the child needs to be considered (see chap. 17).

CHILD-TEACHER INTERACTION. In all cases of severe short stature and in many of the milder ones, it will be necessary to have repeated contacts with the key teachers and counselors in school to prevent the teacher's-pet syndrome or an undue relaxation of expectations and demands. Most of the school contacts can be restricted to brief instructive and supportive counseling over the phone. In many cases this will include some limited medical education. A written problem-based list of recommendations is often helpful to the school.

CHILD'S INTERACTION WITH ADULTS OUTSIDE THE HOME. Many short-statured patients as well as their parents develop a habit of avoidance of contact with strangers which may unduly restrict the range of social mobility to stores and facilities in the immediate neighborhood. To prevent and/or overcome such maladjustive habits, assertiveness training may be needed. This starts with encouragement and practice in speaking up in order to be noticed in stores and offices with high counters, etc., and with the simple straightforward technique of "announcing one's purpose" (Drash, 1969), an act that is very difficult for many patients and/or parents. For example, "This is my daughter. She is fourteen and has a growth problem. We would like to see some clothes that are appropriate for her age level" (or for the patient: "I am fourteen . . ."). Patients and parents need to learn how to respond to curious questions and remarks with some ready answers and simple plain statements of facts, and how to counter offensive comments. Drash (1969) gives many examples. Some degree of behavioral rehearsal in the office with subsequent monitoring by diary may be indicated. The older adolescent with short stature should be encouraged to carry an ID card.

CHILD-PEER INTERACTIONS. The child that grows up in a stable neighborhood of a village or small town will encounter relatively fewer problems with peers. City environments and especially moves to new locations with new peer groups tend to make for difficult times of adjustment. Parents should make every attempt to overcome these difficulties by inviting children from the neighborhood, and by plainly stating the growth problem and giving simple explanations to both other parents and other children. The older child and adolescent should be encouraged and, if necessary, trained to do so on his or her own. Entering kindergarten or first grade typically presents a problem only for very severely short-statured children but later changes of school are difficult for less stigmatized ones as well. A consultation with the teacher as well as a preparatory talk with the class—in absence of the short child—about medical and social aspects of short stature (with particular attention to typical misconceptions) will facilitate the adjustment process. School transfer of the short child along with friends from the old school can be of great help.

In our experience, peer relationships represent the most difficult adjustment task for the majority of short-statured children, and prolonged therapy is most frequently needed in this area. For children that have withdrawn from their peers to younger age groups or into isolation, a variety of techniques is available. A plan needs to be developed with the parents that involves a review of interests and skills of the patient that he or she could share—and compete in—with other children, a review of appropriate potential playmates in the neighborhood and school, and a review of organized social activities like youth clubs, etc., that are available and accessible. A systematic gradual increase in peer activities through invitations to the home and through extracurricular programs can then be established.

For children who are very shy or particularly deficient in peer-relationship skills, we have found activity therapy groups to be very useful. Such activity groups need not be restricted to short-statured children but should be limited in the age range. The activity-group sessions typically constitute a mixture of physical activities, game playing, and/or art activities, with talk sessions. Particularly useful are weekly reports of typical difficulties the patients encountered with their peers. The other children in the group are asked for suggestions on how to cope with the difficulties, followed by modeling (by other children and/or the counselor) and behavior rehearsal by the patients themselves. The procedure may be combined with "social" homework assignments. A variety of similar behaviorally oriented treatment programs involving social-skills training for withdrawn and socially unskilled children have been described in recent years (e.g., Ollendick and Cerny, 1981).

The ubiquitous name calling and teasing that short-statured children experience requires special forms of assertiveness training, since the frequent parental recommendation of "just ignore it" is ineffective and tends to increase inferiority feelings and withdrawal on the part of the child. Simple straightforward statements, such as "I have a medical growth problem and it makes me feel bad if you call me such-and-such name," can be helpful at times, but often "reteasing" is necessary to make another child stop (Drash, 1969). In reteasing, the child picks an assumed or visible characteristic of the teasing child (e.g., obesity) and uses this for a counter comment. Typically, such reteasing by a short-statured child will not lead to physical retribution, especially when done in the presence of other peers. Where physical harassment occurs (usually independent of the reteasing technique), an intervention by parents, teachers, or other adults is often necessary. Many short-statured children are able to draw physical protection from coalitions within their own peer group; sometimes, the teacher will assign one or two leaders or strong boys from the peer group to look after a short-statured child.

To increase self-confidence and self-esteem along with physical skills, we like to enroll all short-statured children in karate or similar programs unless there are medical contraindications. Both parents and the school need to foster and encourage specific physical skills and other activities in which the child can compensate for those peer activities in which he or she cannot participate. In particular, there are many types of sports other than body-contact sports that are not dependent on size and weight—for instance, archery, boating, bowling, cycling, diving, fishing, golf, gymnastics, skate boarding, skating, skiing, sledding, and swimming (Phifer, 1979).

PSYCHOSEXUAL DEVELOPMENT. Adolescents and adults, especially males, with severe degrees of short stature usually have a quite limited field of potential mates to select from. Self-help groups as the Human Growth Foundation and the Little People of America provide important opportunities to meet potential marriage partners at their social conventions.

For patients with mild degrees of short stature, shyness and lack of general social skills tend to be a larger problem than the availability of partners. In such adolescents, coed group therapy including behavioral rehearsals of dating skills can be particularly useful.

Some short-statured patients will need some instructive counseling concerning attractive dressing, hairstyles, and use of cosmetics, especially those that also have delayed puberty or failure of puberty and were not part of the early adolescent scene with its informal but ubiquitous rehearsal of heterosocial interactions in all its aspects.

In patients with hereditary forms of short stature, genetic counseling needs to be included. Women with achondroplasia and other forms of skeletal dysplasia must be informed about the necessity of cesarean sections if they plan to bear children.

HORMONAL INDUCTION OF PUBERTY AND SEXUALITY. In syndromes with pubertal delay, e.g., constitutional short stature or isolated growth-hormone deficiency, and with pubertal failure such as Turner's syndrome, puberty may be accelerated or induced by sex-hormone treatment. The few clinical studies available (Taipale, 1979) support a general policy of inducing puberty at the time when the majority of the child's peers go through sexual maturation even though there may be a slight risk of a minor loss of final height. Also, a very recent double-blind study of short-term low-level testosterone treatment of boys with constitutional delay in the early adolescent years (Rosenfeld et al., 1982) has shown very positive social effects in treated as compared to control patients.

Hypopituitary patients with deficiency of both growth hormone and luteinizing hormone (LH) show only a modest feminizing or masculinizing response to sex-hormone treatment (Zachmann and Prader, 1970; Pertzelan et al., 1982) paired with generally low or absent romantic and erotic interests (Money et al., 1980). Recent pilot studies (MacGillivray et al., 1981; Clopper et al., 1981) have indicated promising improvements of the somatic response when sex-hormone treatment is combined with hCG and Pergonal.

A number of short-statured patients, such as females with Turner's syndrome and males with hypopituitarism, are likely to be infertile. The notion of alternate ways of parenthood, such as by adoption or artificial fertilization, should be introduced on the low elementary-school level so that such notions can be built into childhood play rehearsal, and should be stepwise enlarged upon as the child's cognitive development progresses. As a rule, absolute sterility should not be flatly predicted because there are individual cases of Turner's syndrome or hypopituitarism that have proven fertile, and current progress in medical research makes it likely that the percentage of such patients will be increased in the future. Information on alternate forms of parenthood can easily be combined with appropriate sex education; Money (1968) has provided very useful pictorial and narrative material for this purpose. Sex education is particularly important when sex-hormone treatment is begun. Also, the adolescent patient and his or her parents should be part of the decision process of the timing of sex-hormone treatment. In older patients under hormone treatment, very specific counseling has to address the influence of hormones and treatment regimens on sexual libido and sexual functioning in coitus.

Educational-Vocational Development and Goals

Academic problems due to developmental disorders, specific learning disabilities, or nonspecific emotional problems need to be dealt with as in other child psychiatric patients. Short-stature-specific emotional problems are usually taken care of by managing the social problems as described previously.

Decisions to delay school entry or to repeat kindergarten or later grades are all too often based on the short stature of a patient. However, in moderate or severe short stature, the psychologically insignificant benefit from a slight decrease of the height discrepancy between the patient and his or her peers is gained at the cost of an additional year in school and social retardation. Only if academic standing and psychometric testing indicate marked developmental delays and if there are no other remedial options should delay of school entry or repeating a grade be considered. Where "immature" social behavior is a problem, inappropriate socialization by parents or other caretakers (and sometimes by teachers) needs to be ruled out or corrected before the immaturity is taken as a sign of generalized developmental delay.

Special skills, strengths, and interests of a short-statured child should be supported; they may compensate for some of the short-stature-related problems, raise the patient's standing in the eyes of his or her peers, and improve the self-image. They also may prepare the child for career decisions.

A crucial area of short-stature management of adolescents is the preparation for the work world. Here, the educational-vocational counselor has a function of major importance. Both the parents' and the patient's perspective of the wide range of opportunities available needs to be broadened. As early as possible, the adolescent patient should be encouraged to seek age-appropriate job opportunities. This may require some specific assistance from the educational-vocational counselor in terms of contacting prospective employers before the patient goes out for job interviews. Many employers reject moderately to severe short-statured people on first sight because of prejudices, or because they may think the adolescent patient has not reached the minimum required age. If such disappointing experiences are not countered by parental understanding, support, and persistent encouragement to try again, the adolescent patient may easily acquire an attitude of avoidance and resignation. In the older adolescent and adult who is generally discouraged or resigned, or may have totally dropped out of the job search, behavioral rehearsal of job interviews in the office can be of considerable help.

The educational-vocational counselor may be able to establish a network of employers who are attuned to or familiarized with the problems of short-statured patients and are regularly hiring such adolescents or young adults for part-time or full-time jobs. Sometimes, it is even possible to develop a program of educational or job-training stipends for short-statured patients, as was done in Buffalo in cooperation with the local chapter of the Human Growth Foundation. The educational-vocational counselor is also the important resource person for planning the educational-vocational careers beyond high school. Due to the limitations in size and physical strength, many unskilled jobs will not be available to short-statured people.

Self-Help Organizations

The Human Growth Foundation (HGF) originally was established as an organization of parents of short-statured children. The HGF has chapters around the country and has played a major role in the collection of human pituitary glands for the extraction of human growth hormone. Little People of America (LPA) is a nationwide organization limited to severely short-statured people (below 4'10"), mainly adults. Average-sized parents may become part of the Parents' Auxiliary. Both organizations have local or regional as well as national meetings. They provide opportunities to meet fellow human beings and potential marriage partners who have to cope with similar medical conditions, and these groups supply a tremendous amount of valuable information on solutions to everyday living and employment problems. LPA even provides special help to those members who want to adopt severely short-statured children.

Members of these organizations usually report obtaining great benefits from their membership and participation at meetings, so that we recommend strongly that patients and/or their parents join these organizations if local chapters are available. It is important to note, however, that many parents and quite a few patients need to overcome a psychological barrier in meeting other people like themselves or identifying themselves with one of these organizations, and some never return after they have been introduced (Weinberg, 1968; Ablon, 1981; Stace and Danks, 1981b,c).

Useful Literature

HGF distributes booklets on various growth disorders written for the lay person. LPA distributes an extremely useful handbook to members only. An excellent book for both parents and older patients is Kate G. Phifer's book *Growing Up Small* written from the personal experience of the (moderately) short-statured author.

THE MANAGEMENT TEAM

To be effective, the psychosocial management of any chronic physical handicap that does not require institutionalization has to meet a number of criteria. The service should be available where a relatively large number of such patients go for medical treatment, that is—in the case of growth disorders—usually a hospital with a pediatric endocrine clinic. Medical and psychosocial management should be closely associated. The psychosocial service should be available on a long-term basis in order to help the patients master the developmental crises as they come along. Its orientation should include prevention. Preparing the patient and his or her social environment for potential difficulties usually takes less effort than correcting maladaptive habits and attitudes later. Prevention requires a built-in outreach system, since most parents tend to come on their own only after things have gone wrong. Finally, the psychosocial management program should carry patients through adolescence until they are securely anchored in a career that is appropriate for their intellectual and physical potential; consequently, educational-vocational counseling must be part of the program.

The pediatric endocrine clinic coordinates all medical and financial services involved in the case of a given growth-disordered patient, and thus its staff should include medical social workers. The psychosocial liaison service coordinates all mental-health and educational-vocational services involved. Its major tasks are (1) psychosocial-psychiatric evaluation; (2) psychometric testing; (3) medical and sex education; (4) psychosocial-psychiatric counseling and therapy; (5) educational-vocational evaluation and counseling. Various combinations of the different mental-health professions can perform these tasks. Concerning functions (1), (3), and (4), they are not the place for dogmatic analysts, nor for psychologists who primarily rely on personality questionnaires or projective techniques. Important in these areas are: common sense; sensitivity to and experience with the specific psychosocial problems of short-stature; a good understanding of the medical issues; experience in counseling and a variety of therapeutic skills including behavioral, dynamic, and group/family techniques; experience in dealing with sexual issues; ability to communicate with both medical and nonmedical professionals and with schools. As is typical of pediatric-psychosocial liaison work in general, a high level of effectiveness is reached only if the staff can specialize—to some degree—on selected medical disorders.

The effectiveness of the psychosocial service can be greatly enhanced when it is complemented by local chapters of HGF and/or LPA. Their major function is twofold: (1) providing a network of mutual support and help for short-statured persons and their families; (2) establishing a liaison between the professional services and the community at large which may generate the political and financial support necessary to conduct public-information campaigns, find appropriate jobs, and make specialized professional services available to financially needy patients.

Thanks for clinical experience are due to the hundreds of growth-disordered patients who were evaluated and treated at the Program of Psychoendocrinology which the author codirected (together with Anke A. Ehrhardt, Ph.D.) at the Children's Hospital of Buffalo, New York, from 1970 through 1977. Many of the unit's staff members contributed to the development of our clinical work, especially Joel A. Feinman, B. A., Peter H. Lebenbaum, M.A., Marie E. Hassett, B.A., and Elizabeth A. McCauley, Ph.D., who experimented with our group-therapy approach. Marian F. Goodman, M.Ed., was the model educational-vocational counselor. This work would not have been possible without the encouragement and support of the pediatric endocrinologists, Drs. Thomas Aceto, Jr., Margaret H. MacGillivray, and, later, Mary L. Voorhess. A considerable portion of the clinical and research work of the unit was funded by a grant from the Variety Club of Buffalo, Tent No. 7, and the Human Growth Foundation of Western New York (1970–77). The continuation of the clinical work at the Psychoendocrinology Clinic, Department of Pediatric Psychiatry, Columbia-Presbyterian Medical Center, New York City, provided the basis for the methods contained in the Appendix.

REFERENCES

Ablon, J. 1981. Dwarfism and social identity: Self-help group participation. *Soc. Science Med.,* 15B:25–30.

Bailey, J. A. 1973. Psychosocial aspects of short stature. In *Disproportionate short stature: Diagnosis and management.* Philadelphia: W.B. Saunders, pp. 30–35.

Brooks, J., and Lewis, M. 1976. Infants' responses to strangers: Midget, adult, and child. *Child Dev.,* 47:323–332.

Burns, E. C., Tanner, J. M., Preece, M. A., and Cameron, N. 1981. Final height and pubertal development in 55 children with idiopathic growth hormone deficiency, treated for between 2 and 15 years with human growth hormone. *Eur. J. Ped.,* 137:155–164.

Campbell, M., Greeen, W. H., Caplan, R., and David, R. 1982. Psychiatry and endocrinology in children: Early infantile autism and psychosocial dwarfism. In *Handbook of psychiatry and endocrinology,* ed. P. J. V. Beumont and G. D. Burrows, pp. 15–62. Amsterdam, New York, Oxford: Elsevier Biomedical Press.

Caplan, M. E., and Goldman, M. 1981. Personal space violations as a function of height. *J. Soc. Psychol.,* 114:167–172.

Castells, S., Voeller, K. K., Vinas, C., and Lu, C. 1974. Cerebral dwarfism: Association of brain dysfunction with growth retardation. *J. Ped.,* 85:36–42.

Christiansen, N., Mora, J. O., and Herrera, M. G. 1975. Family social characteristics related to physical growth of young children. *Brit. J. Prev. Soc. Med.,* 29:121–130.

Clopper, R. R., Mazur, T., MacGillivray, M. H., and Voorhess, M. L. 1981. Androgen replacement vs gonadotropin (Gn) replacement in four Gn-deficient hypopituitary males: The behavioral benefits of each treatment. *J. Androl.,* 2:10.

Clopper, R. R., Meyer, W. J. III, Udvarhelyi, G. B., Money, J., Aarabi, B., Mulvihill, J. J., and Piasio, M. 1977. Postsurgical IQ and behavioral data on twenty patients with a history of childhood craniopharyngioma. *Psychoneuroendocrin.,* 2:365–372.

Deck, L. P. 1968. Buying brains by the inch. *J. Coll. Univ. Pers. Assoc.,* 19:33–37.

Drash, P. W. 1969. Psychologic counseling: Dwarfism. In *Endocrine and genetic diseases of childhood,* ed. L. I. Gardner, pp. 1014–1022. Philadelphia: W. B. Saunders.

Ehrhardt, A. A., and Meyer-Bahlburg, H. F. L. 1975. Psychological correlates of abnormal pubertal development. In *Disorders of Puberty.* Clin. in Endocrin. and Met., no. 4(1), ed. J. R. Bierich, pp. 207-222. London: W. B. Saunders.

Feldman, S. D. 1975. The presentation of shortness in everyday life—height and heightism in American sociology: Toward a sociology of stature. In *Life styles: Diversity in American society,* ed. S. D. Feldman, pp. 437-442. Boston: Little, Brown.

Folstein, S. E., Weiss, J. O., Mittelman, F., and Ross, D. J. 1981. Impairment, psychiatric symptoms and handicap in dwarfs. *Johns Hop. Med. J.,* 148:273-277.

Galatzer, A., Nofar, E., Beithalachmi, N., Aran, O., Shalit, M., Roitman, A., and Laron, Z. 1981. Intellectual and psychosocial functions of children, adolescents, and young adults before and after operation for craniopharyngioma. *Child Care Health Dev.* 7:307-316.

Garron, D. C. 1977. Intelligence among persons with Turner's syndrome. *Beh. Genet.,* 7:105-127.

Green, W. H., Campbell, M., and David, R. 1984. Psychosocial dwarfism: A critical review of the evidence. *J. Am. Acad. Child Psych.,* 23:39-48.

Hartnett, J. J., Bailey, K. G., and Hartley, C. S. 1974. Body height, position, and sex as determinants of personal space. *J. Psychol.,* 87:129-136.

Holmes, C. S., Hayford, J. T., and Thompson, R. G. 1982. Personality and behavior differences in groups of boys with short stature. *Child Health Care,* 11:61-64.

Lacey, K. A., and Parkin, J. M. 1974. The normal short child. Community study of children in Newcastle upon Tyne. *Arch. Dis. Child.,* 49:417-424.

MacGillivray, M. H., Peterson, R. E., Voorhess, M. L., Clopper, R. R., and Mazur, T. 1981. Advantages of gonadotropin (Gn) over testosterone therapy for virilization of Gn-deficient hypopituitary males. *J. Androl.,* 2:18-19.

Meyer-Bahlburg, H. F. L., Feinman, J. A., MacGillivray, M. H., and Aceto, T., Jr. 1978. Growth hormone deficiency, brain development, and intelligence. *Am. J. Dis. Child.,* 132:565-572.

Money, J. 1964. Two cytogenetic syndromes: Psychologic comparisons. I. Intelligence and specific-factor quotients. *J. Psychiat. Res.,* 2:223-231.

Money, J. 1968. *Sex errors of the body.* Baltimore: Johns Hopkins Press.

Money, J. 1975. Counseling: Syndromes of statural hypoplasia and hyperplasia, precocity and delay. In *Endocrine and genetic diseases of childhood and adolescence,* 2nd ed., ed. L. I. Gardner, pp. 1218-1227. Philadelphia: W. B. Saunders.

Money, J., Clopper, R., and Menefee, J. 1980. Psychosexual development in postpubertal males with idiopathic panhypopituitarism. *J. Sex Res.,* 16:212-225.

Money, J., Drash, P. W., and Lewis, V. 1967. Dwarfism and hypopituitarism: Statural retardation without retardation. *Am. J. Men. Def.,* 72:122-126.

Money, J., and Pollitt, E. 1966. Studies in the psychology of dwarfism. II. Personality maturation and response to growth hormone treatment. *J. Ped.,* 68:381-390.

Money, J., Wolff, G., and Annecillo, C. 1972. Pain agnosia and self-injury in the syndrome of reversible somatotropin deficiency (psychosocial dwarfism). *J. Aut. Child. Schiz.* 2:127-139.

Ollendick, T. H., and Cerny, J. A. 1981. *Clinical behavior therapy with children.* New York, Plenum Press.

Pertzelan, A., Yalon, L., Kauli, R., and Laron, Z. 1982. A comparative study of the effect of oestrogen substitution therapy on breast development in girls with hypo- and hypergonadotrophic hypogonadism. *Clin. Endocrin.,* 16:359-368.

Phifer, K. G. 1979. *Growing up small.* Middlebury, Vt.: Paul S. Eriksson.

Richardson, S. A. 1976. Attitudes and behavior toward the physically handicapped. *Birth Def.* (original article series), 12(4):15-34.

Rogers, J. G., Perry, M. A., and Rosenberg, L. A. 1979. IQ measurement in children with skeletal dysplasia. *Ped.,* 63:894-897.

Rosenfeld, R. G., Northcraft, G. B., and Hintz, R. L. 1982. A prospective, randomized study of testosterone treatment of constitutional delay of growth and development in male adolescents. *Ped.,* 69:681–687.

Rotnem, D., Cohen, D. J., Hintz, R., and Genel, M. 1979. Psychological sequelae of relative "treatment failure" for children receiving human growth hormone replacement. *J. Am. Acad. Child Psych.,* 18:505–520.

Schumacher, A. 1982. On the significance of stature in human society. *J. Human Evolution,* 11:697–701.

Shaffer, J. W. 1962. A specific cognitive deficit observed in gonadal aplasia (Turner's syndrome). *J. Clin. Psychol.,* 18:403–406.

Stace, L., and Danks, D. M. 1981a. A social study of dwarfing conditions. The reactions and questions of parents of children with bone dysplasias. *Austral. Paed. J.,* 17:167–171.

Stace, L., and Danks, D. M. 1981b. A social study of dwarfing conditions. II. The experience of children with bone dysplasias, and of their parents. *Austral. Paed. J.,* 17:172–176.

Stace, L., and Danks, D. M. 1981c. A social study of dwarfing conditions. III. The social and emotional experiences of adults with bone dysplasias. *Austral. Paed. J.,* 17:177–182.

Taipale, V. 1979. *Adolescence in Turner's syndrome.* Helsinki, Finland: Children's Hospital, University of Helsinki.

Todorov, A. B., Scott, C. I., Jr., Warren, A. E., and Leeper, J. D. 1981. Developmental screening tests in achondroplastic children. *Am. J. Med. Genet.,* 9:19–24.

Underwood, L. E., and Van Wyk, J. J. 1981. Hormones in normal and aberrant growth. In *Textbook of endocrinology.* 6th ed., ed. R. H. Williams, pp. 1149–1191. Philadelphia: W. B. Saunders.

Vimpani, G. V., Vimpani, A. F., Pocock, S. J., and Farquhar, J. W. 1981. Differences in physical characteristics, perinatal histories, and social backgrounds between children with growth hormone deficiency and constitutional short stature. *Arch. Dis. Child.,* 56:922–928.

Weinberg, M. S. 1968. The problems of midgets and dwarfs and organizational remedies: A study of the Little People of America. *J. Health Soc. Beh.,* 9:65–71.

Weinraub, M., and Putney, E. 1978. The effects of height on infants' social responses to unfamiliar persons. *Child Dev.,* 49:598–603.

Wilson, P. R. 1968. The perceptual distortion of height as a function of ascribed academic status. *J. Soc. Psychol.,* 74:97–102.

Yamada, H., Nakamura, S., Tajima, M., and Kageyama, N. 1981. Neurological manifestations of pediatric achondroplasia. *J. Neurosurg.,* 54:49–57.

Zachmann, M., and Prader, A. 1970. Anabolic and androgenic effect of testosterone in sexually immature boys and its dependency on growth hormone. *J. Clin. Endocrin.,* 30:85–95.

APPENDIX 1. *ASSESSMENT GUIDE: PSYCHOLOGICAL EFFECTS OF SHORT STATURE**

1. MEDICAL ASPECTS

1.1 *History of the growth problem as experienced by parent(s) and child*

When and how did the parent(s) become aware of the child's growth problem?

History of medical examinations:

---

*Copyright © 1983 Heino F. L. Meyer-Bahlburg

When, by whom, and how were given:
  the final diagnosis;
  explanation of the growth disorder;
  explanation of causes;
  prognosis;
  options.

Initial and later emotional responses and actions of parents and significant other family members; including reactions:
  to physicians (e.g., justified complaints; exaggerated expectations; hostile projections);
  to spouse (e.g., guilt; blame);
  to child (e.g., guilt; feeling sorry; overprotection; attachment; resentment; rejection; neglect; abuse).

Impact of child's growth disorder:
  on parents' marriage;
  on parents' family planning;
  on parents' life in general (use the Impact-on-Family Scale by Stein and Riessman, *Med. Care*, 18:465-472, 1980).

Psychiatric disorder, especially depression, as a parental response to child's growth disorder.

Did parents receive counseling, psychiatric help, etc., in relation to the child's growth disorder?

At what age did the child seem to become aware of a growth problem?

Child's reaction:
  to diagnosis, prognosis;
  to physicians, examinations;
  to parents (e.g., blame).

History of child's physical (including pubertal) development as seen by parents and child.

History of developmental milestones, and parents' interpretation.

History of growth-related treatment: including parents' and patient's expectations and reactions to results.

History of child's psychiatric treatment, counseling, etc.

1.2 *Understanding of medical condition and associated misconceptions, worries, and fears*

What does the name of the specific growth disorder (and alternate terms) mean to the parents, the child?

Mechanism of growth disorder.

Cause of growth disorder (including parents' and child's assumptions, e.g., regarding insufficient food intake by child or pregnancy accidents).

Consequences for parents' own family planning.

Prognostic expectations by parents, child:
  final adult height;
  medical complications, general health;
  life expectancy;
  medical treatment options, including use of appliances, and expectations of outcome;
  physical mobility, participation in sports;
  quality of life: potential for independent living, emotional and social functioning;
  intelligence;
  potential for education;
  potential for employment;
  sexual and psychosexual development, including fertility;
  potential for marriage.

Financial expectations.

Associated behavior/psychological problems (watch for parent's or child's denial).

Have the parents, or the child, seen persons with the same or similar growth disorders; their reaction?

Would they like to meet patients with similar growth disorders or their parents?

1.3 *Child's and parents' coping with medical treatment*

Examinations, needles, etc.: reactions, especially phobic reactions.

Hospitalizations, operations:
    child's preparation;
    child's behavior;
    family support during hospitalization.

Home-administered medications:
    who administers them;
    compliance.

Parental overwhelmedness.

Financial problems.

2. SOCIAL ASPECTS

2.1 *Apparent age of child (by observation and report)*

Height age.

Facial features.

Secondary sex characteristics.

Associated physical stigmata.

Clothing style and shoes.

Hairstyle and facial makeup.

Mimics.

Speech and vocabulary.

General movement style.

Does the patient elicit from professional staff verbal and nonverbal responses that are appropriate for younger children? (How much younger?)
    from individual family members?

Is the child's style of peer interactions at or below age level?

2.2 *Everyday skills and independence*

(Administer the Vineland Social Maturity Scale with a growth-disorder related inquiry concerning any skill delays).

2.3 *Child-family interaction*

Babying/infantilizing by parents (e.g., communication style; calling older child "cute," "adorable"; holding child on lap when too old; having child sleep in parents' bed).

Indications of separation anxiety, clinginess of the patient.

Is there parental overprotection (e.g., inhibition of peer contact)?

Age-inappropriate (under- or over-) demands by parents (e.g., regarding home chores, dressing, help with physical problems).

Age-inappropriate limit setting (contact sports, bike riding, deadlines).

Do the parents or other caretakers show guilt feelings, ambivalence, resentment, rejection, neglect, abuse?

Do parents or other household members engage in teasing or harassing the child? (Referring to which characteristics?)

How do the siblings interact with the patient (e.g., resentment of patient's special role)?

Is there a younger sibling who is about to bypass or has bypassed the patient in height? Patient's reaction (e.g., rivalry, depression)?

What role do the siblings have in the patient's interaction with peers in the neighborhood (e.g., overprotection; fighting his/her battles; avoidance)?

Is the patient inappropriately bossy with younger siblings?

Are there similarly short-statured older adolescent or adult family members who can serve as positive role models?

How much (active) time do the parents spend with the patient?

Do parents and other caretakers show support for patient's complaints and problems?

Is there an atmosphere of openness concerning the patient's growth disorder and related problems in the family?

Overall style of parents'/patient's dealing with short-stature problems, e.g.,
    failure to look for psychological problems;
    denial;
    hiding child/problems from the outside world;
    realism.

2.4 *Child-teacher interaction*

Babying/infantilizing ("teacher's pet"; holding the patient on lap; communication style).

Overprotection; age-inappropriate (under- or over-) demands by teachers; age-inappropriate limit setting.

Teasing/inappropriate derogatory remarks by school personnel?
    Patient's response?

2.5 *Child's interaction with adults outside the home*

How does patient cope with meeting strange adults?

How do parents and patient handle teasing, inappropriate remarks, curious questions, when going to—
    stores for shopping groceries, clothing, etc.;
    movie theaters;
    restaurants;
    other leisure-time facilities;
    public restrooms.

2.6 *Child-peer interactions in neighborhood and school*

Patient is one of the 1/2/3/4/5 shortest in class (elementary school) or grade (junior high or high school) or school.

Patient is one of the 1/2/3/4/5 weakest in gym class or school.

Infantilizing by peers, including lifting the patient up and carrying him/her around? Patient's reactions?

Teasing:
    frequency;
    terms and phrases;
    who does it?
    patient's typical responses:
        "ignoring"/silent withdrawal;
        complaining to adults/teachers;

reteasing;
physical fighting.

Physical harassment:
frequency;
type;
who does it?
patient's response.

Parents' handling of patient's complaints about teasing and physical harassment.

Patient's attitude toward school (e.g., is afraid of/refuses to go to school because of peer teasing/harassment).

Who are the close friends of the patient:
first names; sex; age;
frequency and type of interaction (note: some patients with impaired peer relationships may give lists of "close friends" with whom they hardly have any contact).

Do friends come to the patient's home and vice versa:
frequency;
type of activity.

Does patient belong to any groups:
sports teams;
youth organizations;
social clubs;
hobby clubs;
church/temple clubs.

Peer activities (sports, games, hobbies, etc.):
which activities does the child participate in?
which activities is the child excluded from because of physical limitations?
which activities does the child not join, although there are no physical limitations?
which activities does the child do on his/her own, although they are suitable for peer involvement?

How does the patient handle meeting new peers, joining new groups?

Determine the overall style of peer interactions:
withdrawal: isolation from peers, loner (may include much day dreaming) or preferential association with adults (may include premature adoption of adult mannerisms);
regression to younger age group;
(boys:) association with girls rather than boys;
adoption of the role of mascot, class clown;
aggressiveness;
winning friends by making presents;
use of humor;
age-appropriate interaction.

2.7 *Psychosexual development*

Satisfaction with gender.

(If indicated:) gender history.

Psychosexual milestones: crushes, dating, boy/girlfriends, steadies; holding hands, kissing, necking, petting, intercourse.

Current interest in interaction with the other sex.

Expectations for future relationships and marriage.

(If appropriate:) sexual dysfunctions.

3. *SELF-IMAGE*

In what ways is the child different from other boys/girls?

What are the advantages of being small?

What are the disadvantages of being small?

What is the worst?

Three wishes.

Determine particularly sensitive issues:
    inferiority feelings;
    overcompensation fantasies;
    use of denial.

APPENDIX 2. PHYSICAL ENVIRONMENT CHECKLIST—HOME AND TRANSPORTATION (PECL-H)

Name of Child _____ Age _____ Your Name _____ Relationship _____ Date _____

INSTRUCTIONS: The items below concern problems with the physical environment that many children, adolescents, and adults with marked growth disorders have. Read each item carefully and decide to what degree your child (in case of self-report: you yourself) has found this to be a physical problem compared to other people of the same age but of average height, during the past six months: NOT AT ALL, JUST A LITTLE, PRETTY MUCH, or VERY MUCH. Indicate your choice by placing a check mark (✓) in the appropriate column to the right of each item. Check DOES NOT APPLY if the item is not part of your child's (in case of self-report: your own) environment. Describe your child's (in case of self-report: your own) main ways of coping with each problem in the past six months: Has he/she avoided the problem, or obtained help from other people, or used physical means such as stools and other equipment, or found still other ways? Leave open the last space on the right, RECOMMENDED SOLUTIONS; it is to be filled in by the growth-problem specialist. PLEASE ANSWER ALL ITEMS.

Item	Problem in the past 6 months					Child's way of coping, past 6 months				Recommended solutions
	Does not apply	Not at all	Just a little	Pretty much	Very much	Avoidance	Help by others (who)	Physical means (which)	Other ways (which)	
BUILDING ENTRANCE										
Stairs										
Name board/bells										
Door handle										
Mailbox										
Elevator buttons										
Apartment doorbell										
Other:										
Other:										

Copyright © 1983 Heino F.L. Meyer-Bahlburg

	Problem in the past 6 months				Child's way of coping, past 6 months				Recommended solutions
Item	Does not apply	Not at all	Just a little	Pretty much	Very much	Avoidance	Help by others (who)	Physical means (which)	Other ways (which)	
FOYER, CORRIDOR										
Light switches										
Coat hangers										
Closet rods										
Shelves, drawers										
Mirror										
Other:										
Other:										
LIVING ROOM										
Light switches										
Table & chairs										
Sofa										
Armchairs										
Shelves, drawers										
Other:										
Other:										

Item	Problem in the past 6 months					Child's way of coping, past 6 months				Recommended solutions
	Does not apply	Not at all	Just a little	Pretty much	Very much	Avoidance	Help by others (who)	Physical means (which)	Other ways (which)	
BEDROOM										
Door handle										
Light switches										
Closet rods										
Shelves, drawers										
Table & chairs										
Mirror										
Bed										
Other:										
Other:										
BATHROOM										
Door handle										
Light switches										
Toilet seat										
Shower knobs										
Sink, faucets										
Towel hooks/bars										
Mirror										
Cabinet										
Shelves, drawers										
Other:										
Other:										

Item	Problem in the past 6 months					Child's way of coping, past 6 months				Recommended solutions
	Does not apply	Not at all	Just a little	Pretty much	Very much	Avoidance	Help by others (who)	Physical means (which)	Other ways (which)	
KITCHEN										
Door handle										
Light switches										
Countertops										
Stove top										
Cabinets										
Other shelves										
Refrigerator										
Sink, faucets										
Other:										
Other:										
BASEMENT										
Door handle										
Stairs										
Light switches										
Shelves, drawers										
Other:										
Other:										
Other:										

	Problem in the past 6 months					Child's way of coping, past 6 months				Recommended solutions
Item	Does not apply	Not at all	Just a little	Pretty much	Very much	Avoidance	Help by others (who)	Physical means (which)	Other ways (which)	
ATTIC										
Door handle										
Stairs										
Light switches										
Shelves, drawers										
Other:										
Other:										
Other:										
OTHER ROOM(S)										
Door handle										
Light switches										
Shelves, drawers										
Tables & chairs										
Other:										
Other:										
Other:										

Item	Problem in the past 6 months					Child's way of coping, past 6 months				Recommended solutions
	Does not apply	Not at all	Just a little	Pretty much	Very much	Avoidance	Help by others (who)	Physical means (which)	Other ways (which)	
APPLIANCES										
Washer										
Dryer										
Vacuum cleaner										
Lawn mower										
Other:										
Other:										
Other:										

TRANSPORTATION

Bicycle										
Car										
Public bus										
School bus										
Train										
Other:										
Other:										

APPENDIX 3. PHYSICAL ENVIRONMENT CHECKLIST–SCHOOL (PECL-S)

Name of Child _____ Informant's Name _____ Position _____ Date _____

INSTRUCTIONS: The items below concern problems with the physical environment that many children and adolescents with marked growth disorders have. Please read each item carefully and decide to what degree this child (in case of self-report: you yourself) has found this to be a physical problem compared to other people of the same age but of average height during the past three months; or, in case of newly enrolled students, which of these problems can be expected: NOT AT ALL, JUST A LITTLE, PRETTY MUCH, or VERY MUCH.
Indicate your choice by placing a check mark (✓) in the appropriate column to the right of each item. Check DOES NOT APPLY if the item is not part of this child's (in case of self-report: your own) school environment. Describe this child's (in case of self-report: your own) ways of coping with each problem in the past three months of school (this section does not apply to students who are about to start attendance): has he/she avoided the problem, or obtained help from other people, or used physical means such as stools and other equipment, or found still other ways? Leave open the last section, RECOMMENDED SOLUTIONS; it is to be filled in by the growth-problem specialist. PLEASE ANSWER ALL ITEMS.

Item	Problem in the past 3 months					Child's way of coping, past 3 months				Recommended solutions
	Does not apply	Not at all	Just a little	Pretty much	Very much	Avoidance	Help by others (who)	Physical means (which)	Other ways (which)	
ENTRANCE, CORRIDORS										
Stairs										
Bell buttons										
Door handle										
Elevator buttons										
Drinking fountain										
Lockers										
Other:										
Other:										

Copyright © 1983 Heino F.L. Meyer-Bahlburg

	Problem in the past 3 months					Child's way of coping, past 3 months				Recommended solutions
Item	Does not apply	Not at all	Just a little	Pretty much	Very much	Avoidance	Help by others (who)	Physical means (which)	Other ways (which)	
CLASSROOM(S)										
Door handle										
Light switches										
Desk, chair*										
Shelves, drawers										
Other:										
Other:										
STUDY HALL										
Door handle										
Light switches										
Desk, chair*										
Shelves, drawers										
Other:										
Other:										

* Including foot support (legs should not dangle unsupported).

	Problem in the past 3 months					Child's way of coping, past 3 months				Recommended solutions
Item	Does not apply	Not at all	Just a little	Pretty much	Very much	Avoidance	Help by others (who)	Physical means (which)	Other ways (which)	
BATHROOM(S)										
Door handle										
Light switches										
Sink, faucets										
Mirror										
Toilet seat										
Urinal										
Shelves, drawers										
Other:										
Other:										
GYM, Etc.										
Door handle										
Light switches										
Lockers										
Shower knobs										
Toilet seats										
Urinals										
Mirrors										
Sink, faucets										
Other:										
Other:										
Other:										

7

Abnormal Puberty: Psychological Implications and Treatment Issues

ANKE A. EHRHARDT

ADOLESCENCE IS THE TRANSITION between childhood and adulthood and roughly extends through the entire second decade. This phase is unique because of its magnitude and the rapidity of change of biological and psychosocial events (Katchadourian, 1977). The special needs of adolescents have been recognized with the establishment of special health-care and counseling facilities (see chap. 31).

This chapter will deal with the psychological correlates of abnormal puberty and the implications for assessment and treatment. Since many behavior problems overlap with those of physically normal adolescents, it is appropriate to begin with a brief overview of normal puberty and typical adolescent behavior as well as common disorders.

NORMAL PUBERTY

Several excellent reviews have described the somatic and hormonal changes of puberty (Tanner, 1970, 1974; Katchadourian, 1977; Meyer-Bahlburg, 1980). The physical changes are mediated at four levels of hormonal control. According to current knowledge, the highest level of control takes place in the hypothalamus, influencing the next level, the pituitary gland, which in turn regulates the gonads (ovaries and testes) and the adrenal gland to release the so-called sex hormones that mediate most of the physical changes of puberty.

The specific features of puberty are predictable and uniform enough between individuals to form a standard pattern, although onset and sequence of pubertal events vary greatly between and within the sexes. Therefore, it is customary to report the timing of pubertal events in ranges that usually span over several years. The onset of external manifestations of puberty is reported as eight and a half to thirteen years for girls and nine and a half to fifteen years for boys (Katchadourian, 1977). The sequence of events usually follows a predictable schedule in both girls and boys, although they are by no means immutably fixed and can occur in reverse order. Breast development in girls is typically the first sign, followed by pubic hair and menarche. For boys, puberty gets signaled by testicular growth and scrotal changes, followed by pubic hair and penile growth. The onset of puberty is consistently earlier in girls than in boys with a time lag of about two years (Kulin, 1972) based on the beginning of the height spurt. If one compares breast budding with the onset of testicular growth, the sex difference is only six months.

The hormonal control of puberty on the gonadal level is due to a dramatic increase in the production of androgens, estrogens, and progestins. During childhood the production of gonadal hormones is relatively low, preceded by rapid changes during prenatal embryonic differentiation. Between ten and seventeen years, plasma testosterone, the major androgen which is produced by the testes in males, increases twentyfold (Faiman et al., 1976). Adrenal androgenic hormones also show a marked increase at puberty in both boys and girls.

Estrogen and progesterone are secreted by the ovarian follicles. Low levels of estrogen are present in both sexes during childhood (Winter and Faiman, 1973). At puberty the production of estrogen accelerates in girls and continues to increase after menarche until ovulatory cycles are attained. The increase of estrogen is much smaller for boys, but adolescent and later adult males continue to secrete small amounts of estrogen probably by the adrenal cortex and the testes (O'Connor et al., 1974). Apart from the increased production of the sex hormones, their pattern of secretion also changes. For the female, the cyclical pattern of estrogen and progesterone is the main regulator of the menstrual cycle. Males do not have an analogous monthly cycle, although their androgen levels follow a diurnal rhythm.

Since the duration of puberty spans over four years or so, and the timing of pubertal onset varies greatly, early adolescence is a developmental phase in the human life cycle that includes individuals who look markedly different from one another and exhibit discrepancies between chronological age, physique age, and psychosocial age—the latter of which can be broken down conveniently into academic age, recreational age, and psychosexual age (Money and Clopper, 1974). The great variability of pubertal changes among girls and boys is probably one of the reasons that early adolescence has been described as a particularly stressful developmental phase (Hamburg, 1974), although the entire second decade is marked as a time of change and challenge that profoundly affects subsequent adult adjustment.

It has been shown that the timing as well as the nature of puberty has psychological significance. For instance, some studies have shown that early maturing boys have a slight advantage in personality development (McCandless, 1960). They tend to be more popular, more relaxed, more good-natured, and generally more poised. In contrast, late maturing boys were less self-confident and more anxious (Jones and Bayley, 1950; Mussen and Jones, 1957; Weatherley, 1964). The picture is far less consistent in girls; the differences between early and late maturers seem less marked and vary according to age, with early maturation being sometimes an advantage and sometimes a disadvantage (Jones and Mussen, 1958). Early maturers of both sexes tend to have a higher IQ and higher educational attainment at colleges (Douglas and Ross, 1964).

The reason for the significance of timing of puberty in personality development is not entirely understood, although it makes good sense to conjecture that the superiority of athletic abilities in boys who undergo early puberty, associated with muscular physique, plays an important part (McCandless, 1960; Tanner, 1962). Girls' reactions to early or later puberty are more complex and may be related to self-consciousness due to looking different before any of their peers do, moodiness associated with the menstrual cycle, and having to deal with sexuality at an early age.

Adolescence: Common Behavior Changes and Disturbances

The second decade in human development is also marked by important social changes, e. g., transition to junior high, high school, and eventually a job or college. Environmental expectations increase and the adolescent has to cope with the complexities of new physical, social, and psychological events. The main areas of adolescent behavior, equally relevant to the child who undergoes an abnormal puberty, are (1) psychosexual development, (2) psychopathology, and (3) mental functioning in terms of level of intelligence and patterns of strengths and weaknesses.

Psychosexual Development

Adolescent behavior has its roots, of course, in childhood and does not start as something completely unique with puberty. Regarding psychosexual development, the formation of gender identity starts from infancy on and is typically well established by the age of three and four years (Money and Ehrhardt, 1972). Therefore, the event of puberty usually is a reinforcer of one's sense of gender, rather than of causal significance. In fact, the early experiences of children are typically strong enough to establish gender identity so that even errors of timing in puberty or an unexpected incongruous feature of pubertal development does not profoundly shake most people's identification of being a girl or a boy.

Similarly, sex differences in behavior have their roots much earlier than in adolescence and are probably shaped by an interplay of prenatal hormonal influences (see review by Ehrhardt and Meyer-Bahlburg, 1981), parental sex typing, peer effects, and many other culture-specific rules and models (see overview by Maccoby and Jacklin, 1974). Puberty and adolescence is the transition to adult gender roles. Some of the childhood sex-dimorphic play gives way to adolescent interests, in particular to sexual interests and activities.

The development of sexuality also starts long before puberty. In fact, reactions of the sex organs occur from infancy on—e.g., erection of the penis has been observed from birth (Halverson, 1940). While these erections initially seem to be largely associated with other bodily functions, they subsequently become part of the overall exploration of the body and of pleasant sensation, resulting in masturbation during childhood. Both boys and girls masturbate long before puberty and react in many cases with orgasmlike responses. Children also engage in sexuality with each other throughout the first decade, and the psychoanalytic concept of a sexually latent period between the ages of five/six and puberty is in contrast to the empirical evidence (Rutter, 1971).

While sexual activities in childhood are exploratory and sporadic, in adolescence sexual concerns and behavior become a major part of everyday life and become linked to falling in love, erotic imagery, and involvement with another person (Meyer-Bahlburg, 1980).

Psychopathology

Psychopathology and behavior problems are often believed to be the norm for adolescents. This assumption has been shown to be exaggerated and misleading (Rutter et al., 1976). Most adolescents are not emotionally disturbed. However, mood swings including unhappiness and misery are quite common during the teens (Masterson, 1967; Rutter et al., 1976). Diagnosable psychiatric disorders increase in adolescence compared to childhood. The prevalence rates vary according to the populations studied, but the overall incidence is probably somewhere around 15%. If one includes psychiatric symptomatology experienced by teenagers, but not noticeable to other people such as parents and teachers, the percentage may be closer to 20% (Graham and Rutter, 1977). The most common adolescent psychiatric problems are emotional disorders, such as depression and anxiety, especially for girls. In fact, the sex ratio of depression will eventually be 2:1 favoring women in adulthood (Weissman and Klerman, 1979). This rise in affective disorders during adolescence is paralleled by a rise in the incidence of attempted and completed suicide (Shaffer, 1974). Boys exhibit more conduct disorders and delinquency.

Mental Functioning

A relationship of intellectual development and pubertal maturation has been suggested. The "brain growth spurt" has been conceptualized as an event that is analogous to the statural growth spurt. A few studies have demonstrated an association of early puberty (within the normal range) with advanced mental development (Kohen-Raz, 1974); the data are conflicting with regard to the maintenance of this advancement after puberty. The positive association between early puberty and intellectual advancement could be due to a common independent factor which will influence both (e.g., socioeconomic level, nutrition); the association would be indicative of the existence of a genuine brain and intellectual growth spurt only if it could be demonstrated that the intellectual "growth rate" is highest at the time of maximum body growth, as has been attempted by Ljung (1965) and in a rather sophisticated study by Kohen-Raz (1974) with inconclusive results.

There are well-known sex differences in mental abilities: for instance, on average, females show superiority in verbal ability (verbal fluency, articulation) and perceptual speed, whereas males show superiority in spatial abilities (Maccoby and Jacklin, 1974). These sex differences can be demonstrated much more easily in adolescents than in prepubertal children, and an obvious question is whether puberty has an influence on their accentuation. Various researchers have suggested that these sex differences in cognitive abilities are related to sex differences in the degree of hemispheric specialization or lateralization of cognitive functioning (Buffery and Gray, 1972; Levy, 1976).

BEHAVIOR PROBLEMS ASSOCIATED WITH PUBERTAL ANOMALIES

Children and adolescents who deviate from the usual timetable of pubertal development or unexpectedly exhibit signs of gender-discrepant secondary sex characteristics, such as breast development in boys or hirsutism in girls, dramatically demonstrate the potential effects of hormonal and somatic changes. They also have special needs in health and mental-health care which child psychiatrists and other clinicians should be familiar with. This section will list a number of pubertal anomalies and summarize issues of medical and behavior management. Two syndromes (precocious puberty and Turner's syndrome) will be described in more detail. The principles described for those two clinical entities are also applicable to the other pubertal anomalies and therefore will not be repeated for every specific disorder.

Timing Errors

In errors of pubertal timing, physique age is advanced or retarded in relation to chronological age. It depends largely on the particular environmental social pressures from peers and adults whether or not and to what extent the psychosocial age will coincide with or deviate from the physique age on the one hand and the chronological age on the other. Usually the adolescent will be aware of these discrepancies. The degree of his or her emotional response and the quality of coping will depend to a large extent on support from the outside.

PRECOCIOUS PUBERTY. What controls the timing mechanism of the initiation of puberty is still not fully understood, so that often one does not know why a child or adolescent develops too early and presents signs of precocious puberty (pubertas praecox). In extreme cases, precocious puberty can begin shortly after birth, but occurs more frequently at the age of six to eight years. Precocious puberty can be secondary to various more general medical abnormalities, including a lesion in the brain or the glands. It also can be idiopathic or spontaneous without any other physical disorder, except for the early onset of puberty. Idiopathic sexual precocity sometimes affects only one member of a family, but may affect several members. Sexual precocity is encountered more than twice as frequently in females as in males. In girls, the so-called idiopathic type accounts for 70% of the reported cases, and in boys for 30–40% (Penny, 1982).

The psychological consequences of precocious puberty do not depend on whether the affected young person has the idiopathic or any other type, except that other symptoms may mean an additional emotional burden. Therefore, this discussion will be limited to the impact of early puberty without other known physical abnormalities.

The definition of precocious puberty is somewhat arbitrary. Many pediatric endocrinologists find it desirable that a child of either sex who begins pubertal changes before age nine have detailed medical investigation (van der Werff ten Bosch, 1975). Others take a more radical point of view and agree with Bierich's (1975) definition by which the term sexual precocity is applied to girls if they show signs of sexual maturation before their sixth birthday and to boys if signs of sexual maturity appear before their eighth birthday.

Although the mechanism by which the timing of puberty is regulated is not yet fully understood, much available evidence points to the assumption that it is not primarily peripheral glands or the pituitary but the brain itself, especially the hypothalamus, that is responsible. Originally, this theory was proposed by Hohlweg and Dohrn (1932) on the basis of rat experiments and suggested that puberty was induced by a change in sensitivity to circulating sex steroids of a sexual center in the central nervous system that regulates gonadotropin secretion. A competing theory of the initiation of puberty has been proposed by Odell and Swerdloff (1976), who believe that sexual maturation, at least in subhuman mammals, is predominantly due to maturation at the gonadal level as a result of follicle stimulating hormone (FSH) induction of luteinizing hormone (LH) receptors in the gonads, resulting in increasing gonadal steroid secretion. Children with idiopathic precocious puberty show a hormonal pattern similar to that of normal children during puberty (Radfar et al., 1976), including the pubertal pattern of sleep-associated LH release (Boyar et al., 1973) and in girls an enhanced (in some cases, even exaggerated) gonadotropin response to luteinizing hormone-releasing hormone (LH-RH) administration (Reiter et al., 1975). It is, however, not quite clear whether idiopathic precocious puberty is simply an early timed but otherwise normal puberty: for instance, Bidlingmaier et al. (1977) found considerably lower basal gonadotropin and estrogen levels in girls with precocious puberty than in normally maturing girls of the same developmental stage, although those patients who were examined repeatedly at short intervals showed an almost cyclic pattern of their estradiol levels similar to the pattern of normal pubertal girls before menarche.

Precocious Puberty in Girls. A girl with precocious puberty typically has to cope with an early growth spurt, putting her on the growth level of other children who are two or three years older than her chronological age, so that a six-year-old girl may measure up to somebody who is eight or nine years old. At the same time she will begin to develop pubic and axillary hair, breast enlargement, and eventually menstruation. A child like this first of all requires specialized pediatric endocrine assessment and management and may be referred for preventive or therapeutic counseling for herself and her family.

The child needs to be referred to a pediatrician who has specialized in endocrinology. Typically, a girl will present with one pubertal sign, namely early breast development or early pubic hair development. A checkup may reveal that she has early breast development or pubic hair growth as an isolated phenomenon. In the case of true idiopathic precocious puberty, however, the child is at the beginning of pubertal development and will go through the full sequence of pubertal events at a much earlier age than her peers. During a complete work-up of such a child, a differential diagnosis of idiopathic precocious puberty or early development due to other causes will have to be made. The girl's height and weight will also be carefully recorded. Most pediatric endocrinologists like to follow children with precocious puberty on a six-month basis (Rosenfield, 1982). Most girls who develop early will eventually not be different from their peers, except for being somewhat shorter due to an accelerated growth spurt with premature fusion of the epiphyses. About half of the females with this disorder have been found to reach an adult height of 53 to 59 inches and the remainder 60 to 65.6 inches (Donovan and van der Werff ten Bosch, 1965).

Pediatric endocrinologists prefer not to treat the benign idiopathic precocious puberty with medication. However, if the onset of pubertal development is very early and rapidly progressing and/or if the psychological effects are detrimental, many physicians may attempt to control the early development medically. Yet, one has to be aware that so far there is no satisfactory medical treatment available for idiopathic precocious puberty. The most widely used form of therapy is medroxyprogesterone acetate (Provera) (Kaplan et al., 1968). Provera can be given intramuscularly or orally. The treatment reverses some of the physical changes but does not necessarily reverse the inordinately rapid maturation of the bones. Cyproterone acetate, an antiandrogenic steriod analogue, has been widely used in Europe for the treatment of precocious puberty but is not available in the United States. The beneficial effects of cyproterone acetate are not proven according to current research (Werder et al., 1974; Kauli et al., 1976). A promising potential new treatment for idiopathic sexual precocity is with long-acting gonadotropin-releasing hormone (GnRH) agonists to inhibit gonadotropin release and diminish estrogen levels. These drugs are only available in the United States on an investigational basis; their long-term effects on the clinical course and on follicle and ovarian maturation remains to be determined (Crowley et al., 1981).

Girls who show an isolated sign of early development such as premature thelarche or pubarche do not require any medical intervention except for a thorough diagnostic investigation. The child's early development is simply a matter of a normal stage of puberty occurring early. It is believed to be due either to an incomplete, slow kind of puberty or to increased sensitivity to the trace levels of hormones that are normally present at the child's age. Typically, pubertal development does not progress after one sign has occurred and menstruation can be expected to occur at an appropriate age.

Psychosexual development of girls with precocious puberty is not well researched. In an early medical review, Reuben and Manning (1922, 1923) cited eighty-three cases of pregnancy below age fifteen (thirty of those below age twelve) and claimed that the majority of the young women had a history of precocious puberty; the authors in addition screened their own eight female cases of precocious puberty without pregnancy and claimed that sexual desire was only present in one mentally defective girl. Kinsey et al. (1953) examined cases of precocious puberty and found sexual activities to be in concordance with their chronological age rather than being precocious. In a follow-up study of fifteen girls with idiopathic precocious puberty (ages ten to twenty-five years) by Money and Walker in 1971, masturbation and sex play did not appear to be increased. Premarital intercourse did not occur earlier than normally expected (age seventeen years and up) with the exception of one girl who became pregnant at age eleven.

We recently completed in our own program a follow-up study of sixteen female adolescents, all of whom had had a documented history of idiopathic precocious puberty with an onset of pubertal development before age nine. To our knowledge, this is the first study that compares a patient sample with a closely matched control group who went through puberty at a normal age (Ehrhardt et al., 1984). Our protocol included aspects of psychosexual development, psychopathology, IQ and achievement, and sex-specific mental abilities as well as subsample hormonal assessments during an overnight admission. At the time of the study, the age range of the patient sample was thirteen years, two months to twenty years, ten months. The first pubertal signs were observed by the children's mothers between the ages of two and a half and eight years, with the median around age six and a half. All of them had been investigated by a pediatric endocrinologist and their medical histories had been documented.

Regarding psychosexual development, the important findings (Meyer-Bahlburg et al., 1982) were that there were no differences with regard to the timing of the first crush and the first date. However, patients had their first boyfriend and their first steady relationship about a year earlier than the controls, and they reported having fallen in love about two years earlier than the controls. The differences were even more clear-cut with regard to the initiation of sexual behaviors. In spite of the modest sample sizes, almost all of those categories reached conventional statistical significance: subjects with a history of precocious puberty reported having been about one and a half to two years earlier in their first holding hands, their first kissing games, first romantic kiss, first necking, first breast petting, first genital petting, and first sexual intercourse, with a highly significant difference in the onset of masturbation of about five and a half years earlier. What is important, however, is to keep in mind that while the patient sample was earlier than the normal controls, they still experienced the various aspects of sexual behavior in adolescence and not in childhood concordant with their onset of pubertal development. For instance, while those patients who had started to be sexually active in heterosexual intercourse had done so between the ages of twelve and a half and sixteen and a half, the analogous range for the controls was fourteen and a half to nineteen and a half. There was no difference between patients and controls at the time of study in the number of partners they had had intercourse experience with nor the absolute number of intercourse occasions they had experienced.

Therefore, it seems that adolescents who have developed much earlier than their peers tend to be somewhat earlier in respect to starting their adolescent sex life, although they still remained within the normal range of current standards. Other aspects of the development of gender role behavior were unremarkable in the patient sample compared to the matched control group. It appears from our study and other reported research that the development of adolescent sexual behavior is strongly governed by cultural norms and learning rather than being determined by sex hormones and pubertal development. However, it appears that pubertal factors do play a part and may be responsible for the relatively earlier onset of dating and sexual behavior in some adolescents who have gone through puberty early. It also may have a relatively stronger effect on autoerotic behavior such as masturbation.

The reports on psychopathology in children with precocious puberty on a short-term or long-term basis are mainly limited to clinical case reports (e.g., Ehrhardt and Meyer-

Bahlburg, 1975; Levitsky and Domash, 1978; Solyom et al., 1982) which suggest that a history of precocious puberty may carry with it an increased risk of psychopathology. In addition, Money and Walker (1971) included in their clinical follow-up study on fifteen females with precocious puberty reports on moodiness and depression in a significant number of the patients and concluded that being different in physique for a significant number of years during childhood may take its toll on adjustment and affective stability in adolescence.

Our own long-term follow-up study includes a systematic assessment of psychopathology and behavior adjustment based on reports by the adolescents and their mothers, and compares the patients with controls. While we did not find increased definitive psychiatric disorders more frequently in the patient sample compared to the controls, we did find differences in psychopathology, albeit to a mild degree and not in all behavior areas, favoring a better adjustment in the control group. This slightly increased symptomatology was especially in the areas of conduct problems and psychosomatic complaints usually associated with menstruation in the patient sample. It appears that idiopathic precocious puberty in females is associated with the long-term risk of minor psychopathology and may in individual cases contribute to more severe behavior problems.

IQ and school achievement is typically not negatively affected in precocious puberty. In fact, there is a suggestion of the opposite. A number of studies by Money et al. (1967) have suggested accelerated intellectual development and school achievement. We also found an unusually high number of girls with precocious puberty to have been advanced in school during childhood and early adolescence, although their IQs did not differ from the control group at the time of study. Therefore, it may well be that if there is an advantage in intellectual development associated with early pubertal maturation, it may be temporary rather than long-term.

The assessment and clinical managment of a girl with precocious puberty will depend on whether the family is referred for preventive counseling or for the diagnosis and treatment of an already developed behavior problem. In the case of preventive counseling, parents and child should be initially seen separately. It is important to assess how adequate the parents' understanding is of normal pubertal development and their child's precocious puberty. Since the issue of sex education and frank communication on pubertal development becomes of extreme importance for the early developing child—she is often totally deprived of the usual peer exchange on these issues—it is imperative that the parents are at a level of understanding and comfort to communicate with their child about sex and reproduction at a much earlier age than they had expected. Dependent on the level of sophistication of the parents involved, detailed explanations will be given with the help of pictorial material and illustrations. We also stress to the parents that their daughter is passing through normal puberty several years too early but eventually will look like her peers. The phase of being unusual is temporary until her peers have caught up with her. The parents also need reassurance about the behavior of their child. One of the most common concerns is early sexual development and sexual interest of their daughter. Counseling will be provided on how to teach the young girl about menstrual hygiene and how to handle curious questions by other people.

As part of the initial evaluation of the parents, a developmental history of the child should be taken and a screening interview relating to any behavior problems at home and in school should be included. This can be done with the usual methodology such as by having the parents fill out one of the common symptom checklists (e.g., the Achenbach Child Behavior Checklist, 1981) in addition to participating in a broad-spectrum screening interview. The evaluation should also include a history of school performance (including a teacher's report). If the child's achievement in school is above average and a psychometric evaluation confirms above-average intellectual development, school acceleration has proved to be an effective method of reducing the period of being different from other agemates. In a study of nine girls, for whom school acceleration was recommended and achieved, the adjustment and outcome was in all cases successful (Money and Neill, 1967). The precociously developing girls were able to hold their own with children a year or two older and were capable of catching up academically and socially. Follow-up after several years confirmed the benefit of school acceleration. Academic achievement remained successful and several girls had graduated from college at the time of last contact (Money and Walker, 1971).

Early enrollment in school and school acceleration clearly has to be viewed as a preventive and ameliorative method against the experience of being out of place and different from peers. Typically, precocious children tend to choose their playmates among older children more similar in physical appearance anyway, and school placement into an older group helps to facilitate a psychosocial age closer to their physical age. If their daughter behaves like an older child, parents need to be reassured not to worry about this accelerated maturity, which may be temporary.

In the case of preventive referral, the child with precocious puberty herself needs frank sex education and an explanation of her own physical changes. Obviously, it should be stressed that what she is going through is a normal process although earlier than her peers. While the language needs to be chosen according to the age of the child, it has been found that one can communicate with children of any age about all aspects of reproduction, pubertal development, and sexuality (Money, 1968; Ehrhardt and McCauley, 1975). Apart from an explanation of pubertal development and her own precocious signs, the child with precocious puberty should be evaluated for the usual areas of behavior adjustment of her age such as psychosexual development, peer contacts, academic adjustment, and psychopathology.

Even if no noticeable behavior problems occur during the evaluation, it is best to follow the family twice a year when they come to the pediatric endocrine clinic to assure early discussion and amelioration of any adjustment problems that may develop.

In rare cases, the precocious girl develops serious emotional problems in relationship to her appearance and physical changes. Then, a more extensive counseling or psychotherapy plan is called for. This is particularly true if the parents are unable to openly communicate with their child about her physical development. The emotional problems that do occur are usually related to the child's inability to cope with looking different from her age mates. The experience becomes easily a destructive one to self-image and self-esteem and sometimes results in total withdrawal from peer contact. A central part of emotional difficulties often concerns the body image which may be distorted and may result in severe dislike of one's physique. Another frequent symptom is fluctuation of mood, often comparable to an accentuated premenstrual tension syndrome (which we observed as early as the second year of life in a child who had started to menstruate around her first birthday). Different behavior problems associated with precocious puberty may occur, unspecific in type rather than any specific syndrome, although that is clearly the exception rather than the rule.

Since the question of pharmacological treatment of young girls with idiopathic precocious puberty is controversial, preventive counseling and clinical management of the behavior should always be attempted without the use of drugs. However, in very young children, as in the range of one to five years, menstruation can become a serious psychological hazard and can disrupt normal psychological development to such a degree that a course of treatment with a relatively new pharmacological agent might become the smaller risk to overall well-being.

Precocious Puberty in Boys. Idiopathic precocious puberty occurs less frequently in boys than in girls. In boys, precocious pubertal development can occur in cases of untreated congenital adrenal hyperplasia, although untreated cases have become increasingly rare since early cortisone treatment has been known for thirty years or so to be effective in preventing early physical maturation. Analogous to precocious puberty in girls, boys may experience complete or incomplete sexual precocity. Complete sexual precocity means an abnormality of gonadotropin secretion that results in testicular growth with associated increased testosterone secretion and the accompanying results of testosterone action such as growth of the penis, sexual hair, and skeletal muscle accompanied by accelerated linear growth of skeleton maturation (Rosenfield, 1982). Incomplete sexual precocity reflects an abnormality of the adrenal cortex or testes and results in increased testosterone secretion which is independent of gonadotropin influence. The important thing is that any boy who shows signs of early development should be thoroughly evaluated by a pediatric endocrinologist. The age limit between early normal and abnormal puberty varies, but signs of penile enlargement prior to ten years of age may reflect precocious puberty. It is particularly important for boys with early development to be thoroughly investigated, since more boys than girls have a serious organic disorder as an etiology. Once it is established that the boy has idiopathic sexual precocity, the medical management is very similar to the one for the girl with the same condition. Generally, reassurance of the parents and patient and preventive follow-up every six months is all that is indicated.

Studies of the psychological development of precocious puberty in boys are rare and have shown that overt sexual behavior is typically not in advance of the chronological age, although erotic fantasies and masturbation may occur somewhat earlier than usual. Psychosexual development was found to be normal for boys (Money and Alexander, 1969; Money and Ehrhardt, 1972; Ehrhardt and Baker, 1974). The same principles of clinical and psychological management that we discussed for the girl with precocious puberty apply to the precociously developing boy (Ehrhardt, 1974).

DELAYED ADOLESCENCE. It is somewhat arbitrary where one places the cutoff mark between normal and delayed puberty. Many clinicians agree that the onset of puberty two to three years after the median age justifies concern and the label "delayed puberty." Individuals who are slow in other aspects of development such as in somatic growth and osseous development—constitutional growth delay—are more apt to have delayed adolescence. However, at times adolescents who are of normal statural growth also are delayed in their pubertal development. In contrast to patients with hypopituitary problems, males and females with delayed adolescence have an increase in height of at least two inches per year and have a growth pattern, if plotted on a growth curve, that is below but parallel to that of normal males and females. Gonadotropin concentrations in individuals with delayed adolescence will be low but consistent with the state of sexual development. It is assumed that delayed adolescence is the result of variability in the rate of maturation of the hypothalamic-pituitary set point (Rosenfield, 1982).

If the differential diagnosis has been made of delayed adolescence with no other associated medical problem, no pharmacological treatment is indicated except for those adolescents in whom psychological adjustment is seriously affected. The delayed adolescent boy seems to be more affected by being a slow maturer than the late maturing girl. This is true for delay within the normal range and for the abnormally slow developer. The psychological assessment and treatment of delayed puberty in males who also have short stature has been discussed in detail by Meyer-Bahlburg (see chap. 6). Therefore, it will not be repeated here. All types of psychological problems can occur and may have to be dealt with by a child psychiatrist or psychologist. In severe cases, treatment with testosterone on a temporary basis may be beneficial. Boys who are not developed by age fifteen are often affected enough that a treatment course with androgens is indicated. It is important to keep this as a last resort, however, since testosterone therapy may have a negative effect on growth because of the ultimate height-limiting influence; testosterone usually causes the advancement of skeletal maturation more rapidly than it does the acceleration of linear growth.

Late maturation in girls does not appear to have negative consequences on personality development compared to boys in long-term follow-up (McCandless, 1960). However, clinically one encounters very late developing girls who suffer as much as late maturing boys and therefore may require evaluation and supportive counseling (see for details the later discussion of Turner's syndrome).

Incongruous Pubertal Development

Some adolescents have to cope with unexpected and incongruous pubertal development that is in contrast to their own gender identity. Examples of these types of pubertal discrepancies are breast development, or gynecomastia, in boys and hairiness, or hirsutism, in girls. These are conspicuous deviations from a masculine or feminine body development and often are cause for confusion and shame in the affected adolescent.

GYNECOMASTIA IN BOYS. Some breast development occurs in 70% of boys during adolescence. Breast size can vary greatly and it is usually temporary, although it persists for two years in 27% of the cases and in almost 8% for three years (Nydick et al., 1961). Therefore, if gynecomastia is marked and ongoing, the adolescent boy should be evaluated and any endocrine cause that requires treatment should be ruled out. Typically, adolescent gynecomastia is associated with a decreased testosterone-to-estradiol ratio, presumably resulting from a transient imbalance in testosterone and estrogen production. Hormonal therapy, such as testosterone, makes the condition worse (Penny, 1982). Mastectomy is indicated only when the hyperplasia is very pronounced and persistent and when the gynecomastia causes severe psychological problems.

Boys with marked and persistent gynecomastia usually do not become gender disturbed. However, they may develop a serious body-image problem and secondary behavior disturbances such as withdrawal from their peers, avoiding any exposure of their body, and depression. Psychological assessment should follow a routine evaluation with special focus on psychosexual issues and body image (Money, 1968; Money and Ehrhardt, 1972). Counseling should always include sex education with explanations about sex-hormone production and effects on the body at puberty. Typically, reassurance is sufficient, although sometimes a mastectomy may be of relief and of great benefit to the affected adolescent.

HIRSUTISM IN GIRLS. The counterpart of gynecomastia in the male is hirsutism in the female. While the control of hair development during puberty is not entirely understood, hirsutism is usually taken as a clue to a high level of androgens. The normally much lower levels of androgen production in females result in the so-called female pattern of secondary sexual hair growth during puberty. There is no clear dividing line between the so-called normal female hair distribution and what might be regarded as excessive or more masculine. It is important to know that two types of body hair are distinguished—vellus and terminal. While the vellus hair is soft, short, and usually unpigmented, the terminal hair is longer, coarser, and full of pigment. At puberty in both sexes terminal hair will develop in the pubic area, as axillary hair, and to varying degrees on the limbs. Both genetic factors and levels of androgen will determine the subsequent amount of terminal-hair development in other body areas. Since boys produce a much higher level of androgens, they typically will show much more terminal hair in the beard region, the chest, the upper pubic triangle, and to varying degrees on other body sites. If an adolescent girl develops excessive hairiness, it usually occurs in the areas of masculine body hair sites, such as in the face or on the chest. Hirsutism may be a sign of a number of endocrine conditions such as Cushing's syndrome or the adrenogenital syndrome; therefore, a specialized diagnostic work-up is indicated.

An endocrine evaluation of hirsutism in an adolescent girl has to include a determination of her ethnic background, her family history, and a hormonal work-up. While the total number of hair follicles shows no racial variation, the type of hair produced under the influence of androgen varies for different populations. For example, Caucasians normally have more terminal hair on their bodies than Asians. The prominent body hair growth also varies between different families and with different hair color, for instance, blond and brunette girls often have less prominent body hair than dark-haired girls.

Cultural norms also may affect the perception of hair growth as abnormal. Current attitudes in Western societies equate hairlessness with femininity and hairiness with masculinity. Since most people do not represent the extremes, slight variations may be perceived as abnormal.

If indeed hirsutism is prominent and in the masculine distribution, and if no other endocrine abnormality has been established, the condition is typically called idiopathic hirsutism. Some investigators have stated that the term *idiopathic* is outdated, since a number of hormonal abnormalities have been determined for this condition. Simple hirsutism (Strickler and Warren, 1979) and "benign androgen excess syndrome" (Wise and O'Laughlin, 1978) have been suggested as better descriptive terms for these patients. The endocrinological abnormalities that have been described for hirsutism in females relate to various androgen abnormalities. The abnormality may be in plasma level, in production rate, or in an abnormal peripheral conversion of testosterone to dihydrotestosterone (see review by Callan, 1983). The source of abnormal androgen production may be either in the ovary or in the adrenal cortex. Dependent on the site of abnormal hormone production, different drugs will be used to either suppress excessive adrenal cortex or gonadal activity. Currently, estrogen-progestin combination pills are prescribed to at least in part suppress the gonadotropin release from the hypothalamic-pituitary axis and hence to inhibit ovarian androgen production. This treatment regimen has been reported to improve hirsutism in 70% of patients after six months (Casey, 1975). However, success is typically measured by the assessment of the lowered plasma testosterone level, rather than the disappearance of unwanted hairiness. While testosterone can be quite successfully suppressed, the outward physical appearance of excessive hair is much harder to eliminate. Another drug regimen is corticosteroid therapy. The rationale for the use of this type of drug regimen is the suppression of excessive androgen production from the adrenal cortex. However, also with this type of drug, a discrepancy between clinical response and improvement of the endocrinological measures has been reported. A combination of ovarian and adrenal suppression is also recommended by some endocrinologists.

In Europe the treatment with antiandrogenic drugs that interfere with the action of androgens at their target organs are widely used. Antiandrogenic drugs have been reported as successful in reducing the actual hair growth in 75% of the patients (Hammerstein and Cupceancu, 1969). In a comparative study between cyproterone acetate and oral contraceptives, it was found that the antiandrogenic drugs produced much more pronounced reduction in hair growth (Anderson, 1978). However, the treatment with cyproterone acetate is not available in the United States. All of the hormone drug therapies have side effects that need to be taken into consideration (Callan, 1983). There are a number of cosmetic procedures that are recommended and used by hirsute adolescent and adult women. They include bleaching and various mechanical methods of removing hair either temporarily or permanently (e. g., shaving, waxing, and electrolysis).

Psychologically, the analogous principle, as for gynecomastia in boys, applies for hirsutism in girls. Hormonal and physical masculinization does not masculinize the mind in a predetermined or automatic fashion (v. Zerssen et al., 1960; Money and Ehrhardt, 1972). There is an absence of systematic studies on the psychological effects of hirsutism in girls during adolescence, and there are only a few studies on adult women. Callan et al. (1980) assessed the behavior of hirsute women compared to a control group of women with minor dermatological complaints. No abnormalities in the hirsute group were found with respect to any of the psychological measures including an assessment of androgyny. Callan's study in Melbourne, Australia, agrees with our own clinical impressions, namely that a young girl who is faced with excessive hairiness may be mortified and upset but usually does not doubt her female gender identity or change her gender-appropriate behavior. However, it may be gravely upsetting to her body image and affect her response to other people, including a withdrawal from peer contacts and any relationships with boys. The most extreme reaction may be total self-isolation and avoidance because she is ashamed of exhibiting her body.

Assessment and clinical management of a girl with hirsutism should therefore include a screening for problems of body image, sexuality, and relationships to peers and erotic partners. Treatment has to include reassurance and desensitization if complete preoccupation with the development of excessive hair exists. Ideally, the behavioral management is carried out in close coordination with the endocrine and/or cosmetic therapy. At times, secondary problems develop and require psychotherapy.

Pubertal Failure

In the case of idiopathic precocious and delayed puberty, only timing is in error. The mechanism of pituitary-gonadal-sex hormone interplay is functioning normally, although its action is starting too early or too late. In other cases the defect is more permanent, so that puberty will never occur spontaneously. For those patients, it becomes of utmost importance for their psychological growth and development that puberty be induced by a sex-appropriate hormone regimen. Such patients often have additional problems like sterility, other physical disorders, and sometimes specific mental deficiencies in association with a particular clinical syndrome.

Some conditions of pubertal failure in females are due to a genetic abnormality of the sex chromosomes, as for instance in Turner's syndrome or androgen insensitivity (testicular feminizing) syndrome. In those cases, the child is born with normal female external genitalia and grows up looking like a normal girl throughout childhood, until the time when normal female puberty should occur but remains absent due to either gonadal failure or absence (after surgical removal in case of androgen insensitivity). In boys, pubertal failure occurs due to simple hyporchia or anorchia. This includes a number of clinical conditions with a defect in the gonads. Both boys and girls may require treatment for hypopituitarism if the problem is at the level of the pituitary rather than the ovaries and testes.

All of these conditions require replacement of lacking sex hormones to induce pubertal development. The timing and the type of sex-hormone therapy requires psychological guidance for the affected child and her or his family. Most children with pubertal failure have additional physical problems which also require psychological management (see chap. 6 for discussion of psychological evaluation and management for hypopituitarism and delayed adolescence; for psychological aspects of androgen insensitivity, see Money, 1968; Money and Ehrhardt, 1972; Ehrhardt and Meyer-Bahlburg, 1975; Lewis and Money, 1983; for hypogonadism in males, see chap. 6; Money and Ehrhardt, 1972; Ehrhardt and Meyer-Bahlburg, 1975).

This chapter will emphasize the psychological implications of pubertal failure in girls with Turner's syndrome. Their diagnostic and therapeutic management will be discussed in detail. Many of the same principles apply to the other syndromes of pubertal failure.

TURNER'S SYNDROME. Girls with Turner's syndrome are born with underdeveloped ovaries, but normal female external genitalia. The etiology of the gonadal defect is cytogenetic, and most individuals with Turner's syndrome have a 45, X karyotype or one of the variants of the abnormality in their sex chromosomes such as a mosaic pattern 45,X/46,XX or structural X abnormalities. The incidence of abnormalities in the sex chromosomal karyotype characterized by the loss of all or part of an X chromosome has been variously reported as 1 in 2,000 to 1 in 5,000 live born phenotypic females (Gerald, 1976; Hook and Hamerton, 1977). Since population screenings in the past used cruder methods than today's karyotyping, the incidence was probably frequently underestimated and therefore the incidence of Turner's syndrome is probably closer to the lower end of the range, i.e., 1 in 2,000 live female births.

The first description of the clinical features goes back to Henry Turner, who reported in 1938 seven cases of a rather uniform appearance in women who had short stature, lack of pubertal development, webbing of the neck, low posterior hairline, and increased carrying angle of the elbows (Turner, 1938). The link between these phenotypic descriptions and the X-chromosome defect came only with the introduction of genetic techniques, and today it is known that the clinical phenotype goes together with many X-chromosome abnormalities and the 45,X karyotype may represent only 50 to 60% of all cases (see review of incidence and etiology of the syndrome by Lippe, 1982).

The etiology of this condition is not entirely understood. The number of live births with X-chromosomal abnormalities represents only a small fraction of those who were conceived and spontaneously aborted during embryonic development. It is estimated that most XO embryos do not survive beyond 28 weeks' gestation and that the XO karyotype occurs in one of fifteen spontaneous abortions (Warburton et al., 1980). Etiologic factors for Turner's syndrome that have been examined previously include birth order and sibling sex and twinning. None of these seem to be significantly associated with the syndrome. Turner's syndrome does not seem to affect more than one individual in one family as a rule, although X-chromosome structural malformations that lead to other clinical syndromes may have an increased risk of recurrence. There is also not a significantly increased parental age. The role of potential environmental factors, such as prenatal drug abuse of the parents has to date not been systematically investigated.

Girls with Turner's syndrome may have many abnormalities or only the cardinal features which consist of short stature, lack of spontaneous pubertal development, and infertility. The associated features may include webbing of the neck, cardiovascular anomalies, structural abnormalities of the kidneys, and otitis media. It is important to stress that these secondary features only affect a subgroup and not necessarily the same individual. A thorough work-up of a child with Turner's syndrome, however, should include checkups of these described anomalies.

Most children with Turner's syndrome get diagnosed sometime in middle childhood when they fall behind in statural growth. A few are diagnosed at birth; most of those have one or more of the associated features, such as webbing of the neck or lymphedema of the feet. During childhood many girls with Turner's syndrome only need attention to their growth pattern. Good medical management includes the referral to a pediatric endocrinologist. The cause of the slow growth is not entirely understood, although a component appears to be a lack of the pubertal growth spurt. Untreated patients with Turner's syndrome would not have the normal female pubertal growth spurt but would grow at a slow rate into their late teens. It has become customary at most medical centers to treat girls with Turner's syndrome with a mild androgen before estrogen replacement therapy is instituted to induce secondary sex characteristics. Usually between the ages of ten and twelve years, depending on the degree of short stature and the expression of concern, growth velocity data are reviewed and the patient who is growing at a subnormal rate (less than 5 cm per year) and is more than two standard deviations below the mean in height is typically considered a good candidate for therapy with androgenic steroids. While the beneficial effects of androgenic therapy before estrogen replacement treatment are difficult to assess, there are presently several studies comparing different treatment regimens in Turner's syndrome that have concluded that the patients with a 45,X karyotype who did not receive androgen therapy did not reach as tall an adult height as those who did (Lippe, 1982).

The initiation of estrogen replacement therapy varies from case to case as to age. In the past, estrogen therapy was often delayed in order not to compromise growth. However, most endocrinologists would agree that low-dose estrogen replacement therapy in girls with a bone age of eleven years or more does not significantly compromise ultimate height. Adult height in patients with Turner's syndrome varies but is typically between 4'6" and 5'. Estrogen replacement therapy is initially prescribed continuously, and after about six to nine months when uterine growth and endometrial development has occurred, cyclic therapy is prescribed with both Premarin and the progesterone, Provera. The cycle consists of initially Premarin alone, subsequently Provera (for instance, from the seventeenth to the twenty-third day in conjunction with Premarin). Subsequently both drugs are stopped and menses usually ensues one or two days after and lasts four to five days. The specific protocol of dose and type of estrogen or progesterone varies, but essentially the principle of both sex hormones administered in a cyclic fashion to imitate the normal hormonal menstrual cycle is observed in all treatment approaches.

Sex-hormone replacement therapy induces breast development, monthly menstrual bleeding, and vaginal lubrication. However, it of course does not change the chances for fertility.

Girls with Turner's syndrome typically are followed at regular intervals once the diagnosis has been made, which may be every six months during childhood and more frequently once any sex-hormone treatment has been started. During puberty when secondary sex characteristics and menstruation have been induced, the adolescent girl with Turner's syndrome should continue to be followed by the pediatric endocrinologist or eventually by a gynecologist who does breast examinations and regular pelvic examinations.

Very recently, growth hormone is being used as a treatment for short stature in Turner's syndrome. At this point, no results are reported that document a significant beneficial effect on statural growth.

Psychosexual development in girls with Turner's syndrome does not differ from other girls. Despite the lack of gonadal development with the concomitant lack of exposure to fetal gonadal hormones, female gender identity in childhood develops normally (Shaffer, 1963; Ehrhardt et al., 1970). The primary concern of parents and children with Turner's syndrome is their slow statural growth which, however, does not typically interfere with prepubertal adjustment in a dramatic way leading to marked psychopathology. Girls with Turner's syndrome were found to be interested in the same toys, games, peers, friendships, etc., as matched normal controls. While adolescence, especially if sex-hormone replacement therapy is initiated relatively late, is often a critical time and may lead to more problems in adjustment, psychosexual development remains feminine with no goals and interests different from other females. Our knowledge on adult development in women with Turner's syndrome is incomplete because of lack of long-term studies. The existing evidence comes from a study by Nielsen et al. (1977) in Denmark which suggested that a significant number of patients were still living at home during adulthood and only 28% of all patients who were over age eighteen were married compared to 63% in the unaffected sisters. Systematic data on sexual functioning in adulthood are not available as of yet. The question of the adequacy of sex-hormone replacement therapy in relation to sexual functioning is an important one for future investigation.

From the existing evidence, it appears that psychosexual development can proceed along normal lines in spite of defective gonads, lack of spontaneous gonadal hormone secretion, and infertility.

The second area of interest is behavior adjustment and psychopathology in girls with Turner's syndrome. Obviously it depends on whether the child has to cope with multiple birth defects or predominately with the three cardinal features of being short, having to be treated with pubertal replacement hormones, and infertility. During childhood, girls with Turner's syndrome usually adjust surprisingly well. Short stature may become an issue in middle childhood and may lead to behavior problems as in other slow-growing children (see chap. 6). Money (1976) has referred to the personality style of many girls with Turner's syndrome as "inertia of emotional arousal" and has suggested that their compliance and lack of behavior problems during childhood may be a beneficial trait which enables them to tolerate the adversities of their condition. The same trait was reported in other studies when girls with Turner's syndrome scored low on questionnaires that measure neuroticism, spontaneity, activity, and enthusiasm (Shaffer, 1963: Baekgaard et al., 1978).

The picture changes somewhat during the second decade. It appears that the psychological risks for girls with Turner's syndrome increase markedly at the time when their peers go into spontaneous puberty. The timing of induced puberty is crucial because it will determine how long they will be out of step with their peers regarding their appearance. It appears that having to cope with looking younger and immature in addition to being shorter than one's peers presents a significant additional risk for psychopathology. In a clinical follow-up study of seventy-three girls and women with Turner's syndrome ranging over a wide age span, Money and Mittenthal (1970) stressed the risk of delayed pubertal development on psychological adjustment. They compared two groups of girls between the ages of fourteen and eighteen, one treated with estrogen versus one still untreated, and found that environmental response to the immature group was very different, increasing the risk of behavior problems. Girls with immature appearance were also significantly less likely to begin dating and establishing romantic friendships.

In a prospective study in Finland, twenty-six girls with Turner's syndrome were followed over several years during adolescence. In the older girls, estrogen replacement was given between ages 15.3 and 19.9. Psychological evaluation of patients up to age 12 confirmed earlier clinical impressions that many patients with Turner's syndrome are well-adjusted in childhood. However, a turning point for many was age 13, at which time the patient group started to fall behind in psychological maturation and often became loners or developed more severe pathology. Those patients who still were undeveloped at age 14 were often afflicted with marked anxiety, serious behavior problems, and a tendency to withdraw. The substitution therapy was found to initiate the process of adolescence and to be of emotional help to the girls (Perheentupa et al., 1975; Taipale, 1979).

Psychopathology can express itself in a variety of problems rather than being specific to one particular disorder. An association between anorexia nervosa and Turner's syndrome has been described (Kron et al., 1977). At this point, however, it is not clear whether indeed anorexia nervosa is increased in girls with Turner's syndrome compared to normal girls. The evidence on adult adjustment is mainly based on clinical studies without adequate controls. It has been described that women with Turner's syndrome can fulfill many different types of professional positions, marry, adopt children, and lead productive lives. However, it is unknown what the rates of good versus poor adjustment are. While psychiatric disorders that meet diagnostic criteria may not be increased judging from the evidence by Nielsen et al. (1977) and our own ongoing project (Downey et al., 1983), there seems to be a tendency for Turner's syndrome women to suffer from "negative symptoms," which means that without troubling others in their environment, they still fail to achieve a satisfactory adult adjustment and often lead lonely, isolated lives.

Intelligence and mental functioning in patients with Turner's syndrome has been the topic of many studies. From all available evidence so far, it appears that the intelligence of persons with Turner's syndrome is usually normal rather than in the moderately or severely retarded range. Girls with Turner's syndrome are not more often represented in institutions for the mentally retarded (Ferguson-Smith, 1965; Palmer and Reichmann, 1976); they are also not different in overall intelligence from their unaffected siblings (Garron, 1977). This is in contrast to earlier reports based on clinical case examples and unrepresentative samples.

Turner's syndrome is associated with a specific pattern of strengths and weaknesses in mental functioning. Many patients with this syndrome have difficulties in visual-motor coordination, motor learning (Shaffer, 1962; Money, 1964; Alexander et al., 1966), spatio-temporal processing (Silbert et al., 1977), and sense of direction and perceptual stability (Waber, 1979). These specific difficulties appear more frequently in patients with Turner's syndrome than usually observed but are not obligatory associations with the other clinical features. The specific features of these deficits vary in different studies dependent on the testing instrument and data analysis, but most studies agree that a common pattern in Turner's syndrome patients is a significantly lower nonverbal IQ compared to the patient's verbal IQ (Shaffer, 1962; Money, 1964; Theilgaard, 1972). The data on mental functioning in Turner's syndrome make it mandatory that an individual patient be assessed carefully with standard psychometric testing and the results be evaluated not only from the full-scale IQ alone, but always with special attention to the verbal IQ versus the performance IQ and to specific aspects of mental functioning. Intellectual patterns have not been found to correlate with specific physical stigmata (Money and Granoff, 1965).

Psychological management of Turner's syndrome has to include the patient, her parents, and often her unaffected siblings. Ideally, endocrine patients are managed by a team approach. The child psychiatrist, psychologist, or social worker who works with patients of this type should deal with them in close coordination with the pediatric endocrinologist. In such a setting, the typical referral is at the time of diagnosis. The age of the child at initial diagnosis may, of course, vary and can be as early as the time of birth. More frequently, however, the referral to a specialist is made when the child falls behind in her statural growth and the pediatrician wants to have an expert consultation. If the child is seven, eight, or nine years of age, the diagnosis is typically only communicated to the parents. If in conjunction the parents are seen by a behavioral specialist, preventive counseling can be started immediately. How many sessions are needed will depend on the educational level of the parents and on their own degree of personal stability and strength of coping with the information. It is best to start with their current major concern at the time of referral which is typically their daughter's growth problem. One should reinforce what the endocrinologist already has told them, namely that their daughter will be a slow grower but that hormonal treatment will help to increase statural growth with an ultimate prognosis in the range between 4' 6" and 5'. The various treatment regimens should be explained and discussed. If the parents want to go for one of the currect experimental regimens with growth hormones, it is important to stress that they and their daughter should not get their hopes unduly raised. So far, none of the available hormonal treatments have dramatic effects on growth in the child with Turner's syndrome, and therefore treatment success has to be viewed realistically. An endocrine success, which may be an additional two inches, can be viewed as failure if the parents and the child expected a much more dramatic response. Rotnem et al. (1979) reported that children with hypopituitary growth-hormone deficiency who were treated and then disappointed due to their unrealistic expectations subsequently became angry, pessimistic, and negativistic. We counsel parents on how to deal with teasing and immaturity in their children, very much along the lines of the approach to other children with short stature (see chap. 6).

The psychological aspects of the condition should be discussed as well as the medical diagnosis. It is crucial that the clinician who works with families with children who have chronic diseases be informed about the newest research data and not transmit misinformation, such as outdated and erroneous knowledge on an increased risk of mental retardation. Although reports have been published for twenty years stating that girls with Turner's syndrome typically have normal intelligence, parents are still being told that their child will probably be mentally retarded. This is particularly detrimental if they are given this misinformation at birth because it can affect the parents' behavior toward the child and have negative consequences in terms of a "self-fulfilling prophecy." Exemplifying this principle is the dramatic case of a family who had been told at birth to expect mental retardation. The prediction was never corrected. When the child was tested at age twelve, she scored with a full IQ of slightly above average but behaved like a child who was mildy retarded with no ambition and no confidence in her abilities.

The information on specific strengths and weaknesses is best given to the parents once the child has had a psychometric evaluation. If she shows the usual pattern of better verbal abilities than space-form perception, counseling should include the fact that she might need special help in geometry and assistance with her sense of directon and with other aspects of visual-motor coordination. It is good, though, to stress that the deficit typically is very specific and does not preclude planning for a wide variety of vocational choices.

To make sure that parents and patients understand the information that has been given them by various clinicians, it is very helpful to have them repeat back what they have ᵈ (Money, 1968). Only then will the clinician know what distortion may have been made ⁻ocess of communication. It also may help to detect specific anxieties and doubts that ᵊt been adequately dealt with.

Children with Turner's syndrome who are diagnosed in middle childhood need to be given information that is accurate but age appropriate. Ideally, a rapport is established with the child and maintained in occasional follow-up visits coordinated with the pediatric endocrine follow-up, so that installments of information about Turner's syndrome can be given in small amounts. Usually by age ten or eleven, the child with Turner's syndrome should have received an adequate understanding about her medical condition. It is at this time that her peers will begin to talk about puberty, adolescence, and sexual development. Rather than falling behind in pubertal development and waiting in vain for the first signs of sexual maturation, the child with Turner's syndrome should have an adequate understanding of normal sexual development and knowledge about her particular condition, which includes information about having been born with "underdeveloped ovaries" that do not produce enough hormones to make her breasts grow and have her start to menstruate. This information can be linked to the fact that her doctor will help her achieve these pubertal milestones by estrogen and progesterone treatment.

The timing issue will be discussed with the reassurance that she herself has a part in the decision process. If there is a waiting period, the girl with Turner's syndrome and her parents should be counseled about choosing adequate clothes to make her look more like other adolescents rather than like a child. The installment about most likely becoming a parent by adoption rather than pregnancy may be given somewhat later than the information on hormonal treatment for pubertal development, or it may be linked to the same part of her diagnosis. It is important to stress, however, whenever the issue of parenthood is being dealt with that the patient can expect to have a normal sex life and that many other patients with the same condition have gotten married and have not been rejected because of their particular ovarian problem.

Information about diagnosis should always be linked to guidance on how to talk about it to other people, such as future boyfriends or husbands. Usually it is best for the girl with Turner's syndrome only to confide in close friends or close relatives and boys or men she feels serious enough about to consider marriage. If many people in one's environment know a significant part about one's medical condition, especially if that condition includes the reproductive or sexual organs, a danger of stigmatization exists that may interfere with peer and erotic relationships.

The communication about the diagnosis and preventive counseling for parents follow the same principles if the child is diagnosed during the newborn period rather than in middle childhood. However, it is particularly important not to transmit erroneous information that may influence in a profound way the rearing of their child. It also should be emphasized that giving parents a complete list of all possible stigmata that may occur with Turner's syndrome may be traumatic and not particularly helpful (Lippe, 1982). Some families have gone through the experience of having an overzealous physician give them a slide demonstration of many of the abnormalities associated with Turner's syndrome. If that information is then linked to erroneous predictions about mental retardation and an unfavorable behavior prognosis, some parents may be so traumatized that they will have serious difficulty accepting and raising their child.

In addition to preventive counseling, families may need special treatment for problems that girls with Turner's syndrome may develop, sometimes specific to their growth disturbance or their lack of puberty, and sometimes unrelated or secondary, such as depression, withdrawal, or school problems. Sibling rivalry may become a problem, especially in families with a sister close in age who has no physical stigmata to cope with. On the other hand, the normal sibling may develop concerns about her own normalcy and may envy the attention her sister gets from specialists and her parents. In that case, family therapy can be extremely helpful. Support groups of parents who have children with the same medical problem can be helpful to exchange information and to offer reassurance. Sometimes, however, they can also be anxiety producing and may raise the level of insecurity.

Conclusion

The second decade of human development is marked by many changes, in particular by the event of puberty with its behavioral sequelae. Children and adolescents who have to cope with pubertal anomalies are in need of specialized medical and psychological care which requires up-to-date knowledge of diagnostic and therapeutic facts. Specialized preventive counseling and guidance of families with children who have to cope with pubertal disorders is effective and satisfying, since it often contributes to an appropriate behavior adjustment without the development of psychiatric symptomatology.

References

Achenbach, T. M. 1981. *Child behavior checklist for ages 4 to 16*. Rev. ed. Burlington, Vt.: University of Vermont Associates in Psychiatry.

Alexander, D., Ehrhardt, A. A., and Money, J. 1966. Defective figure drawing, geometric and human, in Turner's syndrome. *J. Nerv. Men. Dis.*, 142:161–167.

Anderson, J. A. R. 1978. An assessment of (1) cyproterone acetate and (2) ethinyloestradiol and lynoestrenol (Minilyn) in the treatment of idiopathic hirsutism. *Brit. J. Derm.*, 99:545–552.

Baekgaard, W., Nyborg, H., and Nielsen, J. 1978. Neuroticism and extraversion in Turner's syndrome. *J. Abnorm. Psychol.*, 87:583–586.

Bidlingmaier, F., Butenandt, O., and Knorr, D. 1977. Plasma gonadotropins and estrogens in girls with idiopathic precocious puberty. *Ped. Res.*, 11:91–94.

Bierich, J. R. 1975. Sexual precocity. In *Disorders of puberty*. Clin. in Endocrin. and Metab., vol. 4, no. 1, ed. J. R. Bierich, pp. 107–142. London: W. B. Saunders.

Boyar, R. M., Finkelstein, J. W., David, R., Roffwarg, H., Kapen, S., Weitzman, E. D., and Hellman, L. 1973. Twenty-four hour patterns of plasma luteinizing hormone and follicle stimulating hormone in sexual precocity. *N. Eng. J. Med.*, 289: 282–286.

Buffery, A. W. H., and Gray, J. A. 1972. Sex differences in the development of spatial and linguistic skills. In *Gender differences: Their ontogeny and significance,* ed. C. Ounsted, and D. C. Taylor, pp. 123–157. Edinburgh: Churchill Livingstone.

Callan, A. W. 1983. Idiopathic hirsutism. In *Handbook of psychosomatic obstetrics and gynaecology,* ed. L. Dennerstein, and G. D. Burrows, pp. 413–443. Amsterdam: Elsevier.

Callan, A. W., Dennerstein, L., Burrows, G. D., and Hyman, G. 1980. The psychoendocrinology of hirsutism. In *Obstetrics, gynaecology, and psychiatry: Proceedings of the Seventh Annual Congress of the Australian Society for Psychosomatic Obstetrics and Gynaecology,* ed. L. Dennerstein, and G. D. Burrows, pp. 43–54. Melbourne, Australia: University of Melbourne.

Casey, J. H. 1975. Chronic treatment regimens for hirsutism in women: Effect on blood production rate of testosterone and hair growth. *Clin. Endocrin.*, 4:313–325.

Crowley, W. F., Jr., Comite, F., Vale, W., Rivier, J., Loriaux, D. L., and Cutler, G. B., Jr. 1981. Therapeutic use of pituitary desensitization with a long-acting LHRH agonist: A potential new treatment for idiopathic precocious puberty. *J. Clin. Endocrin. Metab.*, 52: 370–372.

Donovan, B. T., and van der Werff ten Bosch, J. J. 1965. *Physiology of puberty.* London: Edward Arnold.

Douglas, J. W. B., and Ross, J. M. 1964. Age of puberty related to educational ability, attainment, and school leaving age. *J. Child Psychol. Psych.,* 5:185-195.

Downey, J. I., Ehrhardt, A. A., Morishima, A., and Bell, J. J. 1983. Psychosexual milestones in women with congenital estrogen deficiency, gonadal dysgenesis, and infertility. Paper presented at the ninth annual meeting of the International Academy of Sex Research, November 22-26, Arden House, Harriman, N.Y.

Ehrhardt, A. A. 1974. What precautions should be taken with the sexually precocious boy? *Med. Aspects Hum. Sex.,* 8:147.

Ehrhardt, A. A., and Baker, S. W. 1974. Fetal androgen, human CNS differentiation, and behavior sex differences. In *Sex differences in behavior,* ed. R. C. Friedman, R. M. Richart, and R. L. Vande Wiele, pp. 53-76. New York: Wiley.

Ehrhardt, A. A., Greenberg, N., and Money, J. 1970. Female gender identity and absence of fetal gonadal hormones: Turner's syndrome. *The Johns Hopkins Med. J.,* 126:237-248.

Ehrhardt, A. A., and McCauley, E. 1975. The sexually precocious girl: Brief guide to office counseling. *Med. Aspects Hum. Sex.,* 9:63-64.

Ehrhardt, A. A., and Meyer-Bahlburg, H. F. L. 1975. Psychological correlates of abnormal pubertal development. In *Disorders of puberty.* Clin. in Endocrin. and Metab., vol. 4, ed. J. Bierich, pp. 207-222.

Ehrhardt, A. A., and Meyer-Bahlburg, H. F. L. 1981. The effects of prenatal hormones on gender identity, sex-dimorphic behavior, sexual orientation and cognition. *Science,* 211:1312-1318.

Ehrhardt, A. A., Meyer-Bahlburg, H. F. L., Bell, J. J., Cohen, S. F., Healey, J. M., Stiel, R., Feldman, J. F., Morishima, A., and New, M. I. 1984. Idiopathic precocious puberty in girls: Psychiatric follow-up in adolescence. *J. Am. Acad. Child Psych.,* 23:23-33.

Faiman, C., Winter, J. S. D., and Reyes, F. I. 1976. Patterns of gonadotrophins and gonadal steroids throughout life. *Clin. Obstet. Gynaecol.,* 3:467-483.

Ferguson-Smith, M. A. 1965. Karyotype-phenotype correlations in gonadal dysgenesis and their bearing on the pathogenesis of malformations. *J. Med. Genet.,* 2:142-155.

Garron, D. C. 1977. Intelligence among persons with Turner's syndrome. *Beh. Genet.,* 7:105-127.

Gerald, P. S. 1976. Sex chromosome disorders. *N. Eng. J. Med.,* 294:706-708.

Graham, P., and Rutter, M. 1977. Adolescent disorders. In *Child psychiatry: Modern approaches,* ed. M. Rutter, and L. Hersov, pp. 407-427. Oxford: Blackwell Scientific.

Halverson, H. M. 1940. Genital and sphincter behavior of the male infant. *J. Genet. Psychol.,* 56:95-136.

Hamburg, B. A. 1974. Early adolescence: A specific and stressful stage of the life cycle. In *Coping and adaptation,* ed. G. V. Coelho, D. A. Hamburg, and J. E. Adams, pp. 101-124. New York: Basic Books.

Hammerstein, J., and Cupceancu, B. 1969. The treatment of hirsutism with cyproterone acetate. *Deutsche Medizinische Wochenschrift,* 94:629-634.

Hohlweg, W., and Dohrn, M. 1932. Uber die Beziehungen zwischen Hypophysenvorderlappen und Keimdrüsen. *Klin. Wochenschrift,* 11:233-235.

Hook, E. B., and Hamerton, J. L. 1977. The frequency of chromosomal abnormalities detected in consecutive newborn studies—differences between studies: Results by sex and severity of phenotypic involvement. In *Population cytogenetics,* ed. E. B. Hook, and I. H. Porter, pp. 63-79. New York: Academic Press.

Jones, M. C., and Bayley, M. 1950. Physical maturing among boys as related to behavior. *J. Educat. Psychol.,* 41:129-148.

Jones, M. C., and Mussen, P. H. 1958. Self-conceptions, motivations, and interpersonal attitudes of early and late maturing girls. *Child Dev.,* 29:491-501.

Kaplan, S. A., Ling, S. M., and Irani, N. G. 1968. Idiopathic isosexual precocity: Therapy with Medroxyprogesterone. *Am. J. Dis. Child.,* 116:591-598.

Katchadourian, H. 1977. *The biology of adolescence.* San Francisco: W. H. Freeman.

Kauli, R., Pertzelan, A., Prager-Lewin, R., Grünebaum, M., and Laron, Z. 1976. Cyproterone acetate in treatment of precocious puberty. *Arch. Dis. Child.,* 51:202-208.

Kinsey, A. C., Pomeroy, W. B., Martin, C. E., and Gebhard, P. H. 1953. *Sexual behavior in the human female.* Philadelphia: W. B. Saunders.

Kohen-Raz, R. 1974. Physiological maturation and mental growth at pre-adolescence and puberty. *J. Child Psychol. Psych.,* 15:199-213.

Kron, L., Katz, J. L., Gorzynski, G., and Weiner, H. 1977. Anorexia nervosa and gonadal dysgenesis. Further evidence of a relationship. *Arch. Gen. Psych.,* 34:332-335.

Kulin, H. E. 1972. Endocrine changes at puberty. In *Pediatrics,* ed. H. B. Barnett, and A. H. Einhorn, pp. 1120-1122. New York: Appleton-Century-Crofts.

Levitzky, S. E., and Domash, L. 1978. Psychological maladjustment in a child with premature pubarche. *Mt. Sinai J. Med.,* 45:125-127.

Levy, J. 1976. Cerebral lateralization and spatial ability. *Beh. Genet.,* 6:171-188.

Lewis, V. G., and Money, J. 1983. Gender-identity/role: G-I/R Part A: XY (androgen-insensitivity) syndrome and XX (Rokitansky) syndrome in vaginal atresia compared. In *Handbook of psychosomatic obstetrics and gynaecology,* ed. L. Dennerstein, and G. D. Burrows, pp. 51-60. Amsterdam: Elsevier.

Lippe, B. M. 1982. Primary ovarian failure. In *Clinical pediatric and adolescent endocrinology,* ed. S. A. Kaplan, pp. 269-299. Philadelphia: W. B. Saunders.

Ljung, D. B. 1965. *The adolescent spurt in mental growth.* Uppsala: Almqvist.

Maccoby, E. E., and Jacklin, C. M. 1974. *The psychology of sex differences.* Standford, Calif.: Stanford University Press.

Masterson, J. F. 1967. *The psychiatric dilemma of adolescence.* London: Churchill.

McCandless, B. R. 1960. Rate of development, body build, and personality. *Psychiat. Res. Rep.,* 13:42-57.

Meyer-Bahlburg, H. F. L. 1980. Sexuality in early adolescence. In *Handbook of human sexuality,* ed. B. B. Wolman, and J. Money, pp. 61-82. Englewood Cliffs, N.J.: Prentice-Hall.

Meyer-Bahlburg, H. F. L., and Ehrhardt, A. A. 1982. Prenatal sex hormones and human aggression: Review and new data on progestogen effects. *Aggr. Beh.,* 8:39-62.

Meyer-Bahlburg, H. F. L., Ehrhardt, A. A., Cohen, S. F., Healey, J. M., Bell, J. J., Morishima, A., and New, M. I. 1982. Precocious puberty and female sexuality. Paper presented at the annual meeting of the Society for the Scientific Study of Sex, November 12-14, San Francisco, Calif.

Money, J. 1964. Two cytogenetic syndromes: Psychologic comparisons. 1. Intelligence and specific-factor quotients. *J. Psychiat. Res.,* 2:223-231.

Money, J. 1968. *Sex errors of the body.* Baltimore: John Hopkins Press.

Money, J. 1976. Turner's syndrome: Principles of therapy. *Curr. Psychiat. Ther.,* 16:21-28.

Money, J., and Alexander, D. 1969. Psychosexual development and absence of homosexuality in males with precocious puberty: Review of 18 cases. *J. Nerv. Men. Dis.,* 148:111-123.

Money, J., and Clopper, R. R., Jr. 1974. Psychosocial and psychosexual aspects of errors of pubertal onset and development. *Hum. Bio.,* 46:173-181.

Money, J., and Ehrhardt, A. A. 1972. *Man and woman, boy and girl: The differentiation and dimorphism of gender identity from conception to maturity.* Baltimore: Johns Hopkins University Press.

Money, J., and Granoff, D. 1965. IQ and the somatic stigmata of Turner's syndrome. *Am. J. Men. Def.,* 70:69-77.

Money, J., Lewis, V. G., Ehrhardt, A. A., and Drash, P. W. 1967. IQ impairment and elevation in endocrine and related cytogenetic disorders. In *Psychopathology of mental development,* ed. J. Zubin, and G. A. Jervis, pp. 22-27. New York: Grune and Stratton.

Money, J., and Mittenthal, S. 1970. Lack of personality pathology in Turner's syndrome: Relation to cytogenetics, hormones, and physique. *Beh. Genet.,* 1:43-56.

Money, J., and Neill, J. 1967. Precocious puberty, IQ, and school acceleration. *Clin. Ped.,* 6:277-280.

Money, J., and Walker, P. A. 1971. Psychosexual development, maternalism, nonpromiscuity, and body image in 15 females with precocious puberty. *Arch. Sex. Beh.,* 1:45-60.

Mussen, P. H., and Jones, M. C. 1957. Self-conceptions, motivations, and interpersonal attitudes of late-and early-maturing boys. *Child Dev.,* 28:243-256.

Reiter, E. O., Kaplan, S. L., Conte, F. A., and Grumbach, M. M. 1975. Responsivity of pituitary gonadotropes to luteinizing hormone-releasing factor in idiopathic precocious puberty, precocious thelarche, precocious adrenarche, and in patients treated with medroxyprogesterone acetate. *Ped. Res.,* 9:111-116.

Reiter, E. O., Fuldauer, V. G., and Root, A. W. 1976. Effect of infusion of gonadotropin releasing hormone upon plasma concentrations of sex hormones in prepubertal and pubertal males. *Steroids,* 28:829-835.

Reuben, M. S., and Manning, G. R. 1922. Precocious puberty. *Arch. Ped.,* 39:769-785.

Reuben, M. S., and Manning, G. R. 1923. Precocious puberty. *Arch. Ped.,* 40:27-44.

Rosenfield, R. L. 1982. The ovary and female sexual maturation. In *Clinical pediatric and adolescent endocrinology,* ed. S. A. Kaplan, pp. 217-268. Philadelphia: W. B. Saunders.

Rotnem, D., Cohen, D. J., Hintz, R., and Genel, M. 1979. Psychological sequelae of relative "treatment failure" for children receiving human growth hormone replacement. *J. Am. Acad. Child Psych.,* 18:505-520.

Rutter, M. 1971. Normal psychosexual development. *J. Child Psychol. Psych.,* 11:259-283.

Rutter, M., Graham, P., Chadwick, O. F. D., and Yule, W. 1976. Adolescent turmoil: Fact or fiction? *J. Child Psychol. Psych.,* 17:35-56.

Shaffer, D. 1974. Suicide in childhood and early adolescence. *J. Child Psychol. Psych.,* 15:275-291.

Shaffer, J. W. 1962. A specific cognitive deficit observed in gonadal aplasia (Turner's syndrome). *J. Clin. Psychol.,* 18:403-406.

Shaffer, J. W. 1963. Masculinity-femininity and other personality traits in gonadal aplasia (Turner's syndrome). In *Advances in sex research,* ed. H. Beigel, pp. 219-232. New York: Hoeber.

Silbert, A., Wolff, P. H., and Lilienthal, J. 1977. Spatial and temporal processing in patients with Turner's syndrome. *Beh. Genet.,* 7:11-21.

Solyom, A. E., Austad, C. C., and Bacon, G. E. 1982. Precocious sexual development in girls during the first three years of life. In *The special infant,* ed. J. M. Stack, pp. 17-43. New York: Human Sciences Press.

Strickler, R. C., and Warren, J. C. 1979. Hirsutism: Diagnosis and management. In *Yearbook of obstetrics and gynecology,* ed. R. M. Pitkin, and F. J. Zlatnick, pp. 311-334. Chicago: Yearbook Medical Publishers.

Taipale, V. 1979. *Adolescence in Turner's syndrome.* Helsinki, Finland: Children's Hospital, University of Helsinki.

Tanner, J. M. 1962. *Growth at adolescence.* 2nd ed. Oxford: Blackwell Scientific.

Tanner, J. M. 1970. Physical growth. In *Carmichael's manual of child psychology,* ed. P. H. Mussen. vol. 1, 3rd ed., pp. 77-155. New York: Wiley.

Tanner, J. M. 1974. Sequence and tempo in the somatic changes in puberty. In *The Control of the onset of puberty*, ed. M. M. Grumbach, G. D. Grave, and F. E. Mayer, pp. 448-470. New York: Wiley.

Theilgaard, A. 1972. Cognitive style and gender role in persons with sex chromosome aberrations. *Dan. Med. Bull.*, 19:276-286.

Turner, H. 1938. A syndrome of infantilism, congenital webbed neck, and cubitus valgus. *Endocrin.*, 23:566-574.

van der Werff ten Bosch, J. J. 1975. Isosexual precocity. In *Endocrine and genetic diseases of childhood and adolescence*, 2nd ed., ed. L. I. Gardner, pp. 619-639. Philadelphia: W. B. Saunders.

v. Zerssen, D., Meyer, A. E., and Ahrens, D. 1960. Klinische, biochemische und psychologische Untersuchungen an Patientinnen mit gewöhnlichem Hirsutismus. *Deutsches Archiv für klinische Medizin*, 206:334-360.

Waber, D. P. 1979. Neuropsychological aspects of Turner's syndrome. *Dev. Med. Child Neurol.*, 21:58-70.

Warburton, D., Kline, J., Stein, Z., and Susser, M. 1980. Monosomy X: A chromosomal anomaly associated with young maternal age. *Lancet* 1 (January), 167-169.

Weatherley, D. 1964. Self-perceived rate of physical maturation and personality in late adolescence. *Child Dev.*, 35:1197-1210.

Nielson, J., Nyborg, H., and Dahl, G. 1977. Turner's syndrome. *Acta Jutlandica*, XLV:1-190. Medicine series 21.

Nydick, M., Bustos, J., Dale, J. H., Jr., and Rawson, R. W. 1961. Gynecomastia in adolescent boys. *J. Am. Med. Assoc.*, 178:449-454.

O'Connor, J., Shelley, E. M., and Stern, L. O. 1974. Behavioral rhythms related to the menstrual cycle. In *Biorhythms and human reproduction*, ed. M. Ferin, F. Halberg, R. M. Richart, and R. L. Vande Wiele, pp. 309-324. New York: Wiley.

Odell, W. D., and Swerdloff, R. S. 1976. Etiologies of sexual maturation: A model system based on the sexually maturing rat. *Rec. Prog. Horm. Res.*, 32:245-288.

Palmer, C. G., and Reichmann, A. 1976. Chromosomal and clinical findings in 110 females with Turner syndrome. *Human Genet.*, 35:35-49.

Penny, R. 1982. Disorders of the testes. In *Clinical pediatric and adolescent endocrinology*, ed. S. A. Kaplan, pp. 300-326. Philadelphia: W. B. Saunders.

Perheentupa, J., Lenko, H. L., Nevalainen, I., Niittymäki, M., Söderholm, A., and Taipale, V. 1975. Hormonal treatment of Turner's syndrome. *Acta Paed. Scand.*, 24-25.

Radfar, N., Ansusingha, K., and Kenny, F. M. 1976. Circulating bound and free estradiol and estrone during normal growth and development and in premature thelarche and isosexual precocity. *J. Ped.*, 89:719-723.

Weissman, M. M., and Klerman, G. L. 1979. Sex differences and the epidemiology of depression. In *Gender and disordered behavior*, ed. E. S. Gomberg, and V. Franks, pp. 381-425. New York: Brunner/Mazel.

Werder, E. A., Mürset, G., Zachmann, M., Brook, C. G. D., and Prader, A. 1974. Treatment of precocious puberty with cyproterone acetate. *Ped. Res.*, 8:248-256.

Winter, J. S. D., and Faiman, C. 1973. The development of cyclic pituitary-gonadal function in adolescent females. *J. Clin. Endocrin. Metab.*, 37:714-718.

Wise, P. H., and O'Loughlin, J. A. 1978. *Hirsutism*, ed. bull. no. 3, Royal College of Obstetricians and Gynaecologists, Australian Council.

AFFECTIVE AND EMOTIONAL DISORDERS

8

Situational Fears and Object Phobias

SUZANNE BENNETT JOHNSON

CLINICAL FEATURES

Fear is a normal response to a wide variety of situations. The child soon learns to fear situations and objects that will hurt him and to avoid them. In this fashion, fear is a very healthy or adaptive response that helps protect the child from harm. Yet, fear can become so excessive that it is maladaptive, preventing the youngster from engaging in normal, everyday activities. When fear is (1) excessive to the situation, (2) cannot be reasoned away, (3) is beyond voluntary control, and (4) leads to avoidance of the feared situation, it is called a phobia (Marks, 1969). Phobias are pathological fears that are unrealistic, maladaptive, and generally unresponsive to advice, support, or suggestion.

A child may manifest fear in a number of ways. He may cry, stutter, or say that he is afraid. He may show behavioral signs of fear, shaking or avoiding a particular situation or object. He may have a physiological reaction to the feared object, sweating profusely or experiencing increased heart palpitations. Fear is considered to be a tripartite construct having cognitive, behavioral, and physiological components. Yet a fearful child may not show fear in all three components. For example, a youngster may avoid an object but say he is not afraid. Or, the child may say he is afraid but show no clear avoidant behavior. It is the clinician's task to assess the nature of the youngster's fear and the extent to which it is maladaptive.

EPIDEMIOLOGY AND CONTENT OF CHILDREN'S FEARS

Ninety percent of all children experience one or more situational or object fears during the course of their development (MacFarlane et al., 1954). The number and content of these fears depend upon both the child's age and sex. Younger children and females report more fears than older children and boys. Of course, society is more accepting of fearful behavior in small children and girls, so that older children and boys may be more unwilling to admit to fears they do have (Bauer, 1976).

The content of a child's fears is clearly related to the youngster's developmental level. Infants are afraid of loud noises, depth, and strangers. These fears are replaced by fears of animals in two and three year olds, and fears of the dark, imaginary creatures, and nightmares in four and five year olds (Jersild and Holmes, 1935). While 74% of kindergarteners report fears of monsters, ghosts, and nightmares, sixth graders rarely report these types of fears. Instead, older children fear some type of bodily injury or physical danger—fears that kindergarteners rarely mention (Bauer, 1976).

Although children's fears are often focused on inanimate dangers (e.g., water, darkness), animals, or imaginary creatures, interpersonal fears are also common. Elective mutism in young children is sometimes fear related. School phobia and fears of doctors and dentists are also frequently reported. Miller et al. (1972) used factor analysis to categorize children's fears into three content areas. The first category consisted of fears of physical injury or personal loss (e.g., being kidnapped, having an operation, divorce of parents, death of a family member). The second category included natural and supernatural dangers (e.g., storms, ghosts, the dark). The third category included situations in which the child's performance might be scrutinized and included fears of exams, making mistakes, school, social events, doctors, and dentists.

While the incidence of children's fears is very high, the incidence of maladaptive or excessive fear is much more difficult to assess. It is estimated that phobic disorders account for only 3-4% of all referrals to child psychiatrists (Marks, 1969; Poznanski, 1973). However, a number of studies of behavioral and emotional characteristics of disturbed children have repeatedly identified a cluster of symptoms that include anxiety, self-consciousness, social withdrawal, crying, worrying, hypersensitivity, and seclusiveness (Quay, 1979). These symptoms seem to be describing an overly fearful child for whom avoidance is a primary mode of response. Approximately 25% of youngsters seen in mental-health clinics fit this description (Wolff, 1971; Frommer et al., 1972). In other words, the incidence of very specific situational fears or object phobias in children is quite low, while the incidence of children who suffer from a number of symptoms including excessive withdrawal and anxiety is quite high.

There is very little known as to the course of excessive fears through the child's development. Normal fears appear to be relatively short-lived while excessive fears seem to persist longer (Poznanski, 1973). Nevertheless, phobias in children appear to be more amenable to change than phobias in adults. The more specific and focused the fear, the better the prognosis (Agras et al., 1972).

Etiology

Early theories suggested that phobic behavior was a defense mechanism protecting an inadequate ego. Later, radical behaviorists such as John B. Watson argued that fears were learned through classical conditioning. In an early experiment Watson and Raynor (1920) demonstrated that fear could be learned by pairing an initially fearless object with an aversive event. In this study they exposed a nine-month-old boy, Albert, to a white rat and the child showed no fear. Next, they presented Albert with the rat and followed the presentation with a loud noise that consistently made the child tremble and cry. After several experiences with the rat and the loud noise, little Albert began to show fearful behavior whenever he saw the rat. This fear of the rat continued even when the loud noise no longer occurred. Soon, Albert was showing signs of fear to other "ratlike" objects such as cotton, a white rabbit, and a fur coat. Although the ethics of conducting such a study with a small child are certainly questionable, the authors argued that Albert's behavior clearly indicated that fear is learned.

Some fears probably are learned in much the same way Albert's fear developed. Nevertheless, most phobias probably cannot be explained so simply. When phobic patients are asked about their fears, a precipitating traumatic event leading to the phobia is rarely identified. Furthermore, adult phobic patients seem to differ from normals in a number of respects in addition to their specific phobias. They report more fears in childhood, have higher levels of general anxiety, tension, and dependency, and more often have psychiatric disturbances in their families (Solyom et al., 1974). In other words, phobias are often associated with more than a single aversive learning experience. In fact, many patients have never experienced a traumatic precipitating event.

Currently, several factors are considered important to the development of phobias. A traumatic or aversive experience may cause some fears but is probably not the critical factor. The object or stimulus itself may serve an important role, since some stimuli seem to induce fears more easily than others. This idea of "stimulus prepotency" was suggested by Thorndike as early as 1935 and is supported by the fact that the content of children's fears is highly consistent and age related. Certain objects are more likely to elicit fear at cerain developmental stages. Further support for this theory is found in the early work of English (1929) and Bregman (1934) who used Watson and Raynor's paradigm in an attempt to condition fear to a toy duck, a wooden triangle, a ring, and cloth curtains. No fear developed in the children studied despite repeated pairings of these objects with an aversive event.

The behavior of significant others in the child's environment is another contributing factor to the development of a child's fears. Mothers of phobic patients often have excessive fears themselves (Solyom et al., 1974) and the number and content of children's fears is often related to fears exhibited by the youngsters' mothers (Hagman, 1932; Bandura and Menlove, 1968).

Finally, the youngster's temperament needs to be taken into consideration (Thomas et al., 1963). Some children are easily aroused and bothered by the slightest provocation. These youngsters may be more likely to develop fears than children who show high tolerance of moderate or even high levels of stimulation. Although arousal and habituation patterns have not been extensively studied in children, there are some data that suggest that anxious children have discriminably different physiological patterns than either normals or conduct-disordered youngsters (Quay, 1979).

It is also important to remember that the factors that cause fear and those that maintain fear are not always the same. For example, a three year old may develop a fear of dogs which may be exacerbated by parents who give the younster excessive attention for this fearful behavior.

Differential Diagnosis

There are two issues in making a differential diagnosis. First, the clinician must determine whether the child's fear is excessive, unrealistic, and maladaptive, or whether the youngster is exhibiting fears that are normal for his developmental level. Second, the clinician must determine whether the youngster's fear is highly specific or whether it is part of a more general anxiety disorder. Specific fears are the focus of this chapter and may be effectively treated by a variety of behavioral intervention strategies. These treatment approaches are also appropriate for some cases of general anxiety. However, diffuse fears are often more difficult to treat and usually require additional or more extensive treatment approaches.

Assessment

Clarification of the Problem

First, the clinician must ascertain the exact nature of the problem. What is the child saying or doing that indicates he is afraid? Usually the parent seeks help because the child says he is scared and avoids involvement with specific objects or situations. Occasionally, a child does not report fear but behaves in a fearful manner.

Next, the clinician must assess how specific are the child's fears. For example, a child might be described as animal phobic. Inquiry should be made as to which animals specifically the youngster fears and whether some animals are more fearful than others. Perhaps the child is afraid of animals that bite or very large animals or animals that can move fast. Another child might be described as exhibiting excessive fears of the dentist. Further assessment should be devoted to understanding which aspects of the dental situation are most anxiety provoking to the child. Perhaps the child is afraid of the drill or a particular dentist or all men in white coats. Or perhaps he is afraid of most aspects of a particular dental setting (e.g., the novocaine injections, the drill, the dentist, the dental assistant) but shows no fear outside of this particular dentist's office.

It is especially important to assess whether the youngster's fears are specific fears occurring in an otherwise healthy child or whether they are part of a more general anxiety reaction. The examiner should always give some attention to the general functioning of the child. Inquiry should be made as to parent-child relationships with attention given to how independently or dependently the child functions. Also of interest are the child's social relationships, i.e., whether he seems excessively shy or has trouble making friends. Difficulties sleeping, nightmares, eating problems, or physical complaints are also signs that the child may be suffering from more than a specific fear or object phobia.

Finally, the severity and seriousness of the problem must be determined. How often does the child show fear? Is the child resistant to almost any form of reassurance? Is the child's fear appropriate or inappropriate for the situation? Is the child's fearful behavior extreme in form and prolonged? How does the child's fear interfere with everyday functioning and his normal development?

History of the Problem

Once the nature of the problem has been clarified, some assessment should be made as to when the child's fear was first noticed and how long it has persisted. Fears of long duration are less likely to disappear spontaneously and may require treatment. Usually, the parent or child is questioned as to any precipitating event that may have been associated with the development of the problem. Also of some importance is whether the child's fear seems to have become progressively worse over time and whether there were any specific events or experiences associated with this progressive deterioration.

The parents should also be questioned as to why they are seeking treatment now and how they have handled their child's problem in the past. Finally, some assessment should be made of any fears experienced by the parents or whether any significant individuals in the child's environment exhibit excessive fears.

Psychometric Evaluation

Formal psychodiagnostic testing is not routinely done with all children who have phobias. However, if there is some question as to the child's language or general intellectual ability, intelligence testing may prove helpful. Similarly, if the clinician suspects that the youngster's fear is part of a more general anxiety or neurotic disorder, a more thorough personality assessment may be desirable. Although the utility of children's projective test data is an area of some controversy, a variety of more objective inventories completed by parent, teacher, and child permit the examiner to determine whether the child is perceived as having more problems than his peers (Johnson and Melamed, 1979; O'Leary and Johnson, 1979).

Treatment Planning

In those cases where the fear is relatively circumscribed and yet so excessive that treatment seems appropriate, several additional issues need to be addressed in order to make decisions about how treatment sessions should be conducted.

The clinician will have already gathered substantial information about what objects or situations elicit the youngster's fear. It is also important to assess what follows the child's fearful behavior. Are the parents reassuring? Do they conscientiously help the youngster avoid the feared object or situation? Or do they ridicule or tease him about his fear or try to "force" him to interact with the feared object?

The examiner should learn whether the child's fear is totally the result of concerns about personal harm or injury or whether the child lacks a skill that may be important to overcoming the fear. For example, a child may fear tests in school and this test anxiety may have deleterious effects on school performance. To overcome this problem, the youngster may need to learn how to study and how to take tests successfully. While many fears are anxiety reactions to specific objects and situations which can be treated by teaching the child to be less anxious and fearful in that situation, other fears demand skill training because the child must perform in the feared situation. A careful assessment of what is demanded of the child is critical to successful treatment.

Parental fear behavior must be assessed in planning treatment because children often learn fears from their parents. If a parent continues to exhibit a fear, it may be particularly difficult to change a child's fear. For example, a little girl with leukemia may show high levels of fear and resistant behavior to the regular spinal taps that are necessary for her management. Her mother may be showing similar (although perhaps more subtle) signs of fear whenever the youngster has to undergo this procedure. Treating only the child's anxiety may not be successful as long as her mother continues to exhibit fear whenever a spinal tap is conducted on the daughter.

Similar problems can arise with siblings. Siblings can exacerbate fear by teasing a child with a feared object or they can attempt to undermine a treatment program when jealous of the extra attention their brother or sister is getting. It is important to assess siblings' reactions to the child's fear and to any treatment program initiated. Sometimes, nonfearful siblings can be used to help a youngster overcome a specific fear.

Finally, it is important to assess what parents expect from a treatment program. Often a parent will want to drop a child off at the clinician's office and have the professional talk the child out of his fear. This rarely works and parents are often surprised when asked to participate in a treatment program themselves. It is important to take the time to clarify parental expectations and attitudes about treatment before any approach is undertaken. If necessary, these attitudes and expectations may need to be addressed or changed. In any case, a careful assessment will help assure the selection of a treatment approach that is most likely to be successful.

AVAILABLE TREATMENTS

Reassurance

Reassurance is the recommended approach for dealing with simple fears that the child is likely to outgrow. The parents should be told that the child's fear is normal and that it is best to be reassuring but not overly solicitous of the youngster's fear. For example, a child who is afraid of the dark may be reassured by turning on a special night-light, leaving the bedroom door open a crack, having the family dog sleep in his bedroom, or learning that his mom and dad can hear him through an intercom. It is important that the parents insist that the youngster sleep in his own room and not "give in" to requests to sleep with mommy and daddy.

Counterconditioning methods

Counterconditioning uses a response that is incompatible with fear to counter the child's fear reaction. First, a graded hierarchy specific to the child's fear is developed. For example, suppose a child shows excessive fear of visiting the doctor. The child's hierarchy might include: (1) getting into the car to go to the doctor's office; (2) traveling in the car to the office; (3) getting out of the car in the office parking lot; (4) entering the office waiting area; (5) sitting in the waiting area; (6) walking to the examining room; (7) talking to the nurse; (8) undressing; (9) waiting for the doctor; (10) seeing the doctor; (11) having the doctor examine him; (12) having the doctor administer an injection. Notice that the hierarchy begins with items that are less threatening or fearful and proceeds through more and more fearful events. In this example, the child's fear is related both to the time and distance away from the moment of injection. Many hierarchies can be developed in this fashion; they take the child through a relatively obvious step-by-step approach to an encounter with his worst fear. However, not all fears are characterized by such elements of time and distance. A child who presents with a dog phobia may have fears of other animals as well. The therapist may have to develop a hierarchy of feared animals, beginning with an animal to which the child exhibits no fear and ending with a dog; animals eliciting varying degrees of fear are placed between these two end points of the hierarchy.

Determining the elements in a hierarchy is not always easy to do if the therapist relies solely on the child's self-report. Some children can be induced to give a fairly extensive description of some feared situation. The therapist can then question the child as to the relative fearfulness of various aspects of the description. However, particularly with very young children, reports by adults who have observed the child's reactions can prove invaluable. Direct observation of the child in the feared environment is one of the best methods of hierarchy delineation. For instance, a four-year-old child who was in treatment for a dog phobia, which developed after a serious injury by an attacking dog, was asked to show the therapist all of the animals that lived on his daddy's farm. The youngster wanted very much to show the therapist around the farm and in doing so gave her ample opportunity to observe which animals the child feared the most or the least.

Once a hierarchy is developed, treatment involves pairing each item on the hierarchy, beginning with the least fearful item, with a response that will "counter" fear. Responses that have been successfully used to counter fear include teaching the child to relax (Tasto, 1969; Weinstein, 1976), playing with a special toy (Bentler, 1962; Croghan and Musante, 1975), eating a favorite food (Jones, 1924; Montenegro, 1968), and using "emotive imagery" (Lazarus and Abramovitz, 1962). In emotive imagery, the child incorporates a favorite hero (e.g., Batman or Superman) into his efforts to counter his fears. Selection of a countering response depends very much on the child's capabilities. For very young children, food or play with a favorite toy may be the best approach. Emotive imagery is appropriate for youngsters who have vivid imaginations; they fantasize each step in the hierarchy by including themselves and their hero in each scene. Children as young as eight to ten years can be taught progressive relaxation by asking them to alternately tense and relax various parts of their body (Jacobson, 1938). Another approach is to have the child lie on a couch or easy chair and imagine something very pleasant while the therapist verbalizes suggestions inducing relaxation, calm, and mild fatigue.

Counterconditioning can be carried out either *in vivo* or by having the child imagine the hierarchy scenes. Often it is done first through imagination and then carried out in real life. Treatment using the child's imagination is usually employed when the child can visualize the phobic scenes well and when gradual treatment *in vivo* would be difficult or impossible (e.g., treatment for fear of flying). Otherwise, treatment *in vivo* is probably the more ideal approach.

It is important to move through the treatment hierarchy *gradually*. Most therapists recommend that movement up through the levels of fear be made dependent on the child's exhibiting *no* fear to items lower on the hierarchy. This process usually takes a number of thirty to sixty-minute sessions. When the youngster can be seen daily, treatment seems to progress faster than when weekly sessions are employed.

Implosion Therapy and Flooding

In implosion therapy the child is exposed to extremely anxiety-provoking imaginary scenes presented by the therapist. In flooding, the child is exposed to the actual situation or object that he fears. In either approach the youngster is not allowed to escape no matter how frightened he becomes. The child's fear presumably diminishes when he learns that no real harm will come to him. Implosion therapy or flooding is generally *not* recommended for children. There is little convincing evidence that this form of therapy is particularly effective, and deliberately frightening children when other effective treatment techniques are available seems unnecessary (Graziano, 1975). Further, there is the risk that the phobia will not diminish and instead the child will learn to fear the therapist and refuse to cooperate with treatment.

Operant Approaches

Operant techniques are designed to change the child's phobic pattern by rewarding approach behavior and ignoring fearful behavior. Kennedy (1965) describes such a program for school-phobic youngsters. Treatment involved forcing the child to attend school, praising him for his attendance, and ignoring somatic or other verbal complaints. Youngsters who are school phobic but who exhibit no other signs of general psychiatric disturbance seem to be rapidly and effectively treated with such an approach. Of fifty cases seen and treated, all were successfully reintroduced to school with no subsequent school-phobic episodes reported at yearly follow-up.

In addition to selecting sufficiently powerful verbal or social rewards for nonfearful behavior, operant approaches also rely on shaping, prompting, and stimulus fading. In shaping, the youngster is initially rewarded for even brief periods of nonfearful behavior or for the slightest attempt to approach the feared object or situation. Gradually, the child is rewarded for longer and longer periods of nonfearful behavior or for more and more extensive contact with the phobic object. This procedure is designed to encourage approach behavior by reinforcing successive approximations to the desired behavior. Neisworth et al. (1975) used such an approach to treat a four year old suffering severe separation anxiety. Whenever her mother left her at a preschool, she would cry, scream, and withdraw, refusing to participate in any aspect of the school's activities. A treatment program was developed which shaped the child's nonfearful, approach behavior. At first, the child's mother left her in the preschool for only a few seconds. This time period of "mother absence" was then gradually increased until the child was able to remain in the classroom for the entire three-hour session with no signs of distress. In fact, she became a willing participant in the preschool's daily activities. Shaping is a particularly useful technique because it encourages increased approach behavior while eliciting almost no distress on the part of the child. In this case the youngster showed only ten minutes of distress (i.e., crying, withdrawal) during the course of the entire intervention program.

Sometimes a child cannot be rewarded for a desired behavior because he does not engage in that behavior at all. In such cases the behavior can often be elicited by prompting techniques and then shaped to some desired level. For example, Nordquist and Bradley (1973) had a child initiate or prompt interaction with a socially isolate child who never talked to or played with any of her peers. The teacher then praised any interactions between the "prompting" child and the isolate youngster. Slowly, the withdrawn child's behavior changed; she verbalized more and readily engaged in cooperative play. The use of the "prompting" child was no longer necessary.

Stimulus fading is another technique used to elicit behavior in situations where previously it has never occurred. This approach is most effective when the desired behavior occurs in one situation but not in others. For example, a child might talk to her mother but be afraid to speak to anyone else. The mother, a "stimulus" who is able to elicit verbal behavior, would be gradually "faded out" or removed from the environment while other people (e.g., teachers, peers) would be gradually introduced or "faded in." Wulbert et al. (1973) provide a good example of how such a technique can be used successfully. They were treating a six-year-old electively mute girl who spoke with her mother but who had never uttered a word to her Sunday-school teacher, preschool teacher, or kindergarten teacher. They asked the child and mother to attend an outpatient clinic three times a week. During the sessions the mother was instructed to ask the child to engage in a series of tasks, some of which required verbal responses. No one remained in the room with the mother and child during these initial sessions. After the child was responding readily to the mother's requests, an unfamiliar adult was gradually introduced into the sessions. At first, this adult simply stood at the open door Later, he sat in a chair in the room. The chair was gradually moved closer to the child and finally he began to ask the child to engage in nonverbal tasks and then verbal tasks. When the child was verbally responding to this adult's requests, the child's mother was then gradually removed from the room and another unfamiliar adult was "faded in." The child's teachers and some of her classmates also participated; they were gradually introduced in the clinic sessions where they initiated verbal interaction with the child. Once the child was able to verbally engage her peers and teachers in the clinic sessions, she continued to interact with them verbally outside of the clinic and in the classroom.

All of the previous examples dealt with social anxieties. Operant approaches are not confined to these types of fears. A child with an animal phobia might be treated by playing a penny game in which he must touch a feared animal before he can guess which of the therapist's hands contains a penny. Of course, he gets to keep the penny when he guesses correctly! This operant program intermittently rewards the child for his approach behavior.

Modeling

There has been a great deal of recent interest in the use of models to reduce avoidant behavior. The child watches a nonfearful peer interact with a phobic object. This can done either *in vivo* or through the use of films. There are some data suggesting that the most successful approach is to have the child contact the feared object right after observing the model (Ritter, 1968; Lewis, 1974). It is unclear whether fearless models or models who initially show fear but successfully cope with their fears are the most effective for children to observe (Johnson and Melamed, 1979). However, it is important that a phobic child *not* be exposed to another avoidant youngster displaying a great deal of distress in the feared situation, as this may enhance the phobic child's avoidant responses.

A therapist treating a phobic child might not have a child model available and the therapist may serve in this role instead. For example, in the earlier case of the youngster with leukemia who shows strong aversive behavior to spinal taps, a repeated requirement of her treatment, assessment of the child's aversive reaction may indicate that it is the needle itself that the youngster most fears. Treatment might involve reducing the youngster's needle phobia by having her first observe the therapist model self-injecting with a needle. The child would then be asked to follow the therapist's lead and to self-inject as well. The use of films that depict a child successfully interacting in a fearful situation are usually employed in settings where a number of youngsters have a similar fear (e.g., social isolate children in a preschool; children facing surgery or dental restoration, etc.). Such films are an excellent and efficient way to treat large numbers of children, but are probably not practical for the therapist who sees only a few phobic children every year.

When a child's fear is exacerbated by a skill deficit, modeling may be a particularly effective treatment technique because it can teach new responses as well as reduce fears (Bandura, 1969). Although most studies have focused on the fear-reduction properties of modeling techniques, some have assessed the skill acquisition effects of this approach (Keller and Carlson, 1974; Gilbert et al., 1982). For example, a socially isolate child may fear interactions with peers because he is not sure what to say or how to behave. A test-anxious youngster may need to learn how to study and take a test. A youngster with juvenile diabetes who avoids daily injections needs to reduce his fears as well as learn how to give the injection appropriately. When new behavior must be taught as well as anxieties reduced, modeling may be the treatment of choice. However, it is unclear how much fear needs to be reduced before new learning may be successfully acquired.

Modeling also has been used to prevent the development of excessive fears. Melamed and Siegel (1975) and others have used this approach to prepare youngsters for surgery and other fear-inducing medical or dental procedures. The child who is about to undergo a relatively anxiety-producing experience watches a film depicting a youngster who undergoes a similar procedure. The model in the film describes the procedure, tells how he felt about it, and how he successfully coped. After watching the film, the youngster has a much better idea of what to expect and how to handle the more difficult aspects of the experience. This is a creative approach to help children cope with their fears *before* they reach excessive proportions.

Self-Control Procedures

Self-control procedures involve teaching the child to self-instruct, problem solve, or reward and punish his own behavior. For example, Kanfer et al. (1975) taught children who were afraid of the dark to say to themselves sentences emphasizing their competence, such as, "I'm a brave boy, I can handle myself in the dark." Children taught to self-instruct in this manner were able to stay in the dark longer than youngsters taught to distract themselves by saying nursery rhymes. Although this is an interesting approach, children who participated in this study did not have excessive fears. Consequently, the clinical utility of this treatment with truly phobic youngsters remains to be seen.

Medication

The role of sedatives or tranquilizers in the treatment of anxiety reactions in nonpsychotic children is unclear. However, since other effective treatments are available, pharmacotherapy is not ordinarily indicated (Conners and Werry, 1979).

PRACTICAL GUIDE TO TREATMENT

Advice to the Parent

Parents should be advised that children with maladaptive situational fears or object probias should be treated and that treatment is usually successful. They should understand that treatment will involve a gradual reexposure of the child to the feared situation and that they should refrain from forcing the child into an anxiety-evoking situation before he is sufficiently prepared. Treatment is usually brief, but often intensive, involving frequent contacts with the therapist initially and then more intermittent contacts at follow-up. Parents are often expected to participate in one or more aspects of the treatment program and should be prepared for this role. In particular, they should understand the importance of supporting and praising their child's nonfearful behavior, ignoring his fearful behavior, and avoiding punitive reactions toward the child.

Selecting a Treatment Approach

There are a number of treatment approaches available to the clinician. All of them are designed to gradually expose the child to the feared situation. In fact, repeated *exposure* to the phobic object or situation may be the critical element of each treatment's success (Marks, 1975).

A treatment plan should be developed after a thorough assessment and with the following considerations: (1) the nature of the child's phobic reaction; (2) characteristics of the child; (3) characteristics of the family or other significant others; (4) generalization and maintenance of nonfearful behavior once treatment has ended. Where possible, a graded hierarchy should be developed beginning with the child's least fear-provoking situation and progressing to his most feared experience. This is a useful approach regardless of the treatment selected (e.g., counterconditioning, operant, modeling) and results in the least overall discomfort for the child. The clinician should feel free to combine several approaches (e.g., desensitization and operant procedures) and not be restricted to using a particular technique in isolation.

NATURE OF THE PHOBIC REACTION. In selecting a treatment program, some consideration should be given to the nature and extent of the child's phobic reaction. The electively mute child who talks to no one except his mother will probably not be successfully treated by modeling, counterconditioning, or simple operant procedures. He has watched numerous models talk with their peers and has probably been promised all types of rewards for giving up his silence. Yet, he remains mute. Since he refuses to talk to anyone outside of the home, counterconditioning seems equally inappropriate. In such a case, a stimulus-fading procedure seems essential. If the child's verbal responses were infrequent rather than nonexistent, modeling or rewards made contingent upon verbal behavior might be successful. If speech was anxiety evoking only in certain evaluative contexts (e.g., answering questions in class or delivering a verbal report), relaxation training might teach the youngster an effective coping strategy. Some thought should be given to possible skill deficits, as these may exacerbate a youngster's fears.

CHARACTERISTICS OF THE CHILD. Some children are highly verbal with an excellent imagination and respond very well to relaxation training. Others cannot be easily taught to relax or are so nonverbal that a therapist would have difficulty assessing or treating the child in an office setting. Similarly, some youngsters respond best to social praise, others to material rewards, still others to adult attention, and others to peer appraisals. Understanding the capabilities, limitations, and special desires of the child is an important basis for developing a successful treatment program.

CHARACTERISTICS OF THE FAMILY. The reactions of significant others in the child's life to his phobic behavior is a critical aspect of almost any treatment program. Family members can serve to undermine treatment by continuing to elicit, reward, or model fearful behavior. Or they may serve as important allies for the therapist, giving the child additional practice in his attempts to approach the phobic object. Often, they serve as the primary therapeutic agent, following the advice of the clinician.

If a treatment program is to be successful, the support and cooperation of family members (or other significant individuals) must be developed and solidified. This may require modification of parental fears, reductions in parental solicitation or punishment of fearful behavior in the child, and some consideration of sibling rivalries. Finally, the intervention program itself must be practical, within family members' capabilities, and easily conducted within the context of the family's activities of daily living.

GENERALIZATION AND MAINTENANCE OF BEHAVIOR CHANGE. As with any improved behavior, plans should be made to ensure generalization of treatment effects outside of the therapeutic setting and maintenance of these effects once the treatment is withdrawn. Intervention programs that occur within the office setting under the direction of the therapist are probably the most susceptible to maintenance or generalization problems. Behavior changes must be practiced *in vivo* and supported by persons in the child's everyday environment, even if they are initially learned in the safe haven of a therapist's office. Where possible, the clinician should design the program so that the youngster receives clear, positive consequences for his newly developed approach behavior. For example, a youngster successfully treated for test anxiety might achieve better grades, a child treated for isolative behavior might develop a new friendship, and a youngster treated for fear of dogs might be given his first pet. These "real-life" positive experiences will help maintain and support the child's treatment gains.

REFERENCES

Agras, W., Chapin, H., and Oliveau, D. 1972. The natural history of phobia. *Arch. Gen. Psych.,* 26:315-317.

Bandura, A. 1969. *Principles of behavior modification.* New York: Holt, Rinehart and Winston.

Bandura, A., and Menlove, F. 1968. Factors determining vicarious extinction of avoidance behavior through symbolic modeling. *J. Pers. Soc. Psychol.,* 8:99-108.

Bauer, D. 1976. An exploratory study of developmental changes in children's fears. *J. Child Psychol. Psych.,* 17:69-74.

Bentler, P. 1962. An infant's phobia treated with reciprocal inhibition therapy. *J. Child Psychol. Psych.,* 3:185-189.

Bregman, E. 1934. An attempt to modify the emotional attitudes of infants by the conditioned response technique. *J. Genet. Psychol.,* 45:169-198.

Conners, K., and Werry, J. 1979. Pharmacotherapy. In *Psychopathological disorders of childhood,* ed. H. Quay and J. Werry. New York: Wiley.

Croghan, L., and Musante, G. 1975. The elimination of a boy's high-building phobia by in vivo desensitization and game playing. *J. Beh. Ther. Exp. Psych.,* 6:87-88.

English, H. 1929. Three cases of the "conditioned fear response." *J. Abnor. Soc. Psychol.,* 34:221-225.

Frommer, E., Mendelson, W., and Reid, M. 1972. Differential diagnosis of psychiatric disturbance in pre-school children. *Brit. J. Psych.,* 121:71-74.

Gilbert, B., Johnson, S. B., Spillar, R., McCallum, M., Silverstein, J., and Rosenbloom, A. 1982. The effects of a peer monitoring film on children learning to self-inject insulin. *Beh. Ther.,* 13:186-193.

Graziano, A. 1975. *Behavior therapy with children.* Vol. 2. Chicago: Aldine.

Hagman, E. 1932. A study of fears of children of pre-school age. *J. Exp. Ed.* 1:110-130.

Jacobson, E. 1938. *Progressive relations.* Chicago: University of Chicago Press.

Jersild, A., and Holmes, F. 1935. *Children's fears.* New York: Columbia University Teachers College.

Johnson, S. B. 1979. Children's fears in the classroom setting. *School Psychol. Dig.* 8(4):382-396.

Johnson, S. B., and Melamed, B. G. 1979. The assessment and treatment of children's fears. In *Advances in clinical child psychology,* vol. 2, ed. B. Lahey and A. Kazdin. New York: Plenum Press.

Jones, M. 1924. The elimination of children's fears. *J. Exp. Psychol.* 7:382-390.

Kanfer, F., Karoly, P., and Newman, A. 1975. Reduction of children's fear of the dark by competence-related and situational threat-related verbal cues. *J. Consult. Clin. Psychol.,* 43:251-258.

Keller, M., and Carlson, P. 1974. The use of symbolic modeling to promote skills in pre-school children with low levels of social responsiveness. *Child Dev.,* 45:912-919.

Kennedy, W. 1965. School phobia: Rapid treatment of fifty cases. *J. Abnor. Psychol.,* 70:285-289.

Lazarus, A., and Abramovitz, A. 1962. The use of "emotive imagery" in the treatment of children's phobias. *J. Men. Sci.,* 108:191-195.

Lewis, S. 1974. A comparison of behavior therapy techniques in the reduction of fearful avoidance behavior. *Beh. Ther.,* 5:648-655.

MacFarlane, J., Allen, L., and Honzik, M. 1954. *A developmental study of the behavior problems of normal children.* Berkeley: University of California Press.

Marks, I. 1969. *Fears and phobias.* New York: Academic Press.

Marks, I. 1975. Behavioral treatment of phobic and obsessive-compulsive disorders: A critical appraisal. In *Progress in behavior modification,* ed. M. Hersen, R. Eisler, and P. Miller. New York: Academic Press.

Melamed, B., and Siegel, L. 1975. Reduction of anxiety in children facing hospitalization and surgery by use of filmed modeling. *J. Consult. Clin. Psychol.,* 43:511-521.

Miller, L., Barrett, C., Hampe, E., and Noble, H. 1972. Factor structure of childhood fears. *J. Consult. Clin. Psychol.,* 39:264-268.

Montenegro, H. 1968. Severe separation anxiety in two pre-school children successfully treated by reciprocal inhibition. *J. Child Psychol. Psychiat.,* 9:93-103.

Neisworth, J., Madle, R., and Goeke, K. 1975. "Errorless" elimination of separation anxiety: A case study. *J. Beh. Ther. Exp. Psych.,* 6:79-82.

Nordquist, V., and Bradley, B. 1973. Speech acquistion in a nonverbal isolate child. *J. Exp. Child Psychol.,* 15:149-160.

O'Leary, K. D., and Johnson, S. B. 1979. Psychological assessment. In *Psychopathological disorders of childhood,* ed. H. Quay, and J. Werry. New York: Wiley.

Poznanski, E. 1973. Children with excessive fears. *Am. J. Orthopsych.* 43:428-438.

Quay, H. 1979. Classification. In *Psychopathological disorders of childhood,* ed. H. Quay and J. Werry. New York: Wiley.

Ritter, B. 1968. The group desensitization of children's phobias. *Beh. Res. Ther.,* 6:1-6.

Solyom, I., Beck, P., Solyom, C., and Hugel, R. 1974. Some etiological factors in phobic neurosis. *Can. Psychiat. Assoc. J.,* 19:69-78.

Tasto, D. 1969. Systematic desensitization, muscle relaxation and visual imagery in the counter-conditioning of a four-year-old phobic child. *Beh. Res. Ther.,* 7:409-411.

Thomas, A., Chess, S., Birch, H., Hertzig, M., and Korn, S. 1963. *Behavioral individuality in early childhood.* New York: New York University Press.

Thorndike, E. 1935. *The psychology of wants, interests, and attitudes.* London: Appleton Century.

Watson, J., and Raynor, R. 1920. Conditioned emotional reactions. *J. Exp. Psychol.,* 3:1-14.

Weinstein, D. 1976. Imagery and relaxation with a burn patient. *Beh. Res. Ther.,* 14:48.

Wolff, S. 1971. Dimensions and clusters of symptoms in disturbed children. *Br. J. Psych.,* 118:421-427.

Wulbert, M., Nyman, B., Snow, D., and Owen, Y. 1973. The efficacy of stimulus fading and contingency management in the treatment of elective mutism: A case study. *J. Appl. Beh. Anal.,* 6:435-441.

9

Major Depression in Children and Adolescents

PAUL J. AMBROSINI / JOAQUIM PUIG-ANTICH

CLINICAL FEATURES

Major depressive disorder (MDD) in children is a psychiatric condition. Its main symptomatic characteristics are persistent depressed mood and/or pervasive anhedonia. Around these two symptoms cluster other associated signs and symptoms, including: excessive or inappropriate guilt; fatigue; loss of interest and/or pleasure in usual activities; difficulty concentrating; psychomotor agitation or retardation; sleep and appetite disturbances; and suicidal ideation or attempts. The child can be diagnosed as having a major depressive disorder when (a) either depressed mood or pervasive anhedonia exist concurrently with at least four of the associated symptoms listed above, (b) the condition persists for at least two weeks accompanied by functional impairment, and (c) there is no evidence of schizophrenia.

It is now possible to diagnose MDD in prepubertal and adolescent patients six years and older with the Kiddie-SADS (Schedule for Affective Disorders and Schizophrenia for School-age Children), a reliable semistructured interview technique. This is based on unmodified Research Diagnostic Criteria (RDC) (Spitzer et al., 1978) or *DSM-III* criteria as used with adult patients. We do not know yet if dysthymic disorders (*DSM-III*) or minor (RDC) depressions in children are akin to or different from prepubertal MDDs, or what therapeutic and prognostic value these less severe diagnoses carry.

HISTORICAL DEVELOPMENT, EPIDEMIOLOGY, AND NATURAL HISTORY

The existence of major depression in childhood has been a subject of controversy in the literature. Although adult depressive symptoms were described in adolescents and children during the 1950s and 1960s (Puig-Antich, 1980), this conceptualization was not generally accepted. It was believed initially that a child's limited cognitive and emotional development made it difficult to express feelings of sadness, helplessness, and depression directly; the disorder could only be inferred from symptoms masking the dysphoric mood (Gleser, 1967; Cytryn and McKnew, 1972). Such depressive equivalents included hyperkinesis, somatic complaints, enuresis, conduct problems, aggressive behavior, delinquency, phobias, and underachievement. The problem with this conceptualization was that a reliable set of criteria could not be developed to separate those children whose behavioral signs (e.g., hyperkinesis) masked a depression from children with true attention deficit disorder with hyperkinesis. As more rigorous assessment methods and diagnostic criteria were used to evaluate major depression in children, it became apparent that masked depressive equivalents may be only presenting complaints, not a syndrome (Kovacs and Beck, 1977). Such symptoms should alert the clinician to assess the affective state of the patient.

There are few epidemiologic studies of major depression in childhood. Using total population sampling methods, the Isle of Wight study (Rutter et al., 1970) and its adolescent follow-up (Rutter et al., 1976) found severe depression to be several times more prevalent in adolescence than in prepuberty. These studies were undertaken before the development of RDC or *DSM-III* criteria, and without the benefit of a semistructured interview method which included all symptoms of major depression.

Reviewing clinical samples, Kashani et al. (1981) noted that the prevalence of depression varied greatly with the population studied and diagnostic criteria employed. Carlson and Cantwell (1980) screened 210 children at an outpatient and inpatient child psychiatry service using a self-report inventory. Later, a selected subsample of 102 patients was interviewed and diagnosed using *DSM-III* criteria. They found 60% of all children so screened had depressive symptoms (i.e., depressed mood, low self-esteem, suicidal ideation, withdrawal), but only 27% of those clinically interviewed had the syndrome of depression. Their data also suggested that approximately one-third of those identified on screening as having depressive symptoms actually had a depressive syndrome by interview. Pearce (1977), using cluster-analytic techniques on clinical records of children with depressive mood, found that items of the depressive syndrome tended to cluster with depressive mood. This association grew stronger the older the subsample considered.

Our group has been attempting to further validate the diagnosis of prepubertal major depression by studying these children and appropriate control groups along several psychobiological parameters which are characteristically altered in adult major depressive disorders. These include psychosocial relationships, family prevalence of affective disorders, neuroendocrine rhythms and hormonal responses, response to antidepressant medication, sleep physiology, and natural history. Data already analyzed suggest several patterns:

1. Children with MDD have marked deficiencies in their relationship to mother and peers; the mother/child relationship improves moderately with recovery of the depressive syndrome, but peer relationships remain almost as impaired (Lukens et al., 1979).

2. Cortisol hypersecretion during the acute stage of illness will normalize on recovery (Puig-Antich et al., 1979a). It is found in only 10–15% of prepubertal endogenous cases when measured by serial plasma sampling.

3. Cortisol may not be suppressed by 0.5 mg overnight dexamethasone test dose in approximately 71% of endogenous prepubertal depressives, while 92% of nonendogenous depressives had normal suppression (Poznanski et al., 1982).*

---

* The term "endogenous" has been applied to major affective disorders and refers to a severe subtype particularly responsive to somatic therapies. *DSM-III* avoids use of "endogenous" since it implies the absence of a precipitating stress, a characteristic not always found (APA, 1980).

4. Growth-hormone response to insulin-induced hypoglycemia is blunted in the active stage of prepubertal major depression. It may remain unchanged on recovery and therefore be a marker of predisposition to illness (Puig-Antich et al., 1981).

5. Lifetime morbidity risk for major depressive disorder, alcoholism, and antisocial personality in first-degree biological relatives or prepubertal major depressives is very high even before age correction, indicating that such children are likely to be a highly genetically loaded group.

Ongoing long-term follow-up studies of depressed children and their families will provide very important evidence of the continuity or discontinuity of child or adult major depressive disorders.

Associated Clinical Conditions

In our experience, conduct disorder in boys and separation anxiety are commonly associated conditions in children diagnosed as depressed. These syndromes most frequently appear after the onset of depressed mood. Yet they can often be the presenting complaints that accompany the child to an initial psychiatric contact. The highly visible symptomatology of conduct disorders and separation anxiety, therefore, may divert attention away from the concurrent depression.

We have found no special clinical association between attention deficit disorder with hyperactivity (ADDH) and MDD in prepuberty. Nevertheless, major depressive children can present symptoms of agitation (hyperactivity) and poor concentration (short attention span) which may be misdiagnosed as ADDH if a full systematic assessment is not carried out. The association of prepubertal major depressive disorder with conduct disorder and with separation anxiety, and the misinterpretation of psychomotor agitation and poor concentration as ADDH further confounded recognition of the depressive syndrome in children and fostered the theory of "masked depression." The most common route to this diagnostic confusion is the lack of an adequate psychiatric interview of the child. This differentiation is important because an accurate diagnosis can lead to effective psychopharmacologic and psychotherapeutic intervention. A recent study of prepubertal depressive disorder emphasizes this point: one-third of depressed boys also fit *DSM-III* criteria for conduct disorder, and successful treatment of their mood disorder with antidepressants led to abatement of conduct problems in a majority of cases (Puig-Antich, 1982b).

Anorexia nervosa shows a variable association with major depression in children: some will have both syndromes concurrently, while about one-third will meet criteria for an affective disorder on follow-up after the anorectic episode (Cantwell et al., 1977). Although anorexia nervosa and MDD can coexist in adolescence, anorexia is very rare in prepuberty. Finally, child abuse accompanied by maternal depression as well as prepubertal and adolescent depression may coexist in the same family.

Differential Diagnosis

Manic disorders fitting adult criteria have been described in youngsters by several investigators (Weinberg and Brumback, 1976; Brumback and Weinberg, 1977; Carlson and Strober, 1978). Their occurrence is quite rare in prepuberty, growing more frequent through late adolescence. A more rapid switch between "highs" and "lows" is seen in adolescents with bipolar disorder than in adults with the same illness. Other characteristics appear to be a greater likelihood of affective disease in the families of these children and suggestive evidence of lithium responsiveness.

Less severe clinical affective pictures do exist, especially in adolescents. These include cyclothymic, dysthymic, and atypical affective disorders. Cyclothymia and dysthymia are chronic mood disturbances interspersed with periods of normal mood lasting a few days to a few months. Neither the severity, the duration, nor the number of affective symptoms present are sufficient to meet criteria for major affective illness.

Atypical affective disorders, as defined in *DSM-III*, refer to adult-onset labile mood disturbances that do not meet criteria for either major or minor depressive disorders. This differs from the clinical picture of atypical major depression which we have found in a subgroup of adolescents. Their moods are reactive to environmental stimuli; they overeat and oversleep during depressive episodes. They are likely to be exquisitely sensitive to rejection and have marked difficulties with interpersonal relationships. This pattern resembles the adult atypical major depressive (Liebowitz and Klein, 1979). The importance of these clinical observations is that atypical adult depressives seem to respond much better to monoamine oxidase inhibitors than tricyclic antidepressants, and thus adolescent atypical major depressives may constitute a group responsive to some types of antidepressants but not to others.

Most of these differential diagnostic disorders have not been validated in childhood and are quite uncommon. However, if one follows strict diagnostic criteria, it is possible to separate the child with a major depression from the more transient characterological pathologic states.

Children with major depressive disorder may also present depressive hallucinations (Chambers et al., 1982). All too often hallucinations in childhood are considered pathognomonic of schizophrenia. Yet, major depression, psychotic subtype, is not an uncommon occurrence. These children will experience mood-congruent hallucinations—e.g., denigrating voices, commands to kill oneself, visions of death or deceased relatives—which are temporally related to depressive disorder and clear with proper treatment with antidepressants (Puig-Antich et al., 1979b).

Psychotic depressives are unlikely to present either conversing or commenting auditory hallucinations incongruent with their mood disorder. The presence of these types of hallucinations, as well as any hallucinations or delusions that are not temporally or thematically related to depressed mood, should lead the clinician to consider the diagnosis of schizoaffective disorder, depressed subtype. *DSM-III* does not list diagnostic criteria for this syndrome because there is no consensus on whether this is a variant of schizophrenia or more closely related to the affective disorders. However, Research Diagnostic Criteria (Spitzer et al., 1978) specify that these individuals have an episode of illness fulfilling the criteria for either the manic or depressive syndrome and have at least one of the symptoms suggesting schizophrenia.

As stated previously, conduct disorder is common in depressed boys, yet one must be able to separate those with true conduct disturbances from those with MDD. The child with a conduct disorder may have periods of depression and anhedonia; however, these are usually brief and/or related to being caught or restricted. The conduct-disordered child enjoys the activities in which he engages.

Factitious disorder with psychological features can in some instances mimic the clinical picture of MDD as can histrionic personality disorder. This pattern has been particularly noted in children with hallucinatory features. A careful assessment of symptomatology is required to clarify the diagnosis and may necessitate either an extended outpatient evaluation period or an inpatient admission.

The psychomotor retardation associated with mental retardation may also mimic aspects of MDD. Of course, mental retardates can experience a full-blown clinical depression, so a detailed academic history and psychometric testing is required for diagnosis. The subject of affective disorder in mental retardates has been reviewed (Carlson, 1979).

Endocrinopathies, particularly of the thyroid and adrenal systems, are associated with MDD in adults (Whybrow and Hurwitz, 1976). The existence of affectivelike pictures in childhood endocrinopathies, however, has not been reliably studied. Because neuroendocrine abnormalities occur in prepubertal MDD (Puig-Antich et al., 1979a; Puig-Antich et al., 1981), it would be important to distinguish between such cases and those with a primary endocrinopathy and secondary depression, because the treatment of choice differs. A physical examination will assist in this differential diagnosis and is mandatory in all children meeting criteria for MDD.

Clinical Assessment

Any child presenting with the following verbal complaints or behavioral patterns must be fully assessed for the depressive syndrome: complaints of feeling "sad," "depressed," "gloomy," "down," "bad," "empty," or "like crying"; depressive appearance; suicidal ideation, gestures, attempts; displays of school refusal (school phobia). In our clinical evaluation, the chronology and symptomatic assessment of the present episode can be reliably obtained using the K-SADS. This instrument is designed to record information regarding a child's functioning and symptoms. The emphasis on symptoms necessitates talking with the child as opposed to playing with the child as a means of psychiatric assessment. Play interviews are an excellent means of eliciting preoccupations and symbolic meanings, but they do not assess symptoms and therefore have only a minor role in the diagnostic process of major depression or most other child psychiatric disorders.

The K-SADS is a semistructured interview administered by interviewing the parent(s) first, then the child alone. The clinician arrives at summary ratings which include all sources of information (i.e., parent, child, school, chart, and other). The interview session should begin with a brief unstructured segment in which the examiner explains the purpose of the session to both the child and parent and obtains an overall view of the presenting problems.

The main body of the K-SADS consists of a schedule of questions for the systematic assessment of most symptoms of child and adolescent psychiatric disorders, including not only those relating to the major affective disorders, endogenous and psychotic subtypes, and to schizophrenia, but also symptoms relevant to conduct and emotional disorders. Children with IQs below 60 and/or severe language problems cannot be interviewed in this manner. For a detailed description of the interview technique, the reader is referred to the interview schedule itself (Puig-Antich et al., 1979c).

It is also important to obtain a psychosocial and psychiatric history from the parents. MDD children frequently have discordant peer and intrafamilial relations, and come from families with high prevalence rates for affective disorders, alcoholism, and sociopathy. The Psychosocial Schedule (PSS) is a semistructured interview guide derived from several pre-existing rating scales (Andrews et al., 1979). It is designed to measure and record clinical data including developmental and past symptomatic history, demographics, family functioning, and relationships. The PSS also allows the clinician a means of assessing change in psychosocial functioning with treatment. The family history RDC developed by Andreasen et al. (1977) is also available for systematic assessment of familial patterns of psychiatric diagnoses.

Psychometric testing should be routinely obtained in childhood depressives. In particular, the Wechsler Intelligence Scale for Children—Revised (WISC-R) can be helpful. Its main function is to rule out demoralization secondary to scholastic failure.

Physical Investigation

All children diagnosed as depressed need a general physical examination. It is advisable to routinely check thyroid function. Also, it is mandatory to obtain a baseline EKG before initiating treatment with tricyclic antidepressants (TCA). The EKG is a most sensitive index for assessing tricyclic toxicity during treatment. Tricyclics are contraindicated in children with conduction defects.

Available Treatments

Pharmacotherapy

Recent evidence suggests that pharmacotherapy of prepubertal major depression is likely to be an effective treatment modality (Puig-Antich et al., 1978; Puig-Antich et al., 1979b). In fact, it may be the initial treatment of choice. The indications for drug therapy are a firm diagnosis of MDD using *DSM-III* criteria, and no EKG or other medical abnormalities.

We recommend an initial trial with imipramine (IMI) because most data on tricyclic therapeutic and toxic effects in children with a variety of diagnoses (enuresis, hyperactivity, separation anxiety disorder, and major depression) have been obtained with this drug. We recommend that IMI be administered in three equally divided daily doses. Dosage is calculated on a mg/kg/day schedule and started at 1.5 mg/kg/day. The dose is raised every third day in stepwise fashion from 1.5 to 3, 4, and 5 mg/kg/day. Before each dosage increase, EKG, blood pressure (BP), and other clinical side effects are measured. IMI regularly induces EKG changes in children. If these EKG changes reach certain preestablished (FDA reference) limits, the dose should not be increased. These limits include: a resting heart rate greater than 130/min; P-R interval greater than 0.21 msec; QRS greater than 130% baseline; systolic BP greater than 145 or diastolic BP greater than 95 mm Hg. Of course, if other unacceptable clinical side effects develop, the dose should not be increased further.

Plasma tricyclic levels should be an integral part of treatment. Clinical response is correlated with a threshold plasma level. A given oral dose is not correlated well with plasma levels (Puig-Antich et al., 1979b). Blood samples, therefore, should be obtained once maintenance dose is reached at least eight hours after the prior dose. Venipuncture must be performed with a syringe rather than Vacutainers, whose rubber top red collection tubes interfere with adequate quantitative assay.

The goal in treatment with imipramine is to obtain a combined (IMI + desipramine [DMI]) maintenance plasma level over 200 ng/ml. Imipramine is metabolized to DMI and the combined imipramine and desipramine level predicts clinical response of the depressive syndrome better than the level of either of the two compounds alone, both in adults and in children. In those with psychotic depression with depressive hallucinations, serum levels may need to be higher (over 350 ng/ml) for an adequate clinical response. Adding a phenothiazine (e.g., chlorpromazine 50—300 mg/day) is probably mandatory in delusional depressives and may also be indicated in hallucinating depressives. It should be emphasized that no specific study has been carried out in either children or adolescents with psychotic subtypes of MDD.

Imipramine toxicity can be monitored through serial EKGs because the most frequent indications of toxicity are cardiac conduction defects. Noncardiovascular side effects include dry mouth, abdominal pains, constipation, nightmares, insomnia, urinary retention, headaches, sweating, and drowsiness. They may become troublesome and necessitate lowering or discontinuation of the drug. Particularly bothersome reactions to tricyclics may be orthostatic hypotension, chest pains, a rare syndrome of cognitive impairment, irritability and agitation (imipramine psychotoxicity), and anticholinergic blockade. These situations are relatively uncommon, but if they occur, changing to desipramine can alleviate these problems because it has fewer anticholinergic side effects, less P-R interval effects, but similar QRS effects.

Overdose of tricyclics is a very serious medical emergency because of the drug's low therapeutic-toxicity ratio. Imipramine toxicity produces cardiac arrhythmias, seizures, coma, and death. Management should include: (1) ipecac or gastric lavage up to eighteen hours after ingestion (use large volumes for lavage, since a significant percentage of the circulating drug is secreted in gastric juices); (2) activated charcoal, 50–100 mg in eight ounces of water, administered every two hours by mouth or through a nasogastric tube (use lower amounts for children less than 40 kg); (3) EKG monitoring—the width of the QRS complex being the best gauge of cariotoxicity; (4) IV fluids to maintain volume; (5) 1–3 mg/kg of sodium bicarbonate to reduce tachycardia; (6) seizure precautions; (7) admission to an intensive care unit for a minimum of twenty-four-hour observation period. The following are not helpful: dialysis, since most of the drug is protein bound; induced diuresis; acidification of urine, since acidification increases the risk of cardiac arrhythmia. Finally, it must be emphasized that intravenous physostigmine is not an antidote for tricyclic overdose. It may clear the sensorium if anticholinergic blockade is present, but will have no effect on cardiotoxicity or seizure propensity.

Acute tricyclic withdrawal may be associated with nausea, vomiting, abdominal cramps, drowsiness/fatigue, decreased appetite, tearfulness, apathy/withdrawal, headache, and agitation (Law et al., 1981). A flulike illness with gastrointestinal symptoms may also appear. It will generally abate within one hour after 25 mg of imipramine by mouth. Tapering withdrawal over one to two weeks, therefore, is desirable.

Children with major depression should be treated with antidepressants for five weeks; at that time, the child should be clinically reassessed. Reassessment should not focus on psychosocial functioning but on the symptoms of the depressive syndrome because the tricyclics are efficacious only for the depressive syndrome and will not directly ameliorate the child's psychosocial dysfunction. The child may have become euthymic but still have difficulty initiating interactions with peers and communicating with parents. If the patient is a nonresponder, plasma levels must be checked to insure that levels are adequate and that the child and parents followed the treatment schedule. In our experience all nonpsychotic children who had adequate serum levels responded to tricyclics. Adequate serum levels are paramount. This is apparent from a recently complete double-blind study in prepubertal MDD (Puig-Antich, 1979b). It indicated that IMI does no better than placebo in inducing clinical response. However, when the IMI group is subdivided according to high and low steady-state plasma levels, the response rate in the high plasma level subgroup is 100% while in the low plasma level subgroup it is only 33%.

Nonresponders who are receiving 5 mg/kg/day and have low maintenance plasma levels may be slowly titrated up to 7 mg/kg/day if there are no clinical contraindications, with further EKG and blood monitoring as previously described. If there is no response within another month, reassessment of diagnosis is indicated. Psychotic and schizo-affective subtypes may need antipsychotic medication added at the start of treatment. When the plasma level cannot be raised to an effective range, switching to DMI, nortriptyline, or monoamine oxidase (MAO) inhibitors is indicated.

A prepubertal responder at five weeks should be maintained on tricyclics for three additional months and postpubertals for six months. One month after discontinuation of medicine, each child must be reevaluated for relapse of depressive symptoms. If the syndrome recurs at any later date, tricyclics can be reinstituted following the previous schedule. Most of the information described in this section applies directly to prepuberty. Very little is known at present about the treatment of adolescent major depressives, although controlled studies are ongoing.

Psychotherapy

Psychotherapeutic modalities used in childhood depression include crisis management, parental counseling and/or groups, and individual, group, or family therapy. However, scientifically acceptable evidence is lacking to support the efficacy or lack of efficacy of various child therapies in prepubertal or adolescent major depression. Most depressive youngsters have two components to their clinical depression: the depressive syndrome and interpersonal and social maladaptation. While antidepressants ameliorate the depressive syndrome, they offer little benefit for interpersonal and social difficulties, which are more sensitive to psychotherapy. The effect of psychotherapy may not fully appear until several months of treatment are completed. The latter treatment will be most beneficial if the patient is kept free of depression through the use of antidepressants.

Pharmacotherapy is essential in the acute treatment of childhood depression, but it should be supplemented by a judicious admixture of available psychotherapies. The goal is to develop a working rapport with family and child, and a plan for ongoing therapeutic intervention focused on social and interpersonal skills. The efficacy of the psychotherapies in MDD, however, remains to be evaluated by properly controlled studies.

PRACTICAL GUIDE TO TREATMENT

All children reported with a depressed mood and/or suicidal ideation or gestures, or school refusal must be fully assessed for the associated signs and symptoms of the depressive syndrome. Once the diagnosis of MDD is substantiated, the child requires a physical examination, thyroid function assessment, and an electrocardiogram.

Prior to treatment with antidepressants, the parents must be counseled on: (1) the associated behavioral abnormalities in their child and how they may be related to the depressive illness; (2) what can be expected from pharmacotherapy—i.e., an amelioration of mood but not necessarily improved interpersonal skills, and (3) a full treatment plan regarding risks and management of tricyclic overdose. The parent must retain control of the medication administration, particularly in a suicidal and/or manipulative child. Also, parents frequently have the misperception that these medicines are addicting or must be given for life. The physician should correct such misconceptions. Finally, parents must be told how to identify the signs and symptoms of relapse to insure early detection of any recurrent illness.

The schedule of treatment modalities begins with titration of tricyclic antidepressants and monitoring of serum levels, EKG changes, and side effects. Psychotherapeutic modalities are also indicated in order to focus on interpersonal relationships and social skills, and to manage crises that may emerge during drug therapy. Effective antidepressant treatment should be continued for at least one month past the end of short-term psychotherapy, so as to prevent loss of psychotherapeutic gains from depressive relapse.

Conclusion

As a valid clinical entity, childhood depression is gaining wider acceptance in both prepubertal and adolescent ages. It is an extremely distressing condition for both child and family. Its treatment requires skillful assessment, judicious pharmacotherapy, and a suitable use of available psychotherapeutic modalities. Successful management of the depressed child can have a major positive impact on the patient's current life and further development.

References

American Psychiatric Association. 1980. *Diagnostic and Statistical Manual of Mental Disorders,* third ed., p. 205. Washington, D.C.: APA.

Andreasen, N. C., Endicott, J., Spitzer, R. L., and Winokur, G. 1977. The family history method using diagnostic criteria. *Arch. Gen. Psych.* 34:1229-1235.

Andrews, E., Puig-Antich, J., Tabrizi, M. A., and Behn, J. 1979. Psychosocial schedule for school age children 6 through 16. Interrater and test-retest reliability. Presented at the American Academy of Child Psychiatry, October 1979, in Atlanta, Georgia.

Brumback, R. A., and Weinberg, W. A. 1977. Mania in childhood. *Am. J. Dis. Child.*, 131:1122-1126.

Cantwell, D. P., Sturzenberger, S., Burroughs, J., Salkin, B., and Green, J. K. 1977. Anorexia nervosa: An affective disorder? *Arch. Gen. Psych.*, 34:1087-1093.

Carlson, G. 1979, Affective psychoses in mental retardates. *Psych. Clin. of North Am.*, 2:499-510.

Carlson, G., and Strober, M. 1978. Manic depressive illness in early adolescence. *J. Am. Acad. Child Psych.*, 17:138-153.

Carlson, G. A., and Cantwell, D. P. 1980. A survey of depressive symptoms, syndrome, and disorder in a child psychiatric population. *J. Child Psychol. Psych.*, 21:19-25.

Chambers, W. J., Puig-Antich, J., Tabrizi, M. A., and Davies, M. 1982. Psychotic symptoms in prepubertal major depressive disorder. *Arch. Gen. Psych.*, 39:921-931.

Cytryn, L., and McKnew, D. 1972. Proposed classification of childhood depressions. *Am. J. Psych.*, 129:149-155.

Gleser, K. 1967. Masked depression. *Am. J. Psych.*, 21:565-574.

Kashani, J. D., Husain, A., Shekim, W. O., Hodges, K. K., Cytryn, L., and McKnew, D. H. 1981. Current perspectives on childhood depression: An overview. *Am. J. Psych.*, 138:143-153.

Kovacs, M., and Beck, A. T. 1977. An empirical clinical approach toward a definition of childhood depression. In *Depression in childhood,* ed. J. G. Schulterbrandt and A. Raskin, pp. 1-25. New York: Raven Press.

Law, W., Petti, T., and Kazdin, A. E. 1981. Withdrawal symptoms after graduated cessation of imipramine in children. *Am. J. Psych.,* 138:647-650.

Liebowitz, M. R., and Klein, D. F. 1979. Hysteroid dysphoria. *Psych. Clin. of North Am.,* 2:555-575.

Pearce, J. B. 1977. Childhood depression. In *Child Psychiatry,* ed. M. Rutter, and L. Hersov, p. 448. London: Blackwell Scientific.

Poznanski, E. O., Carroll, B. J., Banegas, M. C., Cook, S. C., and Grossman, J. A. 1982. The dexamethasone suppression test in prepubertal depressed children. *Am. J. Psych.,* 139:321-324.

Puig-Antich, J. 1980. Affective disorders in childhood. *Psych. Clin. of North Am.,* 3:403-424.

Puig-Antich, J. 1984. Antidepressant treatment in children: Current state of the evidence. In *Depression and antidepressants: Implications for cause and treatment,* ed. E. Friedman, S. Gershon, and J. J. Mann. New York: Plenum, in press.

Puig-Antich, J. 1982b. Major depression and conduct disorder in prepuberty. *J. Am. Acad. Child Psych.* 21, 2:118-128.

Puig-Antich, J., Blau, S., Marx, N., Greenhill, L. L., and Chambers, W. 1978. Prepubertal major depressive disorder. *J. Am. Acad. Child Psych.,* 17:695-707.

Puig-Antich, J., Chambers, W. J., Halpern, F., Hanlon, C., and Sachar, E. J. 1979a. Cortisol hypersecretion in prepubertal depressive illness: A preliminary report. *Psychoneuroendocrin.,* 4:191-197.

Puig-Antich, J., Perel, J. M. et al. 1979b. Plasma levels of imipramine (IMI) and desmethylimipramine (DMI) and clinical response in prepubertal major depressive disorder: A preliminary report. *J. Am. Acad. Child Psych.,* 18:616-627.

Puig-Antich, J., Orvaschel, H., Tabrizi, M. A. et al. 1979c. *The schedule for affective disorders and schizophrenia for school-age children (Kiddie-SADS).* Investigators wishing to use this instrument should contact Dr. Puig-Antich at the Department of Child and Adolescent Psychiatry, Western Psychiatric Institute and Clinic, 3811 O'Hara Street, Pittsburgh, Pennsylvania 15213.

Puig-Antich, J., Tabrizi, M. A., Davies, M. et al. 1981. Prepubertal endogenous major depressives hyposecrete growth hormone in response to insulin induced hypoglycemia. *J. Biol. Psych.,* 16:801-818.

Rutter, M., Graham, P., Chadwich, O. F. D., and Yule, W. 1976. Adolescent turmoil: Fact of fiction? *J. Child Psychol. Psych.,* 17:35-56.

Rutter, M., Tizard, J., and Whitmore, K. 1970. *Education, health, and behavior.* London: Longman.

Spitzer, R. L., Endicott, J., and Robins, E. 1978. Research Diagnostic Criteria. *Arch. Gen. Psych.,* 35:773-778.

Weinberg, W. A., and Brumback, R. A. 1976. Mania in childhood. *Am. J. Dis. Child.,* 130:380-384.

Whybrow, P. C., and Hurwitz, T. 1976. Psychological disturbances associated with endocrine disease and hormone therapy. In *Hormones, behavior, and psychopathology,* ed. E. J. Sachar, pp. 125-143. New York: Raven Press.

10

Somatoform Disorders

DANIEL T. WILLIAMS

CLINICAL FEATURES

SOMATOFORM DISORDERS are characterized by physical symptoms suggesting physical disorder for which there are no demonstrable organic findings or known physiological mechanisms, and for which there is positive evidence, or a strong presumption, that the symptoms are linked to psychological factors or conflicts (American Psychiatric Association, 1980). The symptom production in somatoform disorders is not under voluntary control. For the purposes of this chapter, the following subdivisions of somatoform disorders that are most commonly encountered among children and adolescents will be considered in detail:

Conversion Disorder

Conversion disorder, or hysterical neurosis, conversion type, is characterized by *a loss or alteration of physical functioning* that suggests physical disorder but which instead is apparently an expression of a psychological conflict or need. After appropriate investigation, the disturbance cannot be explained by any physical disorder or known pathophysiological mechanism. Psychological factors may be judged to play a primary etiological role in a variety of ways. This may be suggested by a temporal relationship between the onset or worsening of the symptom and the presence of an environmental stimulus that activates a psychological conflict or need. Alternatively, the symptom may be noted to free the patient from the noxious activity or encounter. Finally, the symptom may enable the patient to get support from the environment that otherwise might not be forthcoming. The most common conversion symptoms are those suggesting neurological disease, but the manifestations of conversion disorder are protean and may mimic most of the known bodily diseases.

MOTOR DISTURBANCES. Conversion symptoms presenting as abnormal movements may take a variety of forms, including seizures, coordination difficulties, and dyskinesias.

Conversion paralysis and paresis most often affect the extremities as a monoplegia, hemiplegia, or paraplegia. A localized form of conversion paralysis can occur in the muscles affecting the vocal cords, leading to aphonia.

SENSORY DISTURBANCES. Conversion disturbances of skin sensation may occur in any location, shape, and pattern, but are found most often in the extremities. Disorders of motor function are often accompanied by diminished or totally absent sensation, often involving all modalities. As with motor disorders, the distribution of sensory disturbance follows a pattern determined by the patient's idea of the limb affected, rather than by the pattern of nerve innervation. Hence, the characteristic post-injury stocking-and-glove anesthesia of the hands and feet, and other unphysiologic patterns of sensory deficit, are commonly observed. The special organs of sense may also exhibit a loss of function, leading to varying degrees of deafness and loss of vision. In addition, there may be sensory hallucinations. Although uncommon, visual hallucinations reproducing a past event of emotional significance to the patient may be encountered. Finally, somatic aches and pains may accompany other sensory and motor disturbances in many patients with conversion disorders.

SYMPTOMS SIMULATING PHYSICAL ILLNESS. The symptoms of conversion disorder may simulate bodily disease so closely that diagnosis is difficult to establish. A common form of conversion disorder of this type involves an identification with the symptoms of the illness of a person with whom the patient has a special relationship. This may be, for example, with a parent or close friend who has recently died, and may be accompanied by the signs and symptoms of a pathological grief reaction.

SYMPTOMS COMPLICATING PHYSICAL ILLNESS. The symptoms of physical illness may be protracted or complicated by symptoms resulting from conversion mechanisms. Limb weakness or disuse that begins after an injury, for example, may be prolonged as a conversion symptom long after the initial physical lesion has healed. A patient with documented neurogenic seizures may also demonstrate conversion seizures that can be difficult to differentiate from neurogenic ones. These cases may present perplexing diagnostic problems in sorting out physical versus psychological contributants to symptoms that manifest themselves as a final common pathway of expression for both of these underlying sources of disturbance.

Psychogenic Pain Disorder

Formerly subsumed together with conversion disorders in *DSM-II* under the rubric of hysterical neurosis, conversion type, psychogenic pain disorder is given an independent status in *DSM-III*. The predominant feature in the clinical picture is the *complaint of pain* in the absence of adequate physical findings to explain the pain in physiological terms, and in association with positive evidence of the etiologic role of psychological factors. For the purposes of this chapter, psychogenic pain disorder will be described conjointly with conversion disorder, as the two appear to be phenomenologically closely linked and there is insufficient data regarding differential manifestations or causes on these two disorders among children and adolescents to discuss them separately.

Somatization Disorder

Somatization disorder (hysteria or Briquet's syndrome) is generally diagnosed in young adulthood (before age thirty), but often has its onset during adolescence. The essential features are recurrent and multiple somatic complaints of several years' duration for which medical attention has been sought, but which are apparently not due to any physical disorder (American Psychiatric Association, 1980). Complaints of at least fourteen symptoms for women and twelve for men from the thirty-seven listed in the *DSM-III* must be elicited in order to establish the diagnosis. These include complaints of general and long-standing sickliness, conversion symptoms, gastrointestinal symptoms, female reproductive symptoms, psychosexual symptoms, pain, and cardiorespiratory symptoms.

It has been estimated that approximately 1% of the adult female population has this disorder. It is rarely diagnosed in males. There is a higher incidence of this disorder and antisocial personality disorder among family members of those with somatization disorder than in the general population. The clinical course tends to be chronic but fluctuating, with rare prospect for spontaneous remission.

There are no firmly established data regarding predisposing factors to the development of somatization disorder. Yet clinical experience suggests that untreated, protracted, or recurrent episodes of conversion disorder or psychogenic pain disorder in childhood or adolescence would be likely predisposing factors. Suggestive data supporting this postulation are the observations that conversion disorders are more commonly diagnosed in children and adolescents than in adults, while the reverse is true of somatization disorder. Whether this developmental transformation from conversion disorder is in fact the common route for the emergence of somatization disorder remains to be clarified by further studies.

Hypochondriasis

Hypochondriasis, or hypochondriacal neurosis, is characterized by an unrealistic interpretation of physical signs or sensations as abnormal, leading to preoccupation with the fear or belief of having a serious disease (American Psychiatric Association, 1980). A thorough physical evaluation does not support the diagnosis of any physical disorder than can account for the physical signs or sensations or for the individual's unrealistic interpretation of them. The unrealistic fear or belief of having a physical disease persists despite medical reassurance and causes impairment in social or occupational functioning.

Common associated features include anxiety, depression, compulsive and narcissistic personality traits, as well as a history of many medical consultations. The age at onset is commonly in adolescence. The course is often chronic, with waxing and waning of symptoms. This disorder is commonly seen in general pediatric and medical practice, yet such patients often resist a psychological interpretation of their symptoms and consequently often decline referral for psychiatric treatment.

Clearly, there are close phenomenological contiguities between somatization disorder and hypochondriasis, with some of the nosological differences between them being more those of degree than those of kind. Therefore, similar questions arise regarding the possible role of early, extended experience with conversion disorder, psychogenic pain disorder, and/or true organic disease as predisposing factors to the development of hypochondriasis.

Epidemiology

Literature on the epidemiology of conversion disorders in childhood is sparse and reports vary substantially on its prevalence, reflecting variations in diagnostic criteria, sampling techniques, and populations studied. Thus, Rutter et al. (Hersov, 1977) found no cases of conversion hysteria among ten and eleven year olds on the Isle of Wight, nor were there any new cases seen in a similar general population study of fourteen year olds in London. Goodyear (1981), in a retrospective review of 3,000 cases over a twelve-year period, found only fifteen cases of hyterical conversion reactions among pediatric inpatients at Park Hospital for Children, Oxford, representing 0.5% of the total inpatient population during that time. The author does not state what proportion of patients receiving psychiatric consultation this represented. By contrast, Maloney (1980) found 105 cases of hysterical conversion reactions among pediatric inpatients at the Cincinnati Children's Hospital Medical Center over a three-year period, representing 16.7% of the pediatric inpatients receiving child psychiatry consultations during that time. The incidence relative to the total inpatient population during that period is not stated.

Proctor (1958) reviewed much of the literature prior to 1958 and reported the incidence rates of conversion reactions to be below 5% for outpatient child psychiatry clinics in all studies reviewed. Robins and O'Neal (1953) studied the incidence of childhood hysteria at St. Louis Children's Hospital for a fifteen-year period (1935–50) and found 41 cases, which constituted 4% of all cases with a psychiatric diagnosis. Rock (1971) found the overall incidence of conversion reactions to be 4% of children receiving psychiatric consultation at Tripler General Hospital in Honolulu. Herman and Simmonds (1975) also found an overall incidence rate of 4% of pediatric patients referred to both inpatient and outpatient child psychiatry consultation at the University of Missouri School of Medicine. Yet, in this study, conversion reactions were found to have an incidence of only 1.3% in the child psychiatry outpatient clinic, but 22% among psychiatric consultations on the pediatric inpatient service.

It is sometimes said that conversion disorders are less frequent currently than they were in the last century, yet how much this reflects a true change in incidence, and how much a change in diagnostic propensity with the emergence of the diagnostic entity of "psychophysiologic disorders," is difficult to ascertain. An example of the mutability in these judgments is a study by Rae (1977), who found that the incidence of childhood conversion disorders at three medical settings ranged from 5 to 24% of psychiatric referrals. Furthermore, the incidence of conversion disorder increased threefold over three years at one setting. This was attributed by Rae to greater education and sensitization of the medical staff to the presence of conversion phenomena, probably leading eventually to their being over-diagnosed.

The majority of these studies note a preponderance of conversion disorders among girls in comparison to boys, with the sex difference being small to negligible in childhood, becoming more prominent during adolescence, and remaining so into adulthood.

Differential Diagnosis

Undiagnosed Physical Illness

Undiagnosed physical illness is probably the most common and certainly the most important source of differential diagnostic error encountered when considering the diagnosis of somatoform disorder. It highlights the fact that the diagnosis of somatoform disorder requires more than just the inability to find an organic basis for a given physical symptom on initial medical evaluation. Many serious medical disorders, such as multiple sclerosis, lupus erythematosus, and dystonia musculorum deformans may present with initially subtle, fluctuating, and insidiously progressive physical symptoms that are frequently misdiagnosed early in their course as conversion disorders. Further, patients with true medical disorders may develop secondary conversion disorders as a reactive way of dealing with their anxiety about what they subliminally perceive as an underlying physical derangement, but which they have trouble communicating about directly with those in their environment. Close contact between a mental-health practitioner and a coevaluating pediatrician or other examining physician, as well as keeping the possibility of undiagnosed physical illness in mind during the course of psychological assessment and treatment are the best defense against this common and sometimes treacherous source of diagnostic error.

Factitious Disorder

Factitious disorder is characterized by physical or psychological symptoms that are produced by the individual or are *under voluntary control* (American Psychiatric Association, 1980). The sense of voluntary control is subjective and can only be inferred by an outside observer, hence giving rise to ready diagnostic confusion with somatoform disorders. The clinical judgment that symptoms are voluntarily produced is based on observations of behavior suggesting dissimulation or concealment, after having excluded all other possible causes of the behavior. However, these acts have a compulsive quality and have no readily evident benefit to the individual, other than to assume the patient role. An example would be a child with a spiking fever of unknown etiology, who is eventually found by surreptitious observation to be rubbing the thermometer against the bed sheets to generate the elevated temperature reading. In its more chronic forms, factitious disorder may be associated with either physical symptoms (Munchausen syndrome) or psychological symptoms (Ganser's syndrome, pseudopsychosis, or pseudodementia). These manifestations are generally associated with severe dependent, masochistic, or antisocial personality disorders.

Malingering

Malingering is not considered to be a mental disorder. It is characterized by the voluntary production and presentation of false or grossly exaggerated physical or psychological symptoms. The symptoms are produced in pursuit of a goal that is readily recognizable with an understanding of the individual's circumstances rather than his or her individual psychology (American Psychiatric Association, 1980). Examples of such readily understandable goals include avoidance of work, securing of financial compensation, evasion of criminal prosecution, or acquisition of drugs.

Since determination of a patient's volitional intent is often not possible with certainty by the clinician, and since there are often "secondary gains" (see section on etiology) associated with conversion disorders that may suggest malingering, caution is advisable in this tricky differential diagnostic terrain. The imputation of malingering generally leads to a confrontational stance between clinician and patient, undermining the chances of developing a therapeutic rapport. It is, therefore, best in ambiguous cases to give the patient the benefit of the doubt, so as to preserve the clinician's therapeutic leverage with a view to symptom alleviation.

Psychological Factors Affecting a Physical Condition

Psychological factors affecting a physical condition is a category used in *DSM-III* to describe not only disorders that in the past have been referred to as psychosomatic or psychophysiological, but more broadly, it is used to define any physical condition in which psychological factors are judged to be contributory (American Psychiatric Association, 1980). This judgment requires evidence that psychologically meaningful environmental stimuli are temporally related to the initiation or exacerbation of a physical condition. Furthermore, the physical condition must have either demonstrable organic pathology (e.g., peptic ulcer) or a known pathophysiological process (e.g., migraine headache.).

As an illustration of the differential diagnostic complexity that may prevail in this area, consider a child with uncontrolled seizures who is referred by a neurologist for psychiatric consultation. The referring and consulting clinicians must first decide whether the seizures represent primarily uncontrolled neurogenic seizures, a conversion disorder, a factitious disorder, malingering, or psychogenically precipitated neurogenic seizures (psychological factors affecting a physical condition). The clinicians must also be aware that two or more of these conditions may coexist in the same patient. The result can be and often is a diagnostic puzzle that challenges the resources of even the most seasoned neurologists and psychiatrists (Williams et al., 1978; Williams et al., 1979).

ETIOLOGY

Space limitations preclude a review of the many interesting and seminal historical explanations that have been offered over time for the development of conversion symptoms. For purposes of this chapter, a brief review will be offered of some of the main contemporary conceptional formulations of the genesis of conversion disorders having relevance to the practicing clinician working with children and adolescents. In contrast to obsessive-compulsive disorders (Rapoport et al., 1982), there is no substantial evidence pointing to a biological substrate or concomitant in conversion disorders of children and adolescents. The present summary will, therefore, address various psychological, situational, and social theories that have been proposed to explain the origin and development of conversion disorders. These explanations do not differ substantially in their general application to children versus adolescents versus adults, though the age of an individual obviously will color the particular manifestations of the disorder. These explanations, furthermore, are not mutually exclusive, but rather may be viewed as elucidating different possible contributions to the development of conversion disorders in different individuals.

Psychoanalytic Theory

In this framework, a fixation is postulated in early psychosexual development at the level of the Oedipus complex (Adams, 1979). The failure to relinquish the incestuous tie to the loved parent leads to intrapsychic conflict over the sexual drive because it retains its forbidden incestuous quality. This drive is, therefore, repressed and the energy associated with the drive is *converted* into a psychologically determined physical symptom. The symptom not only protects the patient from conscious awareness of the repressed drive, but simultaneously often provides a psychologically significant symbolic expression of it.

In addition to this *primary gain,* there are often *secondary gains* of the symptom which contribute to its retention. These include the attention, sympathy, and support often provided to the individual as a result of the conversion symptom. The associated disability may also excuse the individual from onerous tasks and responsibilities, thus gratifying dependency needs and reinforcing the perpetuation of the symptom.

Gratification of Dependency Needs

In some instances, gratification of dependency needs may be a primary rather than a secondary determinant of conversion symptoms (Nemiah, 1980). Experiences with psychiatric combat casualties during the world wars disclosed many conversion disorders where the primary motivation of the symptoms was self-preservation rather than oedipal sexual drives. There the symptoms enabled the individual to escape a dangerous situation and to receive protection and support under the rubric of the patient role.

Among children and adolescents, physical illness often is perceived unconsciously as an accessible route of escape from the onerous burdens of school or other competitive social situations about which the youngster feels anxious or inadequate. Faced with a conflict between unconscious dependency needs on the one hand and idealized demands of conscience to be persevering and productive on the other, conversion symptoms can provide an escape hatch. Since the physical symptom is perceived as an affliction over which the patient has no control, it brings relief of school and/or other social burdens and legitimizes the unconsciously coveted dependency status which the youngster cannot honorably request directly.

Reaction to Environmental Stress

Another perspective on the phenomena of conversion disorder is that of learning theory. From this perspective, behavior can be reinforced by the reduction of the intensity of an inner painful psychological drive that predictably follows the behavior. Thus, a conversion symptom may result in a reduction of the painful drive of fear or anxiety, e.g., that associated with being at school. The relief thus obtained reinforces the conversion symptom that produced it and predisposes to a repetition of the same symptom each time the anxiety occurs. In this manner, a pattern of behavior is evolved which may become chronic.

This learning-theory approach to human behavior shifts the focus of attention away from unconscious psychic forces and onto the observable contingencies of reinforcement of behavior. Many of the differences between learning theory and psychodynamic theory in the approach to actual clinical problems may seem more semantic than substantive (Sloane et al., 1975). Yet, the former emphasizes the systematic review of reinforcing contingencies that affect conversion symptoms, and this is often of pragmatic value in dealing with such patients and their families.

The Phenomenon of Dissociation

Janet and Freud used the term *dissociation* in relation to hysteria to refer to the splitting off from consciousness of painful affects and associated ideas (Frankel, 1976). Insofar as our contemporary definition of somatoform disorders continues to highlight the fact that symptom production is not under voluntary control, there remains an intrinsic presumption that the phenomenon of dissociation plays a central role in these disorders. The curious question of how a conversion paralysis can be mediated by the "voluntary" musculature whose innervation is intact, yet not be under the conscious voluntary control of the patient, continues to be a puzzling clinical phenomenon.

Hypnosis, which was integrally tied to Freud's early interest in the study of hysteria, is characterized by the phenomenon of dissociation (Spiegel and Spiegel, 1978). Contemporary studies of hypnosis thus provide a route of inquiry that offers clues to a better understanding of the phenomenology of somatoform disorders and delineates a useful approach to their assessment and treatment.

Diagnosis

Most often, a youngster with suspected somatoform disorder is referred to the mental-health practitioner by a pediatrician or other primary medical practitioner. It is obviously crucial that this referring physician be contacted directly to ascertain the specific physical findings on examination and the results of any laboratory and X-ray studies. As noted previously, the absence of readily diagnosable physical illness at the time of initial evaluation is by itself not a sufficient basis for establishing the diagnosis of somatoform disorder. On the other hand, if the presenting symptom includes features that are clearly nonphysiologic (e.g., the patient talking during an apparent grand mal seizure), the presence of a conversion symptom is definitively established. Yet full assessment of the diagnostic and treatment implications of a conversion symptom requires integration of physical diagnosis with other features of the patient's history and current psychological status.

History

History supporting the impression that a given symptom is a manifestation of a conversion disorder would include the following:

1. The historical data regarding the symptoms are compatible with the primary diagnosis of conversion disorder.
2. There is a history of other symptoms (past or concurrent) that clearly have the characteristics of conversion disorder, such as paralyses or anesthesias. This inquiry should apply not only to the patient, but also to family members, who are a ready source of identification for the patient.
3. There is a history of other overt emotional or behavioral symptoms, such as anxiety, depression, obsessions, phobias, or school-separation anxiety disorder (APA, 1980, p. 50). Again, inquiry with regard to family members is also of relevance.
4. There is a history of a recent death or other loss of a person important to the patient, or some other major psychological stress temporally related to the onset of the symptom.
5. There is a history of a relative, friend, or acquaintance who has had a physical symptom similar to that which the patient now presents and the patient may have some plausible reason to affiliate with this symptom by identification.
6. There is a history of sexual seduction, especially an incestuous one (Herman and Hirschman, 1981).

It should be emphasized that aside from data meeting the requirements of the primary diagnosis of conversion disorder, other supportive historical features noted in the foregoing list may or may not be present in a given individual with the disorder. Space limitations preclude a thorough discussion of the assessment of each of the different types of somatoform disorder among children and adolescents. Therefore, conversion disorder will be taken as a paradigm, with many of its features being relevant to the other somatoform disorders as well.

In this context, one's tactical approach to the patient is of importance in establishing the diagnosis and is thus a starting point for treatment with respect to all somatoform disorders. Since the patient is, by definition, unaware of the relationship between environmental stress or intrapsychic conflict and the appearance of the presenting symptom, a confrontational approach with the patient or parents seeking information on these matters is likely to be counterproductive. Indeed, any inquiries that are perceived by the patient or parents as seeking to establish such connections in an accusatory tone are likely to be met with denial or distortion. A preferable approach is to begin by explaining supportively to both the patient and parents that consultation has been sought by the referring physician because of the possibility that psychological factors may be playing some role in the patient's presenting symptom as they do in many commonly encountered medical problems.

This opens the way for a collaborative dialogue in which the patient and parents will be helping the mental-health practitioner with two difficult tasks: first, understanding the genesis of the symptom, and then, hopefully, enabling the patient to overcome it. If available medical information at the time of referral is not conclusive regarding the presence or absence of physical disease, it is important to clarify that issue and to note that ongoing contact will be maintained with the primary referring physician, as physical and psychological assessments proceed concurrently.

In other respects, history-taking should be as thorough as possible (see chap. 21). The goal is to have a detailed picture of the patient's individual strengths and weaknesses, social relationships, school functioning, and family dynamics. Gathering the necessary information for such a composite picture will often yield additional clues as to whether there exists a combination of intrinsic vulnerabilities in the patient and cumulative stresses in his or her environment that would predispose to the development of a somatoform disorder.

Physical Examination

While physical examinations are not generally the province of the mental-health practitioner, it is relevant to highlight some illustrative findings regarding physical diagnosis in the somatoform disorders for purposes of communication with one's medical colleagues (Weintraub, 1977).

SENSORY DISTURBANCES. As noted previously, disturbances of sensation in somatoform disorders generally follow the individual's lay concept of anatomy rather than known neuroanatomic patterns of sensation. In addition, most patients are unaware that in organic loss there are gradual borders of sensory change at anatomic sites because of the interdigitation of the peripheral nerves. They are thus unaware that paramedian sparing occurs in organically based hemianesthesia. Further, unilateral loss of vibration sensation when tested over the frontal bone or sternum generally points to conversion disorder, since this sensation is bilateral due to bone conduction if the bony skeleton is intact.

If a patient professes complete loss of sensation in an extremity, the examiner can have the patient perform the finger-to-nose or heel-to-shin test. In true sensory damage there is disequilibrium of the fingers or feet, as the patient does not perceive their position in space. In a conversion disorder the patient is able to effectively touch the designated target.

It should be emphasized, however, that despite the presence of numerous sensory complaints and the absence of neurologic findings indicative of organic disease, the presence of some serious organic illnesses cannot be excluded except by repeated physical examinations. Peripheral neuropathies, such as Guillain-Barré syndrome, provide striking examples of how many medical practitioners can be diagnostically fooled by an insidiously progressive organic disease.

MOTOR DISTURBANCES. The examiner can employ numerous tests based on physiologic principles to detect latent strength in cases of suspected conversion paralysis. For example, contraction of agonistic and antagonistic muscles can be tested for by the physician and the response observed when resistance is suddenly withdrawn or increased. Different responses, indicating residual weakness in organically based disorders and residual strength in the case of conversion disorders, can be diagnostic.

Patients with suspected conversion paralysis can also be observed while eating, dressing, or performing other activities, and may be seen to use the affected limb in a way that would be impossible if it were truly paralyzed. Sleep observations may be additionally helpful; hospitalized patients can be observed to move "paralyzed" limbs in their sleep, either spontaneously or in response to a noxious stimulus.

The Hoover test of unilateral leg paresis is based on the principle that when a person in a supine position attempts to lift one leg against resistance, there is normally an associated downward thrust of the other leg, to provide counterbalancing leverage. In the Hoover test, the examiner places one hand under the heel of the weak leg and with the other hand presses down on the unaffected leg. As the patient attempts to raise the unaffected leg, the examiner's hand under the heel of the weak leg detects pressure. This associated pressure occurs when the paralysis is somatoform, but not when it is organic. Conversely, in attempting to raise the weak leg against resistance, a motivated patient with organic deficit will exert downward pressure with the unaffected leg in an effort to implement the requested response. In the patient with conversion paresis, by contrast, no downward pressure with the unaffected leg will be detected during this maneuver, as there is no volitional effort at compliance.

Again, as with sensory disturbances, it should be emphasized that some motor disturbances, particularly movement disorders, may present with initially subtle, fluctuating, and hence clinically unsubstantiatable neurologic findings that only declare themselves more definitely over time. Thus, Lesser and Fahn (1978) reported that thirty-seven out of a series of eighty-four patients who had idiopathic torsion dystonia had been misdiagnosed originally as having primarily psychiatric illness.

OTHER DISTURBANCES. For additional discussion of specific differential diagnostic tests in disturbances of gait, coordination, vision, and other cranial nerve disturbances, the reader is referred to Weintraub (1977). An updated discussion of differential-diagnostic approaches to patients with suspected pseudoseizures is presented by Williams and Mostofsky (1982).

Mental-Status Evaluation

Children and adolescents with conversion disorder are generally alert, oriented, and in effective communication with the examiner. Their mood may be variable. It is advisable for the clinician to make specific inquiry about feelings of depression and associated vegetative signs, though these are usually not present. Thought content is generally not grossly abnormal, nor is there evidence of a primary-process thought disorder or bizarre behavior.

The most frequently described behavioral feature of patients with conversion disorder is "la belle indifference." This refers to the patient's attitude toward the symptom which suggests a relative lack of concern, out of keeping with the significant nature of the impairment. This feature has little diagnostic value, however, since it is also encountered in some seriously ill medical patients who are stoic about their condition. Furthermore, it should be noted that patients with conversion disorder often experience diffuse anxiety and other painful affects concomitant with the presence of conversion symptoms about which they may remain indifferent. Finally, histrionic personality traits may or may not coexist with either a conversion disorder or organic illness.

If any of the parameters of psychosis are present, conversion symptoms should generally be considered secondary to the underlying psychotic or schizophrenic process. However, in patients with recent onset of psychotic behavior associated with severe environmental stress, rapid recompensation, and other conversion symptoms or histrionic personality features, the diagnosis of hysterical psychosis should be considered (Spiegel and Fink, 1979). In such cases, differential diagnosis can be facilitated by using a standardized measure of hypnotic trance capacity. Patients with hysterical psychosis are generally highly hypnotizable while those who are schizophrenic and psychotic have low to zero hypnotizability.

Psychometric Evaluation

In children and adolescents psychometric testing may prove helpful in the disclosure of a learning disability or other intellectual limitation that may not have been recognized previously by the parents, teachers, or the evaluating clinician. In the absence of other clear evidence of an etiologic basis of a conversion symptom, especially if school absence is a by-product of the symptom, delineation of difficulties in learning can be of importance both in understanding the evolution of the symptom and in formulating an appropriate treatment plan.

Projective tests, such as the Rorschach and the Thematic Apperception Test, may add confirmatory observations to the clinician's own impressions, since they represent a special form of clinical interview in a standardized structured format. As compared with patients having other "neurotic" syndromes, those with conversion disorder tend to give test responses that are freer and more imaginative, accompanied by a more labile affect and a tendency toward impulsiveness.

TREATMENT

A variety of treatment techniques have been used in children and adolescents with somatoform disorders. As with most psychotherapeutic interventions (Frank et al., 1978), controlled studies are extremely difficult to structure and implement, and consequently are simply not available at present for this group of disorders. Those therapeutic approaches that clinical experience has suggested may be useful will be considered here. Each of these treatment approaches has some potential value for some patients. Often, different treatments can be combined effectively in the management of a given patient. It is advantageous for the therapist to be as well-informed about as many of these as possible, so as to be able to innovatively structure a treatment plan that most effectively and efficiently meets the unique needs of each patient.

Reassurance, Placebo, and Suggestion

The suggestive approach, in a variety of forms, has been used for centuries, sometimes quite effectively, by religious healers, physicians, and others as a way of relieving conversion symptoms. It involves the use of reassurance, placebo, and/or suggestion to foster symptom relinquishment without a sophisticated grasp, by contemporary theoretical standards, of the symptom's psychogenic determinants. A common format of the current use of intravenous sodium amobarbital also falls under this heading. Such nonspecific modalities, often used by pediatricians and other medical practitioners prior to referral for mental-health consultation, may be effective for acute conversion symptoms arising in response to a short-term and self-limiting environmental stress. If used supportively and sensitively in such a context, this approach may be not only effective but judicious in sparing the patient and family a long and expensive involvement in unnecessary psychotherapy.

Problems arise, however, when such treatment is used indiscriminately for all conversion symptoms, including those with complex, sustained, intrapsychic determinants and/or in the presence of continuing, unmanageable environmental stress. In such situations this approach is counterproductive. It is either totally ineffective or of only short-term benefit, with the prompt emergence of symptom recurrence or symptom substitution. Further, there is a loss of confidence by the patient in the physician or therapist who takes such an approach. This is so because an attempt has been made to remove a symptom that has been serving a defensive function, albeit maladaptively in many instances, without an effort to correct the patient's underlying sources of distress.

Family and Individual Therapies

Family and individual therapies, delineated in chapters 28 and 29 of this text, need not be reviewed in detail here. It should be noted, though, that with reference to treating conversion disorders, these approaches draw primarily upon the conceptual frameworks outlined earlier in this chapter in the section dealing with etiology. Clearly, there are a myriad of variations that may be developed under this broad rubric. For our purposes, some general guidelines of procedure will be discussed.

The first task of the mental-health practitioner is to glean from the data elicited in the course of the history-taking, the basis of a working hypothesis regarding the evolution of a presenting conversion symptom. With this working hypothesis in mind, the therapist's next task is to explore possible ways to mitigate pathogenic environmental influences impinging on the patient and/or augment the patient's capacity for mastering ongoing intrapsychic conflict.

Environmental manipulation is often an important measure and includes working with the patient's immediate family and other close contacts such as teachers. Thus, if marital conflict between the parents involving sexual and/or aggressive themes is apparently contributing to a youngster's somatization, counseling the parents regarding their marital adjustment and the way they communicate with their child about it may be helpful. Similarly, if a "valedictorian syndrome" exists whereby parents, teachers, and/or the patient himself have generated excessive demands for academic achievement relative to the youngster's capacity, then direct, supportive counseling to readjust these frequent contributants to somatization would be appropriate.

Dealing with the apparent dynamics of intrapsychic conflict in youngsters with conversion disorders requires tact and sensitivity. It often helps to view the conversion symptom as a makeshift refuge to which the patient has intuitively and inadvertently retreated under duress. From this standpoint, the challenge to the therapist is to formulate for the patient a safe and palatable route by which the symptom can be seen as an awkward defensive encumbrance which can be relinquished with dignity in favor of a more effective coping method. The ways in which this can be done are manifold, but they generally all include presenting some version of the therapist's working hypothesis to the patient and/or parents as an aid in the process of cognitive, emotional, and behavioral reorientation. The extent to which this process can be "worked through" with the patient in terms of conscious understanding is generally an indication of the amount of "insight" achieved.

In the interest of attaining the therapeutic goals, a number of specialized treatment approaches are often utilized within the context of individual and/or family therapy. Some of these will be briefly enumerated.

PSYCHOANALYSIS. For many years it was believed that psychoanalysis or intensive long-term dynamic psychotherapy was the specific treatment of choice for conversion disorder (Nemiah, 1980). It is now apparent that only a minority of the total number of patients with conversion symptoms are candidates for such therapy. This is true in part because of the combined demands of time, money, and intellectual capacity which most patients and families simply do not have. Equally important, however, is the fact that for many patients other approaches can achieve therapeutic results more rapidly and with much less expense.

For those therapists using a psychoanalytic approach, treatment is aimed at uncovering the presumed neurotic conflict that has led to the conversion symptom and helping the youngster to "reconvert" (Anthony, 1975). In this mode of therapy, the decoding of the unconscious meaning of the conversion symptom through interpretation is said to induce progressive alterations in the transference relationship and in the symptoms, until the work of reconstruction pieces together the historical development of the symptom, making use of dreams and fantasies as an adjunct.

It is obvious that a mental-health clinician working with patients having conversion symptoms must have a sophisticated grasp of the subtle and complex factors operative in the diverse intrapsychic, interpersonal, and environmental fields that involve these patients. It is *not* true, however, that each such patient must be capable of attaining a full level of insight in order to achieve effective and sustained symptom relinquishment. Extended analytic endeavor can certainly add new dimensions of self-understanding to those with the resources to use this approach (Eckstein, 1979). Yet, for the many who cannot utilize this protracted and costly therapy, more supportive and directive methods of treatment are available which are both more efficient and more appropriate.

HYPNOSIS. Freud's interest in developing the technique of psychoanalysis was to a large extent fostered by the shortcomings he observed in his colleagues' use of hypnosis to treat conversion symptoms (Freud, S., 1955a)—shortcomings such as the use of abreaction and suggestion without benefit of the dynamic understanding of symptom formation which Freud was subsequently to develop. It is not commonly appreciated that Freud himself in later years came to foresee how public-health needs would reactivate a role for hypnosis to enable more widespread therapeutic application of psychonalytic insights in a more expeditious manner (Freud, S., 1955b).

In current conceptual terms, hypnosis is best understood as involving features of both dissociation and transference, including an altered state of intense and interpersonal relatedness between the therapist and subject (Spiegel and Spiegel, 1980). There is an associated nonrational submission and relative abandonment of executive control by the subject, which is actively tapped by the hypnotist for therapeutic purposes. This process enhances the patient's concentration on certain thoughts or feelings which can lead to designated therapeutic reorientations. This guided regression can thus become the basis of authoritatively sanctioned relinquishment of a symptom coupled with the concomitant incorporation of a new, more adaptive coping strategy advocated by the therapist.

Detailed considerations regarding the use of hypnosis with children and adolescents are outlined elsewhere (Williams, 1979, 1981). It should be noted, however, that the vast majority of children and adolescents are hypnotizable and are better subjects, comparatively, than adults. Admonitions sometimes expressed against the use of hypnosis with youngsters having conversion symptoms are based on the mistaken assumption that hypnosis always involves the simplistic and heavy-handed use of direct suggestion which was the usual mode of Freud's contemporaries.

Finally, there are some specific therapeutic benefits to enabling a patient and family to discover that the patient's capacity for dissociation can be elicited under controlled therapeutic auspices. In this context, the dissociation that is an essential component in the symptom formation of somatoform disorders can be understood by the patient and family as a tamable psychological attribute which can be channeled, under therapeutic guidance, in the direction of symptom resolution. Teaching the patient a self-hypnosis format is often a useful way of reinforcing a shift of the youngster's attention away from preoccupation with the sick role and toward the mastery experience of returning to normal functioning.

BEHAVIOR MODIFICATION. Any therapeutic strategy oriented toward symptom relief in the somatoform disorders must deal with the secondary gain features of symptoms. With children and adolescents particularly, the long-range benefits of a therapeutic endeavor may be difficult for the patient to appreciate if the immediate benefits of the symptom constitute a substantial deterrent to symptom relinquishment. It is, therefore, essential that any ongoing secondary gain features of a symptom be diminished or eliminated. Indeed, this is critical in order for the symptom's removal to be sustained. Chapter 27 of this text illustrates a number of ways in which behavior modification strategies can be formulated, taking into account the existing contingencies of reinforcement which impinge on the patient.

PHYSICAL THERAPY. While physical therapy includes some features of reassurance, placebo, and suggestion, it has apparent benefit in clinical practice for patients with conversion symptoms involving motor deficits. This is particularly true if the conversion symptom arises as a complication of an actual physical illness or injury. Clearly, to be effective such physical therapy must be combined with a psychological strategy that addresses pertinent psychodynamic issues of intrapsychic conflict and external contingencies of reinforcement that affect the symptom. Yet, if this is done, the physical therapy often provides a face-saving maneuver which the youngster can use as a facilitating bridge to the resumption of normal functioning.

MEDICATIONS. Aside from commonly being used as part of a placebo component of treatment, medication may have a specific role to play when conversion symptoms arise in conjunction with conditions for which medication is particularly indicated. One such condition is school refusal (separation anxiety disorder) (see chap. 8) in which case imipramine is often effective when supportive and directive psychotherapeutic measures alone are insufficient to effect symptom alleviation (Klein et al., 1980). Other conditions that may predispose to and/or accompany conversion disorders are depression (see chap. 9) and pathological grief reactions, in which case tricyclic antidepressant medication should also be considered when initial psychotherapeutic efforts are ineffective.

There is no justifiable basis for using neuroleptic medications in the treatment of conversion symptoms. If there is clearly documented evidence in a youngster of a schizophrenic disorder upon which substrate conversion symptoms may sometimes be superimposed, the schizophrenia itself then becomes the primary focus of therapeutic concern (Klein et al., 1980) with the conversion symptoms being treated as a secondary manifestation.

Conclusion

Somatoform disorders, under various labels and viewed through various conceptual frameworks, have presented challenges in both diagnosis and treatment to physicians and psychotherapists throughout recorded history. Mental-health professionals working with children and adolescents are likely to encounter some instances of this multidetermined group of disorders, with the frequency depending on the nature of one's treatment setting and pattern of referrals. Effective treatment requires a sophisticated assessment of the patient's psychological state and environmental circumstances as well as a capacity to integrate several therapeutic avenues of approach so as to most effectively meet the unique needs of each patient and family.

References

Adams, P. L. 1979. Psychoneuroses. In *Basic handbook of child psychiatry,* vol. 2, ed. J. Noshpitz, pp. 194–234. New York: Basic Books.

American Psychiatric Association. 1980. *Diagnostic and statistical manual of mental disorders—third edition.* Washington, D.C.: APA.

Anthony, E. J. 1975. Neurotic disorders in children. In *Comprehensive textbook of psychiatry,* vol. 2, 2nd ed., ed. A. M. Freedman, H. I. Kaplan, and B. J. Sadock. Baltimore: Williams and Wilkins.

Eckstein, R. 1979. Psychoanalysis. In *Basic handbook of child psychiatry,* vol. 3, ed. S. I. Harrison, and J. Noshpitz, pp. 21–34. New York: Basic Books.

Frank, J. D., Hoehn-Saric, R., Imber, S. D., Liberman, B. L., and Stone, A. R. 1978. *Effective ingredients of successful psychotherapy.* New York: Brunner/Mazel.

Frankel, F. H. 1976. Hypnosis: Trance as a coping mechanism. New York: Plenum Press.

Freud, S. 1955a. Lines of advance in psychoanalytic therapy. In *The standard edition of the complete psychological works of Sigmund Freud,* vol. 17, ed. J. Strachey, pp. 159–168. London: Hogarth Press.

Freud, S. 1955b. An autobiographical study. In *The standard edition of the complete psychological works of Sigmund Freud,* vol. 20, ed. J. Strachey, pp. 3–74. London: Hogarth Press.

Goodyear, I. 1981. Hysterical conversion reactions in childhood. *J. Child Psychol. Psychiat.*, 22:179–188.

Herman, J., and Hirschman, L. 1981. Families at risk for father-daughter incest. *Am. J. Psych.* 138:967–970.

Herman, R. M., and Simmonds, J. R. 1975. Incidence of conversion symptoms in children evaluated psychiatrically. *Missouri Med.,* 72:597–604.

Hersov, L. 1977. Emotional disorders. In *Child psychiatry: Modern approaches,* ed. M. Rutter and L. Hersov. Oxford: Blackwell Scientific.

Klein, D. F., Gittelman, R., Quitkin, F., and Rifkin, A. 1980. *Diagnosis and drug treatment of psychiatric disorders: Adults and children,* 2nd ed. Baltimore: Williams and Wilkins.

Lesser, R. P., and Fahn, S. 1978. Dystonia: A disorder often misdiagnosed as a conversion reaction. *Am. J. Psych.* 135:349–352.

Maloney, M. J. 1980. Diagnosing hysterical conversion reactions in children. *J. Ped.,* 97:1016–1020.

Nemiah, J. C. 1980. Somatoform disorders. In *Comprehensive textbook of psychiatry,* vol. 2, 3rd ed., ed. H. I. Kaplan, A. M. Freeman, and B. J. Sadock, pp. 1525–1543. Baltimore: Williams and Wilkins.

Proctor, J. 1958. Hysteria in childhood. *Am. J. Orthopsych.* 28:394–406.

Rae, W. A. 1977. Childhood conversion reactions: A review of incidence in pediatric settings. *J. Clin. Child Psychol.,* 6:69–72.

Rapoport, J., Elkins, R., Langer, D., Sceery, W., Buchsbaum, M. S., Gillin, C., Murphy, D. L., Zahn, T. P., Lake, R., Ludlow, C., and Mendelson, W. 1981. Childhood obsessive-compulsive disorder. *Am. J. Psych.,* 138:1545–1554.

Robins, E., and O'Neal, P. 1953. Clinical features of hysteria in children with a note on prognosis. *Nerv. Child,* 10:246–271.

Rock, N. L. 1971. Conversion reactions in childhood: A clinical study on childhood neurosis. *J. Am. Acad. Child Psych.,* 10:65–93.

Sloane, R. B., Staples, F. R., Cristol, A. H., Yorkston, N. J., and Whipple, K. 1975. *Psychotherapy vs behavior therapy.* Cambridge, Mass.: Harvard University Press.

Spiegel, D., and Fink, R., 1979. Hysterical psychosis and hypnotizability. *Am. J. Psych.,* 136:77–781.

Spiegel, H., and Spiegel, D. 1978. *Trance and treatment: Clinical uses of hypnosis.* New York: Basic Books.

Spiegel, H., and Spiegel, D. 1980. Hypnosis. In *Comprehensive textbook of psychiatry,* vol. 2., 2nd ed., ed. H. I. Kaplan, A. M. Freedman, and B. J. Sadock, pp. 2168–2177. Baltimore: Williams and Wilkins.

Weintraub, M. I. 1977. *A clinical guide to diagnosis.* Clinical Symposia, vol. 29, no. 6. Summit, N.J.: CIBA.

Williams, D. T. 1979. Hypnosis as a psychotherapeutic adjunct with children. In *Basic handbook of child psychiatry,* vol. 3, ed. S. I. Harrison, and J. Noshpitz, pp. 108–116. New York: Basic Books.

Williams, D. T. 1981. Hypnosis as a psychotherapeutic adjunct with children and adolescents. *Psychiat. Ann.* 11:47–56.

Williams, D. T., Gold, A. P., Shrout, P., Shaffer, D., and Adams, D. 1978. The impact of psychiatric intervention on patients with uncontrolled seizures. *J. Ner. Men. Dis.* 167:626–631.

Williams, D. T., and Mostofsky, D. I. 1982. Psychogenic seizures in children and adolescents. In *Pseudoseizures,* ed. T. Riley and A. Roy, pp. 169–184. Baltimore: Williams and Wilkins.

Williams, D. T., Spiegel, H., and Mostofsky, D. I. 1978. Neurogenic and hysterical seizures in children and adolescents: Differential diagnostic and therapeutic considerations. *Am. J. Psych.* 135:82–86.

11

Childhood Obsessive-Compulsive Disorder

JUDITH L. RAPOPORT

CLINICAL FEATURES

Obsessive-compulsive disorder is a rare childhood psychiatric illness which has been estimated to occur in, at most, 1% of child psychiatric inpatient populations (Judd, 1965; Hollingsworth et al., 1980). It is an illness dominated by obsessions and/or compulsions that create significant and sustained impairment of function and that are not secondary to another psychiatric disorder.

Three essential characteristics of obsessive-compulsive symptoms are: the sense of an inner compelling force, internal resistance to it, and retention of insight. Patterns in childhood symptomatology are remarkably similar to that found in adult patients; rituals typically focus around cleanliness (washing, changing clothes) and warding off danger or sexual thoughts or acts. Ruminations, that is, obsessive thoughts, occasionally concern "meaningless" material, but more typically involve repetitive thoughts about danger to self or others, or forbidden sexual words or ideas. These may occur in the absence of rituals.

Obsessive-compulsive disorder is equally as likely to have an acute as an insidious onset; precipitating events offered by the family are typically unconvincing. The disorder may start at age three or four, although seems more frequent just before or around puberty; typically the pattern is one of waxing and waning severity. Childhood obsessional illness is also typified by familial involvements in rituals, and often by the child's ability to conceal from friends and teachers extremely deviant patterns which take place exclusively at home during the early years of the disorder.

ASSOCIATED CONDITIONS

Because of the rarity of this condition, systematic analysis of epidemiologic studies of large populations is not possible; most of what is known about this illness is through a case-finding approach. Important hints about the disorder have come from studies with adults; Welner et al. (1976) examined 149 adult inpatients who had received a diagnosis of obsessive-compulsive disorder to see what other disorders were also present at the time of follow-up. Only 30 of the patients had obsessions and compulsions as their only symptom, while over 100 had depression either concurrent or secondary to obsessive-compulsive symptoms. (A minority of 16 patients had primary depression with subsequent development of obsessions and compulsions.) Other disorders, relatively rarely associated, were schizophrenia and anorexia nervosa.

Experience with children and adolescents supports the Welner survey; that is, depression is frequent as a concurrent or subsequent disorder, while schizophrenia, anorexia, and even primary depression are relatively rare (although still associated with obsessions to a degree greater than chance). A recent series (Rapoport et al., 1981) found that eleven of eleven obsessive adolescents had a concurrent or secondary depressive episode, as well as sleep EEG similar to that seen in depression. These findings suggest a link between obsessive-compulsive disorder and depression, the nature of which is not understood.

Other conditions that may be particularly associated with childhood obsessive-compulsive disorder are anorexia nervosa, Tourette's syndrome (Nee et al., 1980), and diabetes insipidus (Barton, 1976). These latter associations are problematic, however, as will be discussed later. Children with various types of brain damage, autistic-like syndromes, and retardation may have some features of obsessive disorder but rarely have symptom patterns meeting diagnostic criteria.

As a rule, there are no developmental disorders associated with obsessive-compulsive disorder, perhaps surprising in light of some of the recent findings that suggest a neurobiological component to this problem (discussed later). However, it is a myth that these are always bright students; the coexistence of average scholarship and either hyperactivity and/or reading disability has been reported (Jessner, 1963; Rapoport et al., 1981). Children seem less likely than adults to have compulsive personality styles associated with the disorder.

It is curious that other anxiety disorders (with the exception of phobic aspects of the obsessive symptoms) are not prominent in this condition, which is itself classified as an anxiety disorder, although occasionally mild separation anxiety will be reported (Berg et al., in press).

Differential Diagnosis

Obsessive-compulsive disorder needs to be distinguished from normal developmental phases (such as some preschoolers' adherence to routine, or the grade-school child's superstitious games such as "not stepping on sidewalk cracks," or having lucky numbers). This is usually not a difficult distinction, as the mildness of the symptoms and lack of interference with normal routine is apparent when such behavior is developmentally appropriate. More difficult may be the diagnosis of Tourette's when swearing and preoccupation with possible cursing may be the dominant feature of the disorder. However, multiple motor tics are usually apparent in Tourette's by the time verbal tics are so advanced. Anorexia nervosa will be evident from the history of weight loss or the current evidence of emaciation.

Retarded and brain-damaged children may have repetitive and even obsessional traits. However, these are rarely seen as ego-dystonic by these groups; similarly, schizophrenic and autistic children may have obsessive-compulsive-like symptoms, but the lack of insight into the senselessness of the symptoms usually distinguishes these disorders.

In many cases, there is *some* belief in the validity of the ritual and the diagnostician should not put too fine a point on "100% insight" into the irrational nature of the ritual; these children may describe themselves as "fundamentalists" or "very superstitious." Finally, the distinction between obsessive-compulsive disorder and phobia may be obscure. A child who broods about the presence of dirt, may act phobic about some objects and situations. Another child may avoid exposure to violent scenes (e.g., avoid the room if the TV is on) and might be considered phobic. This distinction does not seem a useful one, as severe obsessive-compulsive disorder, in our experience, always has some phobic features.

Etiology

Obsessive-compulsive disorder is poorly understood and its etiology is probably determined both by biological and social factors. It is striking how severe the illness may be, in spite of relatively intact mental status and often seemingly supportive homes. Moreover, unlike many other childhood disorders, the clinical picture is virtually identical to its adult counterpart, and over half of adult patient populations report the onset of their disorder in childhood.

There are only hints as to etiology, and all are controversial.

Genetic Components

Twin studies suggest that there may be a genetic component at least for some patients, although ideal studies such as systematic comparison of monozygotic and dizygotic twins with obsessional illness are lacking (Elkins et al., 1980); such a comparison has been made for obsessional *personality* (Carey and Gottesman, 1981). Family studies with obsessive children do not support any consistent psychopathology among parents or siblings (Rapoport et al., 1981).

Brain Damage

The association of obsessive disorder with brain damage has a long history (see review in Elkins et al., 1980). There seemed to have been a high incidence of obsessional symptoms as part of a postencephalitic recovery syndrome. Obsessive symptoms are also reported in uremia, diabetes insipidus, and have been reported associated with abnormal birth history. Whether these symptom pictures would actually have been diagnosed as obsessive disorder, however, is unclear. The data are suggestive, however, that some brain damage may be associated with this disorder. Subtle psycholinguistic test data also support a neurological component (Rapoport et al., 1981).

Experiential and Temperamental Factors

Obsessional children tend to be nonaggressive, although they vary considerably as to the degree of outgoing and friendly behavior they demonstrate. It is interesting that Freud's initial interest in obsessional symptomatology focused on the phase-specific nature of several of his cases (Freud, 1958, 1959); symptoms seemed to appear before puberty (ages six to eight), and earlier experiences, in the anal phase of development, were emphasized.

Here, too, the rarity of the disorder makes systematic study difficult. In a study of fourteen children and adolescents seen at the NIMH, there was no consistent developmental phase of onset identified, nor were there any experiential data that appeared causative. However, separation problems, overconscientiousness, high aspirations, have been true for some of the children. Several of these children did not fit this model, however, and two boys and one girl, all in their early teens, would be considered to be impulsive with milder forms of conduct disorder. A further "soft" impression is that these children may become overly close with one parent, often that of the opposite sex, at the expense of the relationship with the parent of the same sex. Here, too, this is difficult to quantify and does not hold for all cases.

History-taking

Diagnosis

It is most important to know, in detail, the pattern of obsessive or compulsive symptoms. Are these clearly thoughts or rituals that the patient is aware of, feels forced to carry out, and realizes (at least for the most part) are senseless? One must determine whether or not the symptoms interfere sufficiently with normal living patterns to constitute a disorder. An important insight into this may be gotten from knowing the effort the patient makes or has made to resist these impulses, to "get through the day."

In addition, it is important to see what other psychopathology there is or has been. For example, obsessive symptoms may be superimposed on psychosis or Tourette's syndrome or anorexia nervosa. Occasionally, a patient has an isolated bizarre conceptual system which seems to be like an obsession, but may actually be a pure paranoia.

Presence of Associated Features

The presence of depression may serve to prevent useful alliance with the patient and may be the most important feature to address therapeutically. It is important to find out which came first, the depressive or obsessive symptoms. These patients vary widely in their depressive response to even severe life restriction from the rituals.

Determine the nature of familial response to symptoms. Is the family split over their approach to the child? How do siblings relate to the child's difficulty? Is there anyone else with similar problems? What was the premorbid history of this child in this family? Who are the child's allies for working with these symptoms?

Find out about possible medical illness in the child or family (Hollingsworth et al., 1980) and (rarely) about learning difficulties the child may have had or is currently having.

Treatment Planning

Obsessive-compulsive disorder is a chronic, waxing-and-waning condition and, therefore, treatment history may be difficult to interpret. It is most important, however, to find out what the family has tried, their feelings about the success or failure of treatments, and what seemed to precipitate change of any sort in the course of the disorder.

Specific treatments will typically have included psychotherapy, psychoanalysis, chemotherapy, and behavioral treatment. The latter term covers a variety of approaches from commonsense "rewards" of good behavior to formal methods of desensitization, thought stopping, etc. It is most important to find out what family responses to these treatments may have hindered or helped their success. For example, a child may have benefited from a behavioral approach during hospitalization, but the parents may have been unable to carry out the follow-up program and/or may have been insufficiently supervised during the postdischarge period.

Unusual problems with regard to treatment of these children occur when one parent becomes overly involved with complying with the rituals "in order to spare the child distress." This compliance may be so strong that unless this can be addressed, no treatment program is possible. One mother, for example, signed her daughter out of the hospital saying that if her daughter had shared a bathroom she would not have had unlimited access to the shower and thus would have been frustrated in her washing ritual.

A further source of problems is parental disagreement over handling of the rituals, and the ability of these children to conceal their disorder during certain times of the day, making the behavior appear to be deliberately provocative.

Parental attitudes toward different treatment modalities will, of course, be important for treatment planning, such as strong feelings against or for medication, psychotherapy, and/or hospitalization.

INVESTIGATIONS

Physical and Neurological Examination

Because of the rare, but important, clinical conditions that may be associated with and/or mistaken for obsessive-compulsive disorder, a physical and neurological examination should be carried out to identify any evidence of frank brain damage, tics, or signs of brain tumor. Part of this work-up should include a clinical EEG, as well as a CAT scan.

Psychometric Evaluation

A psychometric evaluation may be helpful in both the differential diagnosis (brain damage, schizophrenia) and in evaluating associated problems. Subtle cognitive weaknesses may be important in understanding the particular form of these patients' perfectionistic strivings. There is increasing interest in neuropsychological testing with the growing evidence from studies, primarily with adults, that frontal temporal lobe dysfunction may be implicated in this disorder. Theoretically, such hints may be helpful, and practically, the families may gather support from the recognition of some of the organismic features of their child's illness.

Assessment Scales

A most creative scale is the Leyton Obsessional Inventory (Cooper, 1970) which was developed for adult patients but has been adapted by Rapoport and coworkers for use with children. This scale measures not only the number of positive answers to particular symptoms, but also the amount of resistance to these symptoms and the degree of interference with the patient's life. Unfortunately, the scales do not always correlate well with other measures (nurses' ward rating, physician interviews), and it is likely that one measure proves much more useful than the others for following a given patient. Nevertheless, for some patients, the inventory does provide a good measure for longitudinal follow-up and is therefore recommended.

Mental-Status Evaluation

Obsessional children vary widely with respect to associated personality type. There appears to be considerable discontinuity between trait and state. Therefore, the kind of alliance that can be established with the child is not obvious until an evaluation of his or her ability to trust the therapist and to confront the disorder has been made. These patients vary considerably in the degree to which they "disbelieve" their throughts and rituals. Some are still organized around concealing their symptoms even within the hospital setting.

Determine what the child's view of the disorder is, what he or she feels has been helpful in the past, and who in the family is "on my side." Sometimes children feel that another problem, such as rejection by a parent or school difficulty, is actually primary, and this must be attended to simultaneously with the obsessive symptoms.

It is particularly important when planning a treatment for a chronic and debilitating condition that the expectations of the child regarding treatment ("my last hope," etc.) be understood. This must always be done before any drug trial, as the "magical" nature of the treatment may give the patient an "all-or-nothing" attitude which can be destructive. Alternate or concomitant treatments need to be described, and a plan involving several approaches, sequentially or simultaneously, needs to be worked out together with the child and parents.

AVAILABLE TREATMENTS

Psychotherapy

As with other rare conditions, patients derive considerable support just by meeting therapists who have had contact with others having the same disorder, parents tend to form mutual support groups with an intensity that testifies to their need for such interaction, and children and adolescents are relieved to find a peer with whom they can discuss certain aspects of their difficulties. It is, thus, useful to put such families in contact with each other.

Despite the intimate association between psychodynamic theory and early descriptions of obsessional disorder, the efficacy of psychotherapy for this disorder is not known. However, some of the children appear to benefit at least from the supportive and reassuring features of therapy, and associated problems such as depression and family conflict may be helped by it, perhaps indirectly lightening the severity of the burder of the disorder.

In the absence of clear guidelines and careful research, recommendations stem entirely from clinical experience with these children. It seems that in addition to lightening associated problems, therapy may, in a preliminary way, serve to focus on the symptoms and also serve a kind of baseline record-keeping function that may in itself prove helpful in dissipating the frequency of some of the symptoms.

Pharmacotherapy

A variety of agents have been reported as efficacious for treating obsessional disorder and, thus, the subject has been reviewed in detail elsewhere (Elkins et al., 1980; Insel and Murphy, 1981). For most agents, these studies have been uncontrolled and lacking in objective behavioral assessment.

However, several controlled studies of chlorimipramine suggest that this agent may be specifically useful for this disorder, at least in adult patients (Thoren et al., 1980; Insel and Murphy, 1981; Montgomery et al., 1981; Insel et al., 1983). Doses are approximately those used with tricyclics in depression; the clinical response is usually delayed, appearing after two to four weeks.

One study with a small number of adolescents did not indicate significant drug effect; however, individual "responders" within this group suggest that such a trial is worth repeating.

Recently, a controlled trial with clorgyline, an MAO inhibitor (also in adult patients) (Dr. Tom Insel, personal communication), suggests that this agent is effective but that chlorimipramine is probably superior.

Anafranil (chlorimipramine) is currently an investigative drug in this country. In individual cases, however, CIBA-Geigy, the manufacturer, will provide individual support for cases on "humanitarian grounds."

Because of the extremely disabling nature of this disorder, at developmentally crucial stages, severe cases should probably be given both intense behavioral treatment and a trial of chlorimipramine, the most promising drug to date. Locating appropriate facilities for both of these treatments will be the most difficult part of treatment planning and the clinician may need to tread unfamiliar ground to do so.

Behavior Therapy

By far the most extensive and careful studies have been carried out exploring the efficacy of behavior therapy for adults with obsessive-compulsive disorder. The principle work in this area has been in England (Marks, 1981; Marks et al., 1981) and Philadelphia (Foa and Goldstein, 1978). Although the studies have not specifically involved children, individual reports indicate that similar techniques apply (Weiner, 1967; Campbell, 1973). The studies have been carried out almost exclusively with ritualizers rather than ruminators whose pathology is more difficult to qualify and to manipulate experimentally.

The basic principle is exposure of the patient to the evoking stimuli. A series of studies have demonstrated the usefulness of the specific technique of exposing the patient to the situation that precipitates the rituals. The "control" treatment, that of relaxation exercises alone, indicate that muscle relaxation did not reduce rituals.

Exposure treatment can take several forms. One approach is to have the patient imagine the situation that may bring out rituals (such as contact with sticky substances or touching another person) while relaxing. As this process is repeated, it is termed desensitization in fantasy. If the same maneuvers are repeated in real life (such as having honey applied to the skin, or systematically touching people) this is *in vivo* desensitization. More dramatic strategies involve imagining "overwhelming" situations (such as being immersed in a sticky substance or being rubbed with mud); this approach is implosion or flooding (in fantasy or *in vivo*). As is clear, the different terms refer to different rates of exposure. Therapeutic strategy is worked out for each patient on a highly individual basis; the idea is to provoke symptoms while maintaining an alliance with the patient.

Special considerations may be important with obsessional children. For example, children may minimize their symptoms more than adults, as discussed earlier. For this reason, self-counting record keeping may need to enlist the help of parents, teachers, or ward staff; this requires skillful handling, as it introduces unwelcome intrusiveness—a major concern in the treatment of children and adolescents in particular.

An obstacle to active behavioral intervention can stem from the family's own involvement with ritualistic behavior. Ideally, a family member will be a cotherapist, helping with the "homework" part of a desensitization program. However, a common complication is familial overinvolvement with rituals, and periods of hospitalization may be required because of this issue alone. Most of these children have both inclination and a good ability to intellectualize their difficulty, making them good partners for behavioral programs. Individual case reports have indicated that excellent alliance can be maintained with adolescents (Weiner, 1967; Campbell, 1973).

Like Marks, our experience with ruminators is more complex. There is great difficulty in rating the behavior and in specifying evoking stimuli in many cases. Other techniques such as thought stopping and prolonged exposure in imagination for ruminations have been reported (Emmelkamp and Kwee, 1977) but not studied as systematically as has the behavioral approach to rituals.

In summary, treament by exposure with response prevention requires considerable patient cooperation. Because of the ego-dystonic sense of these symptoms, children usually make appropriate subjects. However, the shyness and humiliation that some of the younger children experience in revealing their rituals may make symptom monitoring unusually difficult and a longer preparatory clinical period may be necessary to build the child's trust.

Psychosurgery

Stereotactic psychosurgery for chronic obsessive illness has been reported to be efficacious. Almost all studies and case reports are on adults, and the literature is of poor quality. However, a review of better studies has suggested that in extreme cases, clinically impressive results may occur (reviewed by Elkins et al., 1980). At the present time, it seems unlikely that any pediatric case, no matter how ill, would be a suitable candidate for this approach.

PRACTICAL GUIDE TO TREATMENT

Explanation to Parents

Parents should be told that it is important to treat this condition, but that the etiology is poorly understood and that they are vital in helping the therapist to understand their particular child. Parents need to be educated away from feeling that the child has complete control of his or her symptoms just because of the fluctuating nature of the disorder or the daily routine with some symptom-free hours.

Working with Ward Staff/Family

Inpatient work with obsessive children presents some unique problems. While these patients typically do not resemble conduct-disordered children, some of the issues of limit setting come up around handling of washing (allocation of soap, bedclothes, etc.) and helping these children adhere to some hospital routine. During the initial observation phase, secretiveness on the part of some children may make observation difficult. Comparison of school, parent, day and night staff observations, as well as self-report may be crucial in establishing the severity of the disorder in some cases.

References

Barton, R. 1976. Diabetes insipidus and obsessional neurosis. *Am. J. Psych.,* 133:235-236.

Berg, C., Rapoport, J., and Behar, D. Childhood obsessive-compulsive disorder: An anxiety disorder? In *Anxiety syndromes in children,* ed. R. Gittelman. New York: Guilford Press, in press.

Campbell, L. 1973. A variation of thought stopping in a twelve year old boy: A case report. *J. Beh. Ther. Exp. Psych.,* 4:69-70.

Carey, G., and Gottesman, I. 1981. Twin and family studies of anxiety, phobic and obsessive disorders. In *Anxiety: New research and changing concepts,* ed. E. Rabkin, and D. Klein, pp. 117-136. New York: Raven Press.

Cooper, J. 1970. The Leyton obsessional inventory. *Psychol. Med.,* 1:48-64.

Elkins, R., Rapoport, J., and Lipsky, A. 1980. Obsessive-compulsive disorder of childhood and adolescence. *J. Am. Acad. Child Psych.,* 19:511-524.

Emmelkamp, P., and Kwee, K. G. 1977. Obsessional ruminations: A comparison between thought stopping and prolonged exposure in imagination. *Beh. Res. Ther.,* 8:441-443.

Foa, E., and Goldstein, A. 1978. Continuous exposure and complete response prevention of obsessive-compulsive neurosis. *Beh. Ther.* 9:821-829.

Freud, S. 1955. Notes upon a case of obsessional neurosis. *The standard edition of the complete psychological works of Sigmund Freud,* vol. 10. London: Hogarth Press, pp. 153-318.

Freud, S. 1958. The disposition to obsessional neurosis. *The standard edition of the complete psychological works of Sigmund Freud,* vol. 12. London: Hogarth Press, pp. 311-326.

Hollingsworth, C. E., Tanguay, P. E., Grossman, L., and Pabst, P. 1980. Long-term outcome of obsessive-compulsive disorder in children. *J. Am. Acad. Child Psych.,* 19:134-146.

Insel, T., and Murphy, D. 1981. The psychopharmacological treatment of obsessive-compulsive disorder: A review. *J. Clin. Psychopharm.,* 5:305-311.

Insel, T., Murphy, D., Cohen, R., Alterman, I., Linnoila, M., and Kilts, C. 1983. Obsessional-compulsive disorder: A double-blind trial of chlorimipramine and clorgyline. *Arch. Gen. Psych.,* 40:605-612.

Jessner, L. 1963. The genesis of a compulsive neurosis. *J. Hillside Hosp.,* 12:81-95.

Judd, L. 1965. Obsessive-compulsive neurosis in childhood. *Arch. Gen. Psych.,* 12:136-143.

Leitenberg, H. 1976. Behavioral approaches to the treatment of neurosis. In *Handbook of behavior modification and behavior therapy,* ed. H. Leitenberg, pp. 153-165. Englewood Cliffs, N.J.: Prentice-Hall.

Marks, I. 1981. Behavioral treatment plus drugs in anxiety syndromes. In *Anxiety: New research and changing concepts,* ed. D. F. Klein, and J. Rabkin, pp. 265-290. New York: Raven Press.

Marks, I., Mawson, D., and Ramm, L. 1981. Chlorimipramine and exposure in the treatment of obsessive-compulsive rituals: Two year followup. Paper presented at the III World Congress of Biological Psychiatry, June 1981, Stockholm, Sweden.

Montgomery, S., Braithwaite, S., Rani, J., McAuley, D., and Montgomery, B. 1981. Chlorimipramine plasma levels in obsessional neurosis. Paper presented at the III World Congress of Biological Psychiatry, June 1981, Stockholm, Sweden.

Nee, L. E., Caine, E. D., Polinsky, R. J., Eldridge, R., and Ebert, M. H. 1980. Gilles de la Tourette syndrome: Clinical and family study of 50 cases. *Ann. Neurol.,* 7:41-49.

Rapoport, J., Elkins, R., Langer, D. et al. 1981. Childhood obsessive-compulsive disorder. *Am. J. Psych.,* 138:1545-1554.

Rapoport, J., Elkins, R., Lipsky, A., and Mikkelsen, E. 1980. A pilot trial of chlorimipramine for children with obsessive-compulsive disorder. *Psychopharm. Bull.,* 16:61-63.

Thoren, P., Asberg, M., Cronholm, B., Jornestedt, L., and Traskman, L. 1980. Chlorimipramine treatment of obsessive-compulsive disorder. I. A controlled trial. *Arch. Gen. Psych.,* 37:1281-1289.

Weiner, I. 1967. Behavior therapy in obsessive-compulsive neurosis: Treatment of an adolescent boy. *Psychotherapy: Theory, Research, and Practice,* 4:27-29.

Welner, A., Reich, T., Robins, E., Fishman, R., and Van Doren, J. 1976. Obsessive-compulsive neurosis: Record, follow-up, and family studies. I. Inpatient Record Study. *Compr. Psych.,* 17:527-539.

12

The Diagnosis and Treatment of Anorexia Nervosa

KATHERINE A. HALMI

CLINICAL FEATURES

Anorexia nervosa is a disorder characterized by preoccupation with body weight and food, behavior directed toward losing weight, peculiar patterns of handling food, weight loss, intense fear of gaining weight, disturbance of body image, and amenorrhea.

Anorectic patients constantly think about food and how fat they are. Although they may deny this, one can assume they are preoccupied with the slenderness of their bodies by observing their frequent mirror gazing and by listening to their incessant concerns about looking fat and feeling flabby. They are preoccupied with collecting recipes and preparing elaborate meals for others. Anorectic adolescents lose weight by drastically reducing their total food intake and decreasing the intake of high carbohydrate- and fat-containing foods overproportionately. These adolescents usually refuse to eat with their families or in public places. They exercise often and are overactive. Many of their weight-reducing behaviors make it very difficult for a physician to realize that the weight reduction is actually secondary to a willful, self-induced weight loss regimen.

Unfortunately, the term *anorexia* is a misnomer. The loss of appetite in anorexia nervosa is rare until the patient is emaciated. Some patients cannot exert continuous control over their voluntary restriction of food intake and will engage in episodes of binge eating (eating a large amount of carbohydrate-rich foods in a short period of time). Vomiting is another way in which anorectics attempt to lose weight. It frequently follows a binge-eating episode. Abusing laxatives and diuretics are other purging behaviors. Such purging presents a danger by lowering serum potassium levels, which, in turn, can cause cardiac arrhythmias and, in rare cases, sudden death secondary to a cardiac arrest. Chronic hypokalemia may also produce renal tubular damage (Wigley, 1960). Persistent vomiting is also associated with the development of severe dental problems.

Anorectic adolescents have peculiar ways of handling food. They will hide carbohydrate-rich foods, such as candies and cookies, around the house. They will hoard large quantities of candies and carry them in their pockets and purses. If forced to eat in public, often they will try to dispose of their food surreptitiously to avoid eating. They will spend a great deal of time cutting food into small pieces and rearranging the food on their plates. If confronted about their peculiar behavior, usually they will flatly deny it or refuse to discuss it.

Most anorectic patients come to medical attention when their weight loss is obvious. Physical signs such as hypothermia, dependent edema, brachycardia, hypotension, and lanugo are often present.

All anorectic patients have an intense fear of gaining weight and becoming obese. This fear exists even in the face of increasing cachexia and contributes to the patient's characteristic disinterest and even resistance to treatment.

Anorectics have a disturbance of body image, in that they fail to recognize that their degree of emaciation is "too thin." They regard themselves as being normal weight or even overweight. They all describe the sensation of "feeling fat." There is a relationship between the severity of body-image distortion and the outcome of the illness. It has been shown that patients who most overestimate the width of various body parts are those patients who gain less weight during treatment and who have had a history of failing to improve in previous hospitalizations (Casper et al., 1979).

Often anorectic adolescents are referred to a gynecologist because of amenorrhea, which can appear before noticeable weight loss has occurred. In the emaciated state, anorectic patients have a regressed pattern of luteinizing hormone (LH) secretion found in prepubertal girls. This regressed pattern changes to a more mature one with weight gain (Boyar et al., 1974). Although restoration to a normal body weight is a prerequisite to the resumption of menstruation, factors other than nutritional state, most likely psychological in nature, contribute to the prolonged amenorrhea. The return of normal menstruation was directly associated with a good psychological state and social adjustment in two studies (Halmi and Falk, 1982; Morgan and Russell, 1975).

Certain common physiological changes such as leukopenia, a relative lymphocytosis, hypocellular bone marrow, low fasting glucose level, and elevated serum cholesterol, are all directly associated with the emaciated state of the anorectics and will revert to normal with weight recovery (Halmi and Falk, 1981). A low erythrocyte sedimentation rate may differentiate anorexia nervosa from other infectious states. This will also return to normal with nutritional rehabilitation.

Demographic Features

Anorexia nervosa occurs predominantly in females. The percentage of males in an anorectic population varies between 4 and 6% (Halmi, 1974). Only indirect evidence is available for familial occurrence of this disorder. One study found that the morbidity risk of a sister of an anorectic patient is about 6.6%, greatly exceeding normal expectation (Theander, 1970). In a study of fifty-six families with anorexia nervosa, Kalucy, Crisp, and Harding (1977) found that 16% of the mothers and 23% of the fathers had a history of significant low adolescent weight or weight phobia.

The onset of anorexia nervosa is usually between the ages of ten and thirty, with 85% of all anorectic patients developing the illness between the ages of thirteen and twenty (Halmi,

1974). In a recent study, a bimodal distribution of age onset was found with peaks at fourteen and a half and eighteen years (Halmi et al., 1979a). It is of interest to note that these ages coincide with the time when the adolescent is attempting to become more independent from her family. At age fourteen and a half most adolescents are about to enter high school and at age eighteen they are preparing to leave home for a job or to attend college. At this time in life, young women are concerned about their appearance, since attractiveness is equated with better acceptance from the outside world. Because great emphasis is placed on the association of beauty and thinness in our present culture, almost all young women diet in order to improve their appearance.

There is indirect evidence that the incidence of anorexia nervosa has been increasing in the past ten years. Most of the evidence comes from reports that more patients with this disorder are being diagnosed and treated in clinics and hospitals. The best estimate of occurrence is probably made from a prevalence study done by Crisp, Palmer, and Kalucy (1976). This study reported one severe case of anorexia nervosa in every two-hundred girls between the ages of twelve and eighteen in English boarding schools.

The course of anorexia nervosa varies from spontaneous recovery without treatment, recovery after a single episode with a variety of treatments, a fluctuating course of weight gains followed by relapses, to a gradually deteriorating course resulting in death due to complications of starvation. Studies of large numbers of anorectic patients who were followed for four years or longer have shown mortality rates in the range of 5–21% (Morgan and Russell, 1975; Halmi et al., 1975). It is likely that mortality rates are decreasing with earlier diagnoses of the illness and increased referral to experienced treatment teams.

There are a variety of demographic and behavior characteristics associated with outcome in anorexia nervosa. The most consistent indicator of good outcome is early age onset of the disorder (Halmi et al., 1973), while consistent indicators of poor outcome across studies are late age onset of illness and the number of previous hospitalizations (Morgan and Russell, 1975; Halmi et al., 1979b). Childhood neuroticism, parental conflicts, bulimia, vomiting, laxative abuse, and obsessive-compulsive, hysterical, and depressive symptomatology, somatic complaints, and the denial of symptoms have been related to poor outcome in some studies, but have not been significant in affecting outcome in other studies.

DIFFERENTIAL DIAGNOSIS

The diagnosis of anorexia nervosa should be made only after finding that the patient has the essential features of the illness. These are (1) behavior directed toward losing weight, (2) peculiar patterns of handling food, (3) weight loss, (4) intense fear of gaining weight, (5) disturbance of body image, and (6) amenorrhea (in women). In rare circumstances the patient can have both anorexia nervosa and a medical illness contributing to the weight loss. In such a situation, of course, both the underlying medical condition and the anorexia nervosa must be treated.

Anorectic adolescents must be differentiated from those with depressive disorders. Depressed patients do not become preoccupied with the calorie content of food, nor do they collect recipes or spend an inordinate amount of time cooking and preparing foods. They are not denying the existence of a normal appetite but rather they truly have a decreased appetite. There are some anorectic adolescents who will meet all the criteria for anorexia nervosa and a major depression. In these cases, both diagnoses should be made and both conditions should be treated.

Somatization disorder is a diagnosis that is not frequently made in adolescents, although it can be diagnosed on occasion in the older adolescent group. Weight loss and vomiting can occur in somatization disorder, but generally the weight loss is not as severe as in anorexia nervosa, nor is the patient as preoccupied with losing weight as is the anorectic patient. Amenorrhea is seldom a persistent finding in somatization disorder.

Schizophrenic patients usually have delusions about the food they are eating but are seldom concerned with calorie content. Also, schizophrenic patients are rarely preoccupied with the fear of becoming obese and do not have the hyperactivity that is present in anorectics. However, on occasion an anorectic patient will also meet criteria for schizophrenia and, in that case, both conditions should be diagnosed and treated.

Bulimia (rapid consumption of large amounts of food in a short period of time) is a behavior that is present in about half of anorexia nervosa patients (Hsu et al., 1979). Bulimia, as a diagnostic entity, is differentiated from anorexia nervosa by the fact that bulimic patients maintain their weight within a normal range. In bulimic patients, large fluctuations of weight, as much as forty pounds, can occur, but still they are within the normal weight range. Two recent studies (Casper et al., 1980; Garfinkel et al., 1980) provided substantial evidence that anorectic patients with bulimia form a distinct subgroup among the patients diagnosed as having anorexia nervosa. Self-induced vomiting, laxative abuse, and diuretic abuse were behaviors far more prevalent in the bulimic-anorectic patients than in the exclusively fasting ones. The bulimic group displayed impulsive behavior, such as alcohol and street drug abuse, stealing, suicide attempts, and self-mutilation. Bulimic patients were more extroverted and had less denial of their illness and less denial of a strong appetite. They showed greater anxiety, depression, guilt, interpersonal sensitivity, and had more somatic complaints.

Assessment

It may seem that the essential criteria for making the diagnosis of anorexia nervosa are obvious. However, the diagnosis is frequently difficult to make. One of the major reasons for this is that anorectic patients are not motivated for treatment and deny many of the characteristic symptoms of the disorder. Often it is necessary to obtain the information from family members or friends who have observed the adolescent's behavior. At times, not even the family can provide sufficient information and, then, it is necessary to hospitalize the patient for diagnostic observation. This is especially necessary when anorectic adolescents are effectively surreptitious in their weight-losing behavior and are not surrounded by observant family members. In order to make the diagnosis of anorexia nervosa, the information listed in table 12-1 should be obtained. In addition to obtaining information about the patient's behavior, it is helpful to make specific inquiries about the family history. One may expect to find depressive disorders in family members (Cantwell et al., 1977) as well as alcoholism (Halmi and Loney, 1973). Frequently, the mother and/or the father have had an episode of weight loss during their adolescent or young adult years.

It is important to inquire into the parents' responses to their adolescent's dieting behavior and weight loss. Have they sought previous consultation? Have they tried to force the child to eat? Have they totally ignored the child's behavior, only to be forced into acknowledging it by the insistence of the child's peers?

Frequently, stressful marital conflict is present in the families of the anorectic adolescent. It is not unusual for the adolescent to openly state that her illness is keeping mommy

TABLE 12-1.
Information Necessary for Diagnosis of Anorexia Nervosa

A. Weight History
   1. Greatest weight the patient has ever achieved, age at that time
   2. Least weight the patient has ever achieved, age at that time
   3. Present weight
B. Menstrual History
   1. Age onset of menses
   2. Date of last menstrual period
   3. Regularity of cycles
C. Eating Behavior
   1. Eating pattern with family
   2. Dieting behavior
   3. Binging episodes
D. Purging Behavior
   1. Self-induced vomiting
   2. Laxative abuse
   3. Diuretic abuse
   4. Enemas
E. Preoccupation with and Fear of Weight
   1. Frequency of patient weighing herself
   2. Mirror gazing, comments about being fat
   3. Collecting recipes
   4. Increased interest in cooking and baking or increased interest in being around food
F. Activity
   1. Jogging
   2. Bike riding
   3. Exercising
   4. General overactivity at home
G. Depressive Symptomatology
   1. Sleep disturbance
   2. Irritability
   3. Crying spells
   4. Suicidal thoughts
H. Impulsive Behavior
   1. Drug abuse
   2. Alcohol abuse
   3. Suicide attempts
   4. Self-mutilation

and daddy together. An assessment of the mother's and father's relationship to each other will be helpful in planning the treatment.

It is important to inquire about previous treatment for the eating-disorder problem. If the patient has had several previous hospitalization treatment failures, then she will be far more difficult to treat. The clinician should find out whether the previous treatments have included behavior-therapy techniques, medications (type and dosage), family therapy, psychotherapy (type), or group therapy. An assessment of the parents' and child's attitudes toward the previous treatment attempts should be made in order to effectively persuade the adolescent and parents to cooperate in any future treatment plans.

All possibly anorectic adolescents should have a routine physical examination with special attention paid to blood pressure, pulse rate, evidence of dehydration, salivary gland enlargement, and dependent edema. Adolescents with anorexia nervosa will frequently have a cardiac rate below 50 per minute (brachycardia), a systolic blood pressure below 80 mmHg (hypotension), and fine excessive body hair (lanugo). These are common physical signs of emaciation.

The hematopoietic profile should include a hemoglobin, hematocrit, white-cell count, and white-cell differential count, since leukopenia and relative lymphocytosis are common findings. Serum electrolytes are especially important to obtain, as many anorectics who self-induce vomiting or abuse purgatives and diuretics have a hypokalemic alkalosis. Abnormal serum electrolytes may be the only evidence that the patient is self-inducing vomiting. A fasting serum glucose level should be obtained; it is low in most emaciated anorectics. It is not unusual for serum enzymes, reflecting liver function, especially SGOT and LDH, to be elevated in anorexia nervosa. These enzyme levels may increase during the refeeding period and not return to normal levels until several months after the patient has maintained a normal weight. Occasionally an anorectic adolescent will have an elevated serum cholesterol level, which will return to within normal limits after nutritional rehabilitation. Since an accurate history of behavior signs and symptoms is sometimes difficult to obtain in adolescents with possible anorexia nervosa, it is necessary to do these physiologic assessments.

No specific psychometric evaluation is necessary to make the diagnosis of anorexia nervosa. During the course of treatment, it may be helpful to obtain an IQ determination, since many of these children have unrealistic expectations for their scholastic performance. Often the parents have unrealistic educational and professional goals for their children and may be exerting considerable pressure on the child to perform well academically.

With the mental-status evaluation, the therapist can find out about the child's attitude toward food, eating, and her weight. It is helpful to learn what the adolescent would like to weigh if no one were offering her advice or bothering her. Often anorectics have a great deal of difficulty concentrating on their schoolwork because they are constantly preoccupied with thoughts of food. Is the child having to spend more time doing the same amount of homework compared to before her dieting? It is useful to find out the anorectic adolescent's attitudes about her family, for frequently she will be disgusted at the vulgar behavior of her siblings or she may be very worried about her mother's and father's conflicts. Often the anorectic adolescent has many social and sexual fears, and so should be asked about her attitudes concerning sex and about her peer relationships. Inquiries should be made as to whether the child feels depressed, has a sleep disturbance, and whether she has frequent crying spells.

TREATMENT

The treatment of anorexia nervosa must be a multifaceted endeavor. Medical management and personal, behavioral, and family therapies are all necessary treatment modalities. Most anorectic adolescents are disinterested and even resistant to therapy and are brought to a doctor's office unwillingly by agonizing parents. It is important to emphasize the benefits of treatment, such as a relief of insomnia and depressive symptoms, a decrease in the obsessive thoughts about food and body weight that interfere with her ability to concentrate on other matters, and a restoration of the peer relationships she once had. If the anorectic is extremely emaciated, she will be upset over the fact that she no longer has the energy to be active. Reassurance that her previous activity level can be restored with treatment will also be helpful in persuading the patient to enter a therapy program. The parents' support for the treatment plan is essential, especially when firm recommendations must be carried out.

The immediate aim should be to restore the patient's nutritional state to normal. Mere emaciation or the state of being mildly underweight (15 to 25%) can cause irritability, depression, preoccupation with food, and sleep disturbance. It is exceedingly difficult to accomplish a behavioral change with psychotherapy in a patient who is suffering the psychological effects of emaciation. Admitting the patient to a structured environment in a hospitalized treatment program allows for an efficient nutritional rehabilitation and a more rapid recovery. Outpatient therapy as an initial approach has the best chance for success in adolescents who (1) have had the illness for less then four months, (2) are not binging and vomiting, and (3) have parents who are likely to cooperate and effectively participate in family therapy. Unfortunately, there are no studies in the literature that give us evidence for the effectiveness of initial outpatient treatment programs versus initial hospitalized treatment programs. A few centers will consistently start with outpatient therapy unless the patient is in dire medical condition. Many other centers, both in the United States and Europe, emphasize immediate hospitalization with follow-up outpatient therapy.

Undoubtedly, there has been a selection bias of the more ill patients going to the hospitalized treatment programs. A controlled study is needed to determine how effective initial outpatient treatment is and how many patients who have started with an outpatient program eventually have to be hospitalized.

The more severely ill patients may cause an extremely difficult medical-management problem. They may require daily monitoring of weight, fluid and calorie intake, and urine output. In a patient who is vomiting, frequent assessment of serum electrolytes is necessary. Because these patients are fearful of various types of food, it is easier and more efficient to give all their nutrition in the form of a formula such as Sustacal which contains adequate amounts of vitamins, minerals, proteins, fatty acids, and carbohydrates, all conveniently blended so that the patient cannot selectively disgard any item. Complications, such as edema and distention of the stomach, may occur if the patient is refed too rapidly. To avoid this, the patient should be given a daily caloric intake to maintain her admission weight plus 50% for activity. The daily caloric intake can be increased by 50% every five days. If the formula is given in six equal feedings throughout the day, the patient will not have to ingest a large amount at any one time.

Hospitalization of anorectic adolescents has another advantage. It isolates them from a potentially noxious environment. This factor was recognized over one-hundred years ago by Sir William Gull when he recommended "the patient should be fed at regular intervals, and surrounded by persons who would have more influence over them, relatives and friends being generally the worst attendants" (Gull, 1874). Nursing treatment programs were developed from this principle. In this type of program, the patient is put to bed and must remain in bed until she achieves a normal weight for her age and height. At that time she is allowed more activity as she continues to cooperate and improve psychologically. Obviously, this nursing treatment program which involves forced bed rest is putting behavioral contingencies to work (Crisp, 1965; Russell, 1973). Recently, with the careful study of numerous investigators, the use of the behavioral contingencies has become more sophisticated.

Agras et al. (1974) were able to demonstrate the strong effect of regular feedback of weight and calorie-intake information on weight gain. This finding was surprising to many clinicians. Since anorectics are so fearful of weight gain, it was expected that the knowledge of their daily weight and of the fact that it was increasing would be a setback rather than an aid. Apparently, however, they are more reassured and less anxious knowing what their weight is than they would be by simply being left unaware. Patients should be weighed before breakfast and after urinating in the same hospital gown every morning and should be informed of their weight.

If it is medically feasible (patient's serum electrolytes are normal and she is taking adequate fluid intake), it is preferable to observe the patient for three to five days after hospitalization. During this time an extensive behavioral analysis should be made of the patient so that appropriate positive and negative reinforcements can be selected and placed into a behavior-therapy program. Behavior therapy is most effective in the medical management and nutritional rehabilitation of the patient, although there are times when other target behaviors can be changed with this approach. Positive reinforcements are used, consisting of increased physical activity, visiting privileges, and social activities contingent on weight gain. Other programs have included powerful negative reinforcements, such as bed rest, isolation, and tube feeding. There are some anorectic adolescents who are withdrawn and prefer to spend all their time isolating themselves in their rooms. Obviously, for this type of patient a negative reinforcement would be not to allow her access to her room during the day unless she has made her expected weight gain. The most effective behavior-therapy programs are individualized; that is, a program is set up only after a behavioral analysis of the patient is completed.

The timing of reinforcements is important in behavior therapy. An adolescent needs at least a daily reinforcement for weight increase. A medically safe rate of gain would be one-fourth pound, or one-tenth kilogram, per day. Initially, weight gain, rather than eating behavior, should be reinforced. The reason for this is that patients can eat a normal-sized meal, earn their reward, and then go to the bathroom and induce vomiting, hence never changing their weight status. Making positive reinforcements contingent only on weight gain is helpful in reducing the staff-patient arguments and stressful interactions over how and what the patient is eating, since weight is an objective measure.

Behavior contingencies are widely used in the management of anorectic adolescents, however, often they are not recognized as such. In addition to effectively inducing weight gain, behavior therapy can be used to stop vomiting. A simple and immediately effective way to stop vomiting is to have the adolescent exclusively use a chair commode in her room. The patient is instructed that if she vomits into this commode, she will have to clean it out herself. This practice stops vomiting in all patients except an occasional adolescent who has the diagnosis of schizophrenia as well as anorexia nervosa. After the patient has achieved her target weight and has maintained that for several weeks, then she may be given the privilege of using the regular bathrooms. If the requirement to clean up her own vomitus is not a sufficient negative deterrent to prevent further vomiting, it may be necessary to require the patient to sit in a dayroom area with other patients for two hours after every feeding. Then if she vomits, she will have to do so in front of others, in addition to having to clean up her own vomitus.

The initial hospitalized deprivation state usually provides great incentive for the patient to work her way out of her condition. She does this, of course, by gaining weight. When she reaches a target weight, she should continue with her personal psychotherapy and family therapy, and be helped to maintain her weight.

When the patient comes into the hospital, a normal weight range should be established. The Iowa growth charts, which are corrected for age, height, and sex, are excellent to use for establishing a target weight. There is an advantage to setting a five-pound weight range with the target weight being in the middle of that range. This allows patients to have a more normal flexibility of weight within a narrow range. When patients reach their normal weight, they should be placed on enough calories per day to maintain that weight. All food should be presented on trays and they should be allowed to eat no additional food. In this way, the patient can visually conceptualize a gross amount of food necessary to maintain her in a normal weight range. After a week to ten days of eating from trays, the adolescent should be transferred over to self-selection of food, for she needs to practice choosing her own food and maintaining her weight. The length of the practice period depends on how easily the patient can maintain her weight and how comfortable she is with more normal eating patterns.

Drugs can often be useful adjuncts in the treatment of anorexia nervosa. The first drug used in treating anorectic patients was chlorpromazine (Dally and Sargant, 1960). This medication is especially effective in the severely obsessive-compulsive anorectic patients. There has been no controlled double-blind study to definitely prove the efficacy of chlorpromazine in inducing weight gain in anorectics. In a small patient who is severely emaciated it may be necessary to start chlorpromazine in a dose as low as 30 mg at bedtime. The dosage then can be gradually built up until the appearance of side effects.

Another category of drugs frequently used in the treatment of anorexia nervosa is the antidepressant. Amitriptyline has been shown to be effective in inducing weight gain, and several uncontrolled studies (Mills, 1976; Needleman and Waber, 1977) suggest that it may be effective in the treatment of anorexia nervosa. In these studies the daily dosage varied between 75 and 150 mg.

Cyproheptadine has also been used and is especially attractive because of its relatively benign side effects. In one controlled study, it was found to induce weight gain in a subgroup of anorexia nervosa patients who were more emaciated, had a history of prior treatment failures, and a history of birth delivery complications (Goldberg et al., 1979). Cyproheptadine should be started at 4 mg three times a day and built up to 32 mg/day.

Single case reports of the use of other drugs in treating anorectic patients have appeared in the literature. However, there are no large series of open trial studies or controlled studies with any of these drugs. Lithium is definitely contraindicated in a patient who vomits or abuses laxatives or diuretics because of the possibility of rapid lithium toxicity. The dehydration and sodium loss from vomiting or diuretic use induces renal-based lithium saving, thus rapidly increasing its serum concentration. If an anorectic patient has many depressive signs and symptoms, it is likely she will benefit from an antidepressant medication. It is important to start out the medication in a very low dosage, as low as 10 mg three times a day in a young adolescent who is severely emaciated. The dosage should be raised only with careful monitoring of the blood pressure.

Counseling of family members is a necessary component of any treatment program. There is no evidence that family therapy as the sole form of treatment is effective; rather, it is usually used in conjunction with behavior contingencies and personal psychotherapy. Other than case reports, there has been no systematic assessment of anorectic families reported in the literature.

Each family should be carefully analyzed for problems unique to that family, and therapy should correspond to their needs. In some cases, it is often wise to do marital therapy with the parents and have only a few family-therapy sessions. In others, it is effective to have separate sessions with the mother and daughter or siblings and patient. Considerable variation of maladaptive interactional patterns exist within anorexia nervosa families, and because of this, a treatment strategy for each individual family should be created.

Classical psychodynamically oriented therapy has been regarded as ineffective in treating anorexia nervosa (Rollins and Blackwell, 1968; Bruch, 1970). Individual psychotherapy should focus on making the patient aware of her behavior and the effect it has on maintaining her illness. Attention is directed to the anorectic patient's fear of failure, fear of becoming independent from her family, and fear of accepting the expected responsibilities of a growing adolescent. A therapist must deal with the patient's great denial of her illness and must make the adolescent aware of her need to control her environment through a maladaptive living pattern.

The patient's anxiety and preoccupation with her weight does not disappear after she regains her weight. Continuing outpatient individual therapy for varying periods of time, depending on the severity of the illness, is needed after the hospitalized treatment phase. Oftentimes, a continuation of outpatient family therapy is needed. A behavioral contract can be set up with the patient after she is discharged from the hospital. Usually it is wise to have the adolescent weighed by a physician's nurse or by the school nurse once a week. If she falls below her normal weight range, she can be removed from sports activities at school and from other physical recreational activities. If the patient continues to maintain her weight, a positive reinforcement schedule can be worked out for the patient and her family.

Anorexia nervosa is a disorder with a considerable range of psychopathology from mild to severe and, correspondingly, a considerable range in outcome from complete recovery to death. The latter fortunately has become less common. Most likely early diagnosis and early vigorous intervention has been effective in reducing the mortality rate of this disorder.

REFERENCES

Agras, W. S., Harlow, D. H., Chapin, H. N., Abel, G. G., and Leitenberg, H. 1974. Behavior modification of anorexia nervosa. *Arch. Gen. Psych.*, 30:279-286.

Boyar, R. M., Katz, J., Finkelstein, J. W., Capen, S., Weiner, H., Weitzman, E. D., and Hellman, L. 1974. Immaturity of the 24-hour luteinizing hormone secretory pattern. *N. Eng. J. Med.*, 291:861-865.

Bruch, H. 1970. Psychotherapy and primary anorexia nervosa. *J. Nerv. Men. Dis.*, 150:51-60.

Cantwell, P. D., Sturzenberger, S., and Burroughs, J. 1977. Anorexia nervosa: An affective disorder? *Arch. Gen. Pscyh.*, 34:1087-1093.

Casper, R. C., Eckert, E. D., Halmi, K. A., Goldberg, S. C., and Davis, J. M. 1980. The incidence and clinical significance of bulimia in patients with anorexia nervosa. *Arch. Gen. Psych.*, 37:1030-1035.

Casper, R. C., Halmi, K. A., Goldberg, S. C., Eckert, E. D., and Davis, J. M. 1979. Disturbances in body image estimation as related to other characteristics and outcome in anorexia nervosa. *Brit. J. Psych.*, 134:60-66.

Crisp, A. H. 1965. Clinical and therapeutic aspects of anorexia nervosa: A study of 30 cases. *J. Psychosom. Res.*, 9:67-75.

Crisp, A. H., Palmer, R. L., and Kalucy, R. S. 1976. How common is anorexia nervosa? A prevalent study. *Brit. J. Psych.*, 128:549-554.

Dally, P. G., and Sargant, W. A. 1960. A new treatment of anorexia nervosa. *Brit. Med. J.*, 1:1770-1775.

Garfinkel, P. E., Moldofsky, H., and Garner, D. M. 1980. The heterogeneity of anorexia nervosa. *Arch. Gen. Psych.*, 37:1036-1040.

Goldberg, S. C., Halmi, K. A., Eckert, E. D., Casper, R. C., and Davis, J. M. 1979. Cyproheptadine in anorexia nervosa. *Brit. J. Psych.*, 134:67-70.

Gull, W. 1874. Anorexia nervosa. *Trans. Cline. Soc. Lond.*, 7:22-28.

Halmi, K. A. 1974. Anorexia Nervosa: Demographic and clinical features in 94 cases. *Psychosom. Med.,* 36:18-24.

Halmi, K. A., Brodland, G., and Loney, J. 1973. Prognosis in anorexia nervosa. *Ann. Intern. Med.* 78:907-911.

Halmi, K. A., Brodland, G., and Rigas, C. 1975. A follow-up study of seventy-nine patients with anorexia nervosa: An evaluation of prognostic factors and diagnostic criteria. In *Life history research in psychopathology,* ed. R. D. Wirt, G. Winokur, and M. Roff, vol. 4, pp. 290-300. Minneapolis: University of Minnesota Press.

Halmi, K. A., Casper, R. C., Eckert, E. D., Goldberg, S. C., and Davis, J. M. 1979. Unique features associated wtih age onset of anorexia nervosa. *Psychiat. Res.,* 3:209-215.

Halmi, K. A., Falk, J. R. 1981. Common physiological changes in anorexia nervosa. *Int. J. Eating Disor.,* 1:16-27.

Halmi, K. A., and Falk, J. R. 1982. Dietary and behavioral discriminators of menstrual function in anorexia nervosa. Proceedings of the International Eating Disorders Meeting, 1982.

Halmi, K. A., Goldberg, S. C., Eckert, E. D., and Davis, J. M. 1979. Pretreatment predictors of outcome in anorexia nervosa. *Brit. J. Psych.,* 134:71-78.

Halmi, K. A., and Loney, J. 1973. Familial alcoholism in anorexia nervosa. *Brit. J. Psych.,* 123:53-54.

Hsu, L. K. G., Crisp, A. H., and Harding, B. 1979. Outcome of anorexia nervosa. *Lancet,* 1:65-69.

Kalucy, R. S., Crisp, A. H., and Harding, B. 1977. A study of 56 families with anorexia nervosa. *Brit. J. Med. Psychol.,* 50:32-47.

Mills, I. H. 1976. Amitriptyline therapy in anorexia nervosa. *Lancet,* 2:687.

Morgan, H. G., and Russell, G. F. M. 1975. Value of family background in clinical features as predictors of long term outcome in anorexia nervosa: Four year followup study of 41 patients. *Psychol. Med.,* 5:355-371.

Needleman, H. L., and Waber, D. 1977. Use of amitriptyline in anorexia nervosa. In *Anorexia Nervosa,* ed. R. Vibersky. New York: Raven Press.

Rollins, N., and Blackwell, A. 1968. The treatment of anorexia nervosa in children and adolescents: Stage I. *J. Child Psychol. Psych.,* 9:81.

Russell, G. F. M. 1973. The management of anorexia nervosa. In *Symposium: Anorexia nervosa and obesity.* Royal College of Physicians of Edinburgh, no. 42. Edinburgh: T and A Constable.

Theander, S. 1970. Anorexia nervosa. *Acta Psychiat. Scand.,* 214 (suppl.):29.

Wigley, R. D. 1960. Potassium deficiency in anorexia nervosa with reference to renal tubular vacuolation. *Brit. Med. J.,* 2:110-113.

CONDUCT DISORDERS

13

Aggressive Behavior in Middle Childhood

P. CHAMBERLAIN / G. R. PATTERSON

A WIDE SPECTRUM OF BEHAVIORS are subsumed under the terms *aggressive* and *antisocial* (in this chapter they are used interchangeably) as they are applied to children. The analysis of problems presented by parents during the intake interview for a large sample of children referred for treatment as antisocial showed they shared one thing in common. Eighty-nine percent of the parents complained that these children were disobedient (Patterson, 1982). Both laboratory studies and field observations in the homes showed antisocial children to be roughly one-half as compliant as normal children of the same age (Bernal et al., 1976; Forehand et al., 1978). Typically, the other symptoms identified by parents during the intake interview included problem behavior such as yelling, fighting, teasing, crying, whining, lying, stealing, and fire setting.* Numerous investigations have developed complex behavioral-coding systems designed to study aggressive behavior in families (Patterson et al., 1969; Wahler et al., 1976). For example, the coding system developed by Patterson and Reid (Patterson et al., 1969; Reid, 1978) utilizes twenty-nine distinct behavior-code categories sampling the behavior of the referred child and the behaviors of other family members as they interact with the referred child and with each other. This system is designed for rapid sequential recording of the family members' behaviors. Fourteen negative categories are combined to produce a cluster category measuring Total Aversive Behavior. Levels of aggressive behavior are measured by calculating the rate per minute that aversive behaviors are engaged in. Typical observations are approximately sixty minutes in length (depending on the number of family members) and during a time when all family members are present. Observational measures have also allowed for *in vivo* studies of child behavior in school settings (e.g., Walker and Buckley, 1973). Observations in the homes of samples of antisocial children and comparison samples of normal families have shown significant

---

*Base-rate values obtained from parent reports of problem behaviors at intake from 142 families referred for treatment to the Oregon Social Learning Center for aggression are 89% for noncompliance, 68% for lying, 56% for stealing, and 23% for fire setting.

elevations for the clinical samples on levels of overt aggressive behaviors, such as yelling, hitting, complaining, teasing, crying, whining, humiliating, and noncompliance (Bernal et al., 1976; Patterson, 1976; Snyder, 1977). Interestingly, these studies also agree on the fact that once problem children engage in one of these coercive behaviors, they are significantly more likely than their normal counterparts to continue being coercive.

Differential Diagnosis

It has long been understood that antisocial behavior represents a very heterogeneous collection of problems. The analyses of intake symptoms presented to child-guidance clinics, departments of child psychiatry, and pediatrics began in the 1940s.

Results from factor-analytic studies have consistently identified two general factors relating to childhood aggression (Jenkins and Glickman, 1946; Quay, 1965; Achenbach, 1966): overt, *oppositional behavior* having to do with coercive behavior directed toward persons (e.g., yelling, whining, hitting, teasing, and crying); and *conduct problems* usually involving covert behavior, both rule breaking and violating of property (e.g., vandalism, truancy, stealing, lying, and fire setting). Most children referred for treatment for aggression can be classified into one or the other of these groups.

The oppositional school-age child is usually characterized by (a) a persistent pattern of disobedience, (b) argumentativeness and temper outbursts, (c) poor or erratic academic achievement, (d) poor peer relationships, (e) poor work skills (i.e., does not do chores), and (f) frequent conflicts with siblings, parents, or teachers. These conflicts take place in the home and, in the more severe cases, also at school. For specific diagnostic criteria, see *DSM-III* (American Psychiatric Association, 1980).

Oppositional behavior in the eighteen- to thirty-six-month-old child is part of the normal developmental phase, and unless it is viewed as either extreme in intensity or rate, or the parents seem particularly inept in child-management skills, treatment is probably not required. In schizophrenia and pervasive developmental disorders, persistent oppositional behavior may be observed but not diagnosed in the presence of these other disorders. Attention deficit disorders, mental retardation, chronic organic mental disorders, and specific development disorders are commonly associated diagnoses (*DSM-III*).

The conduct-problem, school-age child is usually characterized by (a) a persistent pattern of disobedience, particularly when not directly supervised, (b) frequent lying, sometimes for no apparent gain, (c) petty theft, sometimes of items that the child either already has or could get legitimately, (d) physical fighting with peers, (e) poor school performance, (f) frequent wandering (i.e., parents do not know of the child's whereabouts or the child is not where he said he would be), (g) lack of appropriate guilt or remorse, (h) poor peer relationships, and (i) conflict with parents, siblings, and teachers.

In severe cases the characteristics may include vandalism, running away from home, physical fighting with adult authority figures, stealing valuable items and/or breaking and entering, drug use, association with older delinquent peers, and repeated school suspensions and/or dropping out. These conflicts may take place in the home and in the community, or primarily in the community, in which case the parents are often unaware of the problem until it is brought to their attention by law-enforcement or school officials. For specific diagnostic criteria, see *DSM-III*.

It is assumed that there are two different family processes associated with covert and overt forms of antisocial child behavior (Patterson, 1982). The implication is not only that the topographies for covert and overt forms of antisocial behavior are different, but that the form of treatment will also vary. The details of these differences will be discussed in a later section.

Common Characteristics

There are certain characteristics that tend to be shared by antisocial children, whether their symptoms are overt or covert in form. Three such characteristics have immediate relevance for the practitioner:

1. There is an emphasis on short-term gains. Antisocial children display a reduced tendency to delay gratification and a greater likelihood of impulsive behaviors than nonreferred children (Weintraub, 1973). They maximize short-term payoffs and ignore long-term costs. Like two year olds, they have not yet been taught to comply with the majority of adult requests or rules. This tendency to maximize short-term gains is usually at the expense of others in their environment (e.g., parents, teachers, peers).
2. There is a lower level of competency in prosocial functioning than displayed by age mates in areas such as establishment of peer relationships, participation in sports and hobbies, academic achievement, job skills, and control over bladder and bowel functioning. Antisocial children have a generally negative view of others. The assumption is that aggressive children do not mature in their ability to employ prosocial strategies, but continue to rely on the use of aversive behaviors to get what they want and avoid doing that which displeases them. In a sense, aggressive children may be thought of as immature and may engage in whining, clinging, dependent behavior. As these children develop, they continue to add a wider range of coercive behaviors to their repertory and to apply these to the wider range of people they come into contact with (e.g., teachers). In so doing, they increase the likelihood of rejection by others in their environment and of becoming increasingly isolated: opportunities for expanding prosocial skills are further reduced.
3. There is an apparent hyporesponsivity to social approval and disapproval (i.e., rewards and punishments)(Phipps-Yonas, 1979). Aggressive children do not learn as well as children from control groups given that the feedback is social, but function at a normal level when contingencies for performance involve instrumental rewards (e.g., food or money)(Marcus, 1972; Herbert et al., 1973) or punishments (e.g., time out or work chores)(White et al., 1972).

Epidemiology

Childhood aggression is a common problem. By 1932 there were over two hundred child-guidance clinics in operation in the United States. From one-half to two-thirds of the problems for which children were referred concerned aggression and antisocial problems. Robins's (1966) review of epidemiological studies noted that 6% of boys aged ten to twelve years could be labeled as aggressive or antisocial.

Age and Aggression

For nonreferred samples, several studies have concluded that the amount of overt aversive behavior in both home and school settings decreases as a function of a child's age (e.g., Goodenough, 1931). Rates of aggressive behavior peak during preschool years, then gradually decline. Observational studies in the home indicate that nonreferred two to four year olds engage in an average of slightly more than one aversive behavior every one and one-half minutes. The norm for early school-age children (five to seven years) is, on the average, one aversive behavior every four minutes, and for eight to ten year olds, one aversive behavior every five minutes. Children ages eight to nine, referred for aggression, have observed levels of aversive behavior comparable with normal two to four year olds (Patterson, 1976; Bernal et al., 1980).

There is some evidence that the base rates for occurrence of different types of aggressive behavior engaged in (e.g., overt versus covert forms) appear to change as a function of age. Achenbach (1978) administered a behavioral checklist to parents of 2,600 children between the ages of four and sixteen years. Incidences of 112 problem behaviors and 20 measures of social competency were obtained for each age. Although not a longitudinal design, the data from this study suggest a shift in the form in which antisocial behavior is manifested from preadolescent to adolescent years. The nature of this shift is a steady decrease in physical aggression and an increase in covert antisocial behavior such as stealing.

Sex and Aggression

More boys than girls are referred for treatment for aggression (Ackerson, 1931; Wolff, 1967). In a recent sample of four- to twelve-year-old children referred to the Oregon Social Learning Center for treatment for aggression, 74% were males and 26% females (Patterson et al., 1982). Although the findings are not always consistent (Henry and Sharpe, 1947), several studies note differences in the type of aggression displayed by boys and girls. Higher rates of physical aggression are reported for boys than for girls (Mischel, 1966; Maccoby and Jacklin, 1974), while girls tend to be more likely to display verbal aggression (e.g., negativity, crying, teasing) (Rutter et al., 1970).

Ordinal Position in the Family

Evidence suggests that many aspects of antisocial behavior are learned as a function of training by siblings. The highly aggressive child tends to be the middle child (49% in the Rutter et al., 1970, sample), while youngest and only children are underrepresented (Anderson, 1969). In keeping with this, a recent analysis of chronic delinquents showed that 22% of the subjects committed at least one court-recorded offense with a sibling. Of those, 77% of the offenses were committed with an older sibling (Reid & Chamberlain, in preparation).

Family Size

Large families are more likely to produce antisocial children even when investigators control for socioeconomic status (Rutter et al., 1970). Significant correlations between family size and amount of physical aggression in the family have been reported (Burgess et al., 1978). These findings may relate to the fact that the relative amount of interaction with siblings increases in large families, while the amount of interaction with parents decreases.

ETIOLOGY

Many theories on the causes of childhood aggression have been proposed. Some of these are the frustration/aggression hypothesis (Dollard et al., 1939), modeling and imitation of aggressive models (Bandura et al., 1963), and more recently, coercion theory (Patterson, 1982), some aspects of which will be discussed later.

Some studies have implicated the presence of a genetic component in antisocial behavior patterns. Robins (1966) found that if the child's father was diagnosed as antisocial, there was an increased likelihood that the child would be diagnosed as antisocial as an adult. Additionally, the children of the third generation in this sample were also characterized by an increased likelihood of being diagnosed as antisocial. Farrington (1978) observed the relationship between criminality of parents and both violent and nonviolent delinquent behavior in juveniles. In a cross-fostering project, Mednick and Christiansen (1977) found that adoptees whose biological father had a criminal history had almost twice the chance of being criminals themselves as did adoptees whose adopted father had a criminal history. Incidentally, if both biological and adoptive fathers were criminals, the child's chance of becoming criminal was three times higher. It is not possible, of course, to sort out the biological and experiential influences: aggression may well be determined by the interaction of both.

Bell (1968) reviewed a number of studies that support the notion of heritability of assertiveness and impulsiveness, and person orientation in infants. He argues that there is a congenital contributor to early responsiveness to social reinforcement. If the child does not respond as well as other infants to early social reinforcement, it would be reasonable to expect his or her later behavior to be less adequately controlled by the use of love-oriented techniques that depend on the strength of the social bond between the parent and the child.

Data from observational studies (Loeber, 1980) suggest that the child's aggressive behaviors displayed at home are a direct reaction to the immediate social environment: a child's high rate of aversive behavior reflects the fact that she or he lives in a world of irritable people. Studies comparing family members of referred children to family members of nonreferred children consistently show that mothers, fathers, and siblings of referred samples display significantly higher rates of aggressive behavior in their interactions with each other (Bernal et al., 1976; Patterson, 1976, 1982; Snyder, 1977). The problem child plays a special role within the family in these aggressive interactions. A study by Patterson (1982) compared interactions between parents and siblings from normal and clinical samples. When the parents interacted with the siblings of the problem child or with each other, their level of aggressive behavior fell within the normal range. However, when the siblings were observed to interact alone and outside the presence of the problem child, they were significantly more aggressive than siblings from normal families. In effect, the parents allowed the siblings to behave aggressively with each other as long as the aggression was not directed toward the parent. The number of aggressive interchanges occurring between the parents and the problem child were significantly elevated. The problem child appears to serve as a focus, eliciting deviant reactions from both parents. Data from this study suggest that there are repeated episodes in which three or more family members are involved simultaneously in aggressive interchanges: a kind of vortex effect.

Futhermore, these aversive, irritable reactions among family members are a major determinant for the amount of overt aggressive behavior which the problem child engages in. The irritable reactions of the mother, father, and siblings were significantly correlated with the amount of aggressive behavior that the child performed in a sample of 103 preadolescent children (Patterson, 1982). If the child resides in a family in which the irritable reactions are extremely likely, then the level at which the child is observed to perform fighting, temper tantrums, and other overt attacks will be commensurately high. From the practitioner's viewpoint, the implication is that two-pronged treatment approach is indicated, focusing on reducing both the irritable reactions of the family members to the problem child, and the level of the problem child's coercive initiations to family members.

Patterson (1982) asserts that the parents' irritable reactions are related to disruptions in child-rearing practices. It is assumed that effective child-rearing practices include a set of four interrelated parenting skills: (1) the parents and family members agree on a set of clearly defined house rules; (2) the parents track, or monitor, antisocial behavior occurring both within and outside the home; (3) the parents are able to use an effective, nonviolent punishment that will reduce the likelihood of future occurrences of problem behaviors; and (4) the parents possess problem-solving skills that can be used to deal effectively with conflicts within the family and the crises impinging from outside. If the parents have had poor training in one or more of these skills, or are under severe stress such as divorce, unemployment, or illness which disrupts child-rearing practices, likelihood increases that the child will become antisocial. It is assumed that disruption in child rearing will be associated with increased irritability on the part of one or more family members, placing the child, in turn, at risk for increased social aggression.

Different patterns of familial disruption are associated with covert and overt forms of antisocial child behavior (Patterson, 1982). Examination of observation data collected in homes of matched samples of nonreferred children, children referred for overt oppositional behavior problems, and children referred for covert behavior problems (i.e., stealing) reveals some differences for these groups.

Parents of the oppositional child tend to be more irritable than parents of either normal or conduct-problem children, while parents of children referred for conduct disorders tend to be distant and unfriendly (Reid and Hendricks, 1973). They talk with each other less than do normals (although when they do, they are also more irritable) and frequently behave as if the other person has not interacted with them when, in fact, they have (i.e., they tend to ignore initiations of other family members).

In most families, by the time children are five or six years old, the parents have taught them to respect the property rights of others (i.e., not to take others' possessions)(MacFarlane et al., 1954). If children between the ages of six and twelve years steal regularly from family, neighbors, or peers, they are likely to be "caught" often. The reaction of the parents to this activity appears to be a crucial variable in terms of how the children are "trained."

Reid and Patterson (1976) note that parents of childen who were referred for treatment because of persistent patterns of stealing share a common distaste for using the term *steal*. This word is reserved for instances when the child was proven guilty of the offense. They often do not accept the word of a teacher, neighbor, or storekeeper as proof that their child had stolen. They are reluctant to confront the child in the absence of substantial evidence. The clinical impression of these authors was that the parents do not adopt this stance as a means of protecting the child, but rather because they are unattached to their teaching role as parents, to the values of society, and are relatively unattached to their child. Unlike parents of oppositional children who are motivated to change their child's generally aversive behavior patterns, parents of conduct-problem children tend to deny the existence of the problem, and drop out of treatment relatively more often (Holleran, unpublished).

In a multivariate prediction-of-delinquency study carried out at the Oregon Social

Learning Center, 210 boys and their families were assessed on numerous measures of family process, school performance, and behavior variables. These variables were investigated in relation to the occurrence of covert and overt behavior problems. Preliminary analyses suggest that covert antisocial problems, such as stealing or lying, are associated with disruption in parental monitoring and punishment provided for rule-breaking behaviors occurring outside the home. Physical fighting and other forms of overt aggression are related to the parents' inability to effectively punish face-to-face aggressive behavior and to adequately use problem-solving skills (Patterson & Stouthamer-Loeber, 1984). As noted in the previous section, there appears to be a shift in the topography of aggressive behavior as a function of the child's age. It is hypothesized that at around the ages of ten, eleven, and twelve, the parents of the problem child become disrupted in their monitoring of the child's whereabouts and actitivites outside the home. It is at this point that society's rules for parental responsibility become somewhat ambiguous. The child takes advantage of this, and the disruption in parental monitoring is followed by a steady increase in rule-breaking behavior on the part of the child when he or she is in the community (Patterson & Stouthamer-Loeber, 1984). From the viewpoint of the practitioner, this would suggest that the point of emphasis during the treatment of the younger antisocial child might be different from that taken with the adolescent (e.g., different parental practices are being disrupted in each case).

History for Diagnosis and Treatment Planning

Interview the parents and obtain an estimate of the frequency of each of the symptoms occurring currently and the setting in which they occur. Of particular relevance for treatment is whether the majority of these behaviors occur within or outside the presence of the parent or teacher. Use the Parent Daily Report (PDR) checklist, figure 13-1, as a guide. Next, ask the parents to target those behaviors on the checklist that they consider to be currently most problematic.

In a normative study, Chamberlain (1980) found that parents of nonreferred children targeted between two and four checklist behaviors as being problematic, while parents of clinic referrals targeted—on the average—between eight and ten checklist behaviors (Lorber, 1981). Determine how long-standing each of the symptoms has been. Obtain a history of school problems, if any (specifically if problems relate to academic or behavioral performance, or both), as well as parental permission to contact the child's teacher. If further clarification is required, contact the child's teacher and review the PDR checklist with him or her. Ask the parents to provide a brief developmental history of the child, including the following information: any critical or focal event given as the cause of the current problems, the theory or style of child rearing the parents have used, parental agreement or disagreement on child rearing.

Treatment for parents who disagree about child-rearing philosophies should focus on negotiation of a common strategy for reacting to both problem and prosocial child behaviors. Determine what methods the parents have used in the past, specifically concerning methods of discipline and encouragement. Ask why the parents are seeking treatment now. If they are pressured by an outside agency (e.g., school, law-enforcement officials), it is probable they will be less motivated for treatment than if self-referred. Ask them about previous treatments.

Behavioral treatments will often have been used without expert consultation or guidance, and will have been abandoned after a short trial period. It is most common for par-

Behavioral Information

This is a list of common problem behaviors parents have with their children. Read through the entire list of thirty-nine behaviors and ask the parent whether or not that behavior is a problem with the target child in home, at school, or in the community. If yes, check the appropriate box; if no, leave blank.

Specific behaviors	Setting H	S	C		Specific behaviors	Setting H	S	C
1. Aggressiveness					21. Pouting			
2. Arguing					22. Running around			
3. Bed-wetting					23. Running away			
4. Competitiveness					24. Sadness			
5. Complaining					25. Soiling			
6. Crying					26. Stealing			
7. Defiance					27. Talking back to adult			
8. Destructiveness					28. Teasing			
9. Fearfulness					29. Temper tantrum			
10. Fighting w/sibs (hitting)					30. Whining			
11. Fire setting					31. Yelling			
12. Hitting others					32. Police contact			
13. Hyperactivity					33. School contact			
14. Irritability					34. Parents hitting child			
15. Lying					35. Drug use			
16. Negativism					36. Vandalism			
17. Noisiness					37. Whereabouts unknown			
18. Noncomplying					38. Other			
19. Not eating (meals)					39. Other			
20. Pants wetting								

Fig. 13-1. PARENT DAILY REPORT CHECKLIST

ents to have tried, neither consistently nor for a reasonable amount of time (i.e., more than two months), a number of different approaches before seeking professional help. Obtain information on how much time the parents and child are typically together each day, and what periods of the day are especially problematic (e.g., bedtime, mealtime). If parents and/or teachers report learning difficulties, achievement levels in reading, arithmetic, and spelling should be assessed, as well as IQ, to determine if special educational planning is required.

AVAILABLE TREATMENTS: SOCIAL-LEARNING APPROACH

Controlled studies have shown that treatment of the aggressive child individually through psychotherapy (Guttman, 1963; Sowles and Gill 1970), supportive casework (Romig, 1978), or institutionalization (Redl and Wineman, 1951) is not effective in altering the child's aggressive behavior patterns in family or community settings. In fact, treatments encouraging self-exploration or expression of aggressive feelings are associated with increased levels of aggression (Truax et al., 1970). Effective treatments focus on changing the reaction of the environment to the child's aggression through alteration of consequences for specific aggressive and prosocial behaviors in the relevant settings (e.g., family, school).

During the past fifteen years, a good deal of research has been conducted evaluating the effectiveness of social-learning treatments for families of aggressive, preadolescent children. An effective treatment strategy should result in reduced rates of deviant behavior for the referred child and an accompanying increase in positive perceptions of the child by significant adults (e.g., parents, teachers) with whom the child has daily contact. Several studies have demonstrated these changes (Patterson, 1974; Wahler et al., 1977; Weinrott et al., 1979) in 60 to 75% of the referred cases. These treatments have typically focused on teaching parents to observe specific prosocial and aggressive child behaviors, and to set appropriate social and nonsocial consequences for these behaviors. Results from studies evaluating social-learning treatments using inexperienced therapists (e.g., graduate students) and time-limited formats have been less positive (Eyberg and Johnson, 1974; Bernal et al., 1980) than those using experienced therapists and unlimited-time formats (the amount of professional time required averages seventeen hours per family, with a range of five to fifty hours).

Assessment

Social-learning treatment approaches are characterized by a reliance on the use of systematically collected data on the behavior of both the referred child and his or her family members. These data are obtained at baseline, during treatment, and after treatment, and provide the therapist with ongoing information for evaluating the effectiveness of interventions. Observation data collected by trained observers in the home and school setting are thought to be the most reliable means for evaluating day-to-day levels of aggressive behavior. Displays of aggressive behavior lend themselves particularly well to observation techniques because of the overt, easily definable, nature of the problem. It is recommended that clinicians frequently treating children referred for aggression problems devise a simple, efficient observation system for monitoring and evaluating purposes; one such system is described by Ried (1978). Systems utilizing parent reports of symptom occurrence constitute the next most reliable means of assessment. Two methods for obtaining parent-report data will be described here: telephone-interview data and parent-observation data.

TELEPHONE-INTERVIEW DATA. The PDR checklist and similar instruments have been used for screening and evaluating aggressive children in several studies (Patterson et al., 1978). Although interviews with parents have been the traditional means of gathering information for treatment evaluation, several studies have found that global parent-report data correspond poorly with observation data collected in the home (Walters and Gilmore, 1973) or in the classroom (Schelle, 1974). Parents with problem children in particular seem prone to report positive changes in their child's behavior when, in fact, none has been observed (Clement and Milne, 1967). Three characteristics of the PDR checklist are thought to make it a more reliable and sensitive measure than global parent reports: (a) parents are asked to make a binary judgment (yes/no) about the occurrence of behaviors; (b) the behaviors parents are asked about are specific; and (c) parents are asked to recall if these specific behaviors have occurred over the just prior twenty-four-hour time interval. Studies comparing observer-collected data and PDR checklist data have shown reliable correspondence between the two measures (Patterson et al., 1978; Forgatch and Toobert, 1979). For example, in a sample of thirty-five children referred for aggressive behavior, PDR checklist data collected at treatment termination reliably corresponded to observation data collected during follow-up (i.e., four to eight months after termination).

It is recommended that this instrument be administered by telephone each day (Monday to Friday) for a one- to two-week period during baseline, three times per week during treatment, daily (Monday to Friday) for a one- to two-week period at treatment termination, and daily one week per month for a six-month follow-up period.

These telephone interviews should be conducted by other than the treating therapist (e.g., a secretary, aide, or colleague). The caller should be cautioned not to discuss clinical concerns with parents during these calls; instead, the therapist should be notified to contact the parents. Each call should be completed in less than five minutes.

PARENT-OBSERVATION DATA. Following the intake interview and a one- to two-week assessment period, during which PDR data is collected on a second visit, parents should be instructed to collect observation data for a one-hour period each day. To aid the parents in doing this, during the second visit the therapist should (1) pinpoint or operationally define one or two of the child's most frequently occurring problem behaviors and the prosocial opposite behaviors (e.g., not minding/minding; fighting with siblings/playing compatibly with siblings), and (2) instruct the parents to begin observing the child and collecting data on the occurrence of both problem and prosocial behaviors for one hour per day when the problem behaviors are most likely to occur (e.g., mealtime, bedtime) (see fig. 13-2 for a sample of a common target behavior, its definitions, and the observational record sheet). The specific behaviors selected and their definitions will vary depending on the circumstances of the individual family. Two primary functions are served through this process: baseline levels of symptom occurrence rates are established; and parent attention is focused on the specific behaviors of the child, the site of future intervention, and away from global child characteristics.

Successful treatment generally involves two primary factors: reduction of the child's output of overt or covert aggressive behaviors, and concurrently, alteration of the parents' typically irritable reactions and negative view of the child. Research suggests that a key component facilitating abandonment of parental negative stereotyping is a change in their focus away from global descriptors of the child's behavior (e.g., "he has a bad attitude") to a focus on the occurrence of specific problem behaviors (Wahler and Leske, 1973). Early in the development of the behavior-modification technology, Lindsey (1966) suggested that

| Child _____ | Week of _____ to _____ |
| Parent _____ | |

		M	Tu	W	Th	F	Sa	Su
Behavior	Definition							
Minding	Doing what you are asked within 15 seconds							
Behavior	Definition							
Not minding	Not doing what you are asked within 15 seconds							
Behavior	Definition							
Fighting with siblings while playing	Any hitting, crying, whining, or shouting							
Behavior	Definition							
Playing cooperatively with siblings	Absence of any of the above behaviors (Mark one for each ten-minute period with no fighting)							
Actual time observing:	Ms. From / To							
	Mr. From / To							

Fig. 13-2. WEEKLY OBSERVING SHEET

training parents to observe specific behaviors and to collect data on them would not only increase the accuracy of parent judgment of the child, but would likely produce changes in the child's behavior as well. Peine (1970) showed that simply having the parent observe and record child behavior produced reductions in the child's output of deviant behavior, but that the improvement did not maintain over time.

Encourage the parents to select one or two behaviors for observation that are likely to occur frequently (i.e., at least twice during the observation hour) and are easily observable. Stealing and lying are usually poor choices because they are covert and not easily definable or observable. If symptoms are comprised of primarily covert behaviors, encourage the parents to select one or two other behaviors occurring at a high rate as targets for observation. Noncompliance-compliance is often an ideal behavior to begin with for several reasons: noncompliance is often the first problem behavior occurring early in a chain or series of coercive behaviors, it often occurs in samples of children referred for aggression, and it is easily tracked by the parent because of its relationship to the parent's requests or commands.

Treatment: Overt Oppositional Problems

REINFORCEMENT OF PROSOCIAL BEHAVIOR. Numerous studies have noted that aggressive children are less responsive to common social rewards such as adult approval (Herbert et al., 1973). However, antisocial children seem to learn well when nonsocial, tangible rewards such as food or money are used (Marcus, 1972). These children apparently are not as highly motivated by social feedback as their normal counterparts. Additionally, observation data show that parents of aggressive children tend to reinforce deviant child behavior (Sallows, 1972). The use of a prosthetic system (i.e., a point contract) to restructure the family's reinforcement patterns has a twofold advantage. First, rewards for the child's prosocial behavior are made more salient, and second, the parents are systematically taught to reinforce prosocial behavior. Reinforcement of prosocial behaviors with tangible rewards has been shown to be effective in increasing the occurrence of those behaviors. Use of point charts or tokens that earn daily rewards for specific behavior is recommended.

Typically, the aggressive child does not engage in age-appropriate work or self-maintenance behavior at home. Parents are often eager for the child to perform these tasks but have given up pressuring the child to follow through. Specify two or three chores and one prosocial behavior (e.g., minding) to include on a point chart. Define the specific components of each task and establish a time of day when the parent will check them. Set the minimum number of points necessary for the child to earn a reward. This should be fairly low at first, so the child is likely to succeed. Discuss with the parents the awarding of partial points for a job half done. This gives the child some encouragement, but indicates the need for improvement.

The parents and child together should generate a list of small rewards the child can pick from daily if enough points are earned. Caution the parents against selecting costly rewards they may resent giving the child. Special activities with one or both parents—such as playing a special game for fifteen minutes, reading a story, or helping with the cooking—are often effective rewards (see fig. 13-3 for a sample point chart). Parents should be instructed to systematically combine encouragement and praise with points as a means of teaching their child to be responsive to social reinforcement.

In approximately 50% of cases, problems occur around implementation of a reward system. Common problems include:

CHILD _____ WEEK OF _____ to _____

Chores/Behavior	Description	Value	Mon	Tues	Wed	Thur	Fri	Sat	Sun
		Totals							
Clean bedroom by 8:00 A.M.	1) Put toys into box	1							
	2) Put dirty clothes in hamper	1	3						
	3) Make bed with bedspread	1							
Empty garbage by 7:00 P.M.	1) Carry kitchen can to outside garbage and empty	1							
	2) Check for spills	1	3						
	3) Replace plastic liner	1							
Minding	Doing what you are asked within 15 seconds	1 each time							
		Must make: 9	Total	Total	Total	Total	Total	Total	Total

Rewards (select one):
1 Play cards with dad for 15 minutes   4 2¢ per point (if over 9 points)
2 Stay up 15 minutes later   5 Hot chocolate before bed
3 Make dessert for the family with mom   6 Choose a game for the whole family to play for 30 minutes

(#3 can be chosen one per week only)

Fig. 13-3. POINT-INCENTIVE CHART

1. *Parents are concerned that special attention given to the target child will result in unfairness to siblings.* In this situation, parents should be encouraged to think of eventually involving siblings in a similar manner, especially because the data suggest that siblings are likely to share similar behavior problems with the target child (although not as pronounced). Most often, it is beneficial for parents to begin this system with one child, work out the bugs, and then implement it with their other children.
2. *Parents are challenged and defeated in attempts to introduce the point system.* The point system should be presented (not negotiated) to the child. Some parents may approach the presentation in a weak, apologetic fashion. This virtually ensures that a debate and argument will ensue, resulting in failure to impose the system. At the other extreme, parents may approach the presentation in a harsh and punitive fashion, also increasing the likelihood of failure. Experience has demonstrated that if parents present the point system in a calm but firm manner, the child generally reacts in a positive way. Undoubtedly, some children will react with suspicion and distrust. Based on past disagreements with parents, this is probably a predictable reaction. Parents should be more concerned with introducing the new system and less concerned about moderate resistance from the child. Tremendous joy and enthusiasm is not required of the child. The only necessity is that the child clearly understand the rules. Participation is ultimately his or her choice. Parents experiencing difficulty in imposing the system require additional consultation. The therapist should role play with parents the presentation to the child and should monitor their progress. Through this process, the difficulties can generally be pinpointed and resolved.
3. *The child fails to work for or earn any points initially.* Some children may agree to participate in the point system, then fail to earn the required number of points. Inferences regarding the intent of the child's behavior should be minimized, and parents should follow through on prescribed contingencies. Even if the child has earned zero points for the day, parents should calmly review the program at the end of the day and simply state the failure to earn the reward. Beyond that, no further discussion is required. If parents engage in a debate, rearrange the point system, yield to the child's promise of a better day tomorrow, and provide the reinforcer, the point system is defeated.
4. *The child achieves criterion too easily.* Some children may achieve the criterion number of points necessary for obtaining the reward early in the day, and express to the parents—verbally or behaviorally—that they have earned the prescribed reward, implying that good behavior the remainder of the day is unnecessary. This presents a difficult situation for the parents: they are seeing an improvement in specific child behavior, but are likely to fall back into a negative global perception of the child being bad or manipulative. Parents should be encouraged to remain pleasant and positive, providing praise for the child's efforts when appropriate, but should take notes on the occurrence of aversive behaviors. The therapist should make note of these problem behaviors for possible inclusion in programs during subsequent weeks. If the child reached criterion early in three successive days, it may mean that the criterion is too low, in which case the point system may need adjustment by either adding more chores or behaviors to those on the list, moving the criterion up 10%, or both. Another possible solution is to maintain the criterion, but select a chore that can only be completed late in the day, such as washing the supper dishes, picking up toys, etc.

PUNISHMENT FOR AVERSIVE BEHAVIOR. Parents of antisocial children use punishment more often and less effectively than their normal counterparts (Patterson, 1977). Two patterns of parental styles relative to punishment have been associated with childhood aggression: harsh, erratic, or extreme physical punishment (Eron et al., 1963; Farrington, 1978) or laissez-faire permissive styles, usually emphasizing lecturing or scolding with no effective follow-through that stops the child's negative behavior (Patterson, 1976). Studies in the classroom demonstrate that "rule giving" with no backup contingency does not change behavior (Becker et al., 1967). Physical punishment has the advantage of stopping the child's aversive behavior for the moment, but has obvious disadvantages. Physical punishment provides a model of aggressive behavior to family members. Also parents tend to hit the child only *after* she or he has displayed either a number of aversive behaviors or an extremely serious behavior. Parke (1970) reviewed a number of studies regarding parental punishment styles and concluded that punishment for events that occurred early in a sequence of coercive behaviors were more effective in suppressing problem behavior than punishment for events occurring late in the sequence. Particulary ineffective were low-intensity (e.g., scolding) punishments that occurred *late* in a coercive sequence.

The use of *time out,* a procedure in which the occurrence of an aversive behavior is followed by a brief period of isolation, has been shown to be effective in reducing the frequency and intensity of problem behaviors in several studies (Tyler and Brown, 1968; Patterson et al., 1973). For maximum impact, the following procedures are recommended. Parents should begin by selecting one or two frequently occurring child problem behaviors and targeting them for time out. Noncompliance is a recommended behavior to begin with. Parent should select a room for time out that is away from other family members and without interesting things to do (e.g., bathroom, laundry room). Parents should explain the time-out procedure to the child (e.g., "Each time I ask you to do something and you don't do it, you will be sent to time out") and practice with the child (e.g., "Now, I'll ask you to do something and you don't do it"), so the child will know what to expect. It is important, especially in the beginning, to use time out consistently, that is, after each occurrence of the targeted behavior. Parents often develop a pattern of threatening time out as they may have previously threatened spanking. Instruct parents to keep records of how many time outs they use each day, and who (mother or father) administers them. The child typically earns numerous time outs during the first week of implementation—from five to ten per day. Parents reporting low use of time out should be cautioned about consistency. Drops in the occurrence of the targeted problem behavior and use of time out are usually observed by the end of week two. Studies show that a brief period of time out (e.g., five minutes) is as effective as longer periods for reducing the occurrence of problem behaviors (White et al., 1972).

Despite the simplicity of this procedure, the parents should be aware of numerous problems that usually occur:

1. *If children refuse to go to time out,* parents are instructed to respond to the refusal by adding one minute to the time out for each incident of arguing. When nine minutes of time out have been accumulated, the parent should inform children that if they do not go now, they will lose a privilege. Before beginning the time out procedure, parents should generate a list of privileges that could potentially be removed. Parents should be cautioned against engaging in arguments with children about the fairness or appropriateness of time out, especially after they have told them to go.
2. *If children are destructive in time out,* parents should be instructed to have them

clean up any mess they make before leaving time out. Parents should remove any dangerous or valuable items from the room before beginning time out.
3. Parents should initially be encouraged to use time out at home only and to treat the problem behavior as usual in other settings. Once the procedure is working effectively at home, parents are instructed to tell the child she or he has a time out and either administer it immediately upon returning home or remove the child from the setting in which the problem behavior occurred (e.g., use the car, a room at a friend's house) for a brief period.
4. *If misbehavior typically occurs in a given setting* (e.g., restaurants), the parent is instructed to plan a "teaching experience" for the child: this involves taking the child to the problem setting and planning ahead how to use time out.
5. *If the child claims to like time out or refuses to come out* when the time is up, the parents are instructed to ignore the child.

Treatment: Covert Conduct Problems

Approximately 50% of children referred for child-management problems also engage in serious indirect, covert problem behaviors such as stealing (Reid and Hendricks, 1973). The basic conditions characterizing most successful applications of social-learning interventions (i.e., that the problem behavior is easily detected and defined, and that consequences can be applied quickly and consistently) are seldom present when the child is engaging in covert problem behaviors. Typically, such behavior is seldom observed directly, and many incidences are never detected. The problem is further complicated by two factors: most children will lie about behaviors such as stealing when confronted, and parents of children engaging in predelinquent behaviors tend not to closely supervise their child.

An intervention strategy designed to take these problems into account was described by Reid and Patterson (1976). The treatment is broken down into two phases. In the first phase, parents are taught general child-management procedures (operationally defining behavior, observation and keeping track of behavior, point incentive systems, and the use of mild punishment procedures such as time out). This phase is designed, first, to familiarize the parents with general social-learning child-management procedures and, second, to help them deal with overt aggressive conduct problems. In the second phase, the covert problem behavior is redefined so that it is observable. The emphasis is taken off the actual behavior itself. For stealing, the target behavior is described either as the child's possession of anything for which he or she cannot account, an accusation of stealing by an informed other that the parent has reason to believe, or the parents' clear and considered suspicion that the child has taken something. Second, the parents are the sole judge of the occurrence or nonoccurrence of this target behavior. Parents are instructed not to argue with the child in dealing with such an event, but to simply say they have reason to believe a stealing event has taken place. The parents are instructed to admit to the child that "I may be wrong but I suspect . . . ," and not to insist the child confess to the misdeed, so that the child is put in a position where lying would be a functional behavior. In other words, since the emphasis is not on the stealing behavior itself but only the report of the stealing behavior, a child's denial of the act itself is irrelevant.

Third, a mild consequence is instituted given the occurrence of the target behavior (i.e., suspected stealing). The recommended consequence consists of one hour of hard work around the home for reported events involving the suspected theft of objects under $1.00 in value, and two hours of work for events involving values of more than $1.00. The consequence is kept at a mild level because in some cases the child will be unjustly accused. Parents initially find it very difficult to apply even a mild consequence if they are not totally sure the child is the culprit. Prior to implementing this system, parents should explain it so the child knows what to expect. In those cases in which supervision is a problem (e.g., when the parents allow the child to wander outside the home unmonitored for significant periods of time), the parents are instructed to institute a check-in system, the schedule of which depends on the age of the child and the circumstances of the parent. Each time the child fails to comply with the check-in system, a mild, prenegotiated consequence such as a work detail should be enforced.

For some behaviors (e.g., stealing or coming home late) time out is not an appropriate consequence. Parents usually rely on long periods of "grounding" in these situations. However, this consequence has disadvantages. The parent is also grounded, in that they must insure that the child does not leave the house. Children are often extremely coercive during this period, making the grounding as much a punishment for the parent as it is for them. In general, this consequence is not practical. Work details, varying in length depending on the seriousness of the misbehavior or the number of hours of misbehavior, are recommended. Work details have the advantage of being implemented in a relatively short period of time. The parent is instructed to generate a list of various jobs around the house, and estimate the approximate length of time each job requires. This list of consequences is discussed with the child before the parent has reason to implement a work detail. The child is told that given the occurrence of the targeted behavior (e.g., suspicion of stealing), they will be assigned a chore from this list. As with using time out, the parent is instructed to add extra time to the job if the child refuses to work. The parent is cautioned not to interact with the child during the work detail, but to tell the child that the length of the job will depend in part on how hard he or she works at it. The job must be completed to the parent's satisfaction. It is helpful for the parent to indicate what specifically are the parts to the job and what are the criteria for completion.

SUMMARY GUIDE TO TREATMENT

Initial Treatment Interview with the Parent(s)

Communicate to the parents that (a) they can change their child's problem-behavior patterns, (b) the most effective way to do this is in a systematic step-by-step fashion, focusing on specific child behaviors, (c) the family members will do the work of change through doing assignments that will require them to do a little work each day, and (d) the therapist will act as a consultant to them during this process.

Inform the parents that the length of treatment varies depending on the consistency of their work at home and, if there are two parents, on how well they work together. The average treatment time required is four and a half months.

Point out that, in trying to change things at home, they will find some things work well and some things do not; it will be important for them to inform the therapist about these details so that the treatment is effective for their family.

OBSERVATION AND RECORD KEEPING. After selecting and operationally defining one or two frequently occurring, easily observable problem behaviors, introduce the parent observation record sheet and tell them to observe the child for one hour each day when the problem behaviors are likely to occur. Have the parents keep this sheet with them during the observation hour, and make a slash in the appropriate box each time one of the problem or prosocial behaviors occur. It is often helpful to "role play" this step with the parents.

REWARDING PROSOCIAL BEHAVIOR. In most instances, it is preferable to begin by restructuring the parents' reaction to the child's prosocial behaviors rather than focusing on the negative behaviors, with one notable exception: when the parents are reacting in an excessively punitive manner to negative child behavior, and this is interpreted by the therapist as potentially being physically dangerous to the child. In these cases, parents are often resistant to an initial emphasis on positive behavior, and instruction in nonphysical punishment methods (i.e., time out) is a priority.

Details of construction of an initial point contract include: reviewing the parent observation data assessing the baseline levels of occurrence of targeted problem and prosocial behaviors; operationally defining the components of one or two household chores and/or self-maintenance behaviors; assigning point values to these tasks as well as to one of the parent-observed prosocial behaviors (e.g., minding); setting the point criterion required for obtaining a small daily reward—the criterion should be low initially so the child has a good opportunity for success; generating a menu of four to six rewards the child can choose from daily; explaining this system to the child; and reviewing the point contract daily. Instructions pertaining to daily review should include discussing the award of partial points for a chore partially completed and emphasizing that the focus of the review is to attend to those things the child did right and to minimize failures. Role playing with parents is often helpful here to determine how they are likely to behave counterproductively and to caution them against these pitfalls.

In disorganized, chaotic, or inconsistent families, two or three additional visits are often required to establish a point system parents can implement consistently at home. It is recommended that the therapist make telephone contact with the parents between visits once or twice a week to assist with problems the system may have developed and motivate parents to apply the program consistently.

PUNISHMENT OF PROBLEM BEHAVIOR. Although thought to be the "backbone" of the social-learning treatment, time out often meets resistance from parents in one of two ways. In some cases the parent feels sending the child to time out is not enough of a punishment and that it will not make an impression sufficient enough to change the child's behavior. It is important to point out to the parent that time out should be used for small misbehaviors usually occurring early in a coercive sequence (e.g., not minding or the first time the child sasses).

Other times the parent feels time out is too harsh a punishment for a small misbehavior, and would rather wait until the child does something substantially aversive before intervening. Discuss with the parent that, in teaching the child to be better behaved, it is important the punishment be related to the *child's* behavior rather than to the parent's own level of irritation.

In both cases, emphasize the importance of early intervention and consistency in using time out. After explaining the basic procedure, selecting a time-out room, determining what behavior to begin using time out for (it is recommended that only one previously observed behavior be selected initially), and determining what privileges should be withdrawn if the child refuses to go, it is usually helpful for the therapist to act as a troubleshooter in anticipating problems the parent is likely to encounter when implementing the system. Discussion of all the potential problems the parents and therapist anticipate maximizes the chances of success. Prepare the parent for role playing time out with the child before implementation at home.

Telephone contact with the parent for problem solving and giving support is desirable after introducing time out. This procedure rarely works without difficulty during the first week.

Later Treatment: Expanding the Point Contract

As treatment progresses, the point contract should be altered by adding new prosocial behaviors and chores, dropping off behaviors that are no long problematic, altering the criterion points required to obtain a reward, and lengthening the amount of time between the administration of the point and the obtaining of the reward. This process is often best begun by encouraging the parents and child to negotiate a larger reward that will be given in addition to smaller rewards if the child makes the criterion number of points on a certain number of days of the week (e.g., going to a movie on the weekend, getting a weekly allowance). Once this sytem is working effectively, the daily rewards can be dropped. The therapist should be increasingly less involved in these negotiations over the course of treatment as the parents' ability to incorporate this problem-solving framework increases. If the family members remain dependent on the therapist to operationally define problems and generate contingencies for change, training in problem solving and communication skills are indicated.

CONCLUSION

Negative coercive behavior patterns are characteristic of the aggressive child. Parents can change these patterns by changing their reactions to both the child's prosocial and problem behaviors. For some families in which treatment progresses smoothly, the therapist's role is primarily didactic. In disorganized or overly stressed families, the therapist must apply psychotherapeutic as well as behavioral skills. By convincing the parents to consistently alter negative or ineffective interaction patterns, the prognosis for treatment is good.

REFERENCES

Achenbach, T. M. 1966. The classification of children's psychiatric symptoms: A factor analytic study. *Pschol. Monogr.,* 80 (7, whole no. 615).

Achenbach, T. M. 1978. The child behavior profile. I. Boys aged 6 through 11. *J. Consult. Clin. Psychol.,* 46(3):478-488.

Ackerson, L. 1931. *Children's behavior problems.* vol. 1. Chicago: University of Chicago Press.

American Psychiatric Association. 1980. *Diagnostic and statistical manual of mental disorders—third edition (DSM-III).* Washington, D.C.: APA.

Anderson, L. M. 1969. Personality characteristics of parents of neurotic, aggressive, and normal preadolescent boys. *J. Consult. Clin. Psychol.,* 33(5):575-581.

Bandura, A., Ross, D., and Ross, S. A. 1963. Imitation of film-mediated aggressive models. *J. Abnorm. Soc. Psychol.,* 66:3-11.

Becker, W. C., Madsen, C. H., Arnold, C. R., and Thomas, D. R. 1967. The contingent use of teacher attention and praise in reducing classroom behavior problems. *J. Spec. Ed.,* 1:287-307.
Bell, R. Q. 1968. A reinterpretation of the direction of effects in studies of socialization. *Psychol. Rev.,* 75:81-95.
Bernal, M. E., Delfini, L. F., North, J. A., and Kreutzer, S. L. 1976. Comparison of boys' behavior in homes and classrooms. In *Behavior modification and families,* ed. E. Mash, L. Handy, and L. Hamerlynck. New York: Brunner/Mazel.
Bernal, M. E., Klinnert, M. D., and Schultz, L. A. 1980. Outcome evaluation of behavioral parent training and client-centered parent counseling for children with conduct problems. *J. Appl. Beh. Anal.,* 13:677-691.
Burgess, J. M., Kimball, U. H., and Burgess, R. L. 1978. Family interaction as a function of family size. Paper presented at the Southeastern Conference on Human Development.
Chamberlain, P. 1980. Standardization of a parent report measure. Doctoral dissertation, University of Oregon.
Clement, P. W., and Milne, D. C. 1967. Group play therapy and tangible reinforcers used to modify the behavior of eight-year-old boys. *Beh. Res. Ther.,* 5:301-312.
Dollard, J., Miller, N. E., Doob, L. W., Mowrer, O. H., and Sears, R. R. 1939. *Frustration and aggression.* New Haven, Conn.: Yale University Press.
Eron, L. D., Walder, L. O. Toigo, R., and Lefkowitz, M. M. 1963. Social class, parental punishment for aggression, and child aggression. *Child Dev.,* 34:849-867.
Eyberg, S. M., and Johnson, S. M. 1974. Multiple assessment of behavior modification with families: Effects of contingency contracting and order of treated problems. *J. Consult. Clin. Psychol.,* 42(4):594-606.
Farrington, D. P. 1978. The family background of aggressive youths. In *Aggression and antisocial behavior in childhood and adolescence,* ed. L. A. Hersov, M. Berger, and D. Shaffer. Oxford: Pergamon Press.
Forehand, R., Wells, K., and Sturgis, E. 1978. Predictors of child noncompliant behavior in the home. *J. Consult. Clin. Psychol.,* 46:179.
Forgatch, M. S., and Toobert, D. J. 1979. A cost-effective parent training program for use with normal preschool children. *J. Ped. Psychol.,* 4(2):129-145.
Goodenough, F. L. 1931. *Anger in young children.* Minneapolis: University of Minnesota Press.
Guttman, E. S. 1962. Effects of short-term psychiatric treatment. Research report no. 36. California Youth Authority.
Henry, M. M., and Sharpe, D. F. 1947. Some influential factors in the determination of aggressive behavior in preschool children. *Child Dev.,* 18:11-28.
Herbert, E. W., Pinkston, E. M., Hayden, M. L., Sajwaj, T. E., Pinkston, S., Cordua, G., and Jackson, C. 1973. Adverse effects of differential parental attention. *J. Appl. Beh. Anal.,* 6:15-30.
Holleran, P. A., *Prediction of treatment dropouts for families of children who steal.* Unpublished. Eugene, Oregon: Oregon Social Learning Center, 207 E. 5th, Suite 202.
Jenkins, R. L., and Glickman, S. 1946. Common syndromes in child psychiatry. *Am. J. Orthopsych.,* 16:244-253.
Lindsey, O. R. 1966. An experiment with parents handling behavior at home. *Johnstone Bull.,* 9:27-36.
Loeber, R. 1980. Childhood precursors of assaultive behavior in males. Research proposal submitted to the National Institute of Mental Health, Crime and Delinquency Section, October 1980.
Lorber, R. 1981. Parental tracking of childhood behavior as a function of family stress. Doctoral dissertation, University of Oregon.
Maccoby, E., and Jacklin, C. 1974. *The psychology of sex differences.* Stanford: Stanford University Press.

MacFarlane, J. W., Allen, L., and Honzik, M. 1954. *A developmental study of the behavioral problems of normal children between 21 months and 14 years.* Berkeley: University of California Press.

Marcus, L. M. 1972. Studies of attention in children vulnerable to psychopathology. Doctoral dissertation, University of Minnesota.

Mednick, S. A., and Christiansen, K. O., eds. 1977. *Biosocial bases of criminal behavior.* New York: Gardner Press.

Mischel, W. 1966. A social learning view of sex differences in behavior. In *The development of sex differences,* ed. E. Macoby. Stanford: Stanford University Press.

Parke, R. D. 1970. The role of punishment in the socialization process. In *Early experiences and the process of socialization.* New York: Academic Press.

Patterson, G. R. 1974. Interventions for boys with conduct problems: Multiple settings, treatments, and criteria. *J. Consult. Clin. Psychol.,* 42:471–481.

Patterson, G. R. 1976. The aggressive child: Victim and architect of a coercive system. In *Behavior modification and families: Theory and research,* vol. 1, ed. L. A. Hamerlynck, L. C. Handy, and E. J. Mash. New York: Brunner/Mazel.

Patterson, G. R. 1977. Accelerating stimuli for two classes of coercive behavior. *J. Abnor. Child Psychol.,* 5(4):335–350.

Patterson, G. R. 1982. Siblings: Fellow travelers in coercive family processes. Paper presented at the International Conference on the Development of Anti-social and Pro-social Behavior, July 1982, Voss, Norway.

Patterson, G. R. 1982. *A social learning approach to family intervention: Coercive family processes.* Vol. 3. Eugene, Oreg.: Castalia Publishing Co.

Patterson, G. R., Chamberlain, P., and Reid, J. B. 1982. A comparative evaluation of parent training procedures for families of antisocial children. *Behav. Ther.,* 13:638–650.

Patterson, G. R., Cobb, J. A., and Ray, R. S. 1973. A social engineering technology for retraining the families of aggressive boys. In *Issues and trends in behavior therapy,* ed. H. Adams, and I. Unikel. Springfield, Ill.: Charles C. Thomas. (Also in *Violence in the family,* ed. S. Steinmetz, and M. Strauss. New York: Dodd, Mead, 1974).

Patterson, G. R., Ray, R. S., Shaw, D. A., and Cobb, J. A. 1969. *Manual for coding of family interactions.* New York: Microfische Publications.

Patterson, G. R., Reid, J. B., and Maerov, S. L. 1978. The observation system: Methodological issues and psychometric properties. In *A social learning approach to family intervention: Observation in home settings,* vol. 2, ed. J. B. Reid. Eugene, Oreg.: Castalia Publishing Co.

Patterson, G. R., and Stouthamer-Loeber, M. 1984. The correlation of family management practices and delinquency. *Child Develop.* (in press).

Peine, H. 1970. Behavioral recording by parents and its resultant consequences. Master's thesis, University of Utah.

Phipps-Yonas, S. 1979. Reaction time, peer assessment, and achievement in vulnerable children. Paper presented at the 87th Convention of the American Psychological Association, September 1979, New York.

Quay, H. C. 1965. Personality and delinquency. In *Juvenile delinquency research and theory,* ed. H. C. Quay. New York: Van Nostrand Reinhold Co.

Redl, F. and Wineman, D. 1951. *Children who hate.* New York: Free Press.

Reid, J. B., ed. 1978. *A social learning approach to family intervention: Observation in home settings.* Vol. 2. Eugene, Oreg.: Castalia Publishing Co.

Reid, J. B., and Chamberlain, P. *Treatment of chronic delinquents: An outcome evaluation.* (in preparation)

Reid, J. B., and Hendricks, A. F. C. J. 1973. A preliminary analysis of the effectiveness of direct home intervention for treatment of predelinquent boys who steal. In *Behavior therapy: Methodology, concepts, and practice,* ed. L. Hamerlynck, L. Handy, and E. Mash. Champaign, Ill.: Research Press.

Reid, J. B., and Patterson, G. R. 1976. The modification of aggression and stealing behaviors of boys in the home setting. In *Analysis of delinquency and aggression,* ed. E. Ribes-Inesta, and A. Bandura. Hillsdale, N. J.: Lawrence Erlbaum and Associates.

Robins, L. N. 1966. *Deviant children grown up: A sociological and psychiatric study of sociopathic personality.* Baltimore: Williams and Wilkins.

Romig, D. A. 1978. *Justice for children.* Lexington, Mass.: D. C. Heath.

Rutter, M., Tizard, J., and Whitmore, R. 1970. *Education, health, and behavior.* New York: John Wiley.

Sallows, G. 1972. Comparative responsiveness of normal and deviant children to naturally occurring consequences. Doctoral dissertation, University of Oregon.

Schelle, J. 1974. A brief report on invalidity of parent evaluations of behavior change. *J. Appl. Beh. Anal.,* 7:341-343.

Snyder, J. J. 1977. A reinforcement analysis of interaction in problem and nonproblem families. *J. Abnorm. Psychol.,* 86(5):528-535.

Sowles, R. C., and Gill, J. H. 1970. Institutional and community adjustment of delinquents following counseling. *J. Consult. Clin. Psychol.,* 34:398-402.

Truax, C. B., Wargo, M. J., and Volksdorf, F. R. 1970. Antecedents to outcome in group counseling with institutionalized juvenile delinquents. *J. Abnorm. Psychol.,* 76:235-242.

Tyler, V., and Brown, G. 1968. Token reinforcement of academic performance with institutionalized delinquent boys. *J. Ed. Psychol.,* 57:164-168.

Wahler, R. G., House, A. E., and Stambaugh, E. E. 1976. *Ecological assessment of child problem behavior: A clinical package for home, school, and institutional settings.* New York: Pergamon Press.

Wahler, R. G., and Leske, G. 1973. Accurate and inaccurate observer summary reports: Reinforcement theory interpretation and investigation. *J. Nerv. Men. Dis.,* 156:386-394.

Wahler, R. G., Leske, G., and Rogers, E. 1977. The insular family: A deviance support system for oppositional children. Paper presented at the Banff International Conference on Behavior Modification.

Walker, H. M., and Buckley, N. K. 1973. Teacher attention to appropriate and inappropriate classroom behavior: An individual case study. *Focus on Exceptional Children,* May, 5:5-11.

Walter, H. I., and Gilmore, S. K. 1973. Placebo versus social learning effects in parent training procedures designed to alter the behaviors of aggressive boys. *Beh. Ther.,* 4:361-377.

Weinrott, M., Bauske, B., and Patterson, G. R. 1979. Systematic replication of a social learning approach. In *Trends in behavior therapy,* ed. P. O. Sjoden, S. Bates, and W. S. Dockens. New York: Academic Press.

Weintraub, S. A. 1973. Self control as a correlate of an internalizing-externalizing symptom dimension. *J. Abnorm. Psychol.,* 86(5):528-535.

White, G. D., Nielsen, G., and Johnson, S. M. 1972. Time out duration and the suppression of deviant behavior in children. *J. Appl. Beh. Anal.,* 5:111-120.

Wolff, S. 1967. Behavioral characteristics of primary school children referred to a psychiatric department. *Brit. J. Psych.,* 113:885-893.

14

The Hyperkinetic Syndrome

LAURENCE L. GREENHILL

SINCE THE LATE 1960s hyperkinesis has grown into one of the most popular diagnostic clinical concepts in American child psychiatry and, as such, it has become a catchall. In this chapter, the most recent, specific *DSM-III* definitions (American Psychiatric Association, 1980) will be critically applied to enable the clinician to diagnose such children more accurately. In addition, global rating forms, structured interview techniques, and behavioral observation cues will be presented to aid the pediatrician, teacher, or child psychiatrist in identifying hyperkinetic children and tracking their progress during treatment. Finally, the relative merits of drug therapy, counseling, behavior modification, and educational methods employed in the treatment of this syndrome will be surveyed.

CLINICAL POINTERS

Diagnostic Subtypes

Two predominant "core" clinical signs characterize the disorder, namely the developmentally *inappropriate inattention* and the *impulsivity*. Overactivity may or may not be consistently present as a sign. It serves to distinguish the two childhood subtypes: attention deficit disorder with hyperactivity (ADD+H) and the attention deficit disorder without hyperactivity (ADD-H). When individuals continue to manifest the inattentive and impulsive features of the disorder, without the motor component, past eighteen years of age, they can be classified as exhibiting signs of the residual syndrome.

Basic Clinical Features

The attention deficit disorders characterize behaviors that are exaggerations of normal childhood inattentiveness, impulsivity, and overactivity. These behavioral traits often exhibit a protean quality, interacting with the environmental setting. In addition, age must also be considered; children with this disorder exhibit patterns of behavioral deviancy when compared to other children of the same age.

The younger "hyperkinetic" (this term being less cumbersome that the longer attentive deficit disorder with hyperactivity) child will prove to be more overactive and impulsive in all settings. Whether he is viewed in the nursery classroom, in his own home, or at the clinic, the preschooler with the disorder exhibits a motor drivenness. He rapidly moves about the room, getting into everything in a chaotic, haphazard manner. He climbs, jumps, and runs and is often described as being "driven by a motor."

The school-age child often shows more variability in impulsivity and overactivity. In school, group situations bring out the highest levels of inattention and impulsivity. Teachers report that these children appear to be "not listening" or daydreaming when sitting in the classroom. Sloppy handwriting, careless errors, and messy papers may lead to academic performance well below their aptitude level. Signs of overactivity emerge as fidgeting and squirming in the seat. At home the attentional problems interfere with follow-through of parental requests to complete structured tasks. Homework does not get finished without constant adult supervision. The child cannot even stick to play activities for age-appropriate periods of time. Some parents report that their children frequently are unable to entertain themselves in play situations.

The *variability* of the signs within a given child must be emphasized. Even a moderately severe case of hyperkinetic disorder may show age-appropriate behavior in a one-to-one setting with a professional. Out on the playground, he may resemble his normal peers who allow themselves to shout, climb, run, and show some aggressiveness. These nonaffected peers, however, possess the capacity to inhibit and modulate their energy in the classroom, where the hyperkinetic cannot. Group peer situations involving self-paced work (Whalen et al., 1979) exert the greatest stress for such a child. Even so, it is the rare child who reliably displays all the signs of the hyperkinetic syndrome in all settings. (American Psychiatric Association, 1980).

Epidemiology and Natural Hints

Prevalence in the Population

Various estimates suggest that the hyperkinetic syndrome afflicts between 3 and 5% of the primary-school population (Wender, 1971). The Collaborative Perinatal Project follow-up identified a much lower prevalence figure for hyperactive children of 0.25% in the U.S. primary-school population (Rieder and Nichols, 1979), but based its data on a single office visit without the benefit of teacher's reports. Clearly, the hyperkinetic syndrome appears commonly in American psychiatric practice, even though the experts cannot agree on its exact frequency.

Sex Ratio

Males present with this disorder ten times more often than females. This is in keeping with the higher prepubertal male risk for prematurity and childhood psychiatric disorders in general.

Age of Onset

Most children come to professional attention during their primary-school years. Carefully taken histories may reveal that these same children had already displayed most of the hyperkinetic disorder's signs by the age of three. It seems that the academic setting is necessary to truly identify these behaviors as pathological. Although *DSM-III* requires a brief duration criterion of six months, one recent diagnostic interview schedule, the Kiddie-SADS-E (Puig-Antich et al., 1980), requires the signs to have appeared prior to the age of seven. Most clinicians suggest that a several-year history of impulsivity, overactivity, and inattention helps validate the diagnosis. Typically, mothers recall that the hyperkinetic child displayed more activity *in utero* than did his siblings, was more irritable as an infant, was apt to have suffered colic, and clearly did more climbing and running once he became a toddler than did other youngsters.

Course

DSM-III suggests that three clinical courses exist, but cites no studies documenting either predictors or the relative incidences of such outcomes. For one type of course, the child retains the same level of impulsivity, overactivity, and inattention into the adult years that he first demonstrated at age six. In the second outcome, more characteristic of the residual disorder, the overactivity spontaneously remits while the restlessness, impulsivity, and attentional problems persist into adulthood. Finally, there are the children who appear to completely overcome their fidgetiness and inattention during the pubertal years. The relationships among severity of disorder, treatment responsiveness, and type of course are completely unknown.

Family Patterns

Clustering in families tends to occur in the hyperkinetic syndrome. Cantwell (1972) has described an increased incidence of hyperkinesis in the fathers of these children, and alcoholism and sociopathy in secondary, earlier generation relatives. Rapoport reported a relationship among overactivity in infants, the appearance of minor physical anomalies, and past histories of hyperkinesis in the fathers (Rapoport et al., 1977). The exact balance of social and genetic influences in the transmission of the disorder remains unknown. In some instances, the signs of hyperkinesis become identified as a family male temperamental trait rather than a disorder, so fathers may show resistance to having their children treated.

ASSOCIATED CONDITIONS

Personality Features

While the age of the child influences the exact personality style, certain characteristics commonly emerge. Hyperkinetic children often get labeled as "spoiled," "immature," and "bratty" because of their impulsivity, short attention spans, and low frustration tolerance. The core temperamental signs of the disorder in children seem to produce negative, irritable, or labile emotional reactions. Frequent temper outbursts and occasional full-blown tantrums are common, even in older children. They respond poorly to discipline, seem immune to punishment, and condition poorly (Wender, 1971). They will vary between appearing the "happy extrovert" with peers and displaying low-esteem with teachers. In peer-group situations, as noted later, the hyperkinetic child will display bossiness.

Poor Peer Relationships

Peer relationships for hyperkinetic children are marked by friction (Klein et al., 1980). The impulsivity, low frustration tolerance, and overactivity makes these children a nuisance to their peer groups. Hyperkinetic children want to play games by their own rules and will not wait their turns. Furthermore, the peer group has no more success at limit setting than do parents or teachers. Children with this disorder are driven to interact with peers, so their lack of success is not due to any lack of contact with other children.

Poor Academic Performance

Schoolwork becomes a constant trial for many hyperkinetic children. They often peform poorly on classroom tests, in spite of normal or above-average IQs. Attentional problems interfere with the concentration necessary to learn, and lack of follow-through interferes with tasks that require time in preparation. This style in the classroom leads to spotty performance. Even when motivated, hyperkinetic children make careless mistakes, turn in sloppy papers, and show an inability to organize themselves or carry out self-paced assignments. Weingartner et al. (1981) have suggested that these children employ immature learning strategies for storing and retrieving information, as shown by the paired associates test of semantic and acoustic recall. Drug therapies with stimulants did not modify hyperkinetic children's basic strategies in Weingartner's lab. Some large-scale, prospective follow-up studies strongly suggest that academic failure may continue in spite of successful behavior management with medication alone (Weiss et al., 1979).

Hyperkinetic children display characteristically maladaptive behavioral styles in the classroom, perhaps as a result of their frustration and failure. Direct observational studies by Abikoff et al. (1977) and Whalen et al. (1978) have validated teacher's anecdotal impressions that hyperkinetic boys show higher classroom rates of negative verbalizations, noise making, physical contact, social initiation, and disruptiveness than do nonhyperactive peers. In addition, hyperkinetic children spend much class time off assigned tasks, interfering with other children, soliciting the teacher's attention, and showing continuous minor and gross motor movements, even while sitting.

Specific Learning Disabilities

Children with the syndrome may perform two or more years behind on standardized achievement tests, such as the Wide Range Achievement Test (WRAT) or the Peabody Individual Achievement Test (PIAT). Reading and arithmetic skills are often hardest hit. These learning disabilities will not be found in every hyperkinetic child who underachieves. Academic failure may also be due to inattention and misapplication of skills.

Clumsiness

Hyperkinetic children may present as immature because of their innate clumsiness and lack of grace. Lack of skill in sports adds to the problems with the peer group. Many of these children will find noncompetitive, nonteam activities, like horseback riding or swimming, more rewarding, where gross motor skills are more important than precise hand-eye coordination.

Aggressive Outbursts

Fights with other children, either at home or at school, are not unusual. Upon investigation, the aggression most often is found to be reactive and unpremeditated. Awkward, ostracized boys who are abrasive to others often get teased; thus hyperkinetic children are a favorite mark for other children. In contrast, aggression from children with conduct disorder has a planned, sadistic quality and may be accompanied by other problems, such as stealing and oppositionalism. In some cases, however, it may be difficult to differentiate hyperkinetic children with a serious conduct *problem* from overactive children with chronic conduct *disorder*.

Moodiness and Irritability

Hyperkinetic children present major management problems because of their disruptiveness, unresponsiveness to limit setting, and emotional lability. Ten- or eleven-year-old hyperkinetic children can get "jazzed up," overexcited, and loud. Low frustration tolerance drives them into fits of mild rage when tasks do not go smoothly or they do not get their way. Easy disappointment, rapid mood swings, and frequent irritability gives these children the quality of being "spoiled."

Minor Physical Anomalies

Rapoport et al. (1977) reported an increased incidence of minor physical abnormalities in overactive infants. These anomalies consisted of partial or full epicanthal folds, low-set ears, high-arched palate, hypertelorism, bilateral or unilateral simian palmar creases, short, incurving fifth fingers, and an unusually large gap between the large toe and second toes of the foot. While scoring systems have been devised to quantify the severity of these physical findings (Waldrop and Halverson, 1971), a high score does not necessarily put a given infant at risk for the later development of the full hyperkinetic syndrome.

ETIOLOGICAL THEORIES

Brain Damage

During the two last decades the hyperkinetic syndrome has been classified as a central nervous system (CNS) disorder requiring medical treatment. Various authorities writing in the early 1970s conceptualized hyperkinesis as a result of biological brain malfunction. The diverse group of child classroom misbehaviors were merged under a common etiological rubric, named *minimal brain dysfunction* (MBD). In a critique, Shaffer and Greenhill (1979) noted that advocates of the MBD concept implied that the hyperkinetic behavior pattern was part of a diffuse, mild neurological disorder even though lesion could not be documented. Conceptually, the MBD syndrome identified a highly heterogeneous group of children, quite dissimilar in their etiological precedents and their current clinical features. These broad MBD diagnostic criteria lacked validity. They were too vague to predict a characteristic response to treatment, or predict outcome for the treated or untreated group in the future. Thus, an etiological mechanism of brain dysfunction was confused with a quite tentative syndromal description of behavior. Poor construct validity and low interrater reliability further hurt this diagnostic concept.

As Shaffer and Greenhill note (1979), a specific etiological link between frank brain damage and the hyperkinetic syndrome has not been supported by diverse lines of evidence. Factor-analytic studies have failed to find relationships between overactivity or inattentiveness and brain damage (Werry et al., 1972). Both population surveys (Rutter et al., 1970) and direct measurement studies of brain-damaged children (Shaffer et al., 1974) showed no disproportionate incidence of inattention, motor activity, or impulsiveness in brain-damaged children over rates seen in children with psychiatric disorders but who have no brain damage.

Environmental Correlates

Although the exact causal relationships are not apparent, certain factors have been associated with signs of the hyperkinetic disorder. Leading the list are social disadvantage, large family size, and overcrowding. Rutter and colleagues reported these correlates to overactivity and inattention in the classic Isle of Wight epidemiologic study (Rutter et al., 1970). These social factors should be inquired about during any diagnostic investigation. Treatment outcome may be hampered by social factors, reducing the efficacy of drugs or of special therapeutic classroom placements.

Catecholamine Hypothesis

The hyperkinetic syndrome has joined other major psychiatric diagnostic entities as subjects for biochemical speculation. Schizophrenia has been conceptionalized as a disease of dopamine hypersecretion or dopamine postsynaptic receptor hypersensitivity. Depression, in turn, has been explained as relative deficiency of catecholamines, since low norepinephrine and serotonin metabolites have been found in depressed patients' urine and cerebrospinal fluid. Biochemical models of hyperkinesis have been developed as well. Early studies of selectively dopamine-depleted rat pups showed increased overactivity over saline-treated litter mates (Shaywitz et al., 1976), with a calming response to amphetamines. In controlled human studies Shaywitz found lowered metabolites of dopamine and serotonin in hyperkinetic children's spinal fluid (Shaywitz et al., 1977). Wender (1971) theorized that hyperkinetic disorder resulted from a selective deficiency of dopamine in the central nervous system.

There are several problems with this hypothesis. Although the stimulants are dopamine agonists, simply increasing CNS dopamine concentrations does not alleviate the clinical syndrome. Experimental trials with pure dopamine agonists such as L-dopa and Piribedil only make hyperkinetic children nauseous without modifying their behavior. In addition, this dopamine-deficiency hypothesis would predict that dopamine-blocking drugs should worsen the clinical picture. Yet chlorpromazine and thioridazine, well-known postsynaptic dopamine-blocking agents, actually ameliorate the overactive and impulsive behaviors, and show no evidence of worsening the condition (Gittelman-Klein et al., 1976b). Shekim's investigations into the changes in urinary catecholamine metabolites during treatment with d-amphetamine have yielded inconsistent results. Various nonspecific shifts in the relative turnover of dopamine and norepinephrine may occur during successful stimulant treatment (Shekim et al., 1979). These results do not directly support the catecholamine hypothesis of hyperkinesis.

Heritability

Preliminary evidence that hyperkinesis may be transmitted on a genetic basis comes from the finding that there is a clustering of the same or similar disturbances among the close relations of the affected child. Cantwell et al. (1972) have described higher than expected rates of antisocial behavior in the fathers and Briquet's syndrome in the mothers of hyperactive children. Family studies cannot separate the effects of genetics and environment. As a result, Morrison and Stewart (1973) and Cantwell et al. (1972) have utilized the adoptive parents' research technique, by which one examines the mental status of adoptive parents (index parents) who have reared a child who later developed hyperkinesis. Controls included the natural parents of other hyperkinetic children, and a third parental group with natural children affected by another disorder. The natural parents of hyperkinetic children were found to display the most psychopathology, namely alcoholism and Briquet's disorder in the mothers, and sociopathy and a history of hyperkinesis in the fathers. Unfortunately, these studies were flawed, since the interviewers were not blind as to the parent's status. In addition, the adopting parents, who proved to have significantly lower rates of psychopathology, had been prescreened for health by adoption agencies.

Safer (1973) examined the psychiatric status of the full and half siblings of hyperkinetic children, all having been raised in foster care. There was genetically predicted gradation of hyperkinetic behaviors, increasing in level from foster siblings (lowest), to half siblings (higher), and on to full siblings (highest). As was noted, these genetic studies are only suggestive, having been flawed by weak controls, lack of blindness in the interviewers, and small numbers. Still, it behooves the clinician to inquire about the family history of the affected child.

Minimally Elevated Lead Levels

David (1978) has advanced the intriguing hypothesis that lead, at levels below those considered dangerous, may exert toxic effects in the central nervous systems of vulnerable children. His studies reject the threshold model of lead-induced brain damage and assert a continuum of damage; in effect, this hypothesis links an identified form of "minimal brain damage" with abnormal behavior. It differs from the broader, vaguer MBD notion in its etiological specificity. Studying children with minimally elevated lead levels is complicated by the fact that a given lead level may exert differential effects, depending entirely on the host's resistance to lead. David points out that a 100 μg/dl level may kill some children, but "fully 35% will show no discernible symptomatology" (David, 1978). The true impact of lead as the etiological agent in hyperkinesis awaits further work.

Food Additives

Feingold (1975) has hypothesized that artificial food dyes serve as pharmacologically active agents, exacerbating hyperkinetic signs in children. His claims have been criticized, since they are based on uncontrolled parental and clinical observations of elimination diets given the children and were thus subject to placebo effects. As Sobotka (1978) noted in his review, two basic types of studies have emerged to examine Feingold's observation: the dietary crossover design and the specific challenge design. In crossover studies, carefully diagnosed hyperkinetic children were randomly assigned to either a control dietary program or to a specific elimination diet, and then switched to the opposite diet. Crossover studies by Conners et al. (1976) and by Harley et al. (1978) failed to show conclusive advantages for the elimination diet.

More recently, a variety of investigators (Sobotka, 1978) have employed specific food-additive challenges. Hyperkinetic children, selected for behavioral improvement by open trials of elimination diets, were placed on long-term dietary programs and given either the challenge additive or a placebo vehicle by a double-blind, random-order design. Most of the studies employed challenge cookies or drinks supplied by the nutrition foundation or by Nabisco Corporation. The concentration of additives in the challenge vehicle was kept low in most studies. Overall, the effect of dyes, even in sensitive children, has been shown to be a fleeting and minor one, and could not account for the large amount of hyperkinetic behavior reported in American children.

Abnormalities in Cortical Arousal

The etiological theory regarding cortical arousal draws upon a large body of physiological data, including reaction-time studies, galvanic skin responses, EEG-activation data, and evoked-potential work collected on hyperactive children, on and off stimulant drugs. As reviewed by Barkley and Jackson (1977), the theory proposes that stimulants work by activating cortical inhibitory systems. Overall, the physiological data appears equivocal, with untreated hyperkinetic children appearing underaroused in some studies and overaroused in others, when compared to normals or to hyperkinetic children on stimulants. Klein et al. (1980) suggest that our present methods for tapping the relevant aspects of cortical arousal may not be adequate to test this hypothesis.

Dysregulation of Attention as a Core Dysfunction

Virginia Douglas, in her paper intriguingly titled "Stop, look, and listen: The problem of sustained attention and impulse control in hyperactive and normal children" (1972), puts forth a powerful heuristic concept. It maintains that hyperkinetic children possess a *basic primary deficit* which makes it impossible for them to sustain attention. Impulsive behavior and hyperactivity then develop *pari passu* as secondary complications of a primary cognitive impairment. The current diagnostic category of attention deficit disorder with or without hyperactivity seems to emphasize a core attentional handicap leading to social dysfunction. Rather, Klein et al. (1980) believe that the three signs in the hyperkinetic syndrome (impulsivity, inattentiveness, and overactivity) are probably somewhat independent dimensions, with complex causal interrelationships. The central defect may be a "problem in the regulation of appetitive behaviors" which leads these children to a characteristically impulse-ridden behavioral style (Klein et al., 1980). This dysregulation, in turn, creates an inability to maintain attention for any period of time without experiencing habituation and boredom.

Other Factors

Many other theories have been put forward to explain the appearance of hyperkinetic signs in the school-age population. They will be mentioned here for the sake of completeness. Besides the theories of general central nervous system dysfunction (Silver, 1971), chromosomal irregularities (Waldrop and Goering, 1971) and birth complications (Pasamanick and Knobloch, 1959) have been evoked. Social-learning effects were implicated by other workers, including the traumatic influences of severe family discord (Grinspoon and Singer, 1973).

Differential Diagnosis

Age-appropriate overactivity may occur in children who show no impulsive or attentional problems. It can be distinguished from the activity seen in the hyperkinetic syndrome because it shows little of the severely non-goal-directed quality found in the latter condition. Second, overactive and inattentive children who come from chaotic, disadvantaged, and crowded homes may be displaying more of state-dependent behavior than a true hyperkinetic syndrome. Third, children with primary *conduct disorders* may show many of the signs of the hyperkinetic syndrome, due to an overlap in *DSM-III* diagnoses. A child can receive both diagnoses. As mentioned before, the impulsivity of the conduct-disordered child has a calculating, premeditated quality not found in the reactive and impulsive misbehaviors of the hyperkinetic child.

Other conditions are clearly excluded from the attention deficit disorder category in *DSM-III*. Severe and profoundly mentally retarded children may exhibit all the signs of the hyperkinetic syndrome. *DSM-III* excludes such children from the latter diagnosis. Treatment response to stimulants in retardates resembles the response of hyperkinetic children (Bruening, 1982). Children with schizophrenia and affective disorders with manic features display impulsivity, overactivity, and inattentiveness, but only secondarily to the primary illness; again the management and prognosis differs greatly from primary hyperkinetic syndrome. For those children who show less gross motor activity, certain conditions must be excluded before a diagnosis of attention deficit disorder without hyperactivity can be made. Adjustment disorder will produce impulsivity and inattentiveness in children, but there will be a close temporal relationship within six months between the onset of hyperkinetic behavior and the psychosocial stressor. The negative, uncooperative child with oppositional disorder may also resemble the attention deficit disordered child.

Extreme care should be exercised before making the diagnosis of attention deficit disorder, residual type. Such individuals present as late adolescents or adults. First and foremost, the clinician must rule out a substance-abuse disorder involving amphetamine or similarly acting sympathomimetics. Such individuals will gladly fabricate a full history of hyperkinetic syndrome to obtain new supplies of stimulants. Second, and almost as serious, patients with schizophrenia or schizotypal or borderline personality disorders can show all signs of impulsivity and inattentiveness necessary to fulfill criteria. Stimulant treatment of such schizophrenic-spectrum patients, however, can induce a psychotic episode. Finally, adult patients with conduct disorders may be brought in by hopeful parents who would like to believe that their children actually have the potentially treatable diagnosis of attention deficit disorder, residual type.

Investigation of the Hyperkinetic Child

History

The validity of a diagnostic disorder can be strengthened by requiring it to be present for a minimum length of time, thus separating long-term stable hyperkinetic traits from brief adjustment reactions. *DSM-III* requires the signs to be present for at least six months; certain research studies in addition, require the disorder to have been present before age seven. Klein et al. (1980) suggest that the clinician determine if the signs were present in the toddler years. Even with the liabilities of parents' retrospective recall, most clinicians find that children with severe hyperkinetic syndrome showed overactive and impulsive behavior by age two.

The clinician's optimal history-taking approach works best when the inquiry touches upon the positive signs of the disorder, exclusion conditions, severity measures, associated conditions, and family history. Such information can best be collected for the history if both parents are present.

Positive histories of hyperkinesis in first- and second-degree relatives can strengthen the diagnostic conviction of the clinician, since most experts agree that the syndrome aggregates in families. Inquire about the parent's own primary-school education. Fathers often spontaneously state, "I was just like Johnny when I was in third grade; there's nothing wrong with him." With this, the clinician obtains a positive history and a hint that treatment may not be supported by the father. Siblings should also be inquired after, particularly for difficulties with academic work or conduct problems. Siblings can provide a control for the child who presents with the hyperkinetic syndrome from a chaotic, disadvantaged household; if they are not hyperkinetic, then the patient's behavior difficulties may indeed be hyperkinesis and not an adjustment response to poor living conditions. Finally, the clinician should ask about other relatives who might have had trouble with the law or have had multiple operations. The Cantwell (1972) observation that the adult relatives suffer increased rates of sociopathy and Briquet's disorder may provide important leads for validating the child's diagnosis.

Gross motor overactivity may subside at an early age, leaving a child with a developmentally short attention span, impulsivity, and restlessness. One should begin by taking a developmental history of inattentiveness. The age of the patient will determine the approach. For the preschooler, parental home observations will provide the best data. Can the child entertain himself for half an hour looking through a book or building block castles? Hyperkinetic preschoolers will race through all activities, finishing none, and beg for attention from the parent, all within several minutes. School-age children display inattentiveness at home by not completing homework or chores, or by not seeming to listen. Classically, the hyperactive school-age child forgets what he was sent upstairs for. In addition, he may have difficulty carrying out multistep tasks, such as building models, finishing needlepoint or cooking projects. During these times, parents report that they must literally stand over their children, refocusing their wandering attention, or else the task is never completed.

In particular, behavior during homework may be the most revealing of the hyperkinetic child's "invisible handicap" (Taft, 1975). Even bright children with this disorder report the rapid onset of terrible boredom during homework. Unsupervised, such a child will start three other activities and end up finishing neither the schoolwork nor the other projects. Secondary behavior patterns often develop around the homework struggle, particularly avoidance routines, such as "forgetting" assignments, leaving important books at school, and even dashing through the homework unconcerned about errors. Parents quickly get discouraged, taking much of their leisure weektime evening hours to hover over the child, constantly directing them to check the paper once completed, and occasionally doing the work themselves.

School provides the optimal provocative test for attentional deficits. Although biased, the parents are often capable of rendering a very complete academic history. It is important to ascertain which teachers did well or did poorly with the child and why. The current teacher's name, attitude toward the child, and relationship with the parents should be obtained. Particular behaviors in the classroom that have caused trouble over the years should be listed. Parents can facilitate information gathering from the teacher as well. As part of the initial interview, self-addressed envelopes, containing teacher's rating forms, should be handed to the parents. Once the teacher has completed these reports on the child, the papers should be returned directly to the clinician by mail. A set of teacher's ratings should contain the thirty-nine-item Conners Teacher Questionnaire (CTQ) and Achenbach Teacher's Report Form (Achenbach and Edelbrock, 1980). Achenbach's lengthier rating instrument covers attentional, academic, impulsive, and prosocial behaviors, and appeals to teachers because of its comprehensive view of the child. It yields a visual profile, akin to the MMPI, and the scoring sheets contain built-in norms.

ATTENTIONAL DEFICIT. *DSM-III* attempts to operationalize the criterion of *inattention*. It should be noted that there is no empirical data to support the validity of the *DSM-III* ADDH diagnosis, nor is there a portable laboratory tool, with norms, for measuring inattention. Still, experts believe that children most likely are significantly inattentive if the history is positive for three of the four following questions:

— Does the child often fail to finish things he or she starts?
— Does the child often seem not to listen?
— Is the child easily distracted?
— Does the child often have difficulty on schoolwork or other tasks requiring sustained attention?

IMPULSIVITY. Impulsivity represents the mischievous, "Peck's bad boy" behaviors often seen in this disorder. Acting without forethought of the consequences, appearing to "know no danger," and taking dares are often reported during the history. During the early years this impulsivity drives toddlers from one toy to the next disrupting all the objects in their path; during school-age years, low frustration tolerance pushes them to constantly interrupt others and to refuse to await their turn in games. The thoughtless, non-premeditated quality of the hyperkinetic child's rule breaking often leads such children to get caught "holding the bag," while the real instigators are long gone. With characteristically poor judgment, the child then denies that he has the stolen object he has been caught with! As a result, hyperkinetic youths find themselves in mild to moderate conduct-problem situations.

Following *DSM-III* guidelines, the impulsive criterion will be operationally satisfied if three of the following six questions are positively answered:

— Does the child often act before thinking?
— Does the child shift excessively from one activity to another?
— Does the child have difficulty organizing work (without it being due to a cognitive impairment)?
— Does the child need almost constant supervision (cannot be left alone)?
— Does the teacher complain the child frequently calls out in class?
— Does the child have difficulty awaiting turn in games or in group situations?

OVERACTIVITY. Overactivity forms the final part of the clinical triad necessary for the ADDH syndrome. Inquire about activities in which the child must employ some type of motor inhibition to complete the age-appropriate task. Avoid those routine pursuits that are not well structured, such as asking about seated behavior during TV watching or during meals. A more tedious chore, such as practicing the piano, would give a better indication of ability to control activity. At its worst, the motor overactivity makes the hyperkinetic child so restless that he appears to "never tire." Parents complain that they, in turn, are "run ragged."

The overactivity criterion requires that two of the following five questions be answered in the affirmative:

— Does the child run about or climb on things excessively?
— Does the child have difficulty sitting still, so that he or she fidgets excessively?
— Can the child even stay in the seat for a brief period?
— Does the child move about excessively during sleep?
— Is the child always "on the go" or acting as if "driven by a motor"?

DECISION PROCESS. These historical items can be used as necessary and sufficient conditions to make a diagnosis of ADDH, if need be. To summarize, then, the child must have had the problem at least six months, and not have shown signs of major affective disorder, schizophrenia, or profound or severe mental retardation. In addition, he or she must satisfy the three signs of the disorder, namely, inattentiveness, impulsivity, and overactivity. Finally, it would be wise to require that the child show these three cardinal signs in at least two different situations, such as school and at home, to rule out those classroom disorders that are not ADDH. Most clinicians insist on speaking with teachers and receiving their reports prior to any diagnostic decision. Multiple observers reporting similar behaviors in more than one situation for the patient truly raises the confidence level in the diagnostic process.

PRESENCE OF ASSOCIATED CONDITIONS. It is good medical practice to investigate the associated conditions, even though they will not help in ruling in or out a specific diagnosis. They can be the source of future trouble, and, as such, may be susceptible to early intervention. Poor academic perfomance often accompanies the hyperkinetic syndrome and appears to remain a stable characteristic of the disorder; tutoring may be indicated. Satterfield et al. (1980) have shown that an individual, multimodality treatment plan involving tutoring and medication produces better outcomes than simply prescribing medication with no counseling, during a prospective three-year follow-up of ADDH children. Specific learning disabilites may also be revealed during history-taking. Questions regarding impulsivity may reveal more fights with peers than one would anticipate in a child who does not have a primary conduct disorder. Poor coordination may also be compained about during the interview. The clinician may eventually advise the parents to enroll the child in swimming and horseback-riding programs which emphasize gross motor skills over fine ones. Finally, the clinician may be able to explain the child's irritability and mood lability as an aspect of the syndrome, which may be ameliorated by stimulant treatment.

APPROPRIATE TREATMENT PLANNING. The timing of the referral should always be investigated. Did the school simply process the referral at the end of a regular marking period, as an administrative reaction to a chronic, unchanging process? Or did the child's hyperkinesis suddenly worsen with the occurrence of a new stressor at home? Had the school been ignoring signs of serious impulsive behavior until some almost irrevocable threshold had been crossed, like setting a fire in the boy's bathroom?

Inquire about the previous environmental approaches employed by the school and by the parents. Was the hyperkinetic patient referred to a smaller structured class or a resource room where there was increased supervision? Or did the teacher move the child's seat up to the front of the class to lower distractions and increase ability to manage him? Was he sent home when he became too disruptive in class? Was he given a special working desk, with built-in "blinders" to help him concentrate? Did any of these techniques prove helpful in any situation?

At home, were the parents consistent in their limit setting? Was the household routine kept regular and predictable or was it "every man for himself"? Did they respond to the hyperkinetic child's behaviors with time outs and by ignoring negative behaviors? There is evidence that consistent behavioral modification techniques, which reinforce calm, controlled behaviors, can help a hyperkinetic child at home. In addition, if the child's room is kept simple, uncluttered, and organized by the use of easily accessible storage boxes, the child will himself be less prone to get wild. Finally, if there are regular, immediate, and consistent responses by both parents to the child's positive and negative behaviors, he will be easier to manage.

Previous treatment regimes, both with medication and behavioral modification, must be looked into. What drugs did the child take and what were the doses? The most common reason for treatment failure with medication comes from *poor compliance* and *underdosing*. Occasionally, a child will receive a stimulant at a young age and show an equivocal response, only to do very well on the same dose several years later. Tolerance also may explain the failure of previous drug treatments with methylphenidate or d-amphetamine, given a suitable dosage level and no history of adverse side effects. Reinstitution of the previously successful drug to which the child had become tolerant may prove helpful, if several months have elapsed.

Side effects can also interdict an otherwise successful stimulant medication program. Inquire carefully about headaches, stomachaches, weight loss, and insomnia. Did the parents become worried about a particular reaction and stop the medication without telling the physician or returning for appointments? Even though a dosage adjustment might have solved the entire problem, the family may have been chagrined about taking matters into their own hands and hesitated to follow through with the child's doctor. In such circumstances, they may initially be reluctant to reveal a former treatment failure.

Previous special treatments are most valuable to investigate. Were megavitamins or special elimination diets employed? Although the bulk of research data suggests that the Feingold additive-free diets produce no significant benefits in controlled studies (Conners, 1980a), individuals can show powerful positive placebo effects, particularly when the entire family rallies behind the diet. If the parents did carry out the full dietary program, it indicates a willingness to follow a professional's instructions in detail, even at some inconvenience to the household. Shopping around, i.e., compulsively trying out a number of new, exotic, yet unproven, treatment programs in quick succession, may turn up as a pattern of seeking help for certain parents. From the beginning, the professional must address such a pattern if it is discovered, but in a tactful, supportive manner. The parents can be advised to stick to the treatment program for a minimum period before moving on to the next doctor, and a written contract might prove helpful in helping them cope with impatience, anxiety, and the pressure for instant results.

Other data that will help to plan the treatment should also be obtained from the parents.

Does the child staunchly refuse to take pills? He may require a liquid form of medication (available for d-amphetamine). Will the school be cooperative with midday medication and with behavioral-modification programs? Another area to explore is the presence of drug abuse in other family members. A physician should carefully account for number of pills prescribed if someone in the household has had a drug-addiction problem. In that case, the physician probably should begin treatment with pemoline, a mediation that has little street exchange value and has proven to be a compound of low abuse potential.

Finally, and most crucial, will be the parent's attitude toward treatment. Many adults today are deeply worried about the use of psychoactive drugs and their impact on physical and neurological development. Even if questions are not raised by them, parents should be engaged in an open discussion concerning their attitudes toward medication and behavior modification. Do they fear that such interventions will suppress their child's natural spontaneity, creativity, or enthusiasm? They may harbor fears of drug dependence, addiction, or developing the "habit of turning to pills instead of solving one's problems." Extensive follow-up data by Laufer (1971) and more recent work by Kramer and Loney (1981) have shown no increase in drug abuse in hyperkinetic children treated previously with stimulants. Direct observation studies by Abikoff et al. (1977) and by Whalen et al. (1979) show no decrease in the spontaneous rate of classroom interactions for hyperkinetic children treated with stimulants, compared to untreated controls. These facts will prove helpful during discussions with the parents, but, most important, one should let them completely ventilate their fears and anxieties concerning drug treatment before handing them a prescription.

Mental-Status Evaluation

WARM-UP TASK. A "warm-up" activity to reduce the child's anxiety may facilitate your interaction with him and allow you to observe him carrying out verbal instructions. Some children do well starting out with the standard draw-a-person task (DAP). Hand the patient a #2 lead pencil and three sheets of blank white paper. The instructions require the child to draw a person on the first sheet, and then sign his name (in script), and mark the date —if he is eight years or older. The second sheet should be used for drawing a person of the sex opposite to that portrayed on the first. The third piece of paper should be reserved for a self-portrait. Several valuable observations may emerge from this task. Can the child complete the task without frequent reminders? Does he sit still while carrying out the drawing in a self-paced manner, or does he squirm, fidget, or even leave his seat? Examine the quality of the drawing; is it age appropriate or does it show developmental lags? Scoring manuals exist to derive a more exact mental-age score. The quality of the handwriting and the accuracy of the date listed should also be observed. Finally, does the child seem to become anxious doing the task, stating "I don't like to draw people," as some schizoid children might, or does he seem anxious about the quality of performance? All such reactions provide leads for further exploration about the child's feeling about himself, his performance in school, and his own body image or self-esteem.

OBSERVATION OF THE CHILD. Much can be learned by simply recording visual impressions. Many hyperkinetic children appear unkept, with zippers and laces undone and shirttails hanging out. The child's physical appearance may be mildly stigmatized, perhaps due to the presence of minor physical anomalies. The child may talk in an immature manner, using poor syntax. Coordination may be poor, giving the younster an awkward, graceless appearance. Activity levels may be quite high, with the child wandering about the room—even as one is talking to him—touching all the toys, climbing on the chairs, and flicking the lights on and off. This chaotic, disorganized appearance and behavior in a new environment can confirm the historical signs of the disorder. But it will not rule out exclusionary conditions.

COGNITIVE SCREEN. The clinician must not leave the examining room without some notion as to the child's intelligence and the presence or absence of psychotic features. Starting with general orientation questions (date, time, place, person), the interview should cover questions of general information. Inquire about well-known current events, names of local sports teams, or the names of the characters on popular television shows. Ask the child to perform simple change-making operations on purchases without the use of paper and pencil. From such diverse types of mental functions, with special note to their speed, accuracy, and the vocabulary used by the child, one should be able to determine whether the child is bright, average, dull, or retarded.

Psychosis may be investigated by observing deviant thought patterns and asking about the presence or absence of daytime auditory or visual hallucinations. Inquire further to determine whether the patient is or has been delusional or suicidal. Psychosis, retardation (if moderate to severe), and severe affective disorders rule out a diagnosis of hyperkinetic syndrome and are contraindications to the use of stimulant treatments.

CHILD'S ATTITUDE TOWARDS HYPERKINESIS. Determine what the child has been told about his problem, including the reason for his visit with you. Perhaps the child will deny that there is much of a problem. Some hyperkinetic children will agree that school may be giving them trouble. These patients will claim that the teacher gives boring lessons and imposes impossible demands to sit still and to complete inherently dull work. Explore whether the child views himself in constant conflict with peers, teachers, parents, or kids on the block. Does he feel that he is an easy mark for teasing? What do the other children say that really makes him angry? Has this particular child heard about hyperactivity, a condition that makes some children very restless, and has anyone told him that he has it? Determine what he knows about its causes, the treatment, and the prognosis. Inquire if he has ever taken medicine for any condition and how it made him feel to have to swallow pills? Some children believe that taking stimulant medication certifies them as totally insane, and feel that peers will reject and ridicule them.

INTERVIEW RESULTS. Many hyperkinetic children who are unreservedly hyperkinetic at school and at home, often display none of their characteristic deviant behaviors in the one-to-one situation in a professional's office. Yet, as indicated previously, the child's fidgetiness, inability to stay seated, poor capacity to follow conversation, and general anxiety level can be observed during the interview. Many hyperkinetic children will comment, if asked, that they tend to overreact to trivial provocations, as if they had little control over themselves.

Psychometric Tests

Psychometric examinations can be used to document moderate mental retardation and its severity, an exclusion criterion for the diagnosis of hyperkinesis. Some clinicians have used "organicity" descriptors on the Bender-Gestalt and on the DAP to validate the diagnosis. Minimal brain damage as an etiology for hyperkinesis has not been supported by the epidemiological evidence (Shaffer and Greenhill, 1979). Wide interest subscale score scatter on the Wechsler Intelligence Scale for Children—Revised (WISC-R) has been used to justify a hyperkinetic diagnosis. This, too, has not proven to be a reliable or necessary criterion for the disorder. The main value of psychometrics does not figure in the diagnostic stage, but rather in the identification of associated conditions. Academic problems, specific learning disabilities, and developmental delays can be documented on these test batteries.

Neurological Examination and Electroencephalogram

In the heyday of the MBD diagnosis, the neurological examination served to locate minor and major signs of central nervous system dysfunction, which, in turn, validated the behavioral-disorder diagnosis. Imbalances in reflex findings, nonlocalizing signs of minor choreoathetoid movements, inability to carry out rapid alternating movements, and generally poor coordination all became known as "soft signs" and were used by certain clinicians to make the diagnosis of MBD. Soft signs, however, proved to show great intertest and interrater unreliability, and, to date, their prognostic significance is unclear (Shaffer, 1978). Other than ruling in or out the diagnosis of epilepsy, the neurological examination will have little impact during the diagnostic work-up or treatment planning for hyperkinetic children. The electroencephalogram (EEG) has the same problems as the neurological exam. Although the incidence of abnormal EEGs in the hyperkinetic population exceeds that of the normal group, findings in a specific patient do not help with diagnosis, do not predict treatment response, and have no bearing on prognosis.

Global Rating Forms

Conners has developed several global rating forms for research on hyperkinetic children (Guy, 1976). One scale, the Conners Parent Questionnaire (CPQ), consists of 93 items, and is administered to parents. It can be useful during history gathering for assessing the severity of and variety of a particular patient's symptomatology. Repeated use of the course of treatment becomes impractical due to this rating scale's length. The Connors Teacher Questionnaire (CTQ) also is very useful. Factor analysis with principal components analysis yielded four main factors (Guy, 1976). Since the CTQ appears to be sensitive to drug effects (Sprague et al., 1974), particularly demonstrating changes in factor 4 (hyperactivity), much work has centered around tracking factor 4 during treatment. Early epidemiological work suggests that factor 4 may prove useful as an early screening tool, when administered by teachers using the CTQ.

One may use the CTQ in the following manner. Answers to each question can be scored according to item weights. A check in the "Not at All" column should be weighed as 0, a check in the "Just a Little" column receives a weight of 1, "Pretty Much" gets a 2, and "Very Much" gets a 3. To arrive at the factor 4 score, just add the weighted scores of questions 1, 2, 5, 6, 14 and 29, then divide by 6 to obtain the average. Since the mean score of males in the primary school system without psychiatric diagnoses is 0.56 ± 0.65, a score of 1.5 or more has been taken as 2 standard deviations from the norm and held to be significantly deviant. For screening purposes, however, it is probably safer to use a score of 2.2 or more, to reduce the false positives (Trites et al., 1979). During treatment, a factor 4 score which drops 0.5 below the baseline score generally heralds success. One more point: take at least two CTQs on the same child during the pretreatment phase. The factor 4 score tends to drop spontaneously due to scoring changes, and this could be mistaken as a treatment response. During longer periods of maintenance drug therapy, it probably would be wise to collect CTQs trimonthly.

Conners also developed an Abbreviated Symptom Questionnaire (Guy, 1976) (CASQ) that includes ten items that are common to both the CTQ (items 1, 3, 5, 6, 7, 8, 13, 14, 16, and 21) and the Conners Parent Questionnaire. The CASQ has been used by Conners as a repeatable rating scale and has proven treatment sensitive in controlled studies when administered weekly to parents, teachers, and ward personnel. It can be quickly filled out and scored. Dividing the sum by ten to obtain the average, yields a number comparable to factor 4. The CASQ probably should be used with parents on a weekly basis during dose-adjustment periods, then trimonthly during maintenance.

Since these rating scales have shown sensitivity to treatment in controlled studies and also demonstrate interest reliability, the clinician can employ them as a convenience to attain greater rigor in his or her practice. When the treatment effects a drop in CASQ score or in factor 4 CTQ score, and when these numbers remain low throughout therapy, the professional can be confident that this measure is tracking a real change.

AVAILABLE TREATMENTS

Pharmacotherapy

Many different types of psychoactive preparations have proven useful for treating the hyperkinetic syndrome (Klein et al., 1980). Stimulants have become the most common form of treatment for these children, paradoxically inhibiting impulsivity and hyperactivity, while generally improving their performance on attentional measures (Rapoport et al., 1980). Some claim that the use of psychostimulants is controversial and undesirable. Stimulant treatment is criticized for: directing the focus of intervention away from improving the school or home environment; drugging children with classroom disorders who do not have the ADDH syndrome; exposing children with developing nervous systems to the long-term risks of constant dopamine stimulation. Nevertheless, in those cases where rapid intervention is necessary to prevent school dismissal, stimulants may be employed more often than the other main treatment approach, namely, behavior modification.

DEXTROAMPHETAMINE SULFATE. Dextroamphetamine sulfate has had the longest usage, beginning back in 1937 with the open studies of Bradley (1941). More recent studies since 1960, using the appropriate placebo controls, have shown this drug to be highly effective in reducing impulsivity and inattentiveness. Available in liquid suspension, tablet, or slow-release capsule (spansule), d-amphetamine shows a five- to six-hour duration of action, due to its plasma half-life of 10.5 hours in children. The drug usually can be given in a dose range of 10-40 mg/day in divided doses. The stimulant side effects of anorexia, insomnia, and mild increases in blood pressure and pulse rate occur most often with d-amphetamine, since its action occurs throughout the body. Adult abuse of the amphetamine derivatives, particularly methamphetamine ("speed") and the drug's poor performance in controlling adult weight problems have led to FDA restrictions on use of this drug. Currently, indications are limited to the childhood hyperkinetic syndrome and to narcolepsy. The prescriptions must be written on triplicate controlled-drug forms.

METHYLPHENIDATE. Methylphenidate (Ritalin) has become the most popular psychostimulant used in the United States, although it too must be prescribed on a triplicate controlled-drug form. The methyl ester of ritalinic acid, methylphenidate enters the plasma in minute amounts but is highly effective in low plasma concentrations. The parent compound is metabolized to ritalinic acid in the gastrointestinal tract and in the liver. Many controlled treatment studies have shown methylphenidate to be highly effective in the treatment of hyperkinetic children (Weiss et al., 1971) and to work in both moderate doses (Rapoport, 1974) and in high doses (60 mg/day)(Schain and Reynard, 1975). More recent reports by Gittelman-Klein et al. (1976b) and by Conners et al. (1980b) have shown that parents, teachers, and professionals blindly rate over three-fourths of the children as improved while on active Ritalin for at least four weeks. If a favorable response occurs, it does so within the first ten days of treatment; the clinician can begin most children on 5 mg twice a day, at 8:00 A.M. and at noon, and increase the drug by 5 mg per dose every three days. The range of dosage extends from a total daily intake of 20 mg up to a maximum of 60 mg. Currently, Ritalin is dispensed in 5 and 10 mg tablets; a liquid formulation has not been available. Twenty mg sustained-release (SR) tablets, which peak at 4.7 hours and show a disappearance half-life of 8 hours are now available (Whitehouse et al., 1980). This formulation avoids involvement of school personnel in medication administration, and this is the preferred formulation for maintenance.

Ritalin's site of action tends to be the central nervous system, so that blood pressure and pulse changes are less marked than with d-amphetamine; still, children will develop anorexia and insomnia on the drug. Tolerance to Ritalin may develop if treatment extends much past one year. This lack of response should be treated with a switch to another psychostimulant.

MAGNESIUM PEMOLINE. Magnesium pemoline (Cylert) is a dopamine agonist with proven psychostimulant effects in hyperkinetic children. A relatively long half-life of twelve hours in children means that once-a-day administration is possible; since Cylert is not a controlled drug, it may be prescribed using regular forms. Both these features make the drug a promising clinical tool. A large, controlled, lengthy study of 238 children by Page et al. (1974) showed that Cylert begins to exert its strongest action by the third week and later. Cylert's dosage has been set by the manufacturer in pills of chewable tablets in multiples of the 18.75 mg lowest-dose tablet. Treatment follows a regimen of weekly increases through the range up to 112.5 mg/day. Children often begin to show improvement at dose levels above 50mg/day. Some irritability, insomnia, and anorexia may be seen on the drug; rare reports of elevated liver enzymes suggest that the clinician should carry our routine liver function tests and complete blood counts every six months. Cylert's ability to be given once per day makes it an ideal drug for hyperkinetic children who may be teased by classmates for taking pills in school, may have trouble with drug rebound, or may have difficulty with insomnia from late afternoon stimulant doses.

OTHER STIMULANTS. Deanol has been given in several controlled studies, but seems to have minimal therapeutic activity in hyperkinesis. Caffeine does show specific effects on attention span, but has failed to control the impulsive or hyperactive behaviors that cause hyperkinetic children difficulty in the classroom. According to the five out of seven controlled studies, no effect was seen with caffeine treatment.

ANTIPSYCHOTIC MEDICATIONS. Overall, the neuroleptic drugs do reduce the cardinal signs of the hyperactive syndrome in children. Studies by Gittelman-Klein et al. (1976b), Werry et al. (1966), Weiss et al. (1971), and Greenberg et al. (1972) have shown positive treatment responses, particularly in the area of motor hyperactivity. Clinicians as a group, however, hesitate to use neuroleptics because of a concern about the drug's sedating side effects interfering with cognitive activities in school. They also are concerned about involuntary motor problems. These side effects may be transient, as are the withdrawal emergent symptoms seen with sudden discontinuation of high-dose neuroleptic medication. More persistent late-appearing buccal-lingual-masticatory symptoms have been reported in adults (tardive dyskinesia) and may be irreversible in certain cases.

Behavior Modification

The use of behavior modification to treat the hyperkinetic child has been advocated in order to avoid immediate physical side effects and the long-term risks of psychostimulants. There is not a great deal of evidence for the efficacy of behavior modification alone in the treatment of hyperkinesis. Gittelman-Klein et al. (1976a) has compared an eight-week course of behavior modification alone to combined medication and behavior-modification therapies. Ritalin alone, behavior modification alone, and behavior modification with Ritalin all were significantly better than placebo. The children on combined treatment were nondistinguishable from normals, according to the blind observers, while those children treated with Ritalin could be easily separated from nonafflicted classmates. One should consider behavior modification in those cases where the children have shown excessive troublesome side effects to drug treatment or where the parents object to drug treatment. Behavior modification requires much professional time to be effective, and this can be costly in comparison to medication alone. Also, the teacher must devote a great deal of time and effort to any behavior modification program for it to be successful, and this is not always possible.

Other Psychological Therapies

Psychotherapy has often been recommended for the hyperkinetic child, but there is little evidence to support its efficacy. More focused psychological interventions have included the "stop, look, and listen" approach used by Douglas (1972) to teach hyperkinetic children to refocus attention and the cognitive behavior modification (CBM) system, as advocated by Meichenbaum (1979). This latter technique teaches troubled children to use self-verbalization and self-instruction to help themselves focus on the problem and develop better coping styles. Some evidence exists indicating that CBM may be a promising technique, for it has been used successfully to treat the disruptive behavior of hyperactive boys, aggressive children, and unruly preschoolers.

Tutoring and remediation may help some of the academic difficulties that occur in hyperactive children, but the training does not generalize into the behavioral area. A final approach involves parent education, and Dubey and Kaufman (1979) have set up successful ten-week, two-hour workshops to teach behavior modification management techniques to parent groups. This approach, which has reached over two-thousand parents, still requires evaluation.

PRACTICAL GUIDE TO TREATMENT

Assessment of Severity

The clinician must first assess the severity of the disorder. For those children with the mild form, environmental manipulation would be the first approach. Such steps involve appropriate class placement in small, structured academic settings with a teacher who can deliver a good deal of structured supervision and close one-to-one attention. In addition, the parent should be counseled in parental management techniques involving the establishment of a regular, consistent home routine for the child, as well as consistent parental responses to good behaviors (praise and attention) and to undesirable behaviors (ignore, take away reinforcer, or use time out). These techniques may be taught in a parental workshop or in individual office visits.

The child might enter into a behavior modification program whose aim is the reduction of certain target behaviors. Parental counseling will also help the clinician evaluate the strengths of the parent-child relationship, relieve feelings of guilt in the parent, and help the parent to view the difficulties more objectively. For those children with moderate to severe disorders, the treatment plan should be supplemented with pharmacotherapy.

Assessment for Pharmacotherapy

First and foremost, one should learn the parent's attitudes toward the use of medications for their child. An open discussion of risks and benefits might lead the way to a sharing of the parents' fears and misconceptions about drugs. One should also take a drug history, gathering data on past treatment for behavior problems, looking particularly for unfavorable reactions to stimulants, allergic reactions, and a history of severe exacerbation of hyperactivity after being given phenobarbital. The latter drug reaction often occurs in children who will respond well to stimulants.

Explanation to the Patient

Finally, time should be set aside to explain the treatment plan to the child. If there is to be a class change, this must be negotiated with the patient who may be initially against it. He may not understand the need for remediation or the need for increased focus on and tracking of his behaviors for behavior modification plans. In addition, he may have strong feelings about medication. Often it is helpful to explain that the medication is a "crutch" which will enable him to do classwork when *he* wants to, but does not control him. The timing of doses frequently becomes critical for compliance, for a child may decide unilaterally to stop his school-time doses if he is ridiculed by the other children; here, Ritaline SR or Cylert therapy is recommended.

Initiating Drug Therapy

Starting doses for all the stimulants are minimal, and consist of a once-daily, early morning ingestion of 10 mg of Ritalin, 5mg of d-amphetamine, or 18.75 mg of Cylert. Have the parent begin the medication on the weekend, so the onset of action and the duratin of action can be recorded over a week's time. Then, as dosing increments occur, the timing of that crucial early morning dose can be worked optimally to cover the toughest times (getting dressed, getting on the bus, or getting down to work at school). It is probably wise to give the first, and any additional doses, immediately after a meal, to minimize anorexia. Doses are generally titrated up to the maximum (60 mg of Ritalin, 40 mg of d-amphetamine, and 112.5 mg of Cylert) or to the point of troublesome side effects, whichever occurs first. One should switch to a maintenance dose of Ritalin SR as soon as possible to avoid midday doses.

Management of Drug Treatment

Drug rebound can occur either on arising in the morning or during the late afternoon, and is characterized by a withdrawal-like state in which the child becomes unusually irritable and hyperactive. This can be managed by giving an additional small dose on arising or when the child first comes home. Ritalin SR may avoid rebound because of its prolonged action.

Tolerance can develop with chronic psychostimulant therapy and shows itself when the child becomes quickly unresponsive to ever-increasing doses of medication after a long stable period of drug response. This can be handled by switching to another stimulant.

Combination drug therapies can fight anorexia and insomnia side effects; a 25 or 50 mg dose of Mellaril around dinnertime can help greatly with the next day's appetite and with that night's sleep. Monitoring the child's progress is best done through teacher reports, both in the form of rating scales like the CTQ and through direct phone contact with teachers to assess the child's: progress in academics and in peer relationships; distractibility and inattentiveness, impulsiveness and gross motor hyperactivity; and ability to respond to limit setting and to do unsupervised tasks. Teachers will provide the information needed in planning medication changes—both dose level and timing of each dose—by noting the time of classroom behavioral deterioration and type of deterioration. Teacher's reports will also be invaluable for placebo trials during the school year, as they should be the first to detect a major change in behavior off active drug.

Drug Vacations

Children should be withdrawn from psychostimulants at least one time a year, preferably during the summer. They can then be observed in a more active summer camp program at a time when they have the maximum growth period and can catch up any height and weight losses that may have occured. A subgroup of hyperkinetic children have been shown to be sensitive to the growth-inhibiting effect of the stimulants, particularly d-amphetamine (Greenhill et al., 1981). Withdrawal should involve decreasing doses over one week's time to avoid the rebound from a one-day discontinuation. Before reinstituting medication, wait for a three-week period to ascertain whether or not the child still demonstrates enough behavior problems in the new class to merit continued drug therapy. Follow-up should occur even if the child does not currently meet criteria for medication, since the need for continued support and guidance will go on throughout the school year.

General Rules for Successful Management

Hyperkinetic children are best handled by a multi-disciplinary team, consisting of an M.D., a psychologist, a social worker, and an educational specialist, to provide for the many needs these children have (Satterfield et al., 1980). Psychostimulants are the drugs of choice, and chronic drug threapy should be carried out with once-a-day dosing, if possible. Close communication with school personnel is absolutely necessary to work out the dosage and time of administration, both of which must be tailored to each individual case. Drug vacations, preferably placebo controlled, should be regularly planned to evaluate the need for continuation and to allow for physical growth. Tutoring may be necessary to teach children compensatory skills if learning disabilities are present. Children should be followed after the medications are stopped.

Telling Parents about the Future

There has been some evidence that a proportion of hyperkinetic children go on to become inattentive, labile, impulsive adults with psychiatric problems. Unfortunately, it is impossible to predict the future for each individual child. The unknown outcome of the attention deficit disorder can be helpful in persuading the family to maintain follow-up on a regular yearly basis, even if the drugs are stopped.

REFERENCES

Abikoff, H., Gittelman-Klein, R., and Klein, D. F. 1977. Validation of a classroom observation code for hyperactive children. *J. Consult. Clin. Psychol.,* 45(5):722-783.

Achenbach, T. M., and Edelbrock, C. 1980. Child behavior checklist—teacher's report form. For forms, scoring profiles, instructions, and templates, write: Thomas Achenbach, Child Psychiatry, University of Vermont, South Prospect Street, Burlington, Vermont 05401.

American Psychiatric Association. 1980. *Diagnostic and statistical manual of mental disorders—third edition (DSM-III).* Washington, D.C.: APA.

Barkley, R. A., and Jackson, T. L., Jr. 1977. Hyperkinesis, autonomic nervous system activity, and stimulant drug effects. *J. Child Psychol. Psych.,* 18:347-357.

Bradley, C. 1941. Amphetamine (benzedrine) therapy of children's behavior disorders. *J. Orthopsychiatry,* 11:92.

Bruening, S. 1982. Pediatric psychopharmacology: New issues and special populations. Paper presented at the 29th annual meeting of the American Academy of Child Psychiatry, October 21, Washington, D.C.

Cantwell, D. P. 1972. Psychiatric illness in the families of hyperactive children. *Arch. Gen. Psych.,* 27:414-417

Conners, C. K. 1980a. *Food additives and hyperactive children.* Plenum Press: New York.

Conners, C. K., Goyette, C. H., Southwick, D. A., Lees, J. M., and Andrulonis, P. A. 1976. Food additives and hyperkinesis: A controlled double-blind experiment. *Ped.,* 58:154-166.

Conners, C. K., and Taylor, E. 1980b. Pemoline, methylphenidate, and placebo in children with minimal brain dysfunction. *Arch. Gen. Psych.,* 37:922-930.

David, O. 1978. Central effects of minimally elevated lead levels. In *Proceedings of the National Institute of Mental Health on the hyperkinetic behavior syndrome,* ed. N. Reatig, pp. 14-18. Doc. no. PB-297804 (code A12). Springfield, Va.: National Technical Information Service.

Douglas, V. I. 1972. Stop, look, and listen: The problem of sustained attention and impulse control in hyperactive and normal children. *Com. J. Beh. Sci.,* 4:259-282.

Dubey, D. R., and Kaufman, K. F. 1979. Training parents of hyperactive children in behavior management. *Int. J. Men. Health,* 8(1):110-120.

Feingold, B. F. 1975. *Why your child is hyperactive.* New York: Random House.

Gittelman-Klein, R., Klein, D. F., Abikoff, H., Katz, S., Gloiston, A. C., and Kates, W. 1976a. Relative efficacy of methylphenidate and behavior modification in hyperactive children: An interim report. *J. Abnorm. Child Psychol.,* 4(4):361-377.

Gittelman-Klein, R., Klein, D. F., Katz, S., Saraf, K., and Pollack, E. 1976b. Comparative effects of methylphenidate and thioridazine in hyperkinetic children. *Arch. Gen. Psych.,* 33:1217-1231.

Greenberg, L. M., Deem, M. A., and McMahon, S. 1972. Effects of dextroamphetamine, chlorpromazine, hydroxyzine on behavior and performance in hyperactive children. *Am. J. Psych.,* 129:532–539.

Greenhill, L. L., Puig-Antich, J., Chambers, W., Rubinstein, B., Halpern, F., and Sachar, E. J. 1981. Growth hormone, prolactin, and growth responses in hyperkinetic males treated with d-amphetamine. *J. Acad. Child Psych.,* 20(1):71–84.

Grinspoon, L., and Singer, S. B. 1973. Amphetmaines in the treatment of hyperactive children. *Harv. Ed. Rev.,* 43:515–555.

Guy, W. 1976. *ECDEU assessment manual for psychopharmacology,* Rev. ed. U.S. Dept. of Health, Education, and Welfare, DHEW pub. no. (ADM) 76-338.

Harley, J. P., Ray, R. S., Termasi, L., Eictrman, P. L., Matthews, C. G., Chun, R., Cleeland, C. S., and Traitman, E. 1978. Hyperkinesis and food additives: Testing the Feingold hypothesis, *Ped.,* 61:818–828.

Klein, D. F., Gittelman, R., Quitkin, F., and Rifkin, A. 1980. *Diagnosis and drug treatment of psychiatric disorders: Adults and children.* Baltimore: Williams and Wilkins.

Kramer, J., and Loney, J. 1981. Childhood hyperactivity and substance abuse: A review of the literature. In *Advances in learning and behavior disabilities,* vol. 1, ed. K. Gadow, and I. Bialer. Greenwich, Conn.: JAI Press.

Laufer, M. W. 1971. Long-term management and some follow-up findings on the use of drugs with minimal cerebral syndromes. *J. Learn. Disabil.,* 153:518–522.

Meichenbaum, D. 1979. Application of cognitive-behavior modification procedures to hyperactive children. *Int. J. Men. Health,* 8(1):83–93.

Morrison, J. R., and Stewart, M. A. 1973. The psychiatric status of the legal families of adopted hyperactive children. *Arch. Gen. Psych.,* 28:888–891.

Page, J. G., Bernstein, J. E., Janicki, R. S., and Mitchelli, F. A. 1974. A multi-clinic trial of pemoline in childhood hyperkinesis. In *Clinical use of stimulant drugs in children,* ed. C. K. Conners, pp. 98–124. Amsterdam: Excerpta-Medica.

Pasamanick, B., and Knobloch, H. 1959. Syndrome of minimal cerebral damage in infancy. *J.A.M.A.,* 170:1384–1387.

Puig-Antich, J., Orvaschel, H., Tabrizi, M., and Chambers, W. J. 1980. Schedule for affective disorders and schizophrenia for school-age children—epidemiology version (Kiddie-SADS-E). Investigators wishing to use this instrument should contact Dr. J. Puig-Antich at the Department of Child and Adolescent Psychiatry, New York State Psychiatric Institute, 722 West 168th Street, New York, New York 10032.

Rapoport, J. L., Ruchsbaum, M. S., Weingartner, H., Zahn, T., Ludlow, C., Mikkelsen, E. J., Langer, D., and Bunney, W. E. 1980. Dextroamphetamine: Its cognitive and behavioral effects in normal and hyperactive boys and normal men. *Arch. Gen. Psych.,* 37:933–943.

Rapoport, J. L., Panoloni, C. H., Reafield, M., Lake, R., and Ziegler, M. G. 1977. Newborn dopamine-B hydroxylase, minor physical anomalies, and infant temperament. *Am. J. Psych.,* 134:676–679.

Rapoport, J. L., Quinn, P. O., and Lamprecht, F. 1974. Minor physical anomalies and plasma dopamine-B hydroxylase activity in hyperactive boys. *Am. J. Psych.,* 131(4):386–390.

Rieder, R. O., and Nichols, P. L. 1979. Offsprings of schizophrenics. III. Hyperactivity and neurological soft signs. *Arch. of Gen. Psych.,* 36:665–674.

Rutter, M., Tizard, J., and Whitmore, K. 1970. *Education, health, and behavior: Psychological and medical study of childhood development.* London: Longman Group. Distributed by John Wiley and Sons, New York.

Safer, D. 1973. A familial factor in minimal brain dysfunction. *Beh. Genet.,* 3(2):175–186.

Satterfield, J. H., Satterfield, B. T., and Cantwell, D. P. 1980. Multimodality treatment: A two year evaluation of 61 hyperactive boys. *Arch. Gen. Psych.,* 37:915–919.

Schain, R. J., and Reynard, C. L. 1975. Observations on effects of a central stimulant drug (methylphenidate) in children with hyperactive behavior, *Ped.*, 55:709-716.

Shaffer, D. 1978. "Soft" neurological signs and later psychiatric disorder—a review. *J. Child Psychol. Psych.*, 19(1):63-66.

Shaffer, D., and Greenhill, L. 1979. A critical note on the predictive validity of the "hyperkinetic syndrome." *J. Child Pyschol. Psych.*, 20:61-72.

Shaffer, D., McNamara, N., and Pincus, J. H. 1974. Controlled observations on patterns of activity, attention, and impulsivity in brain-damaged and psychiatrically disturbed boys. *J. Psychol. Med.*, 4(1):14-18.

Shaywitz, B. A., Cohen, D. J., and Bowers, M. B., Jr. 1977. CSF monoamine metabolites in children with minimal brain dysfunction: Evidence for alteration of brain dopamine—a preliminary report. *J Ped.*, 90(1):67-71.

Shaywitz, B. A., Klopper, J. H., Yager, R. D., and Gordon, J. W. 1976. A paradoxical response to amphetamine in developing rats treated with 6-hydroxydopamine. *Neurol.*, 26(4):363-364.

Shekim, W. O., Dekirmenjian, H., Chapel, J. L., Javoid, J., and Davis, J. M. 1979. Norepinephrine metabolism and clinical response to dextroamphetamine in hyperactive boys. *J. Ped.*, 95(3):389-394.

Silver, L. B. 1971. A proposed view on the etiology of the neurological learning disability syndrome. *J. Learn. Disabil.*, 4:123-133.

Sobotka, T. J. 1978. Update on studies of the relationship between hyperkinesis in children and food additives. In *Proceedings of the National Institute of Mental Health on the hyperkinetic behavior syndrome*, ed. N. Reatig, pp. 39-47. Doc. no. PB-297804 (code A12). Springfield, Va.: National Technical Information Service.

Sprague, R. L., Christensen, D. E., and Werry, J. S. 1974. Experimental psychology and stimulant drugs. In *Clinical use of stimulant drugs in children,* ed. C. K. Conners, pp. 141-164. Amsterdam: Excerpta-Medica.

Taft, L. 1975. Personal communication.

Trites, R. L., Dugas, E., Lynch, G., and Ferguson, H. B. 1979. Prevalence of hyperactivity. *J. Ped. Psychol.*, 4(2):179-188.

Waldrop, M. F., and Halverson, C. F. 1971. Minor physical anomalies and hyperactive behavior in young children. In *The exceptional infant,* ed. J. Helmuth. New York: Brunner and Mazel.

Waldrop, M. F., and Goering, J. D. 1971. Hyperactivity and minor physical anomalies in elementary school children. *Am. J. Orthopsych.*, 41:602-607.

Weingartner, H., Rapoport, J. L., Buchsbaum, M. S., Bunney, W. E., Jr., Ebert, M. H., Mikkelson, E. J., and Caine, E. D. 1980. Cognitive processes in normal and hyperactive children and their response to amphetamine treatment. *J. Abnorm. Psycol.*, 89:25-37.

Weiss, G., Hechtman, L., Pentman, T., Hopkins, J., and Werner, A. 1979. Hyperactives as young adults. *Arch. Gen. Psych.*, 36(6):675-681.

Weiss, G., Minde, K., Douglas, V., Werry, J., and Sykes, D. 1971. Comparison of the effects of chlorpromazine, dextroamphetamine, and methylphenidate on the behavior and intellectual functioning of hyperactive children. *Can. Med. Assoc. J.*, 104:20-25.

Wender, P. H. 1971. *Minimal brain dysfunction in children.* New York: Wiley.

Werry, J., Minde, K., Guzman, A., Weiss, G., Dosan, K., and Hoy, E. 1972. Neurological status compared with neurotic and normal children. *Am. J. Ortho. Psych.*, 42:441-451.

Werry, J. S., Weiss, G., Douglas, V., and Martin, J. 1966. Studies on the hyperactive child. III. The effect of chlorpromazine upon behavior and learning ability. *J. Am. Acad. Child Psych.*, 5:292-312.

Whalen, C. K., Collins, B. E., Henker, B., Alkus, S. R., Adams, D., and Stapp, J. 1978. Behavior observations of hyperactive children in systematically structured classroom environments: Now you see them, now you don't. *J. Ped. Psychol.,* 3(4):177–187.

Whalen, C. K., Henker, B., Collins, B., McAuliffe, S., and Vaux, A. 1979. Peer interaction in a structured communication task: Comparisons of normal and hyperactive boys and methyphenidate (Ritalin) and placebo effects. *Child Dev.,* 50:388–401.

Whitehouse, D., Shah, U., and Palmer F. 1980. Comparison of sustained release and standard methyphenidate in the treatment of minimal brain dysfunction. *J. Clin. Psych.,* 4(8):282–285.

15

Juvenile Delinquency

DOROTHY OTNOW LEWIS

THE CONCEPT OF DELINQUENCY

The term *delinquency* covers a multitude of sins as well as a multitude of more or less serious psychiatric symptoms and deviant behaviors. *Delinquent* is a legal term rather than a diagnosis and, in the United States, refers to a child or adolescent who has been found guilty by a juvenile or family court of having engaged in some sort of proscribed behavior. The offenses can include a wide range of problems. The child might have been truant from school or might have run away from home. On the other hand, a child of twelve who has committed a murder may also be found "delinquent" by the court.

For purposes of treatment and other dispositions, the courts have recently made a distinction between status offenses and other kinds of delinquent acts. Status offenses refer to those behaviors, such as drinking liquor before age eighteen, being difficult to manage at home, running away, or being truant from school, that are offenses only because of a youngster's status as a child. Adults are free to drink, avoid school, or leave home without legal sanctions. The term delinquent has therefore come to designate a child who has been found guilty of an act that, were he an adult, would be considered to be against the law. These acts range from breach of the peace to rape and murder. Thus, the term delinquent gives no clue either to the severity of an offense or to the characteristics of the individual young offender.

Nevertheless, delinquency, in the minds of laypersons and professionals alike, has come to connote sociopathy or its multitude of synonyms (e.g., unsocialized aggressive reaction, antisocial personality). Its current psychiatric synonym, "conduct disorder," while ostensibly less judgmental than its predecessors, still designates "repetitive and persistent patterns of antisocial behavior that violate the rights of others" (American Psychiatric Association, 1980, p. 47). *DSM-III* attempts to subdivide the disorder into aggressive and unaggressive, and socialized and undersocialized categories.

West (1976), in an English text, pulls no punches, saying, "The classic delinquent personality, with all the traits of aggressiveness, egocentricity, impulsiveness, antisocial attitudes, and lack of conscience is virtually identical with the so-called sociopathic personality'' (p. 518). Clearly, the designations delinquent and conduct disorder are often used more as pejorative epithets than useful diagnoses. It is important to appreciate the distinction between judgment and diagnosis, since the former rarely leads to treatment whereas the whole purpose of the latter is to treat appropriately. This chapter will explore the multiplicity of biopsychosocial vulnerabilities underlying delinquency. It will outline the kind of diagnostic assessment necessary to bring these vulnerabilities to light and finally consider treatment implications.

Epidemiology

Estimates of the prevalence of delinquent behaviors are especially difficult to make because of differing criteria in different cultures and because there is evidence that social and family factors influence whether or not particular antisocial acts performed by particular children will be prosecuted through the courts or handled more informally. According to Meeks (1980, p. 2631), general-population surveys suggest that betweeen 5 and 15% of all children have conduct problems of one sort or another. In contrast, an English report (Power et al., 1972) indicates that up to 25% of all working-class boys are convicted at least once as juveniles. Of this group, half go on to have a second conviction and over a quarter experience further conflict with the law. These data are consistent with the large body of information indicating that crime and delinquency are more prevalent in socioeconomically disadvantaged populations than in affluent populations. There are many theories explaining this association. Whatever the explanation, poverty and delinquency are often (not always) associated with each other.

There is little agreement regarding the relationship of mental illness and delinquency. A 1964 public-health report from the District of Columbia asserted that the behavior of more than 10% of delinquents warranted psychiatric evaluations. In a follow-up study of former child-guidance-clinic patients, Robins (1966) found that of those seen as children for delinquent behaviors (e.g., thievery, incorrigibility, aggression) over a quarter were subsequently diagnosed sociopathic as adults. Robins also found, however, that many so-called antisocial children suffered later from psychotic and neurotic disturbances. In fact, 37% of the formerly antisocial children, when interviewed as adults, reported nine or more nonantisocial symptoms such as anxiety, conversion symptoms, and depression. Of the antisocial children known to the court (i.e., delinquent), 6% were later diagnosed psychotic; of the antisocial children who never reached the juvenile court, fully 30% were later deemed psychotic.

Given these many neurotic and psychotic outcomes, we must ask whether the failure to identify anxiety and psychosis in delinquents is more a reflection of our own clinical insensitivity than the child's lack of symptomatology. It is vital to remember these adverse psychiatric outcomes as we continue, in this chapter, to explore the kinds of psychopathology manifested by seriously delinquent, often violent, juveniles, and as we explore issues of diagnosis and treatment.

Correlates of Delinquency

Medical Correlates

Earlier studies of delinquents reported that they were, on the whole, a healthy group. For example, the Gluecks (1950) were convinced that significant medical problems were rare in delinquents and that delinquents tended to be muscular and robust. Gibbens (1963), in his study of Borstal boys in England, found 18% to suffer from a major disease or defect and 22% from a minor disorder. These proportions were high compared with general population statistics for a similar age group.

More recently we have begun to appreciate the extraordinarily adverse medical histories of delinquents compared to demographically similar nondelinquents. In a study (Lewis and Shanok, 1977) comparing the medical histories of a random sample of youngsters coming through the juvenile court with a nondelinquent sample matched for age, sex, race, geographic area, and approximate socioeconomic status, delinquents were found to have significantly more hospital visits throughout childhood and adolescence than nondelinquents. They made more clinic and emergency-room visits and had more pediatric hospitalizations. Their medical histories indicated they had sustained more accidents and injuries and were treated for more minor illnesses as well. In a comparison of the medical histories of seriously delinquent, violent, incarcerated adolescents with the medical histories of less seriously delinquent youngsters, the more violent group was found to have significantly more perinatal problems, head and face injuries, and was more likely to have been physically abused. (Lewis et al., 1979b; Shanok and Lewis, 1981). It will be important to keep these facts in mind as we consider the kind of diagnostic evaluation necessary to elicit this kind of medical information.

Neurological Correlates

An increasing body of knowledge indicates that many delinquents suffer from a variety of major and minor neurological signs and symptoms. The most common neurological disorder associated with delinquency is hyperactivity or what we now call "attention deficit disorder." In a follow-up study of hyperactive children, Mendelson et al. (1971) found that as teenagers more than half of his sample had been involved in stealing, fighting, and other destructive behaviors and more than a third had threatened to kill their parents.

In a recent clinical study of incarcerated seriously delinquent boys (Lewis et al., 1979c), 46% of the most violent boys had one or more major neurologial abnormalities, and almost the entire group of very violent boys had one or more minor (i.e., soft) neurological abnormalities. Of the most violent delinquents, 29% had abnormal EEGs and/or a history of epilepsy. Psychomotor epileptic symptoms were also extremely prevalent in the very violent youngsters. Most important, the neurological vulnerabilities of these delinquent youngsters seemed to contribute to their impulsivity, violence, poor school functioning, and overall maladaptation.

Psychiatric Correlates

The debate as to whether antisocial behavior is or is not associated with serious psychopathology other than sociopathy continues to flourish. Many investigators (Guze et al., 1969; Cloninger and Guze, 1970a, 1970b; Schuckit et al., 1977) insist that schizophrenia is a rare phenomenon in criminals. Similarly, Kloek (1968) reported that only 1 of 500 delinquents he studied was flamboyantly psychotic, although 30 were thought possibly to be schizophrenic. This figure is six times the estimate of the prevalence of schizophrenia in the general population.

On the other hand, many investigators who have immersed themselves in the clinical study of delinquents and criminals have been impressed by the severity of psychopathology they have encountered (Healy, 1920; Oltman and Friedman, 1941). Heston (1970, 1977) has alluded to the aggressive, antisocial, periodically psychotic states characteristic of the first-degree relatives of schizophrenics and has advocated the use of the term "schizoid psychopath."

Our own study (Lewis et al., 1979c) of the psychiatric symptomatology of especially violent delinquent incarcerated boys revealed that 60% were loose, rambling, and illogical, 30% had had visual hallucinations, 43% had had auditory hallucinations, and 82% had manifested paranoid symptoms. In fact, more than half of these boys had previously been patients in psychiatric hospitals and/or psychiatric residential treatment centers (Lewis and Shanok, 1980a). The fact that the majority of extremely violent incarcerated delinquents had previously been psychiatric inpatients would seem to be objective, independent evidence of the severity of their psychopathology during childhood.

Psychoeducational Correlates

Numerous studies have reported associations between learning deficits and social maladaptation (Murray, 1976; Gagné, 1977). Rutter and his colleagues (1970) in their Isle of Wight study found severe reading retardation to be highly correlated with antisocial problems. Our own studies of learning disabilities in more and less violent delinquents indicated that degree of violence and degree of reading retardation were strongly associated (Lewis et al., 1980b). The term *learning disabilities* has for the most part been used by educators to connote specific learning dysfunctions in the absence of detectable psychiatric or neurological problems. When attempting to understand the problems of seriously delinquent children, such a definition is too restrictive. Many seriously delinquent youngsters suffer from a variety of neuropsychiatric disorders such as attentional problems, periodic psychotic states, and epilepsy. They often, in addition, have specific identifiable learning disabilities. Even after their particular neurological or psychiatric disorders are treated, they may still suffer from specific learning problems requiring specific remediation.

Parental Psychopathology

The association between delinquency and broken homes has long been recognized. The etiological implications of this association, however, are far from clear. According to Rutter and Madge (1976), the association of delinquency and broken homes is greatest when the family has been disrupted because of separation or divorce rather than by the death of a parent. Offord and his colleagues (1978) suggest that it is not the breakup of the home itself that promotes delinquency, but the family discord and disharmony that precedes the breakup.

There is an increasing body of knowledge suggesting that the parents of delinquents themselves manifest serious psychopathology (Glueck and Glueck, 1950; West and Farrington, 1973; Lewis and Balla, 1976; Offord et al., 1978). These kinds of data are difficult to assess because, as Offord and his colleagues point out, the criteria for and definitions of parental psychopathology are often imprecise.

Traditionally, explanations for the association of parental psychopathology and delinquency in their children have been psychodynamic. The concept of superego lacunae (i.e., the parent communicating his or her own unconscious antisocial impulses to the child who then internalizes them and acts them out) was formulated by Johnson and Szurek (1952) and influenced the thinking of a generation of psychiatrists. More recently, West and Farrington (1973) attributed delinquent behaviors in the children of criminal parents to the failure of these parents to supervise their children appropriately. This conceptualization is reminiscent of the early work of the Gluecks (1950), who focused on the failure of the parents of delinquents to discipline their children properly.

With the more recent recognition of the genetic components of schizophrenia, manic-depressive illness, epilepsy, and possibly hyperactivity has come an appreciation of possible inherent vulnerabilities to maladaptive behaviors. There is evidence that delinquency is more likely to occur in the children of schizophrenics (Lewis and Balla, 1976; Lewis and Shanok, 1978) than in the children of nonschizophrenics of the same socioeconomic status. Similarly, family studies of hyperkinetic children suggest familial and environmental variables associated with antisocial behavior (Cantwell, 1978). Mendelson et al. (1971) found that extremely antisocial children tended to have fathers who had learning and behavior disorders as children and who had been arrested as adults.

It must be emphasized that the family studies of delinquent children that suggest possible associations between parental psychopathology and delinquency in children fail to delineate the mode of transmission. It is reasonable to hypothesize that an interaction of biological and environmental factors affects delinquent outcome in the children of seriously disturbed parents. For example, many seriously delinquent children have witnessed violence and have been physically abused by their psychiatrically disturbed parents. One might hypothesize that in some of these cases the effects of modeling, central nervous system trauma, diminished impulse control, displacement of rage, and possible inherent vulnerabilities to disordered thought processes combine to create serious, often violent, delinquent behavior in children.

Social Factors and Race Bias

Delinquency and socioeconomic deprivation are so closely intertwined that no sensible person could discount their association. The majority of incarcerated delinquents come from the most economically deprived sectors of our society. Moreover, the overwhelming majority of incarcerated adults come from racial minorities, and most in the United States are black. The explanations for these phenomena are far from clear. While some sociologists have asserted that poor black children are more likely to be apprehended and sentenced than are wealthy whites for identical behaviors (Nye and Short, 1957), there are other possible explanations. For example, mental illness manifested by socially unacceptable behavior in black children is often dismissed as culturally induced and even as environmentally appropriate whereas comparable behaviors in whites are recognized as pathological. Similarly, child abuse, often leading to central nervous system dysfunction and poor impulse control in black children, is often overlooked by white clinicians for a variety of reasons (Lewis et al., 1979a). Furthermore, there is evidence that psychiatrically impaired black children and adults may have greater difficulty gaining access to appropriate treatment than psychiatrically impaired whites, making it more likely for blacks to be "treated" in (or, better, treated *to*) the penal system. It is also harder to gain foster-home placement and/or adoptive homes for black children, making multiple placements and the adverse psychiatric consequences of such changes more likely for them.

Others (Shaw and McKay, 1942) have asserted that the laws of the street contribute heavily to black delinquency. In fact, there are sociologists who have long insisted that antisocial behavior may be adaptive and acceptable to socioeconomically deprived individuals (Cohen, 1955; Merton, 1957). Such reasoning often leads mental-health professionals to the erroneous assumption that an extremely paranoid outlook coupled with the use of dangerous weapons constitutes normal black behavior. However, most black children are not violent, delinquent, or paranoid. Therefore, any child, black or white, who constantly gets into difficulties with the law or who feels the need to carry or use a dangerous weapon must be assessed carefully (Lewis et al., 1980c). In our own study of an entire population of adolescents from a single community sent in a given year either to corrections or to a state psychiatric hospital, we found that the hospitalized and incarcerated youngsters were similarly violent and similarly psychiatrically impaired. The most important factor distinguishing the groups was race. Violent, psychiatrically impaired white children were hospitalized. Violent, psychiatrically impaired black children were incarcerated. We have found that mental-health workers often dismiss as culturally appropriate in black children behaviors and symptoms such as hallucinations that in white children would be recognized as signs of possible psychopathology and evaluated more thoroughly.

DIAGNOSTIC EVALUATION

The diagnostic evaluation of the juvenile offender is not a search for simple causes. It is, rather, an exploration of vulnerabilities. As evidenced in our earlier exploration of neuropsychiatric and environmental correlates of delinquency, antisocial behaviors are rarely singly determined. Biological, psychodynamic, intrafamilial, and social factors in combination affect what we do. Therefore, no evaluation is complete that fails to take into account the multiple determinants of a child's antisocial behavior.

Psychiatric Evaluation

The psychiatrist requested to evaluate a delinquent child has a special responsibility, greater even than the responsibility of the child-guidance-clinic psychiatrist or the private practitioner. His or her report may be used to determine the child's capacity to stand trial, the child's culpability, the treatment or lack of treatment allotted the child, and whether or not the child will be sent home or incarcerated. The increasingly punitive developments in the handling of children (i.e., lowering the age at which a child can be tried and punished as an adult) increase the psychiatrist's responsibility.

The usual twenty- to sixty-minute court-requested psychiatric interviews with delinquent children, particularly in the absence of other psychiatric, medical, and social information, almost invariably afford inadequate opportunities to make accurate psychiatric diagnoses. The consequences of venturing a psychiatric opinion on the basis of a single brief interview can be disastrous. Rather than capitulate to unreasonable time limitations (based usually on limitations of funds to pay for evaluations), the psychiatrist must insist on adequate time in which to perform the evaluation. If forced to make a statement after one short interview, the psychiatrist is well advised to use the brief contact with the child to assess what further diagnostic measures and what medical and school records are required before an accurate psychiatric assessment can be furnished; this should be indicated in the report.

Interviewing a Parent or Relative

In addition to interviewing the child, it is important to interview a parent or relative. A parent can furnish information about perinatal factors, early life experiences, and medical events about which a child has no information. Furthermore, a parent can provide information regarding the mental health of other family members which can shed light on the psychiatric status of the child.

Naturally, if the child has been raised in a household with a psychotic relative, this experience can be expected to have influenced the child's thinking and behavior in particular ways. A paranoid mother may convey to the child a sense of pervasive danger and even teach the youngster to be wary and to carry weapons at all times. A brain-damaged, violent father may not only set an example of impulsiveness, but may also batter the child and inflict central nervous system damage which will contribute further to the child's antisocial adaptation. Asking about child abuse requires skill. We have found it helpful to acknowledge to parents that we know their child can be very difficult at times. We ask, "Has he ever made you lose your cool? What have you done? What about his dad? Does he ever lose his cool? What has he done then?"

As we have mentioned, psychiatrists are beginning to appreciate more and more the hereditary predisposition to certain kinds of psychiatric disorders. Family members can furnish invaluable clues to the understanding of certain aberrant child behaviors, such as schizophrenia, affective disorders, hyperactivity, and epilepsy. The discovery that a child has a paranoid schizophrenic parent may shed light on the physiological underpinnings of his inordinately suspicious, sometimes violent and bizarre, behaviors. Similarly, the knowledge that an adolescent who is periodically out of control, destructive, and verbally and physically abusive has a manic-depressive parent should encourage the psychiatrist to explore the possibility that such a disorder contributes to the behavior that called the child to the attention of the police. Most important, knowledge of heritable psychiatric disorders in family members has implications for possible effective treatment for the child. Behaviors previously dismissed by the psychiatrist as simply characterological may, with the benefit of an accurate family history, be recognized as manifestations of other kinds of effectively treatable psychopathology.

It is common practice in child-guidance clinics and juvenile courts to have parents interviewed by probation officers and to have only the child seen by a clinician. Many of the children who come to juvenile court have parents who suffer from serious psychopathology. In addition to furnishing information regarding relatives, interviews with parents by skilled clinicians permit an assessment of parental medical and psychiatric status. It is, therefore, advisable that the individual who interviews the parents, whatever his or her discipline, have expertise in psychiatric interviewing and diagnostic evaluation. Otherwise, there is the real danger that the psychotic or organically impaired parent who, for example, has been incarcerated, will be dismissed as merely sociopathic, or that the extremely depressed parent who frequently drinks to excess will be dismissed as simply alcoholic. The recognition of the nature of parental psychopathology underlying the incarceration or alcoholism has implications not only for understanding and treating the child, but also for arranging effective treatment for the parent to enable the parent to function more appropriately and provide a supportive environment for the child.

Medical History

As we have seen, many delinquent children, particularly those who have committed numerous and serious antisocial acts, have extremely poor medical histories. In the case of violent juveniles, medical problems are often characteristic of their entire lives, beginning with perinatal problems and continuing throughout childhood and adolescence. Because of the multiplicity of biopsychosocial factors affecting the lives of delinquent children, it is often impossible to determine the contribution of particular medical events. Sometimes, however, it is possible to document the onset of deviant behaviors following paritcular trauma to the central nervous system. For example, one boy who had remained out of trouble with the law became extremely violent and paranoid and actually raped and assaulted several women following a car accident in which he sustained severe head injury. Another boy became assaultive and unmanageable following an episode of encephalitis at age five. Yet another youngster, a teenage girl who had been considered her "mother's angel," became involved in a multiplicity of antisocial acts and began to experience episodes of violent behaviors for which she had no memory following an episode of meningitis.

All of these children came from multiproblem families. Prior to central nervous system trauma, however, they had been able to cope adequately with their adverse environments. The discovery of adverse medical events is especially important, since in some cases the information may lead to new treatment strategies. For example, the child who suffered encephalitis at age five responded positively to low-dosage amphetamine and barbiturate medication and was able to function in a therapeutic setting where he had previously been unwelcome. Treating medical problems affecting behavior is a time-consuming individualized procedure. Initial trials of medication may be unsuccessful. In many instances, however, the careful identification and treatment of specific medical vulnerabilities means the difference between appropriate adaptation and a lifetime of incarceration.

Optimally, medical histories should be obtained from children, parents, and hospital or clinic records. Hospital records frequently contain vital information that children and parents are either unaware of or are reluctant to disclose. Similarly, children and their parents may recount symptoms and medical events that have not been recorded in medical charts.

Psychiatric Interview with the Child

One might anticipate that children interviewed in the context of a juvenile court or correctional setting (many from ethnic or racial minorities) would be reluctant to talk with middle-class professionals. Psychiatrists might be especially suspect. Such is not necessarily the case. In fact we have found that most children and families welcome that opportunity to participate in the evaluation. The examiner's concerns about possible communication barriers and confidentiality may be greater than the children's or their parents'. Because most delinquent children are eager to communicate, it is important for the examiner to be aware of issues of confidentiality. A child and family must be informed with whom information will be shared in instances where the purpose is adjudication or disposition (i.e., sentencing). If the psychiatrist is working for the court, his role is different from what it would be were he engaged by the child's family.

It almost goes without saying that a major aspect of the psychiatric interview concerns psychodynamic issues. Anger and its expression obviously are major themes, particularly for violent adolescents. Of note, although the majority of violent incarcerated children have come from families in which they have witnessed and been the victims of violence, many abused children are not conscious of their rage toward parents or siblings. It is important that the evaluating psychiatrist who does not have responsibility for treatment appreciate the strength of the child's denial of anger and refrain from premature interpretations, the consequences of which he will not be available to discuss and work through with the child. Children in detention and correctional schools are more aware of their loneliness and sadness than of their rage at neglectful or abusive parents.

Children can furnish surprisingly useful information about pregnancy, delivery, and developmental milestones. Only the child can describe lapses of consciousness, hallucinatory episodes, and a wide variety of subjective experiences of which parents are totally unaware. Frequently parents have forgotten or have been unaware of important events affecting a child's functioning, including serious falls from high places, loss of consciousness, and car accidents (not to mention drug usage and alcohol usage and their effects). Most important, a child can furnish what is in some cases a "blow-by-blow" account of the act with which he is charged. Such information is especially useful when the delinquent act has been violent.

The following questions need to be clarified. Does the youngster frequently have trouble controlling his temper? Once he starts to fight is he unable to stop? Is there, in addition, a long history of impulsivity, hyperactivity, and other signs often associated with organic impairment and/or psychosis? It is also important to ascertain whether or not the child recalls the act and whether or not his recollection conforms to what other people witnessed. Was the child drunk, under the influence of drugs, or experiencing a psychomotor epileptic episode? Is his inability to remember a result of hysterical blocking or are there physiological explanations for his memory impairment? A useful way to explore the question of a psychomotor seizure is to ascertain whether or not the child could somehow tell in advance that he was about to lose control (e.g., did he feel sweaty, peculiar, as though he were in a dream, dizzy, etc.?). Is the child's memory of the act accurate or somewhat distorted? After the event did he feel dizzy? sleepy? sick? Did he actually fall asleep? Finally, has the child ever experienced other episodes, violent or nonviolent, for which his memory was impaired? Does he have a history of severe head injury? of previous seizures? Do close family members have seizure disorders?

Similarly, the child—and only the child—can furnish information regarding his state of mind during the violent act. Did he feel inordinately threatened in the absence of any threat? Did he think had had been called a bad name or that his mother had been insulted? Has he previously been belligerent because he thought someone had made a comment that really had not been made? And, of course, did he think that a person or a voice had commanded him to perform a particular act?

Mental-Status Examination

No matter how obvious the social and psychodynamic forces influencing a child's antisocial behaviors, the psychiatrist who focuses exclusively on these kinds of issues will often fail to uncover other equally important factors affecting behavior. It is as important for the psychiatrist to perform a meticulous mental-status evaluation as it is to explore family relationships. Even the most astute clinician cannot be expected to discern whether or not a child is well oriented, has experienced hallucinations, is delusional, or has an impaired short-term memory unless he focuses deliberately on these issues. Appearances are often deceiving. The fact that children may appear to be socially appropriate does not mean necesarily that they are of normal intelligence, or that they do not hallucinate or suffer from perceptual-motor problems that are not evident in the course of ordinary conversation.

The sensitive clinician can ask, in a context that is nonthreatening, the kinds of questions that might ordinarily be anxiety provoking. For example, assessing the presence or absence of hallucinatory experience can be accomplished in the course of taking a medical history. After discussing family, friends, school, sports, and perhaps some of the difficulties surrounding the behaviors that brought the child to court, the interviewer can introduce an ostensibly different set of questions. "How is your health? Have you ever been in the hospital? Any accidents?" After inquiring about loss of consciousness, headaches, and dizziness, the clinician may ask, "How are your eyes? Do you wear glasses? Have your eyes ever played tricks on you? What was that like?" Questions may be asked about things looking far away or very near, objects becoming blurry or changing shapes. The invitation to discuss visual experiences often enables children to describe episodes that have puzzled or frightened them but about which they have never spoken. Several children reported episodes when they were reading and the print seemed to disappear and the pages seemed blank. One child described watching television and experiencing the sensation that the screen was getting smaller and smaller. Another, looking out the window, perceived faraway buildings loom large before his eyes. These kinds of symptoms, along with multiple episodes of *déjà vu*, falling spells, or acts for which memory is impaired or absent, are sometimes clues to the existence of psychomotor epilepsy.

The medical interview can continue with such questions as, "How are your ears? Do you ever get earaches? Have your ears ever played tricks on you? What was that like? Have you ever had the experience of thinking someone said something to you and you were mistaken? What was that like?" Many paranoid children will recount episodes in which they thought a person called them an obscenity (or, worse, called their mother a bad name!) and they wheeled around and attacked perfectly innocent bystanders.

The same technique described for visual and auditory assessments can be used for olfactory ("Do you get colds much? Do you get nosebleeds? Do you ever have the experience of smelling something and no one else smells it?"), gustatory, and tactile experiences. When questions regarding hallucinations are asked this way, many children will reveal episodes they were previously afraid to share for fear of being thought crazy. It helps, then, to reassure a child that he is not "crazy," that many people have had similar experiences, and that, what is more, you may be able to help the child get rid of these experiences.

The assessment of paranoid thinking is among the most difficult tasks that confront the psychiatrist evaluating delinquent children. A wariness of the interviewer is certainly to be expected in light of the possible consequence of the interview. The precise point at which wariness moves into inordinate suspiciousness is a clinical judgment that must be made, and the reasons for making such a judgment must be well documented in any report. It is, however, a mistake for the interviewer to assume that carrying dangerous weapons or being ready at all times to be attacked is a normal concomitant of lower socioeconomic class existence. A child can be from a tough part of town and still not feel the need to carry large knives, crowbars, or loaded guns.

It is tempting for the psychiatrist who sees many delinquents to dismiss as normal behaviors those indicative of paranoid delusions. Many violent delinquents will assert that they carry weapons because they have been attacked. Careful interviewing may reveal that they have repeatedly invited attack and thereby have justified their own wariness and need to be armed. One must keep in mind the difference between a penknife and a carving knife.

Especially violent delinquent children teach us the usefulness of asking in detail about feelings of endangerment or persecution. Paranoid symptomatology exists if a child not only reports feelings of endangerment and persecution by a wide variety of different persons, but also either acts in response to these feelings (e.g., attacking another individual out of the blue, secreting multiple weapons) or feels seriously troubled by them.

For most delinquents, the most threatening parts of the mental-status evaluation are not the assessment of hallucinations, delusions, or paranoia, but rather the testing of the child's ability to work with numbers and to remember digits forward and backward. These aspects are probably threatening both because of their association with schoolwork and because they tend to reveal impairments of which the child is vaguely aware. Difficulties with these kinds of tasks, while not pathognomonic of any particular disorders, may suggest to the clinician possible short-term memory deficits, impulse disorders, attentional disorders, and learning disabilities, all of which can then be explored further in psychological, educational, and neurological assessments.

Suffice it to say that the psychiatrist who fails to perform a detailed mental-status evaluation will miss discovering a variety of potentially treatable disorders. Many of these disorders, left untreated, contribute to a delinquent child's social maladaptation.

Psychological Testing

It is erroneous to assume that even the most meticulous and sophisticated interview can bring to light all of the problems of personality and cognitive functioning that are tapped by psychological testing. In fact, psychotic thought processes and intellectual retardation, aspects of functioning that one might expect to be most easily recognized by means of psychiatric interviewing, unless the psychosis or retardation is flamboyant, are often far from obvious and among the most difficult aspects of functioning to assess. The wary, paranoid youngster may reveal disorders of thinking on a Rorschach protocol that he had concealed easily during psychiatric interviews. Even extremely intellectually limited youngsters often are able to conduct themselves in socially appropriate ways, giving the psychiatric interviewer little indication that serious intellectual deficits, elucidated through testing, do exist. And, of course, psychological testing can often reveal perceptual-motor disturbances rarely elicited during psychiatric interviews.

The choice of psychological tests, their administration, and the interpretation of results are topics of greater scope than can be encompassed in this chapter (see chap. 24). Suffice it to say that the Wechsler Intelligence Scale for Children (WISC) is useful not only for assessing intelligence, but also for assessing many different aspects of thinking, behavior, perception, and attention. In addition to providing clues to perceptual problems and cognitive difficulties, the WISC is a valuable tool for documenting fluctuating states of attention. Many children vary markedly in their performance within individual subtests, answering difficult questions with ease and being totally unable from time to time to respond to much easier questions. Moreover, at one moment some children are able to repeat six digits backward, while at the next moment they are unable to recall three digits in reverse. This quality of performance, while sometimes evident during testing, often comes to light only at the time the test is scored. Many children with this kind of intrasubtest pattern also have other symptoms suggestive of attentional disorders and/or epilepsy. Thus, differences among individual subtest scores do not always convey adequately the quality of a child's difficulties. In other words, final scores do not necessarily reflect the ways in which tasks are approached and accomplished.

Responses on the Rorschach test, in addition to contributing to the understanding of psychodynamic issues, are useful as indicators of a child's internal controls and ability to organize thoughts coherently. Perseveration, bizarre percepts, impulsivity, or marked disorganization on the Rorschach often suggest the existence of central nervous system dysfunction or latent psychosis which has previously been overlooked. On the other hand, hardly a single Rorschach report fails to comment on latent anger, unconscious rage, and violent fantasies, most of which can be deduced from the situation of the population being tested and from psychiatric interviews.

Psychological testing is most useful when it brings to light hitherto overlooked disorders. When, however, a child's performance on psychological testing fails to reveal any evidence of emotional or cognitive disturbance, it is imperative that the psychologist indicate in his or her report the limitations of psychological test results and that testing is not a substitute for complete psychiatric, neurological, educational, and social evaluations.

For the child's well-being, it is important that the psychologist make explicit the fact that psychological tests (like other kinds of brief evaluations) reflect only the functioning of a given child at a given point in time.

Educational Assessments

As we have said, it is well established that many delinquent children have learning disabilities. Especially violent delinquents have even more serious learning disorders than do less violent delinquents.

Neither standard psychiatric nor standard psychological evaluations assess the kinds of skills that educational testing is designed to measure. Again, which tests to use and the interpretation of specific tests are topics beyond the scope of this chapter.

Obviously, reading and mathematical abilities should be evaluated. But more information than scores on reading or mathematical tests is required if programs are to be designed to meet the specific needs of individual delinquent children. Problems in auditory discrimination and/or comprehension, visual discrimination and/or comprehension, and sequencing may exist separately or may coexist. Programs to remedy one kind of learning disorder may be completely inappropriate for another.

Again, discrete learning disabilities may exist concurrently with serious emotional problems or in the presence of identifiable neurological disorders. The psychiatrist cannot assume that a borderline psychotic delinquent child's poor school performance is necessarily a reflection of the psychotic disorder alone. Nor can he or she be certain that, for example, the poor school performance of an epileptic child is necessarily a function of the epilepsy. In other words, treatment of a neurotic, psychotic, or neurological disorder, while of benefit to aspects of a given child's functioning, may not improve reading or mathematical performance or functioning in other areas of social adaptation.

Institutions caring for delinquent children must be prepared to treat psychiatric and educational disorders. Our work with extremely violent incarcerated delinquent children suggests that it is especially common for seriously delinquent children to suffer from combinations of psychiatric, neurological, and learning disorders.

Neurological Evaluation

Obvious neurological deficits such as grand mal epilepsy or hemiparesis are unlikely to be seen often in the delinquent population (although a history of grand mal seizures is not uncommon). Flamboyantly neurologically impaired antisocial children, like flamboyantly psychotic delinquents, are likely to be recognized as "sick" and channeled to therapeutic facilities during early childhood. A meticulous neurological assessment, however, is likely in many instances to reveal subtle neurological impairment, particularly in seriously delinquent violent youngsters.

Even more important than the neurological physical findings are the findings obtained from detailed neurological histories. The neurologist would do well to assume that he or she may be the only clinician who will take an adequate history, an assumption that in most cases is probably legitimate. Questions about illnesses, accidents, injuries, headaches, dizziness, blackouts, reactions to alcohol and drug abuse, *déjà vu,* macropsia, micropsia, and visual, auditory, olfactory, gustatory, and tactile misperceptions or hallucinations should be an integral part of the neurological assessment. In the case of violent delinquents, questions regarding precipitants of violence, memory for violent and nonviolent behaviors, ability to cease fighting, lapses of fully conscious contact with reality, and whether or not fatigue or sleep follow these kinds of experiences should be ascertained. It is important to recognize that all violent acts performed by the same child may not have identical causes. In a recent study of violent juveniles with psychomotor epilepsy (Lewis et al., 1982), we found that those children who were violent during a seizure were often aggressive at other interictal times as well.

The same kinds of questions asked by the psychiatrist should also be covered by the neurologist. Even questions related to inordinate suspiciousness are essential to the neurological evaluation. It has been reported in a number of publications that paranoid ideation is often associated with psychomotor epilepsy (Pond, 1957; Glaser et al., 1963; Treffert, 1964; Small et al., 1966).

Methods for approaching these kinds of questions have already been discussed in the section on the psychiatric evaluation. They are as applicable to the neurological as to the psychiatric interview. The neurologist must remember (as must the psychiatrist) that his or her certification depends on expertise in both neurology and psychiatry.

Although an EEG is an obvious component of the neurological evaluation, the results of these tests at this time are more often confusing than helpful. Even sleep EEGs in children add little to a diagnosis such as psychomotor epilepsy, for the diagnosis is clinical. A normal EEG does not preclude the existence of epilepsy. Whether or not sleep EEGs in children are more revealing of psychopathology than waking EEGs remains a question. Sometimes a trial of antiepileptic medication in delinquent children with psychomotor epileptic symptoms is more useful than these tests. There is evidence, however, that most of the aggressive acts performed by delinquents with psychomotor epilepsy occur interictally (Lewis et al., 1982). Some acts seem motivated by the pervasive paranoid orientation of the delinquent with psychomotor symptoms. Others resemble the impulsive acts of brain-damaged youngsters. Thus, while antiepileptic medication may reduce certain kinds of outbursts, it may be ineffective in reducing other aggressive behaviors related more to psychotic symptoms or generalized brain dysfunction. There are times when combinations of antiepileptic and antipsychotic or stimulant medication will be more effective than either medication alone.

A problem in evaluating the juvenile delinquent with neurological signs of impairment arises from the fact that the majority of such children come from families in which psychiatric and social problems abound and could possibly, in and of themselves, explain deviance. Neurologists must therefore try to make sure that their knowledge of the psychosocial factors affecting the children not blind them to the possible contribution of neurological impairment.

Treatment

A wide variety of treatment modalities has been undertaken, ranging from residential treatment (Cornish and Clarke, 1975), parental training in behavior modification (Patterson, 1971), to psychopharmacologic interventions (Maletzky, 1974). However, delinquency is not a single entity. It does not have a single cause, nor is there a single treatment for it. Therefore it is not surprising that reviews of the efficacy of particular modalities for "treating delinquency" or "treating criminality" tend to be pessimistic (Craft et al., 1964; Lipton et al., 1975; Martinson et al., 1976). From our exploration of the biological, psychological, intrafamilial, and social factors associated with delinquency, we can infer that no single method can be expected to be helpful to all or even most offenders. For example, remedial educational programs to improve the competence and self-esteem of learning-disabled delinquents may not even meet the needs of delinquents with learning disabilities plus attentional problems, much less meet the needs of borderline psychotic youngsters. Behavior modification may have little effect on a delinquent whose violence springs from paranoid ideation. Similarly, a psychotherapeutic program that ignores social stresses, educational disabilities, and medical (particularly neurological) problems cannot hope to succeed with the majority of multiply handicapped seriously delinquent children.

The issue of treatment is complicated further by the fact that adolescents who engage in antisocial acts, no matter how psychiatrically disturbed, are by and large unwelcome in the mental-health system. It therefore falls upon the juvenile justice system to arrange for the care of these youngsters.

The mood of this country, at the time of the writing of this chapter, has swung from an earlier optimistic belief in rehabilitation to a pessimism regarding the efficacy of treatment. This pessimism is reflected in the decision of many state legislatures to lower from sixteen years to thirteen years the age at which a child can be tried in an adult court for certain acts.

Nevertheless, a few states, such as Minnesota, California, Massachusetts, Illinois, Pennsylvania, and North Carolina, have established programs designed to try to meet the needs of seriously disturbed, often violent, offenders. These programs tend to rely on combinations of milieu therapy, group therapy, and individual psychotherapy. In addition, all incorporate educational and recreational components. Of note, programs and treatment teams within programs are, by and large, headed by psychologists and social workers. Medical personnel such as psychiatrists function for the most part as consultants, prescribing and monitoring medication.

Results of these multifaceted programs are not yet available. Their weakest component, however, is an inability to provide follow-up care for the youngsters they have served; for one reason or another no consistent supports are provided following discharge. Thus it is likely that even the best of such programs may appear ineffective if judged by the long-term functioning of their clients.

Having examined both the vulnerabilites of seriously delinquent youngsters and some of the programs designed to treat them, we can at least speculate about what kinds of interventions have a reasonable chance of success. First, a potentially successful program must have clinicians with the expertise to discern the existence of medical, educational, psychiatric, and intrafamilial vulnerabilities. It is essential to know whether a child has sustained central nervous sytem trauma, has experienced even fleeting psychotic symptoms, has been hampered by intellectual problems or learning disabilities, or has been the victim of or witnessed extreme physical abuse. Often all of these vulnerabilities will be identified in an individual child. Each must be addressed if a youngster is to function adequately within a treatment program—much less after discharge. Medication must not be the primary or sole treatment modality. Used judiciously, however, appropriate medication (be it antipsychotic, stimulant, antiepileptic, or antidepressant) will often enable an individual child to take advantage of the psychotherapeutic, educational, and recreational components of a program. Without appropriate medication, many vulnerable delinquents may be unable to make use of even the best psychodynamic, social, and educational interventions.

There is evidence that even the finest residential program will fail if it lacks the ability to support its clients following discharge (Lewis, M. et al., 1980). Work with families while a child is in residential treatment as well as after discharge is obviously important when a child has a family to which he or she can return. Unfortunately, many of the most seriously disturbed delinquent youngsters come from equally disturbed households. Parents who require recurrent psychiatric hospitalization or who are repeatedly incarcerated themselves are unlikely, on their own, to be able to sustain the gains their children have made while in residential treatment. Therefore it makes no sense to provide a troubled adolescent with sophisticated medical, psychological, and educational assistance while in residence only to deprive him of these supports following discharge to the community. If a program is to succeed, it must be designed to provide continuing supports through adolescence and possibly into young adulthood. Programs that incorporate a spectrum of ongoing treatment facilities ranging from secure to open are far more likely to be successful than those which abandon the youngster at the gate.

We can appreciate the ongoing needs of seriously delinquent youngsters when we look at our own upbringings. Most of the readers of this book have not sustained the kinds of physical and psychological traumata characteristic of the lives of violent delinquents. Nevertheless we have had the support of institutions and family well into the third decade of life (e.g., college, graduate school, medical school, etc.). Surely if most of us required ongoing structure and the caring relationship of family, teachers, guidance counselors, and physicians, we cannot expect the multiply handicapped delinquent child to require less.

References

American Psychiatric Association. 1980. *Diagnostic and statistical manual of mental disorders—third edition (DSM-III)*. Washington, D.C.: APA, p. 47.

Cantwell, D. P. 1978. Hyperactivity and antisocial behavior. *J. Am. Acad. Child Psych.*, 17:252-262.

Clarke, R. V. G., and Cornish, D. B. 1978. The effectiveness of residential treatment for delinquents. In *Aggression and antisocial behavior in childhood and adolescence*, ed. L. A. Hershov, M. Berger, and D. Shaffer, pp. 143-159. Oxford: Pergamon Press.

Cloninger, C. R., and Guze, S. B. 1970a. Female criminals. *Arch. Gen. Psych.*, 23:554-558.

Cloninger, C. R., and Guze, S. B. 1970b. Psychiatric illness and female criminality. *Am. J. Psych.*, 127:303-311.

Cohen, A. K. 1955. The origin and nature of the delinquent subculture. In *Delinquent boys: The culture of the gang,* ed. A. K. Cohen. New York: Free Press.

Cornish, D. B., and Clarke, R. V. G. 1975. *Residential treatment and its effects on delinquency.* London: HMSO.

Craft, M., Stephenson, G., and Granger, C. 1964. A controlled trial of authoritarian and self-governing regimes with adolescent psychopaths. *Am. J. Orthopsych.*, 34:543-554.

District of Columbia Department of Public Health. 1964. Mental health needs of juvenile delinquents.

Gagné, E. E. 1977. Educating delinquents: A review of research. *J. Spec. Ed.*, 11:13-27.

Gibbens, T. C. N. 1963. *Psychiatric studies of Borsta lads.* Institute of Psychiatry, Maudsley monographs no. 11. London: Oxford University Press.

Glaser, G. H., Newman, R. J., and Schafer, R. 1963. Interictal psychosis in psychomotor-temporal lobe epilepsy: An EEG-psychological study. In *EEG and behavior,* ed. G. H. Glaser, pp. 345-365. New York: Basic Books.

Glueck, S., and Glueck, E. 1950. *Unraveling juvenile delinquency.* New York: Commonwealth Fund.

Guze, S. B., Goodwin, D. W., and Crane, J. B. 1969. Criminality and psychiatric disorders. *Arch. Gen. Psych.,* 20:583–591.

Healy, W. 1920. *The individual delinquent.* Boston: Little, Brown.

Heston, L. L. 1970. The genetics of schizophrenia and schizoid disease. *Science,* 167:249–256.

Heston, L. L. 1977. Schizophrenia: Genetic factors. *Hosp. Pract.,* June, pp. 43–46.

Johnson, A. M., and Szurek, S. A. 1952. The genesis of antisocial acting out in children and adults. *Psychoanal. Quart.,* 21:323.

Kloek, J. 1968. Schizophrenia and delinquency. *Int. Psychiat. Clin.,* 5:19–34.

Lewis, D. O., and Balla, D. A. 1976. *Delinquency and psychopathology.* New York: Grune and Stratton.

Lewis, D. O., Balla, D., and Shanok, S. S. 1979a. Some evidence of race bias in the diagnosis and treatment of the juvenile offender. *Am. J. Orthopsych.,* 49:53–61.

Lewis, D. O., Pincus, J. H., Shanok, S. S., and Glaser, G. H. 1982. Psychomotor epilepsy and violence in an incarcerated adolescent population. *Am. J. Psych.,* 138:882–887.

Lewis, D. O., and Shanok, S. S. 1977. Medical histories of delinquent and nondelinquent children. *Am. J. Psych.,* 134:1020–1025.

Lewis, D. O., and Shanok, S. S. 1978. Delinquent and the schizophrenic spectrum of disorders. *J. Am. Acad. Child Psych.,* 17:263–276.

Lewis, D. O., and Shanok, S. S. 1980a. The use of a correctional setting for follow-up care of psychiatrically disturbed adolescents. *Am. J. Psych.,* 137:953–955.

Lewis, D. O., Shanok, S. S., and Balla, D. A. 1979b. Parental criminality and medical histories of delinquent children. *Am. J. Psych.,* 136:288–292.

Lewis, D. O., Shanok, S. S., Balla D. A., and Bard, B. 1980b. Psychiatric correlates of severe reading disabilities in an incarcerated delinquent population. *J. Am. Acad. Child. Psych.,* 19:611–622.

Lewis, D. O., Shanok, S. S., Cohen, R., Kligfeld, M., and Frisone, G. 1980c. Race bias in the diagnosis and disposition of violent adolescents. *Am. J. Psych.,* 137:1211–1216.

Lewis, D. O., Shanok, S. S., Pincus, J. H., and Glaser, G. H. 1979c. Violent juvenile delinquents: Psychiatric, neurological, psychological, and abuse factors. *J. Am. Child Psych.,* 18:307–319.

Lewis, M., Lewis, D. O., Shanok, S. S., Klatskin, E., and Osborne, J. R. 1980. The undoing of residential treatment: A follow-up study of 51 adolescents. *J. Am. Acad. Child Psych.,* 19:160–171.

Lipton, D., Martinson, R., and Wilks, J. 1975. *The effectiveness of correctional treatment: A survey of treatment evaluation studies.* New York: Praeger Publishers.

Maletzky, B. M. 1974. d-Amphetamine and delinquency: Hyperkinesis persisting? *Dis. Nerv. Sys.,* 35:543–547.

Martinson, R., Palmer, T., and Adams, S. 1976. *Rehabilitation, recidivism, and research.* Hackensack, N.J.: National Council on Crime and Delinquency.

Meeks, J. E. 1980. Conduct disorders. In *Comprehensive textbook of psychiatry,* vol. 3, 3rd ed., ed. H. I. Kaplan, A. M. Freeman, and B. J. Sadock. Baltimore: Williams and Wilkins.

Mendelson, W., Johnson, N., and Steward, M. A. 1971. Hyperactive children as teenagers: A follow-up study. *J. Nerv. Men. Dis.,* 153:273–279.

Merton, R. K. 1957. *Social theory and social structure.* Rev. ed. New York: Free Press.

Murray, C. A. 1976. The link between learning disabilities and juvenile delinquency: Current theory and knowledge. Executive summary prepared for the National Institute for Juvenile Justice and Delinquency Prevention Office of the Law Enforcement Assistance Administration.

Nye, F. I., and Short, J. F., Jr. 1957. Scaling delinquent behavior. *Am. Soc. Rev.,* 22:326–331.

Offord, D. R., Allen, N., and Abrams, N. 1978. Parental psychiatric illness, broken homes, and delinquency. *J. Am. Acad. Child Psych.,* 17:224–238.

Oltman, J. E., and Friedman, S. 1941. A psychiatric study of 100 criminals with particular reference to the psychological determinants of crime. *J. Nerv. Men. Dis.,* 93:16–41.

Patterson, G. R. 1971. *Families: Applications of social learning theory to family life.* Champaign, Ill.: Research Press.

Pond, D. A. 1957. Psychiatric aspects of epilepsy. *J. Indian Med. Assoc.,* 3:1441–1451.

Power, M. J., Benn, R. T., and Morris, J. N. 1972. Neighborhood, school, and juveniles before the courts. *Brit. J. Criminol.,* 12:111–132.

Robins, L. 1966. *Deviant children grown up.* Baltimore: Williams and Wilkins.

Rutter, M. L., Graham, P. J., and Yule, W. 1970. *A neuropsychiatric study in childhood.* Clin. in Dev. Med., nos. 35/36. London: Heinemann.

Rutter, M. and Madge, N. 1976. *Cycles of disadvantage.* London: Heinemann.

Schuckit, M. A., Herrman, G., and Schuckit, J. J. 1977. The importance of psychiatric illness in newly arrested prisoners. *J. Nerv. Men. Dis.,* 165:118–127.

Shanok, S. S., and Lewis D. O. 1981. Medical histories of delinquent children. In *Vulnerabilities to delinqueny,* ed. D. O. Lewis, pp. 221–240. New York: Spectrum.

Shaw, C. R., and McKay, M. D. 1942. *Juvenile delinquency and urban areas.* Chicago: University of Chicago Press.

Small, J. G., Small I. F., and Hayden, M. P. 1966. Further psychiatric investigations of patients with temporal and nontemporal lobe epilepsy. *Am. J. Psych.,* 123:303–310.

Treffert, D. A. 1964. The psychiatric patient with an EEG temporal lobe focus. *Am. J. Psych.,* 120:765–771.

West, D. J., and Farrington, D. P. 1973. *Who becomes delinquent?* London: Heinemann.

West, D. J. 1976. Delinquency. In *Child psychiatry: Modern approaches.* ed. M. Rutter and L. Hersov, pp. 510–523. Oxford: Blackwell Scientific.

16

Disturbance in School

Mark A. Stewart

Prevalence of Disturbance

Rutter and his colleagues found that 7% of ten-year-old children in a semirural area of England had definite psychiatric disorders and twice as many were affected in an inner-city population (Rutter et al., 1970; Rutter et al., 1975). Almost all of the children identified in these studies had either neurotic or conduct disorders. Psychoses and syndromes associated with brain damage accounted for only 3% of the total. These figures do not include children who were simply retarded, those who had specific learning disabilities, or those with developmental problems like enuresis.

Rutter et al. went on to rate the seriousness of problems among the children with psychiatric disorder and found that 35% of those with neurotic or conduct disorders were seriously handicapped. The rate of severe disorder in their whole population was 2.4% of ten and eleven year olds in the Isle of Wight and twice that proportion in the inner London borough. Langner et al. (1974) made a similar study of 1,034 children between the ages of six and eighteen in Manhattan and found an overall rate of serious psychiatric disorder of 1.4%. The two estimates are remarkably close, considering that one deals with a narrow and the other with a broad spread of age.

Applying these findings to a typical grade school with 300 pupils, we would expect that 20 to 40 of the children would have significant neurotic or conduct disorders and 7 to 14 would have serious psychiatric problems. This calculation implies that teachers work with a small but steady flow of disturbed children. It is important to add, too, that there are many more troubled children in schools than those who have a specific psychiatric disorder. These are the children whose lives are made miserable by abuse, neglect, and lack of love. Clegg and Megson (1968) have described the problems presented to the schools by "children in distress" all too vividly. Such children are victims of their parents' personality problems, ill health, inability to find work, poor housing, and social isolation.

This brief introduction gives some idea of the extent to which psychiatric disorder affects children and teachers in school. In the remainder of the chapter, I will describe the specific ways in which neurotic and conduct disorders affect children's behavior in the classroom, how these problems can best be defined and measured, and what should be done about them.

The Problems

School problems can be generally divided into disruptive behavior such as fighting or clowning, emotional problems such as anxiety and depression, and those that do not fit into any tidy category such as odd, asocial behavior and ideas of persecution. An outline of the types of problems is shown in table 16-1.

TABLE 16-1.
Problems Seen in the Classroom

Problem	Description	"Syndrome"
Disruptive children	a. Aggressive, disobedient, loud, impulsive, irritable, destructive, mean, restless, not interested in written work.	Aggressive conduct disorder
	b. Restless, unable to concentrate, silly, prone to get attention by playing the fool.	Pure hyperactivity
	c. Lying, cheating, stealing, stirring up trouble in sneaky ways.	Socialized conduct disorder
Shy or withdrawn children	a. Anxious, fearful, tense, self-conscious, diffident, prone to physical complaints, unduly compliant.	Anxiety
	b. Depressed, apathetic, withdrawn, irritable, fearful, tired.	Depression
	c. Working below potential, not well liked by peers, anxious, not able to stand up for self, self-centered.	Low self-esteem
Asocial children	a. Uninterested in other children, not understanding others' feelings, preoccupied with unusual ideas or particular activities, rigid and single-minded.	Schizoid personality
	b. Hallucinations, ideas of influence or reference, believes he has special powers, delusions of persecution, flat or inappropriate affect, disorganized thinking or conversation, unusual movements or postures.	Schizophrenia

Behavior Disorders

Openly disruptive behavior in the classroom comes chiefly in two guises. In one, a child may fight with his classmates, rebel against the teacher's authority, and refuse to do his work. He may be restless, inattentive, and try to get attention by clowning and silly behavior. On the other hand, a child may be subtly disruptive by lying, cheating, and getting others into trouble.

Probably the most common behavior problem in classrooms is that of the boy who is physically and verbally aggressive and defies the teacher's efforts at discipline. It has been estimated that between 3 and 7% of children show this pattern of behavior (Werner et al., 1968; Shepherd et al., 1971), but it is difficult to establish how many children are affected, because the aggressiveness and noncompliance almost certainly exist on a continuum. Schoolchildren with this pattern of behavior provoke their teachers by shouting out, sassy talk, and keeping the class in commotion. They are belligerent and rebellious, want to be the center of attention, tease their classmates, and have tantrums when corrected. They have little interest in doing their work and tend to be distractible and restless. Out on the playground they get into physical fights, are extremely competitive, and are poor losers. They make friends quickly but cannot keep them because of their bossy, self-centered ways and their constant disruption of the class.

This pattern of behavior was first defined by Hewitt and Jenkins (1946) and in *DSM-III* is labeled undersocialized conduct disorder of the aggressive type. As described by Hewitt and Jenkins and later investigators (Achenbach, 1978; Stewart et al., 1980), its principal components are aggressiveness, noncompliance, destructiveness, and quarrelsomeness. Most children who show this pattern appear egocentric with little obvious sensitivity for others and without a readily identifiable sense of guilt. They may be jealous and possessive, impulsive, impatient, and unable to handle frustration. They are often overactive and inattentive in class, but the latter seems to be due to a lack of interest rather than an inability to concentrate (Loney and Milich 1982). Finally, a proportion, perhaps half, of these children are involved in specific antisocial behavior such as lying and stealing.

Unusual aggressiveness appears early in life. It has been systematically observed in nursery-school children (Patterson et al., 1967), and signs of the problem may be seen even earlier in the form of repeated accidents. A number of studies (e.g., Manheimer and Mellinger, 1967) have suggested that aggressive, daring, and impulsive children are unusually prone to accidents. Aggressiveness seems to be remarkably stable through childhood and at least into early adult life (Olweus, 1979). Nylander (1979) and Kellam et al. (1980) found that high levels of aggressiveness in boys predict heavy drinking in adult life, and Robins (1978) found that this trait predicts antisocial personality in men. A substantial minority, perhaps 30-40%, of aggressive boys have such poor fates.

Another disruptive type of behavior, although irritating to teachers, is less serious or troublesome than aggressive conduct disorder. It may be quite common in classrooms, but there are no estimates of its prevalence. This pattern resembles the first in that the children are restless and inattentive. Often they seem to need a lot of attention and try to get it by clowning. They provoke the anger and dislike of classmates who see them as immature, uncontrolled, and silly. The difference between this group and the one described earlier is that children of the latter kind do not flout the rules in school deliberately. The trouble they create in the class appears to stem from lack of self-control rather than design or ill will.

The little we know about these children suggests that they are a heterogeneous group

(August and Stewart, 1982). They have in common their overactivity and distractibility, impulsivity and excitability. Otherwise there seem to be no distinguishing features except a higher prevalence of various learning disabilities, ranging from reading disability to mild retardation. There are hints that learning disabilities are more common in their immediate relatives too.

Given that they seem to be heterogeneous and so little else is known about them, it seems presumptuous to give these children a name, but to distinguish them from the aggressive conduct disorder group my colleagues and I have called them "purely hyperactive." Another important feature that may distinguish them from the conduct disorder group is that these hyperactive children seem to be willing to concentrate on schoolwork but are unable to do so, in contrast to the other group's ability to concentrate but lack of interest. The work of Weiss et al. (1979) and Loney et al. (1981) suggests that the prognosis for purely hyperactive children is quite benign, another contrast to the children with conduct disorder. They will do less well academically in high school but be hard to distinguish from normal people in early adult life.

The fact that children with aggressive conduct disorder are quite often involved in specific antisocial behaviors such as lying and stealing has already been mentioned. There are a number of other children, we do not know how many, who lie, cheat, and steal but are not openly disruptive in school or at home. This pattern of behavior has been studied less than that of aggressive conduct disorder and its definition remains controversial. Hewitt and Jenkins (1946) described a syndrome, which they called "socialized delinquency," of which the main feature was delinquent behavior in groups. Jenkins has argued that the main difference between such children and those with aggressive conduct disorder lies in the former being capable of loyalty, affection, and sympathy toward others, particularly their peers. Other investigators are skeptical of these categories and believe that the only valid division to be made at present is between delinquents who are aggressive and those who are not (West and Farrington, 1973). However this argument is resolved, there are children who are antisocial but not openly aggressive and rebellious. Such children make trouble in the classroom by taking their classmates' property, taking money out of their teachers' purses, cheating, and lying. They may also be manipulative, mean, and spiteful. Though not openly aggressive, they may be involved in destructive behaviors such as setting fires, sometimes with the purpose of revenge.

Little is known of such children except that their antisocial behavior tends to predict the development of antisocial personality in adult life. As many as a third of such children will suffer this fate (Robins, 1966). Considerably more is known about antisocial adolescents. From their extensive field research, West and Farrington (1977) have written a very detailed picture of juvenile delinquents.

Shy, Withdrawn Children

As many as 10% of children in their later years of grade school are shy and withdrawn (Werner et al., 1968). Only a small proportion of them have specific psychiatric disorders, chiefly anxiety and depression, but the group is swelled by the large number of children who are chronically unhappy or have little confidence in their ability to perform in school and make friends with their classmates. Rutter et al. (1970) found that roughly 1% of ten- to eleven-year-old boys and 1.5% of girls in the Isle of Wight had a neurotic or emotional disorder. In most cases this was an anxiety disorder. Relatively little is known of the natural history of neurotic disorders in children, but in general they seem to have a better prognosis than conduct disorders. Individual neurotic symptoms quite often remit spontaneously over the space of a year of two (Shepherd et al., 1971).

ANXIETY. The symptom of anxiety is usually associated with constant worrying and doubt as to one's ability to cope with everyday living. The child's fear is of a half-expected disaster—that the mother who is late to pick him up from school is dead in a traffic accident, that fire engines that go by are on their way to his house, or that the child sitting next to him has some dread disease which will infect him.

Anxious children are frequently in a state of alert. Their muscles are tense, their pulse races at a loud sound or a threatening look. In school the anxious child is likely to be shy of talking in front of the class, fearful of the rough and tumble in the playground, a victim for bullies, and too well-behaved. Such children become particularly nervous when taking tests, returning to school after vacations, or coming back to school after having been sick. At times they may become so anxious that they have physical symptoms such as stomachaches, nausea, and vomiting. Tension headaches may occur in the evenings after school and they may have difficulty going to sleep at night.

As yet we do not know how many anxious children go on to be anxious adults. In one follow-up study, shy, nervous children were followed up into middle age and discovered to be still shy and inhibited, but they had worked and had established families successfully (Morris et al., 1954). Winokur and Holemon (1963) studied a large group of adults with chronic anxiety and found that many of them had started having their symptoms in childhood.

As with aggressive conduct disorder, Hewitt and Jenkins (1946) were the first to define a syndrome of severe anxiety. They reported that the chief traits were social withdrawal, shyness, apathy, worrying, submissiveness, and oversensitivity. Originally termed "the overinhibited reaction," the syndrome has since been given many names, including overanxious reaction or disorder, and generalized anxiety. Whatever the name, the descriptions resemble each other closely. In clinical practice it is often hard to separate a phobic neurosis centered on separation from parents or going to school from generalized anxiety. Rutter et al. (1970) reported that a third of the children they found to have anxiety disorder had specific fears that were intense enough to be significant handicaps.

DEPRESSION AND UNHAPPINESS. Sad, depressed children are upsetting and frustrating for teachers. In the ordinary course of a school day, it is seldom possible for a teacher to reach such children individually. Even if the teacher spends time out of class talking with these students, they may not reveal what is troubling them. They sit blankly in class, only physically present, and take little part in class activities. They have difficulty getting their work done, not simply because they are distracted but because a lack of energy and ability to concentrate are associated with their low mood.

Unhappy children have little interest in playing or talking with their classmates and become socially isolated, finding it hard to enjoy any activity. They are likely to be irritable and prone to cry over minor upsets and frustration. Attendance at school may slip because these children develop physical symptoms such as headaches, feel reluctant to leave home, and tire easily. The last symptom may be compounded by sleep difficulties.

Many schoolchildren are disturbed by problems at home—bickering between their parents, physical abuse, or extreme poverty. Such students may seem unreachable in class, but they probably do not have a pyschiatric disorder.

Several investigators (e.g., Pearce, 1978; Carlson and Cantwell, 1979) have reported that about a quarter of all children attending a psychiatric clinic meet the criteria for a depression. It is useful to distinguish between primary depression and secondary, the latter being a depression associated with some other psychiatric or medical disorder. Two thirds of the children in psychiatric clinics who are depressed suffer from secondary depressions (Kuperman and Stewart, 1979; Birleson, 1981).

We know next to nothing about depression in children, other than how to diagnose it reliably. We do not know how long it lasts, whether there are common precipitants, or whether there are factors that predispose children to this disorder. It is clear that affective disorders identical to those occurring in adult life do occur in adolescence. One very important and happy fact is that suicide is extraordinarily rare in childhood (Shaffer and Fisher, 1981).

LOW SELF-ESTEEM. The normative distribution of scores on self-esteem inventories for children is skewed to the positive pole, making it hard to define a point at which scores are pathologically low. Piers (1969) found that 5% of schoolchildren scored two standard deviations or more below the mean. Low self-esteem, in a general sense, is one of the most common symptoms seen in a child psychiatry clinic. There are many factors at work here. Emotional, behavioral, and cognitive handicaps may all sap a child's confidence; other influences on children's self-esteem seems to be related to parental child-rearing styles. Coopersmith (1967) has reported that authoritarian, punitive, and inconsistent parents tend to have children with low self-esteem and data from Rosenberg's (1965) study on adolescents support this idea. Parents who adopt this style may have little confidence themselves.

Low self-esteem can be expected to affect children's behavior and performance in school in a number of ways. The child may fall short of his potential because he does not aim high enough or make enough effort (Coopersmith, 1968). He may seem indecisive and unenthusiastic in class discussions, believing that no one is interested in his opinions. This outlook may also affect relationships with classmates and teachers for the child may be diffident and tentative, expecting people not to like him.

Rosenberg (1962) analyzed the behavior of adults with low self-esteem and showed that this trait was strongly related to anxiety, sense of isolation, and loneliness. He argued that the trait led people to have an unstable picture of themselves, to put on poses or fronts when dealing with others, and to be unduly defensive in the face of criticism. Futhermore, they tended to become preoccupied with themselves and to spend more of their time in fantasy than those with a normal level of self-confidence. These traits are all obstacles to forming close relationships and therefore lead to isolation and loneliness. Another way to express the key idea is that low self-esteem tends to create a vicious circle. Expecting failure, the person sets low goals, makes little effort, and objectively experiences failure, which simply reinforces the original attitude to the self. Somerset Maugham, in *The Summing Up,* wrote

> The common idea that success spoils people by making them vain, egotistic, and self-complacent is erroneous; on the contrary, it makes them, for the most part, humble, tolerant, and kind. Failure makes people bitter and cruel.

In addition, children with low self-esteem make dull companions because they are preoccupied with themselves and how they will cope with each day's stresses. Their classmates see them as self-centered and lacking in fun. Second, as Somerset Maugham implied, these people come to resent their sense of failure and become covertly aggressive. Sarcasm, cruel teasing, and other thinly disguised expressions of hostility result. Finally, these children find it difficult to accept praise on the occasions when they do do a good job and find it impossible to admit that they did something well (Piers, 1977).

Asocial Behavior

Asocial behavior is a relatively uncommon problem in the classroom. Lack of interest in social relationships, inability to understand other people's feelings, aloofness, and eccentricity seem to be stable traits in such children. Only 5–10% of the psychiatric clinic population engages in such behavior. These children are handicapped socially, and also tend to have intellectual difficulties with language (Quitkin and Klein, 1969; Wolff and Barlow, 1979), making it hard to distinguish them from the brighter autistic children.

An even rarer problem in the classroom is that of the child who is developing schizophrenia. Such a child is likely to be at least eleven years old and is most likely to come to the teacher's attention for expressing ideas of being spied upon or watched, being influenced in unusual ways, or being harmed by others. These ideas may be associated with the belief that he or she has unusual powers, such as being able to read other people's minds or being possessed by God. Eccentric behavior may follow these delusions; for example, a child may come to school in the summer dressed in a parka, heavy pants, and gloves in order to prevent people from seeing through to his body and influencing him sexually. The natural history of schizophrenia in children has been well described by Kolvin et al. (1971); they point out that most children with this disorder have a history of being somewhat asocial for years before their disorder declares itself. However, others are apparently quite normal until the disease appears. Wolff and Chick (1980) have published a detailed description of schizoid personality with the only follow-up study of such children.

ASSESSMENT

A "problem-oriented" approach is appropriate for several reasons. Present methods of treatment in child psychiatry are designed to deal with specific behavioral or emotional problems rather than syndromes; and teachers, together with their supporting specialists, find this approach more familiar and practical. The plan of assessment described here is intended to define specific problems, to find clues to their origins, and to suggest remedies. What follows is also based on an assumption that the problems have been serious enough to persist over a period of several weeks and that they are seldom, if ever, confined to the child's life in school.

Whether the difficulty lies primarily in the child's behavior, performance, or feelings about school, its proper assessment calls for coordinated collection of data on all three aspects together with a judgment on how well the child's current educational program fits his or her needs. A schema of the essential parts of assessment is shown in table 16–2. Data are taken from the child by interview and tests, from the parents by questionnaire and interview, and from the teacher by questionnaire, interview, and observation. Carrying this out in a reasonable time calls for at least three people: a psychiatrist, a teacher, and a psychome-

300 / THE CLINICAL GUIDE TO CHILD PSYCHIATRY

TABLE 16-2.
Assessment of Children with Problems in the Classroom: The Essentials

Sources	
The child	a. Semistructured interview, covering home and family, friends, interests, school, and the problems.
	b. Physical examination and laboratory tests such as urinalysis, CBC.
	c. Tests of intelligence (e.g., WISC-R), school achievement (e.g., Peabody or Stanford), self-esteem (e.g., Coopersmith), cognitive style (e.g., Kagan's MFF).
	d. Observations of cooperation, concentration, self-confidence, style, etc., during the tests.
	e. Observation of behavior in the classroom and, when possible, systematic counts of specific behaviors.
The parents	a. Semistructured interview to cover: the child's problems; a systematic review of all the common psychiatric symptoms of children; development and medical history; social history of the family; psychiatric and cognitive problems of the child's first- and second-degree relatives. (Cognitive = language, reading, and general performance in school.)
	b. Questionnaires for each parent, covering: identifying data; the parent's main concerns about the child at home, at school, and in the neighborhood and what his or her goals are for treatment; the mother's obstetric and child's medical history; a review of the parent's mood; and a review of the parent's satisfaction with her of his marriage.
The teacher	a. Semistructured interview to cover: the child's problems; academic progress; relationships with teachers and peers; record of attendance, health, and disciplinary actions; and performance in gym. Also the attitudes of the parents to the school and education in general, and the performance of the brothers and sisters, if they have gone to the same school.
	b. Questionnaire to cover: an exact description of the child's classroom; special resources available in the school district; the child's problems in various aspects of school; results of intelligence and school achievement tests; rating the child's present performance in different subjects; texts and teaching materials being used with the child; and a checklist of behavioral and emtional symptoms.

trist. Most child psychiatry clinics involve a social worker to get detailed information on the state of the family.

Even with a full complement of professionals, such an assessment may take three hours or more, the lion's share of time going into interviews with the child, parents, and teacher. This fact has made visits to child psychiatry clinics an endurance test for the child and parents, and one of the world's duller experiences for medical students. However, the interviewing time can be cut significantly by getting parents and teachers to fill out questionnaires beforehand. In these, parents and teachers briefly describe what they see as the child's problems in answers to open-ended questions, and then give an overall picture of the child's behavior in answering a series of structured questions. As an example, the questionnaire sent out to schools by the University of Iowa's Child Psychiatry Clinic is shown at the end of this chapter as an appendix. The reader will see that this is a convenient way to get information on the results of past intelligence and school achievement tests, the type of materials that are being used in the child's classroom, and what sorts of special educational help are available in the child's school district. This alone saves a good deal of time interviewing or telephoning teachers.

Some points need to be stressed. One cannot adequately assess the problems a child is having in school without at least talking with the teacher on the telephone. While it may not be practical for someone in practice to do this regularly, a visit to the child's classroom and a talk with the teacher and the principal is often more worthwhile and revealing than many more hours spent in one's own office trying to grasp the problems. In such visits one can quickly sense the atmosphere of a school and a classroom, learn the teacher's attitude toward a child, and get an idea as to how well the child is understood by people in the school. It is possible, though not likely, that one will see something of the actual problem. It is more likely that children, being forewarned, will be on their best behavior, at least when someone they already know comes to visit.

Some psychiatric clinics and a growing number of special education agencies now collect systematic data on a wide range of specific behaviors (e.g., "off task," "out of seat," "hitting") by sending trained observers to the classroom who count and record these behaviors over several twenty- to thirty minute periods. This system is made a great deal easier by using portable data loggers on which one can record many hours of data which can be transmitted directly to a computer.

A few details follow which I think are important. Probably the best single criterion of whether a child has a significant behavior problem or not is how well liked they are by their classmates. If the clinician doubts the judgment of the teacher, the child's popularity can be measured with a sociogram (Oden and Asher, 1977). Every child in the class is asked to write down his or her top three choices of a classmate to play with; the frequency with which one is nominated is the measure. There are variations allowing for different types of nomination, but the tests can be done unobtrusively as a part of a regular class routine and without singling out any particular child.

Tests of self-esteem are often revealing in what they show of a child's attitude toward himself. They are particularly helpful when, as in the Coopersmith or in the Piers-Harris, the responses can be broken down into different categories such as performance in school, behavior problems, and relations with the family. There is, unfortunately, an aspect of testing self-esteem that is commonly neglected: the difference between the child's subjective report and what outsiders see in his behavior. Coopersmith (1967) designed a questionnaire that could be filled out by parents or teachers and that was designed to be the objective counterpart of the child's self-report. With both reports, a clinician can know which children reveal self-doubt in their actions in addition to expressing it verbally, and which (a relatively small number) describe themselves as successful but are seen by adults as lacking self-confidence.

Again, on the subject of testing, those children who are found to have a serious reading disability as well as some behavioral or emotional problem often need to have their language skills assessed formally. There is a definite association between delayed language development and later difficulties in learning to read (Ingram et al., 1970). Whether programs for developing language skills do anything to improve reading skills is not yet clear, but there is evidence that improving language skills can help a child develop control over physical aggressiveness and impulsivity (Camp, 1977).

Finally, it is important to sound out parents on their attitudes toward the child's school and teachers. Occasionally one meets parents who belittle the importance of education or have strong antagonisms to a particular school or teacher, or who for some unknown reason sabotage teachers' efforts to help a difficult child. Fortunately, these complications are uncommon, but they need to be recognized and dealt with.

TREATMENT

Brophy and Good (1974) analyzed the interactions between children and their teachers and found that teachers tend to ignore the children with behavior problems. They do not call on them to answer questions and they are less likely to notice when these children want to take part in a discussion. Since children with behavior problems are less likely to make an interesting comment and more likely to say something provocative or silly, the teachers' behavior is easy to understand. However, it helps to set up a vicious cycle such as the one that operates in the homes of boys with conduct disorders (Patterson, 1974). Knowing that they are being passed over, the children are more likely to make impudent comments and to disrupt the class in order to get back at the teacher. When a man asked a famous rabbi what he should do about his wicked son, the answer was that he should love him all the more. This is a counsel of perfection, but teachers can at least become aware of their habits and deliberately adopt a policy of complete fairness.

People observing everyday events in the classroom have learned another simple lesson. Teachers generally reserve praise for good academic performance. They tend not to praise children for following the rules or for good social behavior. Rather, they criticize and punish infractions. It follows that children with behavior problems tend to get less praise and more criticism than their classmates. Coaching teachers to catch children being good and to praise them when they are behaving well, if only by accident, and doing this as often as they praise good academic work, has a positive effect on most of the children in the class. The badly behaved and the average children both spend more time at work than they did before. Minor bad behavior can be ignored, but major misbehavior should be dealt with privately rather than publicly.

Self-awareness

Teaching patients to label their behavior and rate its success is a basic part of psychotherapy with adults. Equally, it seems sensible that children, especially those with behavior problems, should be helped to label their behavior, to understand when it does not work and why. It seems particularly important for aggressive children because they have so little ability to control their impulses or responses to frustration. As previously noted, there is some reason to believe that such children are handicapped by poor language skills (Camp, 1977) which may be one reason for their lack of control. Techniques for helping students learn deliberate solutions to social or academic problems are centered on having children instruct themselves out loud as they work (Douglas, et al., 1976).

Other techniques for helping children to label their behavior are transactional analysis, talking over social situations shown on cards ("consequence cards," "sensitivity cards"), and immediate discussion of incidents with other children ("life space interviews"). Playing back videotapes of their natural behavior or of role playing are methods that have a strong impact on children, especially when the tapes are discussed with a teacher well-known and liked by the children. These tapes can be used as a focus for group discussions and problem solving.

Requiring a child to rate his or her own behavior on a simple form during the school day and having the child determine the reinforcement (e.g., points per period) is another technique widely used. As people have become more sophisticated about behavioral therapy, it has become obvious that children should be made responsible for carrying out their own behavior modification whenever possible and as early as possible. External control with strict contingency management is unlikely to help children over the long run. One clear advantage to having children track their own behavior and determine their rewards is that it makes the child practice self-awareness. Another way of doing this is to require the child to keep a detailed diary of each day's progress on the problem behaviors. For example, on the author's ward, children who are being trained in assertiveness record all the angry feelings they have had each day and how they have handled them.

Awareness of Others' Feelings

Attention to the skills involved in becoming aware of other people's feelings follows naturally from work on self-awareness. In role playing and role rehearsal, and in coaching children in specific social skills, the two functions go together. Evidence that self-awareness inhibits antisocial behavior has been reported for adults (Wicklund, 1979) but not as yet for children. On the other hand, Chandler (1973) and Chandler et al. (1974) have published interesting data showing that delinquents and children with behavior problems benefit from short programs of intensive role playing in groups. Moreover, Chandler has established some relatively simple tests with which one can measure a child's awareness of others' feelings and follow the effects of treatment.

Social Skills

Oden and Asher (1977) have reported encouraging results from a relatively brief period of training given to socially isolated children, a group that probably included a proportion of aggressive and antisocial children as well as some that were withdrawn. The target children were chosen on their sociometric scores and these were later used as a criterion for effects of treatment. The coaching consisted of verbal instruction in social skills, practicing the skills and playing with a peer, and a review session after the play. The specific skills taught were how to take part in a game, how to take turns and share, how to talk with and listen to another, and how to help or give attention to another child. Six treatment sessions, each one lasting about twenty-five minutes, were given over a period of about a month. There were two groups of controls, one which had no treatment and one in which subjects played with peers but had no coaching.

The second set of sociometric ratings showed that the coached children made significantly greater gains as "someone I'd like to play with" than the two control groups. The children were rated again a year later and the coached group had continued to gain in popularity. At that point, the once-isolated children who had been coached were only slightly below the mean for their classes, whereas the two other groups remained about one standard deviation below the mean. That this modest course of training in social skills should have a significant and lasting effect on peer relationships in a group of problem children is an exciting lead. Many school districts now have teachers and counselors who are trained in applying this form of treatment, and there are an ever-increasing number of specific programs (Carltedge and Milburn, 1980).

Assertiveness

An interesting body of research has accumulated on the measurement of assertiveness in adults, the relationship of anxiety, depression, and low self-esteem to the inability to assert oneself normally, and on the effects of training (Rathus, 1973; Orenstein et al., 1975; Pachman and Foy, 1978). So far little or no research has been done on the same questions with children. However, my experience is that children and adolescents can be readily trained to be assertive in constuctive ways and that this is helpful for children who are anxious, depressed, or handicapped by low self-esteem as well as for those who are unduly aggressive. A vital part of the training is to get children to express their feelings openly and deliberately, in naturally occurring or engineered challenges. When they can do this successfully, they are able to handle everyday frustrations in a mature way.

An important part of assertiveness training is persuading a child to see himself or herself in a positive light. Two particularly good books to help children see the good things in themselves are *Liking Myself* and the *The Mouse, the Monster, and Me* by Palmer (1977a, 1977b). These are intended to stimulate conversations between parent, teacher, or therapist and the child on reasonable attitudes toward oneself.

Impulse Control and Problem Solving

Training in impulse control and problem solving has its origins in the work of Luria (1961). This distinguished Russian psychologist carried out experiments to find how children of different ages used speech while they performed tasks. He observed that children went through phases of commenting on tasks out loud, directing themselves through tasks, and finally thinking their plans out before starting their tasks. From his findings he argued that children developed control over their behavior by internalizing the directions they have learned from adults. Several groups of investigators have developed treatment programs based on his work.

Two serious tests of this method of treatment have been reported. Douglas et al. (1976) used modeling, self-instruction, and self-reinforcement to teach hyperactive children effective ways of solving various problems. All of the boys involved had been rated as impulsive by their parents and teachers and had low latency scores on the Kagan matching familiar figures test. Training took place in twenty-four one-hour sessions spread over a period of three months. The instructor demonstrated how to solve various problems and talked his or her way through the tasks. The subject then practiced the same approaches. In succeeding sessions subjects were taught to internalize the directions they gave themselves. They were also taught to plan ahead, to remember vital cues, and to take account of other children's feelings when playing with them. At the end of treatment the experimental group (eighteen boys) had made modest but significant improvement in performance on Kagan's matching familiar figures test and the Bender-Gestalt, and gave healthier responses on a story-completion test that was designed to assess children's responses to frustration. The controls (eleven hyperactive boys) had not changed. Subjects' improvment lasted at least to a second assessment done three months later.

Camp et al. (1977) described the results of a similar program, but one that focused more on verbal mediation and self-control. The subjects were twenty-three boys in second grade who had been rated by their teachers as very aggressive; twelve were treated and eleven were controls. A number of standard cognitive tests were given before and after treatment and the subject's speech during the testing was recorded. Half-hour sessions were held every school day for six weeks. The results of the treatment, known as "think aloud," were quite impressive. Irrelevant, self-distracting speech during the testing was reduced and the experimental subjects showed signs of being more reflective. However, there was little evidence that their classroom behavior improved. I believe that these early studies are promising and that it is certainly worthwhile to try them in working with any child who is markedly impulsive, impatient, or lacking in tolerance for frustration.

Physical Approaches

Many shy, anxious children are particularly embarrassed by their failures in gym and sports. Children with conduct disorders, learning disabilities, and other mental or physical handicaps may also suffer from clumsiness or weakness, and not do well in athletics. There are few things that children worry more about than whether they will make a fool of themselves in the fitness tests given in grade school. Individual or small-group training from an activity therapist can boost a child's self-esteem significantly by building confidence in his or her own body. Training can be directed at the usual skills of throwing and catching balls, increasing strength and endurance, or developing special interests such as weight lifting.

Taking this idea further, many young people have experienced an increase of self-confidence from taking a wilderness survival course such as the well-known Outward Bound. In the United States there are five official Outward Bound programs and many other offshoots, all of which involve activities such as white-water canoeing, rappeling, mountain climbing, strenuous backpacking, and solo camping. The idea is to challenge an individual's personal resources and bring out abilities that the young person never knew he or she had. A further benefit, useful for aggressive and antisocial children, is that there is forced training in social skills. For example, young people have to learn to get along well together if they are to rely on each other for security during mountain climbing. There is some evidence that these programs do increase assertiveness and self-esteem (Smith et al., 1975) and that there are short-term effects, at least on recidivism in delinquency (Kelly and Baer, 1971). The Child Psychiatry Service at the University of Iowa has run such courses for seven years. My colleagues and I find that one of the most obvious benefits is that the young people go back to school with a much better attitude toward their work.

Conclusion

Psychological methods for studying children's emotional and behavioral problems in school have become thorough and objective. Many promising but largely untested treatments are available which seem to fit the most troublesome of children's psychiatric handicaps. However, our knowledge of the problems themselves, the patterns in which they occur, their course, and their origins lags far behind.

CONFIDENTIAL TO CHILD PSYCHIATRY SERVICE, PSYCHIATRIC HOSPITAL, IOWA CITY, IOWA 52242

REFERRING SCHOOL REPORT

Please complete the following form. The information you provide will assist in evaluating the child's abilities and handicaps.

Name of Child _____   Date of Report _____

School _____   Age _____ Grade _____

Teacher _____   Principal _____

Report compiled by _____   Position _____

Child's Classroom

( ) a. Self-contained (specify size) _____

( ) b. Departmentalized

( ) c. Ungraded

( ) d. Modular Grouping

( ) e. Special Education (specify type) _____

( ) f. Remedial Assistance (specify areas) _____

( ) g. Other _____

( ) h. Not attending (specify since when and why) _____

Please check resources available to your school, district, or area.

( ) learning disabilities class ( ) or teacher

( ) emotional disabilities class ( ) or teacher

( ) resource room

( ) remedial reading class

( ) strategist

( ) counselor

( ) speech clinician

( ) social worker

List other relevant resources: _____

What problems do you see in this child's schoolwork?

What problems do you see in this child's behavior at school?

What problems do you see in this child's relationships with teachers and other students?

Describe methods which you are trying with this child. How successful are they?

What help would you like from us in further understanding this child or in working with him/her?

Please list or attach results and subtest scores on the following:

Intelligence

Name of Test*	Date	VIQ	PIQ	FSIQ	CA	MA	Examiner

*For most recent testing include scaled scores if available.

Achievement

Name of Test	Date	Grade	Results (subtests and composite raw scores, grade equivalents, percentiles, etc.)

Other (i.e., ITPA, Wepman, Key Math, etc.)

Name of Test	Date	Results

How would you judge the child's academic performance this year?

	Functional Grade Level	Receives Special Help (X if Yes)	Progress (1-5 Scale*)
Reading			
Math			
Spelling			
Handwriting			
Language Arts/English			

*Scale   1-None   2-Unsatisfactory   3-Inconsistent   4-Satisfactory   5-Excellent

Please list all texts and special materials, and the last page worked on, in the areas of reading, math, and language arts.

    1)   Reading Materials   Page

    2)   Mathematics Materials   Page

    3)   Language Arts Materials   Page

If you want to tell us anything else, please use this space.

Your answers to the following questions will help us to understand the child's personality. Please check the statements about him or her as "Definitely true" if they are things that you see often in the child and that you feel are problems. If you see the behavior only some of the time or if you do not feel it is a problem check "No more than most children of the same age." If you think the child is the opposite (for example, doesn't ever worry, has too good an opinion of her/himself, or is inactive) check the third column. If you are not sure which is the right answer check "No more than most children of the same age." Please put one check only against each statement.

	Definitely true	No more than most children of the same age	The opposite
1. Hard to make him/her mind; no method of discipline seems to work.	____	____	____
2. Wants more attention than other children.	____	____	____
3. Does not work long at projects, school work. Often leaves work unfinished.	____	____	____
4. Afraid of new situations, experiences.	____	____	____
5. Has low opinion of self, lacks self-confidence.	____	____	____
6. Bad temper, has tantrums.	____	____	____
7. Shy with other children.	____	____	____
8. Daring, knows no fear.	____	____	____
9. Often fights with other children.	____	____	____
10. Has special fears; for example, of being alone, animals, or water.	____	____	____
11. Not well liked by other children.	____	____	____
12. Worries a lot.	____	____	____
13. Easily upset, cries often.	____	____	____
14. Gets wound up and silly in groups of children.	____	____	____
15. Often does things without thinking.	____	____	____
16. Has a lot of aches, pains, complaints about body.	____	____	____
17. Unhappy most of time.	____	____	____
18. Always in a hurry, easily frustrated.	____	____	____
19. Very active, hardly ever still.	____	____	____
20. Fussy; things have to be "just so."	____	____	____
21. Has to be first or to win.	____	____	____
22. Often destroys property of others.	____	____	____
23. Mean to younger or smaller children.	____	____	____
24. Shouts at or abuses adults.	____	____	____

		Definitely true	No more than most children of the same age	The opposite
25.	Teases other children a lot.	___	___	___
26.	Solitary, keeps to herself/himself.	___	___	___
27.	Often ignored or excluded from group activity by other children.	___	___	___
28.	Appears indifferent to other children's problems.	___	___	___
29.	Does not follow general classroom routine.	___	___	___
30.	Has difficulty concentrating.	___	___	___
31.	Gets back at other children.	___	___	___
32.	Lies to get out of trouble.	___	___	___

How well do you know this child? Very well_____   Fairly well_____   Not well_____

The subject you teach _____

Approximate number of hours per week you have contact with this child _____

REFERENCES

Achenbach, T. M. 1978. The child behavior profile. Boys aged 6–11. *J. Consult. Clin. Psychol.,* 46:478–488.

August, G. J., and Stewart, M. A. 1982. Is there a syndrome of pure hyperactivity? *Brit. J. Psychiat.,* 140:305–311.

Birleson, P. 1981. The validity of depressive disorder in childhood and the development of a self-rating scale: A research report. *J. Child Psychol. Psychiat.,* 22:73–88.

Brophy, J. E., and Good, T. L. 1974. *Teacher-student relationships: Causes and consequences.* New York: Holt, Rinehart and Winston.

Camp, B. W. 1977. Verbal mediation in young aggressive boys. *J. Abnorm. Psychol.,* 86:145–153.

Camp, B. W., Blom, G. E., Hebert, F., and van Doorninck, W. J. 1977. "Think aloud": A program for developing self-control in young aggressive boys. *J. Abnorm. Child Psychol.,* 5:157–169.

Carlson, G. A., and Cantwell, D. P. 1979. A survey of depressive symptoms in a child and adolescent psychiatric population. *J. Am. Acad. Child Psychiat.,* 18:587–599.

Cartledge, G., and Milburn, J. F. 1980. *Teaching social skills to children.* New York: Pergamon Press.

Chandler, M. J. 1973. Egocentrism and antisocial behavior: The assessment and training of social perspective-taking skills. *Dev. Psychol.,* 9:326–332.

Chandler, M. J., Greenspan, S., and Barenboim, C. 1974. Assessment and training of role-taking and referential communication skills in institutionalized emotionally disturbed children. *Dev. Psychol.,* 10:546–553.

Clegg, A., and Megson, B. 1968. *Children in distress.* Baltimore: Penguin Books.

Coopersmith, S. 1967. *The antecedents of self-esteem.* San Francisco: Freeman, W. H.

Coopersmith, S. 1968. Studies in self-esteem. *Scientific American,* 218:96–106.

Douglas, V. I., Parry, P., Marton, P., and Garson, C. 1976. Assessment of a cognitive training program for hyperactive children. *J. Abnorm. Child Psychol.,* 4:389–410.

Hewitt, L., and Jenkins, R. L. 1946. *Fundamental patterns of maladjustment.* State of Illinois, Springfield.

Ingram, T. T. S., Mason, A. W., and Blackburn, I. 1970. A retrospective study of 82 children with reading disability. *Dev. Med. Child Neurol.,* 12:271–281.

Kellam, S. G., Ensminger, M. E., and Simon, M. B. 1980. Mental health in first grade and teenage drug, alcohol, and cigarette use. *Drug Alc. Depend.,* 5:273–304.

Kelly, F. J., and Baer, D. J. 1971. Physical challenge as a treatment for delinquency. *Crime Delinq.* 14:437–445.

Kolvin, I., Ounsted, C., Humphrey, M., and McNay, A. II. 1971. The phenomenology of childhood psychoses. *Brit. J. Psychiat.,* 118:385–395.

Kuperman, S., and Stewart, M. A. 1979. The diagnosis of depression in children. *J. Affect. Dis.,* 1:213–217.

Langner, T. S., Gersten, J. C., Greene, E. L., Eisenberg, J. G., Herson, J. H., and McCarthy, E. D. 1974. Treatment of psychological disorders among urban children. *J. Consult. Clin. Psychol.,* 42:170–179.

Loney, J., Kramer, J., and Milich, R. 1981. The hyperkinetic child grows up: Predictors of symptoms, delinquency, and achievement at follows-up. In *Psychosocial aspects of drug treatment for hyperactivity,* ed. K. Gadow, and J. Loney. Boulder, Colo.: Westview Press.

Loney, J., and Milich, R. 1982. Hyperactivity, inattention, and aggression in clinical practice. In *Advances in behavioral pediatrics,* vol. 2, ed. M. Wolraich, and D. K. Routh, pp. 113–142. Greenwich, Conn.: JAI Press.

Luria, A. R. 1961. *The role of speech in the regulation of normal and abnormal behavior.* New York: Liveright.

Manheimer, D. I., and Mellinger, G. D. 1967. Personality characteristics of the child accident repeater. *Child Dev.,* 38:491–513.

Morris, D. P., Soroker, E., and Burruss, G. 1954. Follow-up studies of shy, withdrawn children. I. Evaluation of later adjustment. *Am. J. Orthopsych.,* 24:743–754.

Nylander, I. 1979. A 20-year prospective follow-up study of 2164 cases at the child guidance clinics in Stockholm. *Acta Paed. Scand.,* 276 (suppl.): 1–45.

Oden, S., and Asher, S. R. 1977. Coaching children in social skills for friendship making. *Child Dev.,* 48:495–506.

Olweus, D. 1979. Stability of aggressive reaction patterns in males: A review. *Psychol. Bull.,* 86:852–875.

Orenstein, H., Orenstein, E., and Carr, J. E. 1975. Assertiveness and anxiety: A correlational study. *J. Beh. Ther. Exp. Psych.,* 6:203–207.

Pachman, J. S., and Foy, D. W. 1978. A correlational investigation of anxiety, self-esteem, and depression: New findings with behavioral measures of assertiveness. *J. Beh. Ther. Exp. Psych.,* 9:97–101.

Palmer, P. 1977a. *Liking myself.* San Luis Obispo, Calif.: Impact Publishers.

Palmer, P. 1977b. *The mouse, the monster, and me.* San Luis Obispo, Calif.: Impact Publishers.

Patterson, G. R. 1974. Retraining of aggressive boys by their parents: Review of recent literature and follow-up evaluation. *Can. Psychiat. Assoc. J.,* 19:142–161.

Patterson, G. R., Littman, R. A., and Bricker, W. 1967. Assertive behavior in children: A step toward a theory of aggression. *Monogr. Soc. Res. Child Dev.,* 32:1–43.

Pearce, J. B. 1978. The recognition of depressive disorder in children. *J. Royal Soc. Med.,* 71:494–500.

Piers, E. V. 1969. *The Piers-Harris children's self-concept scale.* Nashville: Counselor Recordings and Tests.

Piers, E. V. 1977. Children's self-esteem, level of esteem certainty, and responsibility for success and failure. *J. Genet. Psychol.,* 130:295–304.

Quitkin, F., and Klein, D. F. 1969. Two behavioral syndromes in young adults related to possible minimal brain dysfunction. *J. Psychiat. Res.,* 7:131–142.

Rathus, S. A. 1973. A 30-item schedule for assessing assertive behavior. *Beh. Ther.,* 4:398–406.

Robins, L. 1966. *Deviant children grown up.* Baltimore: Williams and Wilkins.

Robins, L. N. 1978. Sturdy childhood predictors of adult antisocial behavior: Replications from longitudinal studies. *Psychol. Med.,* 8:611–622.

Rosenberg, M. 1962. The association between self-esteem and anxiety. *J. Psychiat. Res.,* 1:135–152.

Rosenberg, M. 1965. *Society and the adolescent self-image.* Princeton: Princeton University Press.

Rutter, M., Cox, A., Tupling, C., Berger, M., and Yule, W. 1975. Attainment and adjustment in two geographical areas. I. The prevalence of psychiatric disorder. *Brit. J. Psychiat.,* 126:493–509.

Rutter, M., Tizard, J., and Whitmore, K. 1970. *Education, health, and behavior.* London: Longman.

Shaffer, D., and Fisher, P. 1981. The epidemiology of suicide in children and young adolescents. *J. Am. Acad. Child Psychiat.,* 20:545–565.

Shepherd, M., Oppenheim, B., and Mitchell, S. 1971. *Childhood behavior and mental health.* New York: Grune and Stratton.

Smith, M. L., Gabriel, R., Schott, J., and Padia, W. L. 1975. Evaluation of the effects of Outward Bound. In *Evaluation studies review annual.* Denver: University of Colorado, pp. 400–421.

Stewart, M. A., de Blois, C. S., Meardon, J., and Cummings, C. 1980. Aggressive conduct disorder of children. *J. Nerv. Ment. Dis.,* 168:604–610.

Weiss, G., Hechtman, L., Perlman, T., Hopkins, J., and Wener, A. 1979. Hyperactives as young adults. *Arch. Gen. Psychiat.,* 36:675–681.

Werner, E., Bierman, J. M., French, F. E., Simonian, K., Connor, A., Smith, R. S., and Campbell, M. 1968. Reproductive and environmental casualties: A report on the 10-year follow-up of the children of the Kauai pregnancy study. *Pediat.,* 42:112–126.

West, D. J., and Farrington, D. P. 1973. *Who becomes delinquent?* London: Heinemann.

West, D. J., and Farrington, D. P. 1977. *The delinquent way of life.* London: Heinemann.

Wicklund, R. A. 1979. The influence of self-awareness on human behavior. *Am. Scientist.,* 67:187–193.

Winokur, G., and Holemon, E. 1963. Chronic anxiety neurosis: Clinical and sexual aspects. *Acta Psychiat. Scand.,* 39:384–412.

Wolff, S., and Barlow, A. 1979. Schizoid personality in childhood: A comparative study of schizoid, autistic, and normal children. *J. Child Psychol. Psychiat.,* 20:29–46.

Wolff, S., and Chick, J. 1980. Schizoid personality in childhood: A controlled follow-up study. *Psychol. Med.,* 10:85–100.

SPECIAL SITUATIONS

17

Child Abuse and Neglect

ARTHUR GREEN

DEFINITION OF CHILD ABUSE AND NEGLECT

The definition of child abuse has been continually expanding in recent years. In a classic paper, "The Battered Child Syndrome," Kempe and his collaborators (1962) described child abuse as the infliction of serious injury upon young children by parents and caretakers. The injuries, which included fractures, subdural hematoma, and multiple soft tissue injuries, often resulted in permanent disability and death. Fontana's concept of the "maltreatment syndrome" (1964) viewed child abuse as one end of a spectrum of maltreatment which also included emotional deprivation, neglect, and malnutrition. Helfer (1975) recognized the prevalence of minor injuries resulting from abuse and suspected that abuse might be implicated in 10% of all childhood accidents treated in emergency rooms. Gil (1974) extended the concept of child abuse to include any action that prevents children from achieving their physical and psychological potential.

According to most state laws, child abuse is defined as the infliction of injury on a child by a parent or guardian and encompasses the total range of physical injury. Child abuse is differentiated from child neglect, which usually refers to the failure of the parent or caretaker to provide the child with adequate physical care and supervision. Abandonment of a child also constitutes neglect. The legal definitions of child abuse and neglect stated in the New York State Child Protective Services Act of 1973 are as follows:

> Definition of Child Abuse: An "abused child"' is a child less than 16 years of age whose parent or other person legally responsible for his care:
> 1. inflicts or allows to be inflicted upon the child serious physical injury, or
> 2. creates or allows to be created a substantial risk of serious injury, or
> 3. commits or allows to be committed against the child an act of sexual abuse as defined in the penal law.

Definition of Child Neglect: A "neglected child" is a child, under 18 years of age, impaired as a result of the failure of his parent or other person legally responsible for his care to exercise a minimum degree of care:
1. in supplying the child with adequate food, clothing, shelter, education, medical or surgical care, though financially able to do so or offered financial or other reasonable means to do so, or
2. in providing the child with proper supervision or guardianship, or
3. by reasonably inflicting or allowing to be inflicted harm or a substantial risk thereof, including the infliction of excessive corporal punishment, or
4. by using a drug or drugs, or
5. by using alcoholic beverages to the extent that he loses self-control of his actions, or
6. by any other acts of a similarly serious nature requiring the aid of the family court.

A "neglected child" is also a child, under 18 years of age, who has been abandoned by his parents or other person legally responsible for his care.

DETECTION OF CHILD ABUSE

The possibility of child abuse must be considered in every child who presents with an injury. A careful history and physical evaluation is warranted when one suspects physical abuse. The physical examination should include a routine X-ray survey of all children under five and laboratory tests to rule out the possibility of an abnormal bleeding tendency. The child, of course, should be hospitalized during this diagnostic evaluation.

While there is no single physical finding or diagnostic procedure that can confirm the diagnosis of child abuse with absolute certainty, the presence of some of the following signs and symptoms derived from the history-taking and physical examination is suggestive of an inflicted injury:

History

1. Unexplained delay in bringing the child for treatment following the injury.
2. History is implausible or contradictory.
3. History is incompatible with the physical findings.
4. There is a history of repeated suspicious injuries.
5. The parent blames the injury on a sibling or a third party.
6. The parent maintains that the injury was self-inflicted.
7. The child had been taken to numerous hospitals for the treatment of injuries (hospital "shopping").
8. The child accused the parent or caretaker of injuring him.
9. The parent has a previous history of abuse as a child.
10. The parent has unrealistic and premature expectations of the child.

Physical Findings

1. Pathognomonic "typical" injuries commonly associated with physical punishment, such as bruises on the buttocks and lower back and bruises in the genital area or inner thigh, may be inflicted after the child wets or soils, or is resistant to toilet training. Bruises and soft tissue injuries at different stages of healing are signs of repeated physical abuse. Bruises of a special configuration, such as hand marks, grab marks, pinch marks, and strap marks, usually indicate abuse.

2. Certain types of burns are typically inflicted, e. g., multiple cigarette burns, scalding of hands or feet, burns of perineum and buttocks.
3. Abdominal trauma leading to a ruptured liver or spleen.
4. Subdural hematoma with or without skull fracture.
5. Radiologic signs, such as subperiosteal hemorrhages, epiphyseal separations, metaphyseal fragmentation, periosteal shearing, and periosteal calcifications.
6. Eye injuries, including retinal hemorrhage, dislocated lens, and detached retina.

DIFFERENTIAL DIAGNOSIS

Bone Diseases

Several bone diseases may result in fractures and pathological alterations in the bones which can resemble lesions caused by physical abuse. Some of these are osteogenesis imperfecta, congenital syphilis, scurvy, osteomyelitis, infantile cortical hyperostosis of Caffey, and spina bifida. These diseases may be identified by characteristic radiological findings.

Bleeding Disorders

Some inflicted soft tissue injuries resulting in bleeding and bruising might simulate various forms of purpura or hemophilia. The bleeding disorders may be detected by coagulation studies, including a platelet count, bleeding time, prothrombin time, partial thromboplastin time, and thrombin time.

Accidental Injuries

Although inflicted injuries are often described by the parents as "accidents," true accidental injuries are fairly common in young children. Accidental injuries may usually, but not always, be distinguished from inflicted injuries by the absence of the "typical" abusive history and physical findings outlined previously.

Abuse Committed by Siblings

Infants and toddlers may be seriously injured by older siblings. These attacks are often motivated by rivalry and jealousy of the "baby" who is perceived as the recipient of most of the parent's love and attention. The "abusive" sibling is often the one who had been previously abused or scapegoated by the parent (Green, 1984).

SCOPE OF THE PROBLEM

The classic description of "the battered child syndrome" by Kempe and his associates in 1962 stimulated nationwide interest in child abuse, which soon became recognized as a major pediatric problem. Between 1963 and 1965, the passage of laws by all fifty states requiring medical reporting of all suspected cases of child abuse led to the formation of child protective services throughout the country. Abusing parents were subjected to investigation and legal process, and the first psychological studies of abusing parents were finally carried out during this period. The improved reporting procedures have demonstrated the true magnitude of this problem. The child abuse law in New York State became effective on July 1, 1964. During the first twelve-month period, 313 cases of child abuse were reported in New York City with 16 deaths. New York City statistics from 1982 indicated that 4,228 were reported with 98 deaths. An additional 43,176 children were reported to be neglected. The huge increase in reported cases of child abuse over a seventeen-year period undoubtedly reflects an improvement in reporting procedures as well as an absolute increase in the incidence of child abuse. Yet, according to most experts in this field, there are 15 to 20 actual cases of child abuse for each one reported, so that the statistics only show the "tip of the iceberg." In 1980, 30% of the 58,000 reports of abuse and neglect in New York State involved children under five years of age. Light (1973) estimated an annual nationwide abuse incidence of 200,000 to 500,000, with 1,500,000 cases of maltreatment if severe neglect and sexual abuse were included. This figure is approximately equivalent to an estimate by Douglas Besharov (1975), Director of the National Center of Child Abuse and Neglect. Besharov indicated that 1,600,000 cases of child abuse and neglect occur each year with 2,000 to 4,000 deaths.

Maltreatment is currently regarded as a leading cause of death in children and a major public-health problem. The proliferation of child abuse and neglect might bear some relationship to the alarming general increase in violence in our society, demonstrated by the rising incidence of violent crimes, delinquency, suicide, and lethal accidents.

Characteristics of Abusing Parents

The late 1960s witnessed the growth of a sizable literature on the characteristics of maltreating parents. The quantity and scope of clinical studies in this area has increased dramatically during the current decade and has included observations of abused children and parent-child interaction in maltreating families. The initial studies were impressionistic and naive, and largely consisted of observations of a few abusing parents. Many of the early investigators sought to discover a single personality trait or psychological abnormality that could explain the phenomenon of child abuse. They also failed to include control groups in their studies, which led to faulty conclusions and generalizations. Many of the characteristics ascribed to abusing parents, such as immaturity, impulsivity, social isolation, and a tendency to depend too much on their children were too general and were present in large numbers of nonabusing parents.

Fortunately, the quality of the research in this area has improved during the past few years. The federal government began to actively support research through its National Center on Child Abuse and Neglect which was established in 1974. The more recent research has been based on the theory of multiple causality, focusing on the relative contributions of parental personality factors, demographic data, environmental and socioeconomic variables, and the characteristics of the target children. Many of the studies documented differences for abusing parents. Starr et al. (1978) observed that abusing mothers had significantly lower IQ scores than matched control mothers of children hospitalized for nontraumatic medical emergencies. The abusing mothers also reported significantly more stressful events during the past year and had lower annual incomes. They were more socially isolated than the controls. The abusers also scored higher on "denial of the complexity of child rearing" as measured by the Choler Maternal Attitudes Scale. Wolock and Horowitz (1977) interviewed single-parent welfare mothers who were divided into abuse only, neglect and abuse, neglect only, and nonmaltreating comparison mothers. The abusing mothers differed from the comparisons in that they experienced greater difficulties growing up (poverty, beatings, inadequate food and clothing, etc.), reported less positive attitudes toward their children, and were more socially isolated. The neglecting families were differentiated from comparison families by having larger numbers of children.

Chapa (1978) compared seventy-six families involved with maltreatment (either abuse or neglect) with ninety-two comparison families selected at random from a street directory. The results indicated that two to three times as many maltreaters as controls reported that at times they could not cope with life. Fewer maltreating parents lived with both natural parents and more experienced greater physical punishment as children. With regard to childrearing variables, two to three times as many maltreaters as controls reported feeling inadequate as parents and finding child-care responsibilities too burdensome for them. The maltreating parents were more restrictive and used harsher child-rearing measures than the controls.

Green (1976) compared 60 mothers of abused children with 30 neglecting mothers and 30 normal controls obtained from a pediatric outpatient clinic. The majority of the 120 mothers were black or Hispanic and resided in the inner-city slums. The results indicated that the mothers of the abused children most frequently reported these children to be problems at home and in school. These mothers also reported more marital difficulties than the neglecting and control mothers, and a higher incidence of being beaten by their husbands or boyfriends. A significantly higher percentage of these mothers described a poor relationship with their own parents. The mothers of the neglected children reported the highest percentage of unplanned pregnancies and the absence of a husband or male companion at home. The neglecting mothers also exhibited the highest incidence of alcoholism, psychosis, and chronic physical illness.

It is striking that although fathers share equal responsibility with mothers for child abuse, psychological investigation of male child abusers has been conspicuously absent from the battered-child literature. The only specific characteristics attributed to abusing fathers have been their passivity and tendency to reverse domestic roles with their wives because of lack of employment (Merrill, 1962; Galdston, 1965). Green (1979) studied abusing fathers and father surrogates (stepfathers, mother's boyfriends, etc.) during their participation in a child-abuse treatment program. These men often manifested extreme jealousy of their spouse's attention toward the target child, based upon unresolved sibling rivalry and maternal deprivation experienced during their own childhoods. These fathers typically beat their wives or girlfriends in addition to the children. They were usually unemployed, or vocationally inadequate, and abused alcohol. The abuse was frequently provoked by a sudden or unexpected increase in child-care responsibility, often created by the absence or illness of their wives, and it was often associated with excessive drinking.

Parent-Child Interaction in Abusing Families

The failure to adequately explain the phenomenon of child abuse solely on the basis of parental character traits, predisposing factors in the child, or environmental stress has led to a recent interest in observing parent-child interaction within maltreating families. These observations permit us to study the reciprocal impact of parent and child upon one another during varying levels of stress.

Burgess and Conger (1977) studied daily interaction in abusing, neglecting, and control families. The families were observed in their homes by trained, naive observers. The abusing and neglecting families displayed lower rates of overall interaction. Abusing and neglecting mothers exhibited positive interaction (affectionate and supportive behavior) significantly less frequently than the mothers in the control families. On the other hand, the abusing and neglecting mothers displayed much higher rates of negative behavior (threats and complaints, etc.) toward their children than the control mothers. Reid and Taplin (1977) found that abusive families exhibited significantly higher rates of aversive behavior than did families with no history of abuse. Gaensbauer and Sands (1979) observed that the reciprocity of mother-infant interaction was impaired in cases of child abuse. The infants often failed to respond to their mothers' attempts to initiate interaction, often resulting in parallel play in which sustained reciprocal interactions are rare. When social contact was left to the infant's initiative, proximity seeking to the mother and bids for attention were less frequent than in the normal population. Robison and Solomon (1979) reported avoidance of eye contact between abused toddlers and their mothers in a structured play situation, in contrast to their close physical proximity.

Wasserman et al. (1983) described significant differences in mother-infant interaction between abusing and nonabusing dyads. The abusing mothers displayed less interactive behavior with their infants and often ignored them. When these mothers attempted to initiate play, their infants were less likely to respond. The nonabusing mothers, on the other hand, demonstrated more positive affect and made more frequent attempts to engage the baby in games and other interactions. The nonabused infants played more actively and complied to their mothers' attempts to change and direct their focus. The abusing mothers lacked skills in positively arousing their babies and themselves.

These observations suggest that the abusing dyad might be locked into a mutually reinforcing negative spiral, in which the mother is unable to display the kinds of positive affective behavior required to engage her infant, and the infant, in turn, is less likely to respond to the mother's attempts at initiating play. This might cause the mother to withdraw further. A vicious cycle may ensue, consisting of ineffective or inappropriate maternal responsiveness, discomfort and withdrawal in the infant, and further frustration and lack of confidence in the mother, leading to asynchrony and a lack of reciprocity in the dyadic relationship.

Psychodynamics

On the basis of his extensive therapeutic intervention in abusive families, Green (1980) postulated that the psychodynamics in a given case of child abuse are largely determined by the "abuse-prone" personality traits of the parent while he or she interacts with a "difficult" child in an unsupportive, nongratifying environment. The relationship between the abusing parent and the child is distorted by the cumulative impact of the parent's own traumatic experiences as a child reared in a punitive, unloving environment. Individuals who abuse their children cannot envision any parent-child relationship as a mutually gratifying experience. The task of parenting mobilizes identifications with the parent-aggressor, child-victim dyad of the past. The key psychodynamic elements in child abuse are role reversal, excessive use of denial and projection as defenses, rapidly shifting identifications with the child, and displacement of aggression from frustrating objects onto the child.

Role reversal occurs when the unfulfilled abusing parent seeks dependency gratification —which is unavailable from spouse and family—from the "parentified" child. It is based on an identification with the "child-victim." The child's inability to gratify the parent causes him or her to be unconsciously perceived as the rejecting mother. This intensifies parents' feelings of rejection and worthlessness which threaten their narcissistic equilibrium. These painful feelings are denied and projected onto the child, who then becomes the recipient of the parents' self-directed aggression.

This is accomplished by a shift toward identification with the aggressive parent, terminating the role reversal. By beating the child, the abuser assuages his or her punitive superego and attempts to actively master the traumatic experiences passively endured as a child. The scapegoating process continues as the child becomes the additional target for aggression displaced from various despised and frustrating objects in the parent's current and past life, such as a rejecting mate or lover, a hated sibling rival, or a depriving parent substitute. The objects are unconsciously linked to the original "parent-aggressor."

The choice of a particular child for scapegoating might depend upon accidental factors such as time of birth, physical appearance, temperament, and/or sex, in addition to actual physical or psychological deviancy. It is ultimately based upon the child's capacity to evoke the negatively perceived characteristics of the parents or of significant others.

Characteristics of Abused Children

Elmer (1965) studied the effects of abuse by comparing abused and nonabused children who had been hospitalized for multiple bone injuries. The abused children showed a higher incidence of mental retardation and speech difficulties. Martin (1972) reported a study in which one-third of a sample of abused children were mentally retarded, 43% were neurologically damaged, and 38% exhibited delayed language development. Morse, Sahler, and Friedman (1970) discovered mental deficiency in 70% of a group of children whose injuries resulted from abuse or neglect. Green (1968) documented a high incidence of self-mutilation in schizophrenic children who had been physically abused. Martin and Beezely (1976) observed the following personality characteristics in a group of fifty abused children: impaired capacity for pleasure, low self-esteem, school learning problems, withdrawal, oppositionalism, hypervigilance, compulsivity, and pseudo-mature behavior.

Behavioral observations of abused children have found them to be stubborn, unresponsive, negativistic, and depressed (Johnson and Morse, 1968); fearful, apathetic, and unappealing with a blunting of their appetite for food and human contact (Galdston, 1965); and likely to provoke physical attack from others.

Kempe (1976) observed delays in speech, motor, and social development in a group of thirteen preschool abused children. In relating to adults, they were anxious and fearful and expected punishment or criticism. These children often demonstrated an impaired capacity to play and to make use of toys. Galdston (1971) described puposeless, unpredictable, and unpremeditated violent behavior in a group of abused boys of preschool age at a special day-care treatment center. The abused girls of this age group were less aggressive. They demonstrated more withdrawal and reliance on autoerotic activities. Both the boys and girls exhibited bodily awkwardness and poor motor coordination.

Abused infants have recently become a focus for clinical observations. Kempe (1976) noted that abused infants below six months of age were frequently irritable with a high-pitched irritable cry. These infants also exhibited difficulties with feeding, were hard to satisfy, and began to demonstrate delays in motor and social development. Kempe also described impaired social responsiveness in these infants which became noticeable between six and twelve months of age. These abused infants failed to demonstrate the usual anxiety upon separation from their parents or when they were confronted with strangers. They also exhibited "frozen watchfulness," consisting of intense scanning of the environment accompanied by motor passivity and immobility. Gaensbauer and Sands (1979) documented disturbances in affective communication in a group of abused infants, including social and affective withdrawal, diminished capacity for pleasure, a proneness toward negative affects such as distress, sadness, and anger, and an unpredictability and shallowness in affective expression. The infants demonstrated a weakened attachment to their mothers and caregivers.

Unfortunately, the reliability of these observations must be questioned because of their failure to include nontraumatized normal control groups. However, a recent controlled study by George and Main (1979) revealed similar impairment in social and affective behavior in abused infants and toddlers. These investigators observed that abused children from one to three years of age physically assaulted their peers in a day-care setting twice as often as the nonabused controls. They also harassed their caregivers verbally, and nonverbally, and were the only children who assaulted or threatened to assault them. The abused children were less likely to approach their caregivers in response to friendly overtures. When they did so, they were more likely to approach to the side, to the rear, or by turning about and backstepping.

These observations and studies of abused infants and toddlers suggest that their attachment to their mothers and caregivers is noticeably compromised. The fearfulness, irritability, and distress experienced with their parent(s) appears to be readily generalized and reenacted with subsequent caretakers. This is consistent with clinical observations which describe the pronounced difficulties of abused children in relating to foster parents, day-care personnel, and schoolteachers.

Green et al. (1974a) explored the psychological and emotional sequelae of abuse in sixty school-age battered children at the Downstate Medical Center in Brooklyn, New York. Thirty normal and thirty neglected, nonabused children comparable in age, sex, and socioeconomic level served as controls. Psychiatric evaluation and psychological testing of these children documented the cognitive impairment and psychological disturbances described by others. The abused and neglected children exhibited significantly lower mean IQ scores than the normal controls. Twenty-five percent of the abused children were found to be mentally retarded with IQs of less than 70. These children also demonstrated severe deficits in a wide variety of ego functions, such as impulse control, defense functioning, reality testing, object relations, thought processess, body image, and overall ego competency. The abused children also exhibited a basic mistrust of adults, and a rather typical pattern of depressive affect with low self-esteem, which was often accompanied by self-destructive behavior. They also were preoccupied with aggression and violent fantasies. These abnormalities were attributed to the disruptive impact of physical and emotional trauma on the normal development of the child's cognitive and adaptive ego functions as a consequence of deviant and neglectful parenting. In some cases, however, the defects of the child preceded and precipitated the maltreatment (Sandgrund et al., 1974).

Psychopathology of Abused Children

Impairment in Ego Functioning

Green (1978a) described the most common types of psychopathology and ego impairment encountered in abused children during their involvement in the study and in subsequent psychotherapy.

When viewed globally, the abused children exhibited an overall impairment in ego functioning associated with intellectual and cognitive deficits. They displayed a higher incidence of delayed development and central nervous system (CNS) dysfunction than their nonabused peers. Many were mentally retarded. They were often found to be hyperactive and impulsive with minimal frustration tolerance. Motor activity, rather than verbalization, was the preferred mode of expression. Many abused children manifested aberrant speech and language development. Although these children were of latency age, they failed to demonstrate the progressive ego growth and reorganization characteristic of this stage. There was an absence of typical latency defenses which enable the normal child to bind anxiety from internal and external sources and cope with phase-specific stresses and conflicts. The abused children's preoccupation with external danger and overstimulated drive activity deprived them of the energy necessary for learning and mastery.

"Traumatic" Reaction with Acute Anxiety State

The frightening physical and psychological assault experienced by these children during an abusive episode exposed them to the threat of annihilation and/or abandonment. Many of the children were overwhelmed by both the quality and quantity of the noxious stimulation, which paralyzed ego functioning and resulted in severe panic. This situation resembled Freud's concept of traumatic neurosis and the breaching of the stimulus barrier (1957). The abused children experienced feelings of helplessness, annihilation, and humiliation which were often accompanied by a loss of ego boundaries. The anxiety states occurred prior to or during a beating, or in the anticipation of an attack.

These children exhibited a striking tendency to continually reenact the traumatic situation. Repetition of the trauma was observed in overt behavior and in symbolic activities such as fantasy, play, and artistic productions. It was also encountered in the therapeutic relationship in which the children acted out the role of the "bad child" and sought punishment from the therapist. This "fixation to the trauma" may be considered as a defensive reaction that permits the abused child to actively recreate, master, and control the painful affects and anxiety that otherwise might be instigated by the environment.

Pathological Object Relationships

Early and pervasive exposure to parental rejection, assault, and deprivation had an adverse effect on the development of subsequent object relationships. Potential new objects were regarded with fear and apprehension. The abused children were not able to achieve Erikson's stage of basic trust (1950). They expected similar frustration and maltreatment from other adults on the basis of previous experience. Violence and rejection were regarded as the major ingredients of human encounters. During psychotherapy, a typical abused child initially appeared detached and guarded and was ingratiating in order to please the therapist and avoid punishment. Once he felt safe, he displayed an enormous object hunger. The therapist was overidealized, and the child attempted to incorporate this "good parent" as a source of dependency gratification and as a means of protection against his "bad" parental objects. However, the inevitable frustrations and limitations in the therapeutic relationship incited the child's rage and disillusionment.

The child's increasing anger and provocative behavior led to his anticipation of punishment by the therapist, who was rapidly transformed into the "bad parent." The child's projection of his own rage onto the therapist helped to consolidate this negative image and increase his fear of retaliation. At this point, he adopted the negative self-image of the "bad child," which represented an "identification with the aggressor" (his own violent parent) in the face of increasing anxiety and helplessness in the treatment situation. The child then proceeded to reenact his relationship with the abusing parent with the therapist. He sought to achieve mastery and control over anticipated punishment through provocative and testing behavior.

Primitive Defense Mechanisms

The abused children relied on an excessive use of primitive defenses such as denial, projection, introjection, and splitting in order to cope with threatening external and internalized parental images. They were unable to integrate the loving and hostile aspects of their parents and others. This accounted for the baffling tendency of some of these children to completely support their parent's transparent denials and rationalizations concerning inflicted injuries.

While this need to suppress knowledge of parental wrongdoing was occasionally motivated by fear of additional punishment, it also represented the child's need to protect himself from the awareness of the actual and internalized destructive parent and to safeguard the parent from his own murderous rage. The image of the "bad parent" was subjected to denial and was projected onto some other person, allowing the child to maintain the fantasy of having a "good parent."

Impaired Impulse Control

The abused children were often cited for aggressive and destructive behavior at home and in school. Bullying, fighting, and assaultive behavior were observed in their contacts with peers and siblings. The younger children were frequently restless and hyperactive, while the older children and adolescents were commonly involved in antisocial and delinquent behavior. The origin of this problem was overdetermined. The abused children formed a basic identification with their violent parents, which facilitated the use of "identification with the aggressor" as a major defense against feelings of anxiety and helplessness. Hyperaggressive behavior typically followed incidents of physical abuse. Loss of impulse control was further enhanced by the presence of CNS dysfunction. These children also lacked the usual superego restraints found in normal children during latency due to inadequate superego models and faulty internalization.

Impaired Self-Concept

These children were frequently sad, dejected, and self-depreciatory. Their poor self-concepts were an end result of chronic physical and emotional scarring, humiliation, and scapegoating, compounded and reinforced by each new episode of physical abuse. These children ultimately regarded themselves with the same displeasure and contempt that their parents directed toward them. The young children who were repeatedly punished, beaten, and threatened with abandonment assumed that it was a consequence of their own behavior, regardless of their actual innocence. The loathsome self-image often created such anxiety and discomfort that it became projected or displaced onto others. At times, the poor self-concept was disguised by compensatory fantasies of grandiosity and omnipotence.

Masochistic and Self-Destructive Behavior

Abused children commonly exhibited overt types of self-destructive behavior such as suicide attempts, gestures, and threats, and various forms of self-mutilation. These were often accompanied by more subtle forms of pain-dependent activity in the form of provocative, belligerent, and limit-testing behavior which easily elicited beatings and punishment from parents, adults, and peers. Accident proneness was considered to be another form of self-destructive activity frequently observed in this population. Forty percent of our research population of abused children manifested direct forms of self-destructive behavior, a significantly higher incidence than in the neglected and normal controls (Green, 1978c). In the majority of cases, the self-destructive behavior was precipitated by parental beatings or occurred in response to actual or threatened separation from parental figures. Self-destructive behavior represented the child's compliance with parental wishes for his destruction and/or disappearance.

The abused children often reacted to actual or threatened separation and object loss with intense anxiety. This was frequently traced to numerous experiences of separation and abandonment with parental figures during infancy and early childhood. Hypothetically, chronic physical abuse might have increased the vulnerability of these children to separation because each beating implies the parent's withdrawal of love and wish to be rid of the child. The abused child's frequent lack of object constancy resulting from cognitive impairment and/or cerebral dysfunction was another contributing factor to the separation problems. This interfered with the construction and internalization of the mental representation of the absent object.

Difficulties in School Adjustment

Most of the abused children exhibited major problems in school adjustment. Their limited attention spans, frequent hyperactivity, and cognitive impairment led to deficient academic performance. At times, these children demonstrated specific learning disabilities such as dyslexia, expressive and receptive language disorders, and perceptual-motor dysfunction on the basis of minimal brain dysfunction of maturational lag. Their aggressiveness and poor impulse control contributed to behavior problems with peers and teachers. Their parents were frequently called to school because of their disruptive behavior and learning difficulties, which often led to further abuse. A vicious cycle often ensued, consisting of academic and behavioral problems, parental beatings, and increased disruptiveness in the classroom due to the displacement of anger at the parents onto the teachers.

Central Nervous System Impairment

Most retrospective studies of CNS functioning of abused children have revealed neurological impairment (Elmer and Gregg, 1967; Baron et al., 1970; Morse et al., 1970; Martin et al., 1974; Smith and Hanson, 1974), yet the precise etiology of this impairment has been the subject of controversy. With the exception of obvious cases of massive head trauma resulting in skull fractures with subdural hematomas, as originally described by Kempe et al. (1962), brain damage alone would not appear sufficient to explain CNS impairment. This uncertain impact of child abuse on neurological development has been noted by Martin et al. (1974) who showed that appreciable numbers of abused children with skull fractures and subdural hematomas were neurologically intact, while numerous abused children without head injury exhibited neurological deficits. Because most abused children manifest a variety of soft tissue injuries as opposed to major skull trauma, it is important to clarify this issue.

Several hypotheses have been offered to account for neurological impairment observed in children not known to have sustained massive head injuries. Caffey (1972) described how vigorous shaking of a child's head could result in petechial hemorrhages in the brain. Neglect (Coleman and Provence, 1957), malnutrition (Scrimshaw and Gordon, 1968; Birch, 1972), and maternal deprivation (Spitz, 1945; Bakwin, 1949; Bowlby, 1951) often accompanying child abuse have all been implicated in adverse neurological development. Some observers (Milowe and Lourie, 1964; Sandgrund et al., 1974) have postulated that this impairment may precede and even provoke abuse by rendering these children hyperkinetic and difficult to manage.

Unfortunately, the major weakness thus far in studies documenting neurological problems associated with child abuse has been the failure to compare them with control children from otherwise comparable backgrounds.

A study was carried out at the Downstate Medical Center exploring the relationship between the abusive environment and CNS development (Green et al., 1981). The neurological competency of physically abused children who were not known to have sustained severe head trauma was assessed. The neglect, family disorganization, and emotional deprivation were controlled by including nonabused, neglected, and normal comparison groups. The neurological evaluation of the 120 children (60 abused, 30 neglected, and 30 normal) followed the psychological and psychiatric studies described previously. The children received physical, neurological examinations, including an EEG, and a battery of perceptual-motor tests. On the basis of all available information, the pediatric neurologist assigned each child a global rating of impairment. The results indicated that the abused sample obtained the highest rating of neurological impairment, followed by the neglected and normal controls. Fifty-two percent of the abused children received designations of moderate or severe impairment, as compared to 38% of the neglected children and only 14% of the controls.

The findings that the abused children were not statistically significantly more damaged than their neglected counterparts was contrary to expectation. Similarities in the nature and prevalence of impairment in the two maltreatment groups in contrast to the relative intactness of the controls suggest that the adverse physical and psychological environment associated with maltreatment may be of greater neurological consequence than the physical assault itself. The combination of behavioral and neurological disability in the maltreated child could result from abnormal child rearing, poor prenatal and infant care, nutritional deficiency, inadequate medical care, and abnormal (insufficient or excessive) sensory stimulation.

Environmental Factors Associated with Child Abuse

While environmental stress has often been suggested as a prominent etiological factor in child abuse, the precise definition of this relationship has eluded most investigators. One author has attributed child abuse almost exclusively to socioeconomic determinants (Gil, 1968, 1970), while most researchers agree that environmental stress serves as a catalyst, in some instances, for an abuse-prone personality.

In addition to Gil, economic pressures were important findings in studies by Elmer (1967), Kempe et al. (1962), Young (1964), Johnson and Morse (1968), and Bennie and Sclare (1969). Contrary evidence can be obtained in Paulson and Blake (1969) and Steele and

Pollock (1968) who observed child abuse in economically advantaged populations. These authors and others (Adelson, 1961; Kempe et al., 1962; Simons et al., 1966; Holter and Friedman, 1968; Green et al., 1974b) place far greater emphasis upon personality factors and intrafamily dynamics.

The stress argument has at least in part been predicated on the high percentage of low socioeconomic multiple-problem families in child-abuse registers throughout the country. Gil's 1967 study (1970) revealed that nearly 60% of the families involved in abuse incidents had been on welfare during or prior to 1967, and 37.2% of the abusive families had been receiving public assistance at the time of the incident; 48.4% of the reported families had incomes below $5,000 in 1967 compared with 25.3% of all American families. The American Humane Association's national survey of reported cases of maltreatment in 1977 (1979) indicates that this pattern continues. The median family income of the 1977 families involved in substantiated cases of abuse and neglect was $5,361, only 36% of the United States median income of $16,009. The median family income of neglecting families was even lower, $4,633 or 29% of the median. Forty-four percent of abusing and neglecting families were receiving some form of welfare.

It is probable that reporting procedures themselves have led to the great emphasis on socioeconomic determinants, because of the disproportionate number of deprived persons being served by municipal agencies. The conclusion that Spinetta and Rigler (1972) reach in their review of the literature is far more likely—that environmental stress is neither necessary nor sufficient for child abuse but that it does, in some instances, interact with other factors, such as parent personality variables and child behaviors, to potentiate child battering.

Family size has been recognized as another environmental factor related to child abuse. One might expect that large numbers of children would be stressful for a parent or caretaker, and several observers have documented this relationship between child abuse and large families (Young, 1964; Gil, 1970; Light, 1973).

A number of investigators have cited the importance of unemployement as a contributing factor to child abuse. Gil (1970) reported that only 52.5% of the fathers in his sample were employed throughout the year preceding the abuse incident. Galdston (1965), Young (1964), and Green (1979) also demonstrated a relationship between unemployment and child abuse. In addition to financial problems, the lack of a job poses a threat to the father's self-esteem.

Justice and Duncan (1976) described the contribution of work-related pressures to environmental stress which triggered child abuse. Justice and Justice (1976) were able to document the importance of stress in terms of excessive life changes in child-abusing families by means of the social readjustment rating scale developed by Holmes and Rahe (1967).

The concrete aspects of poverty, i.e., lack of money, inadequate, overcrowded, and unsanitary living conditions, family disorganization, high crime rate, unsafe neighborhoods, etc., exert a stressful impact on family life and parental functioning, and might trigger the onset of abuse; but it is likely that a background of poverty is more intimately related to neglect than physical abuse. Thus, many of the substandard living conditions routinely observed in impoverished inner-city ghettos may be considered "neglectful" by middle-class standards and might be used by protective caseworkers to confirm an otherwise equivocal allegation of neglect.

If we consider the variables of environmental stress, parental personality traits, and characteristics of the child as a complementary series of factors leading to abuse and neglect, one might hypothesize that the combinations of these factors will change as one ascends the socioeconomic ladder. For example, middle-class abusers would be likely to demonstrate more abuse-prone personality traits which might be more easily provoked by a relatively milder stressful condition than a poverty-class population of abusing parents. Middle-class parents are also less likely to be cited for neglect, as they possess the material resources to provide for the basic physical requirements of their children and the capacity to employ substitute caretakers. The aberrant child-rearing practices of these parents might more frequently fall into the category of "emotional" abuse or neglect, which includes more subtle symptoms of maltreatment, such as emotional detachment and indifference, ridiculing and humiliation short of physical abuse, infantilization and overprotection, etc. The inability of middle- and upper-class parents to adequately care for their children on the basis of abuse-prone personality traits derived from their own pathological childhood experiences may be compensated for by delegating primary parenting responsibility to nursemaids, governesses, and boarding schools.

Treatment: Intervention with Abusing Parents

The major goal of treatment is to protect the child from further injury and to strengthen the family and its child-rearing capacity. This should be accompanied by an attempt to modify the pathological personality traits of the abusing parent which interfere with his caretaking ability. Wherever possible, therapeutic intervention with the parents should proceed with the children remaining at home. If the immediate risk for reinjury is considered too great, the parents might be engaged in treatment while the children are temporarily placed out of the home. The primary objectives of the therapeutic contact with the abusing parents are:

1. Providing immediate crisis intervention to alleviate family conflict and environmental stressors.
2. Helping parents establish a trusting, supportive and gratifying relationship with the therapist and other adults.
3. Helping parents improve their chronically devalued self-image.
4. Overcoming parents' social isolation. With the establishment of satisfying contact with others, parents will no longer depend on their children to bolster their self-esteem.
5. Providing parents with a positive child-rearing model for identification.
6. Reversing the parental misperceptions of the child, which contribute to scapegoating.
7. Helping parents develop nonabusive disciplinary and child-rearing techniques.
8. Providing parents with basic information about child rearing and child development, including special counseling regarding physical, emotional, and intellectual limitations of the child.
9. Helping parents to understand the relationship between their misperception and inappropriate handling of the child and their own painful childhood experiences.
10. Enabling parents to derive pleasure from the child.

The traditional outpatient psychiatric intervention must be greatly modified if these objectives are to be attained. A crisis-oriented multidisciplinary treatment program with a strong outreach component is the most appropriate type of intervention for these families. The facility may be hospital or community based, and it should be capable of providing the following comprehensive services.

Supportive Psychotherapy

The therapist (psychiatrist, psychologist, psychiatric social worker, or psychiatric nurse) sees the maltreating parent once or twice weekly, and the psychotherapy is modified to suit the special needs of these parents. The therapist must be supportive and noncritical, in order to overcome the parent's distrust of authority figures. The parent's excessive use of denial and projection, which leads to misperceptions and scapegoating of the abused child, must be gradually interpreted. If the psychotherapy is successful, parents will be able to understand the link between their abusive practices and the maltreatment they endured during childhood.

Counseling

Counseling is available to unsophisticated or poorly motivated parents who are less suitable for psychotherapy. It also might be offered as an initial intervention in preparation for subsequent psychotherapy. Counseling might focus on such important areas as spouse and family relationships, child rearing, and vocational problems. Concrete issues, such as housekeeping, shopping, budgeting, and health care may be effectively managed through a counseling approach.

Parenting Education

A major goal of parenting education is to sensitize the parents to the individual needs of their children, based on a better understanding of the child's physical and psychological development. This educative process attempts to modify parents' misperceptions of their children, which result in inappropriate demands for precocious and premature performance. Parents are also taught routine child- and health-care practices. Parenting education may take place in small parent groups, during individual counseling sessions, or during the observation of parent-child interaction in a therapeutic nursery.

Group Therapy

Group therapy can be beneficial to maltreating parents in several ways. It may act as a bridge to therapeutic involvement in extremely defensive and mistrustful parents who are threatened by a one-to-one relationship. It may also supplement ongoing individual counseling or psychotherapy. The realization that their problems are shared by others diminishes parents' guilt and low self-esteem. The permissive atmosphere of open discussion facilitates the expression of long-suppressed feelings of anger, pain, and distress. Finally, the establishment of personal ties with other group members fosters social contacts outside of the program.

Family Therapy

Family therapy may be utilized with relatively intact maltreating families containing children who are old enough to communicate verbally. Family therapy might be appropriately initiated after preliminary individual treatment of the parents and children. A family systems approach can be extremely useful in identifying and reversing the pathological family interaction and aberrant communication commonly observed in abusing families. This modality is also effective in dealing with the major distortion in the roles of family members in cases of sexual abuse and incest.

Outreach Services and Crisis Intervention

Outreach in the form of home visits and telephone contacts is often necessary to engage a resistant family during the initial phase of treatment. Home visiting can also be carried out during a period of crisis when the parent might be physically or emotionally unable to leave the house. A twenty-four-hour-a-day hotline is also invaluable in such crisis situations as suicidal behavior, impending loss of impulse control, marital violence, and various other psychiatric emergencies. Planned home visiting may be utilized to assess the family's progress in treatment, or to evaluate the degree of risk to the children at any given time.

TREATMENT OBJECTIVES: INTERVENTION WITH ABUSED CHILDREN

Once these children are in a safe environment, every effort should be made to reverse the serious emotional and cognitive impairment associated with their traumatic life experiences. Without therapeutic intervention, the abused child can be expected to perpetuate the traumatic condition by projecting his struggle with internalized bad parents onto new objects in his environment. Therefore, once the abused child's personality is formed, modification of the traumatic conditions at home may not be sufficient to reverse his maladaptive behavior. This is illustrated by the large numbers of abused children whose aggressive and provocative behavior has contributed to their expulsion from foster homes that provided them with adequate parental figures and material supports.

Infants and Preschool Children

A therapeutic nursery for preschool children provides an ideal milieu for observing and improving the pathological parent-child interaction typically described in cases of maltreatment and for enhancing the normal growth and development of the children.

Therapeutic activities designed to remedy the most typical problems and deficits of these children include:

1. Appropriate motor and sensory stimulation to compensate for environmental deprivation.
2. Use of developmentally appropriate toys to promote the child's capacity for play.
3. Providing predictable and gratifying one-to-one contact with staff members to modify the child's fearfulness and mistrust.
4. Use of structured play activities to foster the development of motor and sensory skills.
5. Providing group experiences to enhance the development of peer relationships and cooperative play.

Therapeutic involvement with the parent-child dyad is designed to:

1. Eliminate distortions in the parent's perceptions of the child.
2. Help the parent understand the cues and signals of the child.
3. Identify and change mutually frustrating aspects of the parent-child interaction.

4. Educate the parent about infant/child care and development.
5. Counsel the parent about the child's medical or developmental disabilities.
6. Help the parent to achieve self-confidence and pleasure during the interaction with the child.

School-Age Children

A wide range of psychotherapeutic and educational techniques have proven successful in reducing the deficiencies and symptoms of abused school-age children and adolescents (Green, 1978b). These include psychoanalytically oriented play therapy and psychotherapy, group psychotherapy, and psychoeducational intervention.

Therapeutic intervention must deal with each of the major psychopathological sequelae of child abuse previously outlined. The acute traumatic reactions may be attenuated by allowing the child to master the trauma through a controlled repetition of the event, using symbolic reenactment with dolls, puppets, drawings, etc. Strengthening of ego functions is achieved by containment of impulses and action, and the encouragement of verbalization. The therapist helps the child with reality testing, promotes sublimation, and encourages the development of more adaptive controls and defenses, so the child can eventually experience a latency period free from excessive external and internal stimulation.

Strengthening of defensive functioning may be accomplished by the gradual incorporation of the therapist's attitudes and controls, internalization of superego elements from the therapist, and the encouragement of sublimation. Strengthening of impulse control is enhanced by imposing limits on direct manifestations of aggression such as hitting or destroying toys and play materials. The child should be encouraged to verbalize anger or express it symbolically through play. Limit setting must be clearly defined with respect to entering and leaving the playroom, removing toys and materials, and the length of the sessions. The binding of aggression may also be fostered through the introduction of sublimatory activities and typical "latency" games.

Improvement of self-esteem gradually takes place during the child's exposure to the climate of warmth and acceptance generated by the therapist. The abused child slowly modifies his self-concept to coincide with the therapist's positive view of him. The therapist must be active in challenging the child's readiness to assume the role of the scapegoat. He needs to be told that his beatings resulted from parental problems rather than as a consequence of his "badness."

Strengthening object constancy and the capacity to tolerate separation may be promoted by active reassurance on the part of the therapist concerning his or her ongoing interest in the child in the absence of contact. Interruptions of treatment should be kept at a minimum. Missed sessions, vacations, and changes of therapist must be clearly presented and worked through. If necessary, the child should be allowed to take home token "symbols" of the therapist (drawing, pencils, candy, etc.) to promote internalization of his mental representation during separations.

Improvement of school performance in most abused children requires psychological testing and educational assessment to document current intellectual functioning and learning capacity. The presence of specific learning disabilities or behavior problems might require remedial intervention or placement in a special class. The therapist should maintain contact with the child's teacher and guidance counselor, and act as an intermediary between the child's parents and the school. The child's school adjustment should become a major focus of treatment.

Advantages of a Hospital-Based Treatment Program

A hospital-based program has the capacity to deliver efficiently and to coordinate a wide variety of medical, mental-health, social, and educational services. Duplication of these comprehensive services by a nonmedical agency would require the subcontracting of services to local hospitals and mental-health and child-care centers at much greater cost and would result in the investment of disproportionate efforts for interagency liaison and communication. Decentralization of services would require an unrealistic commitment of the parent's time and energy necessary for extensive multiagency contacts and travel. Patient compliance would be more difficult to monitor, with a predictable increase in dropout rates. The hospital-based program also has the capacity to initiate therapeutic contact with the family as soon as the maltreatment is detected, thus maximizing the potential for successful participation in the program. It is easier and more economical to initiate a hospital-based program because the nucleus of the treatment team can be formed with existing staff from the departments of pediatrics, psychiatry, nursing, and social service.

References

Adelson, L. 1961. Slaughter of the innocent: A study of forty-six homicides in which the victims were children. *N. Eng. J. Med.,* 264:1345–1349.

Bakwin, H. 1949. Emotional deprivation in infants. *J. Ped.,* 35:512–521.

Baron, M. A., Bejar, R. L., and Sheaff, P. J. 1970. Neurological manifestations of the battered child syndrome. *Ped.,* 45:1003–1007.

Bennie, E. H., and Sclare, A. B. 1969. The battered child syndrome. *Am. J. Psych.,* 125:975–979.

Besharov, D. *New York Times,* November 30, 1975.

Birch, H. G. 1972. Malnutrition, learning, and intelligence. *Am. J. Pub. Health,* 62:773–784.

Bowlby, J. 1951. Maternal care and mental health. *Bull. WHO,* 31:355–533.

Burgess, R. L., and Conger, R. D. 1977. Family interaction patterns related to child abuse and neglect: Some preliminary findings. *Child Abuse Neg.,* 1:269–277.

Caffey, J. 1972. On the theory and practice of shaking infants: Its potential residual effects of permanent brain damage and mental retardation. *Am. J. Dis. Child.,* 124:161–169.

Chapa, D. 1978. The relationship between child abuse/neglect and substance abuse contrasting Mexican-American and Anglo families. Interim report. San Antonio Child Abuse Project Civic Organization, February 1978, San Antonio, Texas.

Coleman, R. W., and Provence, S. 1957. Developmental retardation (hospitalism) in infants living in families. *Pediatrics,* 19:285–292.

Elmer, E. 1963. Identification of abused children. *Child.* 10:180–184.

Elmer, E. 1965. The fifty families study: Summary of phase 1: Neglected and abused children and their families. Pittsburgh: Children's Hospital.

Elmer E. 1967. *Children in jeopardy: A study of abused minors and their families.* Pittsburgh: University of Pittsburgh Press.

Elmer, E., and Gregg, C. S. 1967. Developmental characteristics of abused children. *Ped.,* 40:596–602.

Erikson, E. H. 1950. *Childhood and society.* New York: Norton.

Fontana, V. 1964. *The maltreated child.* Springfield, Ill.: Charles C. Thomas.

Freud, S. 1957. Beyond the pleasure principle. *Standard Edition,* vol. 18. London: Hogarth Press, pp. 3–64.

Gaensbauer, T. J., and Sands, K. 1979. Distorted communications in abused/neglected infants and their potential impact on caretakers. *J. Am. Acad. Child Psych.,* 18:236-250.

Galdston, R. 1965. Observations on children who have been physically abused and their parents. *Am. J. Psych..* 122:440-443.

Galdston, R. 1971. Violence begins at home. *J. Am. Acad. Child Psych.,* 10:336-350.

George C., and Main, M. 1979. Social interactions of young abused children: Approach, avoidance, and aggression. *Child Dev.,* 50:306-318.

Gil, D. 1968. Incidence of child abuse and demographic characteristics of persons involved. In *The battered child,* ed. R. E. Helfer, and C. H. Kempe. Chicago: University of Chicago Press.

Gil, D. 1970. *Violence against children.* Cambridge, Mass.: Harvard University Press.

Gil, D. 1974. A holistic perspective on child abuse and its prevention. Paper presented at the Conference on Research on Child Abuse, National Institute of Child Health and Human Development.

Green, A. H. 1968. Self-destructive behavior in physically abused schizophrenic children. *Arch. Gen. Psych.,* 19:171-179.

Green, A. H. 1976. A psychodynamic approach to the study and treatment of child abusing parents. *J. Am. Acad. Child Psych.,* 15:414-429.

Green, A. H. 1978a. Psychopathology of abused children. *J. Am. Acad. Child Psych.,* 17:92-103.

Green, A. H. 1978b. Psychiatric treatment of abused children. *J. Am. Acad. Child Psych.,* 17:356-371.

Green, A. H. 1978c. Self-destructive behavior in battered children. *Am. J. Psych.,* 135:579-586.

Green, A. H. 1979. Child abusing fathers. *J. Am. Acad. Child Psych.,* 18:270-282.

Green, A. H. 1984. Child abuse by siblings. *Child Abuse and Neglect* (in press).

Green, A. H., Sandgrund, A., Gaines, R. W., and Haberfeld, H. 1974a. Psychological sequelae of child abuse and neglect. *Proceedings of the American Psychiatric Association Annual Meeting,* p. 191.

Green, A. H., Gaines, R. W., and Sandgrund, A. 1974b. Child abuse: Pathological syndrome of family interaction. *Am. J. Psych.,* 131:882-886.

Green, A. H., Voeller, K., Gaines, R., and Kubie, J. 1978. Neurological impairment in maltreated children. Paper presented at the annual meeting of the American Academy of Child Psychiatry, October 1978, San Diego, California.

Green, A. H. 1980. Child maltreatment: *A handbook for mental health and child care professionals.* New York: Jason Aronson.

Green, A. H., Voeller, K., Gaines, R., and Kubie, J. 1981. Neurological impairment in battered children. *Child Abuse Neg.,* 5:129-134.

Helfer, R. E. 1975. The diagnostic process and treatment programs. DHEW pub. no. OHD 75-69. Washington, D.C.: U.S. Department of Health, Education, and Welfare, National Center for Child Abuse and Neglect.

Holmes, T., and Rahe, R. 1967. The Social Readjustment Rating Scale. *J. Psychosomatic Med.,* 11:213-218.

Holter, J., and Friedman, S. 1968. Principles of management in child abuse cases. *Am. J. Orthopsych.,* 38:127-136.

Johnson, B., and Morse, H. 1968. Injured children and their parents. *Child.,* 15:147-152.

Justice, B., and Duncan, D. F. 1976. Life crisis as a precursor to child abuse. *Pub. Health Rep.,* 91:110-115.

Justice, B., and Justice, R. 1976. *The abusing family.* New York: Human Sciences Press.

Kempe, C. H., Silverman, F., Steele, B., Droegemueller, W., and Silver, H. 1962. The battered child syndrome. *J. Am. Med. Assoc.,* 181:17-24.

Kempe, R. 1976. Arresting or freezing the developmental process. In *Child abuse and neglect, the family and community,* ed. R. E. Helfer, and C. H. Kempe, pp. 64-73. Cambridge, Mass.: Ballinger Publishing Co.

Light, R. J. 1973. Abused and neglected children in America: A study of alternative policies. *Harv. Ed. Rev.,* 43:556-598.

Martin, H. P. 1972. The child and his development. In *Helping the battered child and his family,* ed. C. H. Kempe, and R. E. Helfer. Philadelphia: J. B. Lippincott Co.

Martin, H. P., Beezely, P., Conway, E. F., and Kempe, C. H. 1974. The development of abused children. *Adv. Ped.,* 21:25-73.

Martin, H. P., and Beezely, P. 1976. Personality of abused children. In *The abused child,* ed. H. P. Martin, pp. 105-111. Cambridge, Mass.: Ballinger Publishing Co.

Merrill, E. 1962. Physical abuse of children: An agency study. In *Protecting the battered child,* ed. V. DeFrancis. Denver: American Humane Association.

Milowe, I. D., and Lourie, R. S. 1964. The child's role in the battered child syndrome. *J. Ped.,* 65:1079-1081.

Morse, W., Sahler, O. J., and Friedman, S. B. 1970. A three-year follow-up study of abused and neglected children. *Am. J. Dis. Child.,* 120:439-446.

New York City Central Registry for Child Abuse, 1980, and New York State Central Registry for Child Abuse, 1980.

Ounsted, C., Oppenheimer, R., and Lindsay, J. 1974. Aspects of bonding failure: The psychopathology and psychotherapeutic treatment of families of battered children. *Dev. Med. Child Neurol.,* 16:446-456.

Paulson, M., and Blake, P. 1969. The physically abused child: A focus on prevention. *Child Welf.,* 48:86-95.

Reid, J. B., and Taplin, P. S. 1977. A social interactional approach to the treatment of abusive children. Unpublished manuscript.

Robison, E., and Solomon, F. 1979. Some further findings on the treatment of the mother-child dyad in child abuse. *Child Abuse Neg.,* 3:247-251.

Sandgrund, A., Gaines, R., and Green, A. H. 1974. Child abuse and mental retardation: A problem of cause and effect. *Am. J. Men. Def.,* 79:327-330.

Scrimshaw, M. S., and Gordon, J. E. 1968. *Malnutrition, learning, and behavior.* Cambridge, Mass.: MIT Press.

Simons, B., Downs, E., Hurster, M., and Archer, M. 1966. Child abuse. *N. Y. S. J. Med.,* 66:2783-2788.

Smith, C. A., and Hanson, R. 1974. 134 battered children: A medical and psychological study. *Brit. Med. J.,* 14:666-670.

Spinetta, J., and Rigler, D. 1972. The child abusing parent: A psychological review. *Psychol. Bull.,* 77:296-304.

Spitz, R. A. 1945. Hospitalism: An inquiry into the genesis of psychiatric conditions of early childhood. In *The psychoanalytic study of the child,* vol. 1. New York: International Universities Press, pp. 53-74..

Starr, R. H., Seresnie, S. J., and Steinlaus, J. 1978. Social and psychological characteristics of abusive mothers. Paper presented at the annual meeting of the Eastern Psychological Association, Washington, D.C., May 1978.

Steele, B., and Pollock, C. A. 1968. A psychiatric study of parents who abuse infants and small children. In *The battered child,* ed. R. E. Helfer, and C. H. Kempe. Chicago: University of Chicago Press.

Wasserman, G., Green, A., and Allen, R. 1983. Going beyond abuse: Maladaptive patterns of interaction in abusing mother-infant pairs. *J. Am. Acad. Child Psych.* 22:245-252.

Wolock, I., and Horowitz, B. 1977. Factors relating to levels of child care among families receiving public assistance in New Jersey: First report. DHEW grant no. 90-c-418, National Center on Child Abuse and Neglect, Office of Child Development.

Young, L. 1964. *Wednesday's children: A study of child neglect and abuse.* New York: McGraw-Hill.

18

Sexual Abuse in Childhood and Adolescence

JUDITH V. BECKER / LINDA J. SKINNER

DEFINING CHARACTERISTICS

Child molestation refers to the sexual abuse of young people by adults and includes the subcategories of pedophilia, hebephilia, and incest. The common thread in all three types of sexual abuse is the lack of consent underlying the interaction, resulting from the victim either being physically forced or verbally coerced to participate or lacking the emotional and cognitive development necessary to give consent. However, these three subcategories of child molestation differ with regard to the age of the victim and relationship of the victim to the offender. While in both pedophilia and hebephilia the victim is unrelated to the offender, the former is the term applied to sexual interactions with a prepubertal child and the latter refers to sexual desires directed at a postupubertal adolescent. In contrast, the defining characteristic of incest is the relationship between the victim and the perpetrator. Included in this subcategory of child molestation are sexual interactions between an offender and a victim who share a familial relationship based on blood or law, or, psychosocially, on a current living pattern and *de facto* relationship, such as stepfather or a male living in the home and assuming the role of father.

PREVALENCE

The national incidence of child molestation is unknown and attempts to ascertain the actual number are greatly complicated by the comparatively low reporting rate for such assaults. Yet, the results of some research studies suggest that the problem of sexual abuse of young people has been and continues to be epidemic. For example, Wells (1958) found that 84% of known rape victims in her jurisdiction were sixteen years of age or younger and 58% were less than thirteen years of age. In a retrospective study of 12,000 college-age females, 26% of the women revealed that they had a sexual experience with an adult before they were thirteen years old (Gagnon, 1965). During a ten-year period in Hennepin County, Minnesota, reports of sexual abuse of children were almost four times more prevalent than reports of physical abuse of children (Jaffe et al., 1975). Based upon their work, Woodbury and Schwartz (1971) hypothesized that 10% of all Americans have been involved in incestuous experiences.

The most comprehensive study of selected sexual crimes against children (De Francis, 1969) investigated all such reported offenses over a five-year period in Brooklyn, New York. During this period, an average of 1,113 cases of child molestation were reported to the Brooklyn police each year and this number did not include pedophilic cases involving victims under the age of seven, hebephilic cases involving victims fifteen years of age or older, and any case of sexual abuse that did not involve physical contact. The high incidence of child molestation is particularly striking when it is compared with the incidence rates for other crimes. Based on the data collected, the reported incidence rate for child molestation in Brooklyn was 149.2 per 100,000 children. In contrast, the national incidence rate for forcible rape was 12.9, and for robbery and aggravated assault the national indices were 78.3 and 118.4, respectively. Clearly, child molestation has a history of being a very significant problem.

Myths about Child Molestation and Their Impact

If a survey were conducted, the sexual abuse of children would undoubtedly be identified as one of the least acceptable behaviors in our society. Yet, in practice, our society has not addressed the problem adequately. In recent years, increased public concern about this long-standing problem has been evidenced. However, three major myths about child molestation continue to limit our response to the sexual abuse of children.

Myth 1. Most parents have warned their children not to take candy from strangers or accept rides from unknown persons in the belief that these admonitions will protect their children from possible sexual abuse. Such warnings are predicated on the myth that, with the exception of incest, the sexual abuse of children is perpetrated by unknown offenders. In reality, however, the majority of pedophilic and hebephilic assaults are carred out by assailants who are known to the victims. In the sexual abuse cases investigated by De Francis (1969), only 25% of the perpetrators were strangers to the children and/or the victim's families. Obviously, a societal response that ignores children's vulnerability to sexual abuse by adults they know is inadequate.

Myth 2. According to this myth, child molesters are a rather passive, unassertive group who usually interact sexually with their victims by mutual consent and who rarely use physical coercion with a child. However, existing data indicate that, in fact, child molesters are frequently very aggressive. Of the 250 child victims studied by De Francis (1969), 50% experienced physical force, with an additional 10% of the children being threatened with bodily harm. The types of physical force used against the children included holding them down, striking them repeatedly, and shaking them violently. In addition, threats to harm, maim, or kill the child and, in some cases, to harm or kill a member of the child's family were made.

Similar results were reported by Christie, Marshall, and Lanthier (1978), who conducted a study of 150 sex offenders, including adult rapists (73%) and child molesters (27%). In addition to using the self-reports of the offenders, these investigators drew extensively from interviews with the medical personnel who examined the victims in the emergency rooms of hospitals, the presentencing reports of probation officers, and trial transcripts. With regard to the degree of aggression used during the perpetration of the crimes, 29% of the child molesters and 7% of the rapists were identified as using no aggression or threat of force, while 12% of the child molesters and 20% of the rapists used verbal threats of force only. However, 59% of the child molesters and 73% of the rapists used physical force. Even more surprising were the consequences of the physical force used. Of the rapists who used force, 39% caused "noticeable injury" to their victims, while 42% of the child molesters using force caused "noticeable injury" to their victims. Thus, regardless of the differences in the percentages of child molesters and rapists using force, both groups of offenders were found to produce similar incidences of injury to their victims.

The use of physical aggression also extends to incestuous assaults. In a project investigating the long-term impact of sexual assault, fifty-seven women who as children had been assaulted by relatives were interviewed about the circumstances surrounding and the consequences of their assaults (Skinner & Becker, 1983). Contrary to the perception of incest as a nonviolent crime, 63.7% of these women indicated that their assailants had used physical aggression in the commission of their assaults.

Despite the existence of such data, the violent component of child molestation is all too frequently overlooked, with the result that the seriousness of the sexual abuse of children may be underestimated. Any societal response to child molestation must consider the physical as well as the emotional well-being of children.

Myth 3. Another common myth that limits our societal response to the problem of child molestation is the belief that, in many cases, the child rather than the adult is the instigator of the sexual interaction. According to this myth, the child molester is the victim of a sexually precocious and provocative child who initiates and willingly participates in the interaction. This myth stems from the erroneous interpretation of a child's behavior in terms of an adult's perception or motives. For example, the apparent consenting participation of a child may actually be compliance to the requests or demands of an adult who has authority over the child. Similarly, in an attempt to explain a child's behavior, an adult desire for sexual satisfaction may be substituted for a child's desire for emotional and/or physical closeness. The attribution of responsibility for the assault to the child is inconsistent with the recognition of the seriousness of child molestation.

These three myths about the sexual abuse of children and adolescents have had a significantly negative impact on the development of an appropriate response to the problem. As these myths have begun to be challenged, however, some improvements in this response have occurred, as evidenced by the establishment of both the National Center on Child Abuse and Neglect and the National Center for the Prevention and Control of Rape, the emergence of organizations such as Parents Anonymous and Parents United, and a significant increase in the amount of research being conducted focusing on the sexual abuse of children and adolescents.

Epidemiology

The Victim

It is not possible to identify the parameters of the population of children and adolescents likely to become victims of sexual abuse, as all children are potential victims, regardless of age, race, and socioeconomic status. The only factor that has been identified to date as being related to such victimization is the sex of the victim. The ratio of female to male victims is estimated to be 10 or 12 to 1 (De Francis, 1969).

The Perpetrator

The child molester is usually characterized as being different from other people. For example, the molester is labeled a sex fiend, sexually inadequate, retarded, psychotic or insane, or suffering from a degenerative disease such as alcoholism, drug addiction, or senility. While these characterizations may make people feel more comfortable and secure in the belief that molesters are unlike themselves, these stereotypic descriptions do not fit the majority of known child molesters but are, rather, the exception. Instead child molesters represent all races, socioeconomic levels, and walks of like. Sex of the molester is the only personal characteristic that can be predicted with any degree of confidence. Our society seems to be more tolerant of deviant sexual behavior by females (Gebhard et al., 1960), with the result that individuals labeled as child molesters are overwhelmingly males.

The Assault

Child molestation covers a broad spectrum of behaviors, including nudity and exposure, kissing, fondling, digital penetration, and oral, vaginal, and/or anal intercourse. Frequently, the behavior engaged in by a molester may progress from less intimate sexual behavior to some form of penetration (Sgroi et al., 1982a). The assault of a child is likely to occur in either the home of the child or of the perpetrator and in the afternoon or at night (De Francis, 1969). Additionally, tangible enticements, coercion, or threats, or the use of physical force are likely to be elements of the abuse (De Francis, 1969).

With regard to incest, while sibling incest may be the most frequently occurring form (Weeks, 1976), father-daughter incest is the most likely form to be reported to police and mental-health professionals (Lester, 1972; Lukianowicz, 1972; Justice and Justice, 1979). Like pedophilic and hebephilic assaults, sexual abuse by a relative can include a variety of sexual behaviors. Contrary to popular belief, some form of penetration is frequently a part of incestuous assaults. In a comparison of samples of incest and rape victims, Skinner and Becker (1983) found the 89.2% of the rape victims and 71.9% of the incest victims reported that their assaults included penetration.

Sexual abuse is most likely to be disclosed to others if the perpetrator is a nonrelative and a stranger, and if the abuse involves physical force (De Francis, 1969). Nevertheless, like victims of other types of sexual assault, many sexually abused children and adolescents do not disclose their assaults to others. In some assaults the offender will threaten to hurt or kill the child or a member of her or his family should the child tell others about the assault, while in many assaults by known adults the perpetrator plays on the child's loyalty, making it extremely difficult for the child to disclose the sexual abuse. In cases of incest, the perpetrator will frequently conduct the abuse under the guise of a special game that will be stopped if others learn about it. In other instances a child will be told by the perpetrator that he might be forced to leave the family or be imprisoned if the sexual activity is made known, with the result that the child is put in the position of being responsible for the consequences of disclosure of the assault. Regardless of the means used by perpetrators to insure the silence of their victims, many child sexual-abuse victims do not tell others about their assaults and, consequently, are unable to obtain needed intervention. Thus, mental-health professionals working with children should be knowledgeable about and sensitive to the particular behaviors of children that may be suggestive of sexual abuse.

Assessment

Behavioral Warning Signs

Numerous behaviors that may suggest that a child is being or has been sexually abused have been identified (Sgroi et al., 1982b). While these behavioral indicators are not in and of themselves conclusive evidence, they can be considered as warning signs of sexual abuse, and any clinician who observes some of these behaviors in a child should investigate the possibility of such abuse.

AGE-INAPPROPRIATE SEXUAL ACTIVITY. Children who make sexual remarks or engage in inappropriate sexual behavior with peers or toys may be sexually abused children. For example, a victimized child may reenact her or his abuse upon a doll or begin to assault younger children. Occasionally, a child's drawings may reflect such victimization, particularly drawings that include nudity or a preponderance of phallic or genitallike objects. Additionally, a child with a history of sexual abuse may display a precocious knowledge about and understanding of sexual behavior.

FEAR OF BEING ALONE. A sexually abused child may express great fear at the prospect of being left alone in a house or even a room. Such a child may appear overly dependent on her or his parents.

REGRESSIVE BEHAVIOR. The stress experienced as a result of sexual abuse may cause a child to exhibit regressive behavior, such as a return to thumbsucking or reliance on a security blanket. Similarly, a child may withdraw into a fantasy world that provides the safety and security missing in the real world.

DEPRESSION. Children who have been sexually abused are at risk for developing a clinical depression and suicidal feelings. It is imperative that a clinician evaluate for suicidal thoughts in child sexual-abuse cases, as young victims are not likely to mention such feelings spontaneously.

SLEEP DISTURBANCES. Difficulty in falling asleep, waking during the night, and the occurrence of nightmares are frequent warning signs of sexual abuse. Victims of incest may attempt to avoid sleep, fearing that they will be molested again should they sleep. Conversely, some child molestation victims may use sleep as a means of escape, sleeping ten or more hours each day.

DIFFICULTY IN TRUSTING OTHERS. The invasion of a child's body, inherent in most sexual abuse, frequently causes the victim to feel that she or he is unable to rely on others for safety and protection and, consequently, to develop the feeling that other people cannot be trusted. As a result, the child may be unable to develop trust relationships. This indicator is particularly prevalent among incest victims who have been betrayed by a parent or close relative.

DECLINE IN SCHOOL PERFORMANCE. As a result of sexual abuse, children may experience great difficulty concentrating or may lose interest in school, with the result that there is a sudden change in school performance. The anxiety and/or depression caused by the abuse may cause the child's grades to remain low for a long period of time.

INAPPROPRIATE RESPONSE TO MALES. If there is a significant change in a female child's behavior toward males, sexual abuse should be suspected. The most frequently reported changes include unusual fear of males or seductive behavior toward males.

While the following behavioral indicators may be manifested by any victim of child molestation, these signs are particularly likely to be observed in incest cases.

OVERLY COMPLIANT BEHAVIOR. As a result of having been assaulted repeatedly by a relative and having the perpetrator control not only the child's body but, often, everyday details of the child's life, an incest victim frequently lacks assertiveness and, instead, demonstrates overly compliant behavior. Such behavior is not restricted to the demands of the perpetrator but may be manifested in response to the requests of any person perceived to be in a position of authority.

ACTING-OUT BEHAVIOR. Rather than being compliant, some incest victims display acting-out or aggressive behavior both at home and at school. This behavioral indicator is most frequently manifested by victims who have attempted to gain assistance from other adults in terminating the incestuous behavior but have been unsuccessful in such efforts.

PSEUDO-MATURE BEHAVIOR. Some incest victims are forced to assume the role of an adult, taking on responsibilities that are generally reserved for parents or caretakers. Such a child displays a level of maturity and sophistication uncharacteristic of her or his age, and this mature facade is frequently reinforced by the perpetrator.

POOR PEER RELATIONSHIPS. Since many incestuous families are insular at the insistence of the perpetrator, incest victims frequently have poor relationships with friends and are unable to make friends easily. The incest offender may not allow the child to associate with peers, and during the child's adolescence may refuse to allow the victim to date. Even if the child is allowed to interact with friends, the victim may perceive herself or himself as being different from other children and, consequently, may have difficulty relating to peers.

CHANGES IN SCHOOL PARTICIPATION. Frequently, children who have experienced incest look for reasons to be away from home in order to escape further sexual abuse and will use school as a legitimate excuse. Thus, these children may arrive at school early and leave late on a regular basis. In addition, they may suddenly become very active in numerous extracurricular school activities in order to delay going home. Conversely, nonparticipation in school and social activities may also be indicative of sexual abuse. The incest offender may insist that the child return home immediately after classes, as any involvement in activities outside the home may be perceived by the perpetrator as a threat to his control over the victim's life.

Physical Symptoms

The list of behavioral indicators is not exhaustive of the signs of child molestation, but it does offer some guidelines for clinicians who routinely work with children. In addition, physical symptoms that are frequently experienced by a child or adolescent who has been sexually abused include headaches, stomachaches, and recurring urinary tract infections. A clinician should consider the possibility of sexual abuse if a child has a history of frequent visits to the school nurse.

Any child suspected of being a victim of sexual abuse should be provided with a complete medical examination (Sgroi, 1978) and abuse should be considered a possibility if any of the following symptoms or signs is found (Sgroi et al., 1982b).

GENITAL OR RECTAL TRAUMA. If the sexual abuse includes some form of penetration, the child may display soft tissue injury or lacerations in the urethral, genital, or rectal openings. Abnormal dilation of these openings may also be suggestive of sexual abuse.

PRESENCE OF FOREIGN BODIES. Some perpetrators will place foreign objects in a child's urethral, genital, and/or rectal openings and, occasionally, a young victim may model the behavior of the assailant, placing objects in her or his own openings. The presence of such objects, as well as possible irritation or trauma caused by the objects, should cause a physician to suspect the possibility of sexual abuse.

TRAUMA TO BODY. Soft tissue damage to a child's breasts, buttocks, thighs, or lower abdomen should be questioned. Since many child molesters use force to subdue the victim, such trauma to the child's body may be observed.

SEXUALLY TRANSMITTED DISEASES. The presence of a sexually transmitted disease, such as herpes, syphilis, or gonorrhea, may be indicative of abuse. The presence of *Candida* or *Trichomonas* should be similarly suggestive.

PREGNANCY. While pregnancy in a child or adolescent may be the result of sexual interaction with a peer, any such case should be further investigated.

Interviewing the Victim and Family

Even if the physician is uncertain whether or not sexual abuse has occurred, the collection of evidence should be undertaken as if the case were to be heard in court. Documentation of evidence is of utmost importance.

Interviewing a child or adolescent who is a victim of sexual abuse serves two primary functions: it provides information about the assault and about the amount of stress the victim and family are experiencing as a result of the assault (Burgess and Holmstrom, 1978). It is imperative in these cases to establish a therapeutic relationship based on trust. At the beginning of the interview, as well as throughout the session, the clinician must demonstrate true interest in the child. Initially, the conversation should be general, focusing on nonthreatening topics such as activities the child enjoys or, in nonincestuous cases, family matters. A casual approach should be used in questioning and a clinician should always be prepared to answer truthfully any questions raised by the child.

A child may be put more at ease if she or he is told that the clinician has talked to many other children who have had similar things happen to them. In addition to establishing credibility, the clinician should clarify the child's expectations of the interview. The interviewing process will be facilitated if the child understands that the clinician is there not only to obtain information but also to provide help.

When the focus of the interview turns to the sexual abuse, the child initially should be encouraged to describe the assault. It is important that children discuss the abuse at their own speed, as this allows them to experience some control and generally fosters participation. General information about the assault should be sought first, with specific details becoming the focus only after an overall picutre of the abuse has been obtained. The following information about the assault should be noted: (a) how the abuse began; (b) who the perpetrator is; (c) what sexual activities were involved; (d) the location of the assault; (e) the time of the abuse; (f) whether or not the abuse has continued over time; (g) who has been told about the abuse; (h) what the child's reasons were for participating in the sexual activity; (i) the type and degree of coercion or force used by the perpetrator; and (j) what prompted the current disclosure.

It is important for the clinician to be aware of the language used by the child when describing the sexual abuse and to use these words during the interview. Additionally, since many victims may not be familiar with standard sexual terms, a clinician should rely heavily on descriptions of body parts and/or sexual activities. Anatomically correct dolls may be used to facilitate the discussion about the sexual activities included in the abuse.

In order to understand the impact of sexual abuse on a child, it is important to have some baseline information against which to compare present behavior (Burgess et al., 1978). Thus, it is necessary to be aware of the child's developmental level prior to the sexual abuse and to know how the child usually responds to stressful situations. The primary caretaker should be able to provide such information.

It is also important to assess the family of the child or adolescent, particularly with respect to the response of family members subsequent to the disclosure of the sexual abuse and how family members view the child. Additional information that should be obtained includes family composition, strength and direction of emotional ties within the family, and the identity of extended family members who may be important to the family. Sgroi (1982a) offers a good outline for assessing the contribution an adult family member can make in helping a child victim recover from sexual abuse. The typical family response to stressful situations should be ascertained as well. Armed with information about the child's developmental status and the integrity of the family, the clinician is in a good position to determine both positive and negative changes in the child's behavior that have occurred following the sexual abuse, as well as what roles, if any, family members may assume in helping the child.

It is imperative that a clinician interviewing a victim of child molestation evaluate the immediate safety of the child or adolescent. In cases of incest and ongoing assaults, a child may be at risk for continued abuse and/or pressure from the perpetrator to withdraw the complaint or deny that the abuse occurred. Consequently, it may be necessary to effect some type of separation, such as removing the offender from the victim and family or separating the child or adolescent from the perpetrator and family. While the former is the preferred type of separation, the latter type should be used with no hesitation if the child's immediate safety is at risk.

Initially, parents of a sexually assaulted child or adolescent may deny that the abuse has occurred or blame the child for the abuse, particularly in the case of incest. Consequently, it is very important that a clinician explain to the parents that a child, frequently failing to understand the nature and consequences of the act, cannot consent to sexual relations. The excuses offered by many incest offenders that the child "did not say no" or "seemed to enjoy it" should not remain unchallenged. A clinician can point out that not only are children taught to obey their elders but also that children are in a power imbalance vis-à-vis adults. Adults hold all the power and children are dependent upon them for material, biological, and emotional needs. Very often, children know intuitively that the behavior is wrong but are not able to say no for fear of being deprived of basic needs. It is imperative that a clinician help parents to understand that their child is truly a victim.

General Comments on the Interview

Prior to agreeing to see a possible victim of child molestation, clinicians should evaluate their ability to work effectively with children and their ease in discussing sexual issues. If a clinician feels any discomfort dealing with children or sex, the child should be referred to someone who has skill and experience working with sexually abused children.

Second, a clinician should never ignore the disclosure of an assault made by a child or adolescent or any of her or his comments about the abuse. Many clinicians have been surprised when what were considered to be unbelievable allegations about sexual abuse were later substantiated. Even if unfounded, the mere fact that such allegations are made is indicative of a problem.

A child should never be held responsible for the sexual abuse to which she or he is subjected. A few children or adolescents may derive some level of pleasure from the sexual involvement and do not disclose the assault for that reason. For some of these children, the attention and physical contact inherent in the abuse is the first or only expression of any type of affection they have recieved from the offender and these children do not want to lose this "affection." For other children, the touching is very pleasurable. Young children do not always differentiate stimulation of their genitals from that of any other part of their bodies. A clinician should take care never to blame children or engage in guilt-inducing behavior if children indicate that they experienced pleasure or enjoyed the "special attention" the offender directed toward them. The important issue is that the child was used for someone else's sexual pleasure and did not have the ability to consent to such behavior. The responsibility for the sexual abuse lies with the perpetrator and any other adult who exposed the child to such abuse and did not respond in a protective fashion.

Finally, a clinician should always respect the child or adolescent being interviewed and the child's feelings. Similarly, a clinician should not act surprised or disgusted by the information, as such a reaction will indicate to the child that it is not safe to talk about the sexual abuse. With the appropriate approach, a clinician can make the interview a therapeutic experience rather than a traumatic one that only compounds the problems a child or adolescent is already experiencing.

TREATMENT OF CHILD MOLESTATION VICTIMS

Levels of Intervention

All victims of child molestation can benefit from crisis intervention. At this level of intervention, the therapist helps the victim and, whenever possible, the family to cope with the immediate needs resulting from disclosure of the abuse, such as coping with the medical and criminal justice systems and working with the child protective services. Additionally, the therapist is able to provide the emotional support needed by the victim and help protect the child from further psychological trauma. Finally, through her or his action, the therapist can provide the victim with the opportunity to establish a trusting relationship, a significant factor for all victims of sexual abuse. Crisis intervention should always be on an individual basis.

The vast majority of child sexual-abuse victims can benefit from intervention extending beyond the crisis phase. During short-term therapy the victim can find a source for the emotional support that will be needed during the recovery process, as well as a safe place to ventilate and work on the many negative feelings stemming from the abuse. Short-term therapy, generally lasting no longer than one year postassault, may be sufficient for many victims who did not experience physical and emotional trauma as a result of the abuse and/or who receive emotional support from family members and significant others. For most incest victims, however, long-term intervention is necessary.

Therapy continuing beyond one year after disclosure of the sexual abuse may be indicated for children who experienced severe physical and emotional trauma or who have not been provided with emotional support by significant others.

Treatment Formats

INDIVIDUAL THERAPY. Recommended for children immediately after disclosure of their sexual abuse, individual therapy provides a child with the opportunity to begin to come to grips with her or his abuse in a safe environment and without the pressure of many people being present. For adolescents, individual therapy should generally be employed as a step toward group therapy; however, this approach may be the preferred treatment for preadolescents.

GROUP THERAPY. Compared to individual therapy, group therapy has the advantage of group influence, a very powerful tool, particularly for adolescents. In this treatment format, a sexual-abuse victim is able to continue working on her or his recovery while aided by the support and suggestions of peers. However, a clinician should take care not to introduce a child or adolescent victim into a group before the victim has recovered sufficient strength to be able to discuss such an emotionally charged topic in the presence of others.

COUNSELING THE PARENTS OF NONINCESTUOUS VICTIMS. It is of utmost importance that the parents of a child victim receive some counseling, since the response of parents and significant others can have a major impact on the victim. Parents who continue over time to react negatively to the abuse most likely prolong the trauma of the child or adolescent, while parents who are able to accept the abuse can greatly facilitate the recovery of the victim.

The parents experience a broad range of emotions, including anger at the perpetrator and/or victim, guilt for their own failure to protect their child, and genuine concern for the welfare of their child. Counseling can help the parents work through their emotional turmoil. A clinician can assist the parents in examining their behavior to determine if they contributed to the assault by failing to protect the child adequately; however, the parents should be helped to understand that a child cannot be watched every minute of the day. Additionally, some parents become overprotective when their child is sexually abused, a postassault response that is not in the best interest of the child and may interfere with the child's natural psychological development. A clinician can point out to the parents the danger of such behavior.

While feeling angry at the child or adolescent for the sexual abuse is not an uncommon response in parents, it certainly does not contribute positively to the recovery of the victim. A therapist should help parents understand that their child is not responsible for the abuse, but instead is the victim, and should help the parents work through such feelings. A therapist should also assist the parents in dealing with their anger toward the perpetrator, since a continued expression of such emotions can also interfere with a child's recovery.

Parents frequently have specific questions related to the sexual abuse. For example, they may be concerned about the sexual orientation of their child subsequent to the abuse or about the child's normal sexual development, or they may not understand the reactions of their child. Thus, a major role of the therapist is to serve as an expert who can provide information needed by the parents.

FAMILY THERAPY IN INCEST CASES. Family therapy is the recommended treatment in incest cases, since all family members played either a direct or indirect role in such abuse (Giarretto et al., 1978; Sgroi, 1982b). The initial step is to conduct a family assessment that focuses on the strengths and weaknesses of each family member, as well as each member's contribution to the sexual abuse. Frequent familial contributory factors which should become issues during therapy include failure to protect, abuse of power, isolation of the family, fear of authority, poor familial communication patterns, denial of family problems and sexual abuse, a lack of empathy from the perpetrator, blurred role boundaries, inadequate parental controls and limit setting, and extreme emotional deprivation and neediness (Sgroi, 1982b).

As would be expected, the success of family treatment will depend in large part on the family's efforts in therapy. If the parents resist, success will be greatly limited. Many members of incestuous families may participate involuntarily in therapy, a situation for which a therapist must be prepared. When working with such a family, it is helpful to employ the unconventional strategies of personal authority, use of leverage to bring about patient participation, aggressive outreach, and the provision of support touching all aspects of a family's functioning (Sgroi, 1982b).

DYAD THERAPY IN INCEST CASES. Porter et al. (1982) suggest that mother-daughter treatment in cases of father-daughter incest is important, as it allows both parties to understand how the sexual abuse was allowed to occur and continue. Additionally, the mother and daughter are able to discuss the various emotions they experienced as a result of the incest. While this therapeutic format may be very difficult for both parties, such an approach can be particularly helpful in building a protective liaison for the victim.

Impact and Treatment Issues

Ten impact and treatment issues related to the sexual abuse of children have been noted by Porter et al, (1982). The first five of these issues may be applicable to any victim of child molestation, while the remaining issues are most likely to affect incest victims. An understanding of these factors serves as a basis for effective treatment.

THE "DAMAGED GOODS" SYNDROME. Almost all children who have been sexually abused feel damaged in some way as a result of their experiences. Additionally, the negative response of society to molested children may reinforce the child's feeling of being damaged. Thus, one therapeutic goal may be helping these children understand that they are not damaged and that if any real *physical* damage has been suffered, they will receive treatment. Additionally, significant others of the child should be helped to respond to the child positively rather than as damaged.

GUILT. Most sexually abused children or adolescents will experience guilt as a result of believing that they are responsible for their abuse, disclosure of the abuse, and/or the disruption of the family subsequent to disclosure. A goal of treatment should be to help erase the belief that the child is responsible for the abuse and its aftermath.

FEAR. A common response to sexual abuse is the development of fears, many of which may be realistic. Consequently, it is necessary to allow children to discuss what is frightening them and help them dispel the unrealistic fears while also assisting them in developing appropriate methods for coping with the realistic fears.

DEPRESSION. Depression is almost a universal consequence of sexual abuse for children, adolescents, and adults. An opportunity to ventilate feelings is often sufficient to alleviate depression. Should the depressed feelings continue, medication and/or hospitalization should be considered.

LOW SELF-ESTEEM AND POOR SOCIAL SKILLS. The various problems experienced by a child victim of sexual abuse may have a significantly negative impact on her or his self-esteem and self-confidence. The low self-esteem may subsequently affect the ability to relate to others. In cases of incest, the lack of adequate social skills may also be the result of restrictions imposed by the perpetrator that limited the child's or adolescent's interactions with peers. Providing the victim with the opportunity to discuss negative self-feelings is an important aspect of treatment. Additionally, social-skills training and/or allowing the child to practice her or his social skills in a group of peers should be considered.

REPRESSED ANGER AND HOSTILITY. Understandably, most children who are sexually abused experience great anger stemming from the abuse itself and/or their treatment by others subsequent to disclosure of the abuse. However, the abuse-related anger is usually repressed, particularly when the perpetrator is a family member. As part of therapy, the child or adolescent should be assured that it is quite natural to feel angry and disappointed when people let you down or hurt you, and needs to be given permission to express anger appropriately in order to deal with the trauma caused by the sexual abuse. Modeling in how to assert both positive and negative feelings is extremely helpful.

INABILITY TO TRUST. Incest victims are particularly likely to feel that they are unable to trust other people as a result of having been betrayed by a significant other. Learning once again to trust people is a long-term process but can be facilitated if the child or adolescent has the opportunity to experience healthy functional relationships, beginning with the bond between therapist and patient. Additionally, the child needs to be told that not all people are like the perpetrator and that, with time, she or he will again regain a sense of trust in others.

ROLE CONFUSION. As a result of having been thrust into the role of an adult sexual partner and, possibly, that of a quasi partner or parent, an incest victim is very likely to experience role confusion. Other family members may share this confusion. The role of the therapist includes aiding the child and parents to delineate appropriate role behaviors for each family member. It is important that the child be allowed to act as a child rather than as an adult.

PSEUDO-MATURITY AND FAILURE TO COMPLETE DEVELOPMENTAL TASKS. The role confusion experienced by incest victims may result in their manifesting pseudo-mature behavior while simultaneously robbing them of the opportunity to complete age-appropriate developmental tasks. The therapist's efforts to assist family members in defining appropriate role behaviors will allow the victim to engage in age-appropriate behaviors and tasks.

CONTROL. Perhaps the most significant impact of sexual abuse is the loss of control over her or his body and life that a victim experiences. It is imperative that the child be allowed to regain a sense self-mastery and control. Family members should be counseled about the importance of providing their child with the opportunity to be responsible for her or his behavior and should be advised to reinforce the child's independent decision making. Within the therapy situation, role playing and modeling will provide the victim with necessary practice. Realistically, an incest victim may be unable to make much progress toward self-mastery and control while living at home unless family therapy is undertaken.

Therapeutic Techniques

The use of psychotherapy in helping a sexual assault victim come to terms with her or his assault is the traditional approach and can be very effective. However, many children and adolescents lack the verbal skills that are necessary for this approach.

Behavior therapy is directed at alleviating specific problems experienced by victims of child molestation, such as fears, eating problems, and self-destructive behavior. Behavioral techniques are particularly effective with children who are either too young and/or nonverbal for other approaches.

Play therapy is most suitable for young children but can also be used effectively with victims through junior-high age. The use of age-related toys or materials provides victims an opportunity to express negative feelings and to act out their trauma. Burgess et al. (1978) discuss play material appropriate for various age levels.

Art therapy has been suggested as a very effective means by which child sexual-assault victims are able to express many of the emotions they are unable or unwilling to verbalize; it is, therefore, useful both in the assessment and treatment of victims (Stember, 1980). Naitove (1982) notes that, in addition to the use of drawing, art therapy with victims of child molestation may include dance, mime, drama, and poetry.

Parents As Therapists

In some cases of child molestation, one of the victim's parents can be trained to serve as the therapist for the child. Under the supervision of the clinician, the parent can learn to monitor specific behaviors and apply the agreed upon contingencies for negative and positive behaviors. Such an approach not only has the advantage of directly assisting the child in recovery, but also allows the parent to assume an active role in the process.

PREVENTION

Primary Prevention

TREATMENT OF CHILD MOLESTERS. The importance of providing treatment to child molesters as a means of preventing future sexual abuse cannot be overstressed. Many studies demonstrating the effectiveness of various treatment interventions with this population have been reported (Brownell and Barlow, 1976; Brownell et al., 1977; Callahan and Leitenberg, 1973; Cautela and Wisocki, 1971; Levin et al., 1977; Little and Curran, 1978; Marshall, 1973; Marshall and Barbaree, 1978; Marshall and Lippens, 1977; Nolan and Sandman, 1978). While not all child molesters may be amenable to treatment or voluntarily enter therapy, more treatment programs for pedophiles, hebephiles, and incest offenders need to be made available and research on the treatment of child molesters must be continued.

CHILD-REARING PRACTICES. Child-rearing practices should be modified so that children are taught they have the right to control their bodies and to tell other people that they have no right to touch their bodies. In our society, so much emphasis is placed on having children obey their elders that the rights of children are frequently overlooked. Not only do children have the right to protect their bodies, but they should be trained to assert this right.

In a related vein, efforts toward nonsexist child rearing are important. Males should not be reared to assume a power position and females must learn that they do not have to acquiesce to the power of males. Instead, respect for the equality and rights of both sexes should be taught.

Another preventative effort would be to provide sex education for all children. By understanding the implications and consequences of sexual behavior, children would be in a better position to refuse to be victims of sexual abuse.

SOCIETAL PERCEPTIONS. Our society needs to change its perception of child molestation and, with it, societal warnings to children and adolescents. To continue to warn children of the possible dangers of strangers only is an injustice to them. Instead, children and adolescents should be told that they may be at risk for sexual abuse by anyone and should be taught how to behave if confronted by possible abuse.

Secondary Prevention

PROGRAMS FOR VICTIMS. There is a dire need for the establishment of many more programs for sexually abused children and adolescents. More importantly, these programs must be made readily available to the victims. A national hotline for sexually abused children and adolescents, similar to that for runaway youths, could be established to help these victims as well as direct them to local sexual-abuse centers. Schools can also play an active role by opening the door to the discussion of sexual abuse. In addition, each school should have a sexual-abuse expert who is readily available for victims and who is able to intercede in continued cases of abuse.

TREATMENT FOR INCESTUOUS FAMILIES. An increased number of treatment programs for families involved in incest is needed. By early and comprehensive treatment, the number of child sexual-abuse victims experiencing long-term problems can be significantly reduced.

Tertiary Prevention

RAPE CRISIS CENTERS. Current rape crisis centers need to continue making their services available to adults who were sexually abused as children. Since many child and adolescent victims never recieve help at the time of their assaults, they continue to have the need to discuss their experiences, and rape crisis centers can meet this need. Additionally, such centers should expand their services to male victims and should provide them with male counselors.

TREATMENT PROGRAMS. Many adults who were sexually abused as children have significant abuse-related problems. Unfortunately, treatment services are seldom available to them. Thus, treatment programs for individuals who are experiencing long-term problems stemming from sexual abuse are needed.

SUMMARY

While child molestation is a most significant problem with a long history, our knowledge about the sexual abuse of children and adolescents is inadequate. To date, no systematic study has investigated the effects of pedophilia, hebephilia, and incest on the victims. Similarly, no controlled research has been conducted studying the efficacy of various treatment approaches in alleviating the problems of sexually abused children and adolescents. Yet, the comparatively little information known about child molestation indicates that, while it is not a problem likely to go away, the emotional and physical trauma to the victims caused by such abuse can be reduced.

REFERENCES

Brownell, K., and Barlow, D. 1976. Measurement and treatment of two sexual deviations in one person. *J. Beh. Ther. Exp. Psych.,* 7:349–354.

Brownell, K., Hayes, S., and Barlow, D. 1977. Patterns of appropriate and deviant sexual arousal: The behavioral treatment of multiple sexual deviations. *J. Consult. Clin. Psychol.,* 45:1144–1155.

Burgess, A. W., and Holmstrom, L. L. 1978. Interviewing young victims. In *Sexual assault of children and adolescents,* ed. A. W. Burgess, A. N. Groth, L. L. Holmstrom, and S. M. Sgroi. Lexington, Mass.: Lexington Books.

Burgess, A. W., Holmstrom, L. L., and McCausland, M. P. 1978. Counseling young victims and their families. In *Sexual assault of children and adolescents,* ed. A. W. Burgess, A. N. Groth, L. L. Holmstrom, and S. M. Sgroi. Lexington, Mass.: Lexington Books.

Callahan, E., and Leitenberg, H. 1973. Aversion therapy for sexual deviation: Contingent shock and covert sensitization. *J. Abnorm. Psychol.,* 81:60–73.

Cautela, J., and Wisocki, P. 1971. Covert sensitization for the treatment of sexual deviation. *Psychol. Rec.,* 21:37–48.

Christie, M., Marshall, W., and Lanthier, R. 1978. "A descriptive study of incarcerated rapists and pedophiles." Unpublished manuscript.

De Francis, V. 1969. *Protecting the child victim of sex crimes committed by adults.* Denver: American Humane Association, Children's Division.

Gagnon, J. 1965. Female child victims of sex offenses. *Soc. Prob.,* 13:176–192.

Gebhard, P. H., Gagnon, J. H., Pomeroy, W. B., and Christensen, C. U. 1960. *Sex offenders.* New York: Harper and Row.

Giarretto, H., Giarretto, A., and Sgroi, S. M. 1978. Coordinated community treatment of incest. In *Sexual assault of children and adolescents,* ed. A. W. Burgess, A. N. Groth, L. L. Holmstrom, and S. M. Sgroi. Lexington, Mass.: Lexington Books.

Hartman, V. 1965. Group psychotherapy with sexually deviant offenders (pedophiles): The peer group as an instrument of mutual control. *Crim. Law Quart.,* 7:464-479.

Jaffe, A. C., Dynneson, L., and Ten Bensel, R. W. 1975. Sexual abuse of children: An epidemiological study. *Am. J. Dis. Child.,* 129:689-692.

Justice, B., and Justice, R. 1979. *The broken taboo: Sex in the family.* New York: Human Sciences Press.

Lester, D. 1972. Incest. *J. Sex Res.,* 8:268-285.

Levin, S. M., Barry, S. M., Ganebaro, S., Wolfensohn, L., and Smith, A. 1977. Variations of covert sensitization in the treatment of pedophilic behavior: A case study. *J. Consult. Clin. Psychol.,* 45:896-907.

Little, L. M., and Curran, J. P. 1978. Covert sensitization: A clinical procedure in need of some explanations. *Psychol. Bull.,* 85:.513-531.

Lukianowicz, N. 1972. Incest. II. Other types of incest. *Brit. J. Psych.,* 120:308-313.

Marshall, W. L. 1973. The modification of sexual fantasies: A combined treatment approach to the reduction of deviant sexual behavior. *Beh. Res. Ther.,* 11:557-564.

Marshall, W. L., and Barbaree, H. E. 1978. The reduction of deviant arousal: Satiation treatment for sexual aggressors. *Crim. Jus. Beh.,* 5:294-303.

Marshall, W. L., and Lippens, K. 1977. The clinical value of boredom: A procedure for reducing inappropriate sexual interests. *J. Nerv. Men. Dis.,* 165:283-287.

Marshall, W. L., and Williams, B. "A behavioral treatment program for incarcerated sex offenders: Some tentative results." Paper presented at the annual meeting of the Association for the Advancement of Behavior Therapy, San Francisco, November 1975.

Naitove, C. E. 1982. Arts therapy with sexually abused children. In *Handbook of clinical intervention in child sexual abuse,* ed. S. M. Sgroi. Lexington, Mass.: Lexington Books.

Nolan, J. D., and Sandman, C. 1978. "Biosyntonic" therapy: Modification of an operant conditioning approach to pedophilia. *J. Consult. Clinc. Psychol.,* 46:1133-1140.

Porter, F. S., Blick, L. C., and Sgroi, S. M. 1982. Treatment of the sexually abused child. *Handbook of clinical intervention in child sexual abuse,* ed. S. M. Sgroi. Lexington, Mass.: Lexington Books.

Resnick, H., and Peters, J. 1967. Outpatient group therapy with convicted pedophiles. *Int. J. Group Psychother.,* 17:151-158.

Quinsey, V. L., Chaplin, J. C., and Carrigan, W. F. 1979. "Sexual preferences among incestuous and nonincestuous child molesters." Unpulished manuscript.

Sgroi, S. M. 1978. Comprehensive examination for child sexual assault: Dianostic, therapeutic, and child protection issues. In *Sexual assault of children and adolescents,* ed. A. W. Burgess, A. N. Groth, L. L. Holmstrom, and S. M. Sgroi. Lexington, Mass.: Lexington Books.

Sgroi, S. M. 1982. An approach to case management. In *Handbook of clinical intervention in child sexual abuse,* ed. S. M. Sgroi. Lexington, Mass.: Lexington Books.

Sgroi, S. M. 1982b. Family treatment. In *Handbook of clinical intervention in child sexual abuse,* ed. S. M. Sgroi. Lexington, Mass.: Lexington Books.

Sgroi, S. M., Blick, L. C., and Porter, F. S. 1982a. A conceptual framework for child sexual abuse. In *Handbook of clinical intervention in child sexual abuse,* ed. S. M. Sgroi. Lexington, Mass.: Lexington Books.

Sgroi, S. M., Porter, F. S., and Blick, L. C. 1982b. Validation of child sexual abuse. In *Handbook of clinical intervention in child sexual abuse.* ed. S. M. Sgroi. Lexington, Mass.: Lexington Books.

Silver, S. 1976. Outpatient treatment for sexual offenders. *Soc. Work,* 21:134–140.

Skinner, L. J., and Becker, J. V. 1983. "Myths underlying societal responses to sexual assaults." Unpublished manuscript.

Stember, C. J. 1980. Art therapy: A new use in the diagnosis and treatment of sexually abused children. In *Sexual abuse of children: Selected readings,* ed. K. MacFarlane. Washington, D. C.: National Center on Child Abuse and Neglect.

Weeks, R. B. 1976. The sexually exploited child. *South. Med. J.,* 69:848–850.

Wells, N. H. 1958. Sexual offenses as seen by a woman police surgeon. *Brit. Med. J.,* 5109:1404–1408.

Woodbury, J. and Schwartz, E. 1971. *The silent sin.* New York: American Library.

19

The Divorcing Family: Its Evaluation and Treatment

ALAN M. LEVY

THE TYPES OF PROBLEMS for which a child psychiatrist's opinion may be sought in cases of the divorcing family are: (1) child-custody determination, (2) visitation arrangements, and (3) whether treatment is necessary. Custody questions to be answered are: (1) should the mother or the father be the custodial parent, (2) should they have joint or shared custody, or (3) should neither parent have custody? Visitation arrangement questions are: (1) how should a new program be determined, or (2) how should an existing one be altered (Levy, 1982)? Questions relative to treatment are: (1) is it for the children or parents or both, (2) do the problems relate specifically to the divorce or are they independent of it, and (3) do the problems predate the divorce, coincide with the divorce, or both?

Epidemiology

While epidemiological data in this area are incomplete, information is available with regard to the number of divorces, the rate of divorce, and the number of children of divorced parents. Over one million divorces occurred in a given twelve-month period (Vital Statistics, 1977). This represented a 200% increase in the number of divorces since 1960, making the rate of divorce for those marrying in 1977 30 to 35% (Olson, 1977). Some 60% of those divorces affected young children (Saxe, 1975). In 1982, divorces in the United States were in excess of one and one-fifth million (U.S. Department of Health and Human Services, 1982).

Other demographic changes have also occurred. These include a rise in the number of children who are under eighteen, who live with a stepparent, who spend time in a one-parent family, and who live with an unmarried couple (Glick, 1979). Though there are no exact records kept, most divorced couples reach their own settlement in regard to custody and visitation issues. While only a small percentage of divorcing couples litigate custody and/or visitation issues, there is no way to determine how often, if at all, psychiatric consultation is sought in both the known litigated and the nonlitigated cases. The number of litigated cases is, however, on the rise (Petlicka, 1978). A small but growing number of these litigated cases receive court-ordered psychiatric consultation. The opinion of a child psychiatrist in these matters is being sought with increasing frequency as there is greater reliance on psychiatric opinion by judges and lawyers, and there are increasing attempts to gain custody by fathers, previously disadvantaged by the presumption that mothers would automatically gain custody.

Clinical Features

Questions regarding custody, visitation, and treatment are presented to the consultant in a variety of ways. Indeed, their timing and scope have clinical relevance. Three such situations may be considered. First, parents having a true interest in the mental-health issues facing them and their children will either alone or together seek a consultation with the child psychiatrist, even before they have consulted an attorney. They wish to explore and learn about a full range of issues and options that lie ahead regarding custody and visitation. They wish to know the possible adverse effects that divorce may have on them and/or their children—especially if these effects may require counseling or treatment. These parents and their children are relatively healthy individuals. The parents' psychopathology is minimal. When present, it tends to focus on the other spouse and not on the children. Acting out is usually absent and these parents tend to have a good relationship with their own parents. Children of these parents tend to have fewer problems relating to the family discord and subsequent divorce. Their loyalty to each parent is generally not conflicted or polarized. Parents in this group favor the consultation room over the courtroom for resolving family problems (Levy, 1978b). The consultant's opportunity to arrive at a therapeutic solution for the family, as opposed to a court-imposed solution, is maximized with this type of parent.

A second group of parents reaches the consultant after they have contacted an attorney regarding divorce, custody, or visitation issues. They seek the consultation at the attorney's recommendation. These parents and their attorney may do so with a true mental-health interest as previously mentioned, or they may do so to seek a tactical advantage for the forthcoming trial. In some cases their motivation for seeking a consultation may represent a combination of these two factors. In any event, a consultation involving only one parent and his or her children will obviously have less mental-health impact and usefulness than one in which the entire family is available. Parents and children in this second group as a rule score higher on all or most of the aforementioned indices; there is more individual psychopathology in the children and/or parents, the parental psychopathology no longer focuses only on the spouse but now envelopes the child, there is more parental acting out, and the parents will show a less positive relationship with their own parents. Children in these families show more problems and greater conflict in regard to parental loyalty. In addition, there is an increase in the other usual problems seen in children of divorce, such as guilt, depression, and anger. Occasionally there is some acting out (running away, turning parent against parent) or somatic symptoms. The chance of such a family resolving the custody and/or visitation issues apart from the courtroom is greatly lessened.

Finally, a consultation may be sought after the two parents have reached the courtroom. A consultation is court ordered or otherwise agreed to by both parents and their attorneys. While this avenue succeeds in having all parties participate in consultation, it does so with less genuine belief by either or both parents in the importance or relevance of mental-health issues to the questions or problems involved in divorce. Parents in this third group usually score the highest on the problem-predicting indices. Their children are the most polarized and traumatized of all. The so-called normal problems seen in separation and divorce are amplified and intensified many times over, as the fighting and bitterness between parents escalates. The parental pull on the children to join one parent or the other becomes unbearable. These children are very prone to act out or develop a variety of psychiatric symptoms—enuresis, school failure, depression, or general regression in functioning. Obviously, all hope for a consultation-room solution has long since faded and a court-imposed "solution" takes its place. These solutions are notoriously fragile and are often only an invitation to further court action.

Associated Conditions

In the Children

Divorce itself is not automatically pathogenic. It is usually the preexisting disturbed relationship between the parents that creates the problems for the children of divorce (Anthony, 1974). Some have related the trauma of divorce to that of death (Sugar, 1970), while others feel it is closer to the impact of abandonment (Anthony, 1974). In any event, the emotional impact of divorce on children, especially when preceded by family stress and emotional conflict between parents, is extensive. Children may show bewilderment, depression, confusion, anger, seeming indifference or anxiety with symptom formation and regression. They may act out, run away, become delinquent, develop somatic complaints or become accident-prone, and do poorly in school (McDermott, 1970; Wallerstein and Kelly, 1980).

The reactions of children to divorce have been studied and described according to age and sex (Wallerstein and Kelly, 1980). For example, in a group of children ages 2½ to 3¼, regression, fretfulness, bewilderment, neediness, and heightened aggression were noted by the authors. Children between the ages of 3 and 3¼ to 4¾ showed problems in self-esteem and self-image, feelings of responsibility for parental separation, and a loss of sense of order and predictability. In the group aged 5 through 6, problems in oedipal resolution and delay in accomplishment of latency-age tasks were noted. In all these preschool children, girls outnumbered boys three to one in their poor adjustment on follow-up.

In the early latency-age group, the following characteristics were observed: sadness and grieving, somatic complaints, avoidance and silence, fear and anxiety, feelings of deprivation, fantasies of responsibility and reconciliation, as well as loyalty conflicts. The late latency-age group was characterized by conscious intense anger, fears and phobias, shaken sense of identity, loyalty conflicts, and alignment with one or the other parent. In addition, there was a profound sense of loneliness and isolation. Finally, Wallerstein and Kelly reported that in the adolescent group, the following features emerged: anxiety about their future marriages, worries about money, a sense of painful experience, precipitously changed perceptions of their parents, accelerated individuation from parents, withdrawal, heightened awareness of their parents as sex objects, and finally interferences with entry into adolescence.

The fantasies that frequently emerge in children of divorce are abandonment, omnipotence relating to their own role in causing the divorce, identification with the aggressor, and rescue (Levy, 1978a). Conflicts revolving around the question of loyalty almost inevitably arise and are frequently intense.

These findings on children's reactions are of special importance both for the clinician and the parents, and taken as a whole they may be referred to as the "normal problems" of children of divorce.

Any psychiatric or developmentally deviant condition seen in the population at large may, of course, be seen as well in children of divorce. Often these independently occurring conditions are aggravated by the divorce and separation. They may be incorrectly used by one parent as an example of how the other parent is neglecting the child. Learning problems or developmental delays are frequently used in this fashion.

In the Parents

Parental reaction to the dissolution of their marriage is often one of a sense of loss and rejection. This can lead to anger, rage, and depression. Parents often feel a heightened need to maintain their identity. They may seek revenge. Each usually views himself or herself as the better parent and may wish to exclude the other parent from the lives of the children—an act of final punishment for the parent's alleged or imagined aggressive actions. Sometimes parents' personal past history will reveal rescue fantasies or specific identifications with childhood figures that will shed some light on their behavior. For example, a father sought custody of his son largely because of an unrecognized rescue fantasy based on the death of a younger brother during his childhood. Some parents' motivation for seeking custody relates to their relationship with their own parents. They may be seeking to avoid humiliation in the eyes of their parents and see their gaining custody as achieving this. Grandparents often fuel their own children's desires for sole custody and/or exclusion of the other parent from the lives of the children. In the case of a remarried parent, the new couple may seek to maintain their own relationship by passively agreeing that whatever is wrong in their marriage is caused by the ex-spouse. Consequently, sole custody may be sought or visitation prevented (American Psychiatric Association, 1982).

Assessment

Format for Interviews

1. A minimum of two clinical interviews with each parent alone.
2. A minimum of two clinical interviews (and/or play sessions) with each child alone.
3. When there is more than one child, see them all together for one session.
4. See each child together with each parent separately for at least one session.
5. If possible, it would be useful to see children together with both parents for one session.
6. See both parents together (if possible) for one session.

History

History-taking can often be somewhat clouded and contradictory due to the self-serving interests of the parent(s) seeking consultation.

PARENTAL HISTORY. One must ascertain the history of the courtship, marriage, marital life, birth of children, role of each parent in child rearing, child-rearing practices and beliefs, relationship between the parent and child, how the present situation arose, including whose initiative led to the divorce or separation. It is important to know the history of the courtship, marriage, and marital life, as these details allow one to examine each parent's conscious and unconscious attitudes and expectations about their marital partner, the marriage itself, and their own role in the marriage (Sager et al., 1971). These same attitudes, expectations, and fantasies often shed light on reasons for the divorce and may relate directly to whether the divorce will be accomplished smoothly or with great bitterness and hatred, as well as how the parents view the issue of the children's custody. For example, a woman who consciously or unconsciously viewed her marriage as a way to be protected, cared for, and adored like an idol will be angry and disappointed when her husband fails to meet these needs. He in turn may have wanted his wife to be assertive and take the leadership in the marriage. When she fails to do so, he may become angry and depressed. Each parent could feel cheated and betrayed, see themselves as the better parent, and feel that the children need to be with him or her as a way to protect them from the harmful other parent and give them what the other parent fails to provide. Thus, the potential for a bitter divorce and custody struggle.

Learning the history of the birth of the children, the role of each parent in child rearing, and their child-rearing practices and beliefs will allow for an evaluation of each parent's interest in and empathy for children, the nature of their understanding of children, and their development as well as their understanding of their role as a parent. One is not looking for the "perfect parent" but rather for a "good enough parent." It is reasonable to expect wide variations in parenting. A parent who was indifferent to the pregnancy and birth of the child, contributed little to the child care in the early years, and believed children should be seen but not heard, will, of course, give a clear picture to the examiner and help to define the parent-child relationship. In contrast, a parent who was happy with the pregnancy and delivery, enjoyed child care, and gives evidence of being pleased by the children's development and maturation paints a different picture of a parent-child relationship.

It is usually valuable to ask who initiated the divorce and how it was done. This may tell us more about the personality of each parent, their assessment of reality, and their reaction to the separation. Often one parent is taken by surprise that there is something wrong in the marriage and will feel rejected and depressed when asked for a divorce. This can lead to a feeling of deprivation for which the custody of the children becomes the only solution.

Additional questions to ask concern the parents' relationship to their own families, the history of their personal lives, their medical, psychiatric, and work histories. Details regarding the parents' relationship with their own parents can relate to their marital choice and even the outcome of their marriage. A parent with a strong unresolved dependent relationship with one or both of his or her own parents may contribute to the failure of a marriage by seeking to fulfill this infantile need. In addition the parents' attitude toward custody of the children may be dictated by a need to please their own parents by presenting them with a substitute child—the grandchild. Questions regarding their personal histories are, of course, routine in evaluating any person's mental health.

CHILDREN'S HISTORY. One must ascertain the following items both in regard to the period of time *before* the separation and divorce and the period of time during or *after* the separation and divorce: daily routine in the family, school performance, peer relationships, medical or psychiatric history, signs or symptoms of developmental difficulties or emotional problems, prior treatment, and any indications of the child's parental preference. These are the usual questions asked when evaluating a child for emotion difficulties. By differentiating the "before" and "after" aspect, one may learn how the divorce or separation affects the child, how the parents interpret this change, and what if anything they wish to do about it. Answers to these questions will reveal a parent's perceptiveness, empathy, and general awareness regarding the family situation. Some parents may claim a vast array of problems existed and relate them only to the divorce and/or their spouse's poor management. Other parents may be more specific and indicate that some problems in their children were always present; still others relate to that period when marital troubles began.

Content and Process of Interviews

If not gathered elsewhere and made available to the consultant, he or she should determine each parent's ability to provide for the material, health, school, and general needs of the child or children.

The primary questions to be addressed by the consultant are (American Psychiatric Association, 1982):

1. The emotional and psychological relationship and attachment between the parents and child or children.
2. The specific needs of the child or children (as they may relate to age, sex, health, and/or disabilities) and the parents' capacities and/or willingness to meet these needs. For example, a learning-disabled or physically handicapped or mentally retarded child will have special needs and requirements that will need to be recognized and planned for by each parent. Preschool children require a lot of physical care, emotional nurturing, help with impulse control, and training of body functions, while latency-age children are seeking to develop a balance between guilt and pleasure, master the learning process in school, and function effectively for long periods of time with peers and adults other than their parents. Children of each sex pass through stages when they feel closer to or more interested in the parent of the opposite sex (ages three to six), only to shift this focus to a predominate need to identify with the same sex parent (ages six to eleven). In addition, boys tend to seek and need more physical and motor activity than girls.
3. Family psychodynamics.
4. The child's custodial preference, if any.

Interview with Each Parent Alone

Accordingly, the consultant's questions and observations would be directed at the following when *interviewing parents alone:*

1. The parent's attitude to parenting.
2. The parent's attitude regarding children's developmental needs and the parental needs. For example, adolescents will wish to break away from their parents and relate more to their peers. This normal process is often accompanied by rebelliousness, provocativeness, and moodiness. Early echoes of these issues are seen in three year olds who are searching for autonomy and self-control. They need guidance, leeway to experiment, and patient parents.
3. A description of the child as a person—to include the expectations the parent has of his or her child, the child's likes and dislikes, as well as a listing of any of the child's special or general needs, especially including whether or not the parent mentions contact with the other parent as an important need.

4. Questions to reveal whether or not the parent views the child as a separate person and to determine if the parent and the child have a healthy or unhealthy sense of autonomy. Exploration of the child-rearing practices and parent-child relations during the separation individuation phase of development (second and third years of life), first school and away-from-home experiences, and the handling of the adolescent years will reveal a great deal. Parents who are overly insecure, ambivalent, overprotective, intrusive or rejecting, rigid, or unemotional may be revealing problems in their own sense of autonomy and are a high risk to pass along their trouble to their children. As they discuss their children and their child-rearing practices, one can note whether they enjoy or fear their child's growing independence and sense of self and just how they cope with it. The evaluation of the children will reveal to what extent they are overly attached and dependent, timid and inhibited, or detached, indifferent, and overly independent.
5. Questions to determine whether the parent considers parental modeling important and useful to a child. For example, inquiries into the child's wish to dress and act like one of the parents, verbal expressions of wishes to grow up and to be like a parent, acquisition of the mannerisms of one parent, can open up the area of identity and modeling. The parents' view of this behavior as appropriate, positive, and conducive to normal development, or as irritating, silly, and only reminding the parent of the hated spouse will have repercussions on the child's future relationships with each parent, as well as on their own self-esteem and identity.
6. Degree and quality of parental involvement and participation in the life of the child.
7. Any detailed plans parents may have regarding their projected lives after the custody and visitation issues have been settled. Often parents have never considered in detail what their lives and those of the children will be once a custody decision has been made, as they have been too engrossed in the struggle to "win." Postdivorce realities are often very grim financially and require dislocation in home and school arrangements. These needs as well as future needs five and ten years hence must be considered and dealt with. Plans to remarry need not be hidden or avoided. Reconstituted families present certain problems as well as positives.
8. Whether or not they are aware of any custodial preference by the child or if they have suggested or implied one to the child.

Parent-Child Interview

The consultant would want to observe the interaction of the parent and the child with regard to both verbal and nonverbal communications. This can be done either when the parent and child are together and performing a task assigned by the consultant or during a free-flowing verbal clinical interview situation. The consultant would want to look for the following in the parent: amount and type of communication, empathy for the child, flexibility in their relationship, physical distance between the two, sense of comfort and cooperativeness, sense of humor, trust, mutuality, anxiety, fear, uncertainty, lack of understanding, anger, punitive behavior or speech, taunting, provocation, or hostility (Levy, 1978a).

This session may also be used to assist the latency-age or adolescent child in asking the parent about the present marital situation, including questions about custody. One wishes to help the child ventilate his or her feelings toward the parent(s) as well as to ask any "unasked questions," such as why did you get a divorce, who wanted it, why are you sad, who will look after me, why do each of you say different things, etc. Parents are also encouraged to ask children questions. The encouragement of an open two-way discussion and even more direct confrontation can be useful. This joint meeting may also serve as additional opportunity to have the parent and child talk about any previously expressed parental preferences.

It is important to note if there are any discrepancies between the child's statements when interviewed alone, and when interviewed together with either parent. Consistency of responses tends to increase the validity of the child's statements. When there are significant discrepancies, however, this may either indicate the child's need to accommodate to the parent with whom he or she is now interviewed and, therefore, to remain "in the middle," or it may represent a sign of true parental influence and/or pressure upon the child (Levy, 1978).

Interview with the Child Alone

The consultant should ascertain if the child understands the reason for the visit and should explain to the child that the role of a therapist is to help the child express feelings in this difficult situation and not to take sides with either the mother or the father. The consultant should emphasize that the child's preferences, if any, are not determinative but that the parents or a judge will make the necessary decision. As in other evaluations of children, the initial part of the interview or the entire first interview may focus on general questions (and/or play if age appropriate) geared to eliciting the child's feelings, fantasies, and ideas. The consultant may ask the child to draw a person or a family or even to complete a drawing of a family doing something together. One should, at the end of the first session or the beginning of the second session, start to ask the child more direct questions about his or her family life, understanding of the current troubles and the events leading up to the present difficulties, perceptions of the parents' personalities and behavior, and assessment of the parents' good and bad points.

Additional questions should be asked about the child's plans and ideas in general, thoughts about any causal relationship between the child and the current events, his or her understanding of what custody implies and, finally, if it has not already come up in relationship to drawings, play, or volunteered statements, an inquiry into the child's parental preference for custody, if indeed there is one (Levy, 1980). This question would not be asked of preschool children. When the search for a preference or lack of it is undertaken, one reiterates that any stated preference on the child's part is not determinative. This should relieve the child's sense of guilt and minimize any sense of omnipotence. To elicit preference, one can begin in a general sense with such questions as, "If your mother and father each had a house on the same block, where would you spend your time?" More direct questions can follow.

Interview with Siblings

When there is more than one child involved in the custody evaluation, each should be seen individually as outlined previously. It is also of value to hold a joint interview with all the children together. This provides an opportunity to observe their interaction and relationships. Such things as rivalry and competition, leadership or subservience, bullying and intimidation, empathy and provocativeness, projection and criticism, can be looked for in the relationships between the children. In some custody cases a question may be asked about the possibility of separating the children. There should be no hard and fast rule in this regard.

The examiner must carefully evaluate the children's interaction, noting, for example, exaggerated dependence on a sibling in place of a failing parental relationship, marked jealousy and excessive fighting accompanied by a sense of relief when they are separated, or a surprisingly mild indifference to the thought of being separated with the statement that they would not mind this arrangement too much, and indeed, could see each other on weekends.

Other Investigations

Specific assigned tasks (storytelling, making or doing something together) can be performed by the parent and preschool or latency-age child together while the consultant observes the interaction. This enhances the assessment process (McDermott et al., 1978). Psychological testing may be obtained in order to shed light on: (a) psychiatric or developmental problems previously known or suspected in regard to the children or parent; (b) the child's unconscious perception of either or both parents, especially as it concerns perceptions of nurturing, trust, or hostility and rejection.

There may be meetings with the attorneys in order to obtain additional information regarding the family and to assist the consultant in evaluating the parents' and attorney's motivation with regard to the consultation. A telephone conversation or a personal visit with the judge in order to get his or her ideas and gain a general sense of the case may prove helpful.

Read all relevant legal and court papers, hospital or clinic records, school reports, treatment or remediation reports, etc. Interview or talk by telephone with any or all "significant others"—grandparents, stepparents, baby-sitter, aunts and uncles, treating physicians, teachers, etc. One must realize of course that all information obtained from other individuals and not obtained directly by oneself constitutes indirect information and is viewed as hearsay in the eyes of the law.

Abbreviated Assessments

The assessment outlined in the preceding represents the "ideal" assessment. A great deal of time and money will have been expended in pursuit of thoroughness and excellence, and in accord with a proper sense of seriousness that these matters demand. On occasion, requests may be made that the evaluation process be curtailed in some fashion due to the pressure of time or limitations of money. We should vigorously resist these attempts, pointing out the serious import of these evaluations to the children and families involved, as well as the fact that shortcuts reduce the reliability of the findings and make opinion formation even more risky than it normally would be. If, in spite of these admonitions exigencies prevail and all parties knowingly accept the inherent risk of a curtailed evaluation, then the abbreviated evaluation could be done by making the following changes. The examiner could schedule single rather than multiple interviews for each or some of the parties involved and the interview sessions could be made shorter. The evaluator could restrict the amount of time utilized in reading reports, letters etc., by only reviewing pertinent clinical reports that were deemed to be of utmost importance. Interviews with significant others could be eliminated or reduced. Telephone calls or telephone time spent with attorneys and/or significant others could be eliminated completely. Psychological tests could be omitted. Attempts to meet together with the parties' attorneys or to hold a telephone conversation with the involved judge could be omitted. The one shortcut that should never be taken is to omit spending time with the child together with each parent separately. This is one of the most crucial parts of the evaluation and should always be retained.

Opinion Formation, Conclusions and Recommendations

Reaching opinions, conclusions, and recommendations in any type of clinical assessment process is always difficult, since we are never dealing with an exact science. The usual hazards we face are incomplete information, countertransference, haste, and finally personal preexisting bias. In forming opinions regarding child custody and visitation, these hazards are magnified and multiplied. We often have incomplete information, as we are coping with an adversarial process (and not necessarily one seeking a therapeutic resolution), self-serving informants, and often a time limit in which we must complete our work. Opportunities for distortion due to countertransference are far greater, for we are dealing with parents, children, grandparents, attorneys, and even a judge. Our own preexisting bias in these assessments is important. It deals with our attitude toward single-parent custody versus joint or shared custody, as well as whether mothers as opposed to fathers are better custodians both in general or specifically at a certain time in the child's life (infancy, latency, or adolescence) (Levy, 1983). Other types of clinical assessment we usually undertake deal with the presence or absence of psychopathology, its extent, and whether intervention is required. These contrasting features in child-custody cases throw us off course and require special self-awareness as we are in the process of formulating opinions and conclusions from our assessment.

Guidelines to Decision Making

No exact description for decision making is possible. Each case is truly different as are the ages of children, sex of children, numbers of children, family situation at time of assessment, degree of emotional or mental illness in one or both parents, etc.

Nonetheless, it is possible to distinguish some general guidelines as follows. Whenever possible one should consider shared or joint custody as preferable to single-parent custody (Beck v. Beck, 1981). The sharing process should involve the time the children spend with each parent as well as participation by parents in the major decisions affecting their children. Next, consideration would be given to single-parent custody rather than to custody by neither parent. When one parent is clearly emotionally ill or physically disabled, custody would generally be awarded to the other parent. When both parents appear to be equally fit in most respects but one parent appears far less flexible and insists on severe limitations in the child's contact with the other parent, then single-parent custody should be selected favoring the more flexible and reasonable parent. When both parents are equally fit and equally flexible and joint custody has been ruled out because of geographic, financial, or other reasons, then decision making becomes very difficult indeed. Also, the needs of the children vary with their ages and sex, so any custody assignment made today may be "outgrown" by next year. The passage of time itself brings about changes and shifts in both parents and children, possibly necessitating a change in custodial arrangements. Therefore, recommendations coming from the assessment should be considered as being for today's needs but not necessarily for the future (Lewis, 1974).

Joint or Shared Custody

Parents, when divorced, can do without each other. But in most cases of post-divorce custody, children need and want a meaningful relationship with both parents (Levy, 1984). Separation and divorce will alter family relationships. They can never be as they had been before. However, these changes can be kept to a minimum and need not be extreme in most cases. It is not simply wish fulfillment or fantasy that acknowledges the continuing needs of growing children and seeks to mend the "fracture" and to make it as close to the original situation as possible. Realistically, we know that *some* fractures will never heal or will do so badly. Equally realistically, we know that *most* fractures can heal with a good approximation of the premorbid status.

The question is often asked, "How can two parents who don't agree on anything share custody?" The answer could be that perfect agreement is not required. Courts impose single-parent custody on disagreeing parents! Why not shared custody? After a trial period of sharing custody, it is amazing how the supposed differences between the parents seem to diminish or disappear.

Others ask, "How can a child shift residence back and forth between parents? What about constancy and predictability as important factors in the child's growth and development? Isn't one stable home better than two shifting residences?" The answer could be that all children differ in regard to their abilities and their vulnerabilities. Each postdivorced situation is different, with the ages of the children involved varying. Why then do we propose a uniform answer to complex issues when the variables are so numerous? Why not try new arrangements before considering them as unworthy of trial based on theoretical grounds? One could look at it in the following way. All custodial decisions have an element of risk. The question then is which situation is less risky. Should you take the risk of weakening or eliminating parental bonds and psychological parenthood with one parent when you assign single-parent custody, or should you take the risk of possibly (and you can always change the arrangements if you need to) threatening the psychological process of constancy and predictability in the child's development? This latter risk often turns out to be minimal in most, although not all, cases.

Clinically, in the evaluation and assessment of most cases of postdivorce custody, we find that the parents are equally fit or equally unfit. This is to say, both are equally healthy and positive or both are equally beset with emotional and psychological problems—neither to such a degree that they are substantially incapacitated. Therefore, in these cases, which represent the majority of cases, one should opt for joint or shared custody. In determining the physical sharing process, one must take into account the proximity of the parent's home, the school district, daily schedule for each parent, etc. The exact percentage of time spent by the child with each parent is secondary to the parent and child being able to feel that each parent is equal and meaningful in their participation in the child's life.

The next most frequent clinical finding is that one or the other parent has a significant personality problem that leads them to polarize the children against the other parent. This has been called brainwashing or pathological identification. Visitations are obstructed and any sense of equilibrium for the child has been destroyed (Levy, 1982). Joint or shared custody in such cases would obviously not work. Custody should be assigned to the parent who is most flexible and has not been seeking a pathological alliance with the child. If and when an equilibrium between the two parents is ever established, the single-parent custody could be altered in favor of shared custody.

The smallest group of cases is that in which one parent has a substantial or major mental or physical illness that makes it impossible to properly care for the child. Single-parent custody is obviously preferred until, if at all, a better equilibrium is established.

All decision making in child custody should be viewed as relative and subject to review and revision. Child development is a dynamic process. The psychological needs of children change. Today's needs might be met by one or both parents. What about tomorrow's? Parents also change. Following divorce, life situations such as remarriage, schools, friends, etc., alter. The assessment should stress the need for flexibility in arrangements and the willingness to reassess the situation with all concerned as time goes by.

Decisions about which parents and which children need treatment is less complex. Almost all need some form of treatment. However, most fail to see this need. Caught in the crises of the divorce process and the rending pull of the adversarial process, decisions for therapy are assigned a low priority. Clearly, treatment is more suitable and has a higher chance of success if it is voluntarily sought out by the parents.

TREATMENT

Child-custody and visitation consultation is most often set within an adversarial framework. Accordingly, more often than not the goal of the consultation is to win something or punish and find fault with someone. A decision regarding custody and/or visitation is required as a practical matter in the divorce process. Rarely does the consultation have a therapeutic aim. Consequently, it behooves the consultant to try to direct the process as much as possible toward a therapeutic outcome (Levy, 1978b). The goals of any treatment undertaken with regard to custody and visitation problems would be to eliminate the abrasive interaction arising from the custody or visitation struggle and to strive for the optimal sharing by parents of their time with the children as well as their mutual participation in decision making.

Available Treatment and Therapeutic Approaches

Individual counseling and psychotherapy for one or both parents is directed at (1) discussions of common problems of parents and children of divorcing families, before, during, and after the divorce, (2) deeper probing into the parents' problems stemming from their own childhood, problems involved in the original selection of the marital partner, parental behavior during the divorce, the parental motivation related to the custody and visitation consultation.

Problems common to parents who are divorcing are not too dissimilar from those confronting their children. They center around themes of loss, rejection, financial uncertainty, threatened identity, dislocation of daily routines, anger, depression, and guilt. These problems are often superimposed on deeper preexisting emotional conflicts in one or both parents. If the parental history has revealed, for example, deep-seated dependency needs by one parent on his or her own parent and a subsequent heightened ambivalence toward the spouse, one could expect that any depressive response to the divorce would be greatly intensified and exceed the "normal." Should parents be especially narcissistic as a result of their own early childhood experiences, then an overprotective reaction to their own child as their self-extension could lead to a demand for sole custody and an insistence that their spouse is unable to parent adequately. Levels of parental pathology that underlie the marriage contract and its dissolution have been beautifully described by Sager (Sager et al., 1971).

Therefore, treatment approaches need to distinguish between "normal" responses to divorce and those responses that come from deeper levels. Often they are mixed. Short-term psychotherapy is useful for "normal" problems, whereas intensive individual treatment is needed for deeper and mixed psychopathology.

Individual counseling and psychotherapy for the child or children must focus on (1) problems common to children in divorcing familes, and (2) deeper problems caused by preexisting psychiatric or developmental problems or more serious problems for the children/family caused by an especially bitter and difficult divorce.

As mentioned earlier, the common and almost ubiquitous problems for children of divorce are: feelings of rejection and abandonment of one or both parents (with the intense anger, rage, and depression this engenders); a false sense of responsibility for the divorce; attempts at repair and restitution of the parental marital state; conflicts over loyalty to one or both parents; and subsequent identification with either the parent perceived to be the aggressor or the one who is now the principal caretaker. Preexisting problems such as attention deficit disorder, anxiety states, personality problems, etc., can be delineated clinically from the "normal" problems superimposed upon them. In cases of especially bitter and prolonged divorces in which the parents are disturbed and polarize the children's loyalty, the psychological trauma and turmoil in these children will be greatly intensified. In these cases it may be difficult to distinguish whether their current psychopathology relates more to the divorce or to predivorce problems.

Therapy should be selected according to the assessment of the genesis of the pathology. Problems common to children of divorce are often best treated by "family-style" approaches such as parent-child discussions directed at clarification and confrontation of issues. This approach can be enhanced by individual brief therapy approaches with parent and child focused on the common themes already enumerated.

Family treatment would be a modified type involving the children and one parent. It would be directed at clarifying the existing situation with regard to the child's new "family life" (having two homes and possibly having a stepparent, etc.). This approach should be considered as potentially useful in almost all cases. It might suffice as the only form of therapy or be assisted by individual treatment for parent and/or child when special attention to individual problems are required. The family approach is especially useful in improving communication between family members and clarifying misinterpreted acts and feelings by each family member. Treatment provides a forum for give and take that is often avoided in everyday family life.

Therapeutically Oriented Consultation

Certain factors favor therapeutically oriented consultation. Some mention of these factors has been made in the discussion of clinical features; a favorable outcome relates to such things as low parental psychopathology, absence of parental acting out, early and independently requested mental-health consultations, and the participation of attorneys who possess a humanistic outlook toward the practice of family law. Specific strategies can enhance the therapeutic potential. From the moment the consultant is first contracted by either the parents or their attorneys, he or she should stress the need to see all parties (including the attorneys) if at all possible, explaining the limited value of a consultation that includes only part of the family. In this fashion the consultant is stressing his or her lack of partisanship and preference for a full clinical evaluation as opposed to a partial one. When all parties do participate in the evaluation, stress the value of explaining the clinical findings of the consultation to both attorneys and the parents, either alone or together. This is a way of using the consultation as a therapeutic instrument rather than a legal one, and a way to obtain feedback from the parents and their attorneys which can be used for additional consideration by the consultant. By explaining the details of the evaluation and clinical findings to the attorneys and parents, one will invite further information or comments from them. It will provide an opportunity to further assess goals, motives, and preferences of parent and attorney. Taken together, all this will stimulate the potential for resolution of the problems in the consultation room and not the courtroom. The consultant's final report and opinions should await the completion of these steps.

When the consultation has been requested by the court, the consultant may talk to the judge prior to completion of the report. This will often provide the consultant with more information, a sense of the judge's views and leanings, and an opportunity to discuss with the judge clinical findings, including family dynamics. The consultant may also discuss with the judge his or her recommendations regarding custody, visitation, and treatment, elaborating on the pros and cons of each option available. The judge will have an opportunity to ask questions and acquaint the consultant with legal issues. Together the judge and consultant can search for a therapeutic/legal outcome.

Since consultation regarding custody and visitation are not undertaken in the same way and for the same reasons as other consultations regarding children and families, the climate for a therapeutic follow-up is distinctly less favorable. In some cases, however, a therapeutic milieu or even therapy itself may commence from the moment of first contact or slowly emerge as the consultation proceeds.

Written Psychiatric Report

Form

In writing a report for a parent, attorney, or judge the following is suggested. Indicate at the onset who requested the report, why it was requested, and what questions are being asked of the consultant. List the individuals interviewed, the date when these interviews took place, the length of each interview, and who was seen in each instance. List and identify all documents received and read, as well as any telephone conversations with individuals related to the case. The style of the report is important. It should be objective in its tone. Direct quotations from the interviews can and should be used freely to illustrate what people felt and said. Findings and conclusions should be stated in simple terms, avoiding the use of theory or argument. Diagnostic terms should be used wherever applicable. However, it is important that the terms should be explained as to meaning and relevance. One should keep in mind who will be reading the report. This will require that a careful balance be struck between the therapeutic aims of the report and the aims of providing information to the reader. In addition, the consultant should be aware that at some subsequent time, he or she may need to testify in court regarding this report. Therefore, one should be prepared to support and document any of its content (American Psychiatric Association, 1982).

Content

The heart of the report should consist of an exposition of the clinical material obtained, as it addresses the four core questions: (1) the emotional and psychological relationship and attachment between the parents and child or children; (2) the specific needs of the child or children (as they may relate to age, sex, health, and/or disabilities), and the parents' capacities and/or willingness to meet these needs; (3) family psychodynamics; and (4) the child's custodial preference, if any. Accordingly, one will find that each participant in the evaluation should be clinically described as a separate person and also in relationship to the other family members as these four questions are answered.

Opinions should be stated clearly and all pronouncements should be supported by directly observed behavior and statements made during the clinical assessment process. The clinician's interpretation of the meaning of these observations should be stated, together with the reasons for this opinion. If a clear-cut opinion cannot be offered, a range of options with pros and cons should be discussed, as well as the reasons for failing to put forth a definitive opinion. When additional evaluation might be required before reaching an opinion, this should be stated. If treatment is necessary, state for whom and why. If a reevaluation of the recommendations should be made after a period of time, state when, who should be included, and who should be evaluated.

Conclusion

Family dissolution leading to questions of child custody, visitation, and treatment is creating an increased demand for child psychiatric consultation. This type of consultation differs from that usually dealt with by the child psychiatrist. The aim or goal of the consultation may be less therapeutic and more related to legal strategy and partisan advantage than the ordinary type of consultation. Special problems arise in history-taking and evaluation of the parents and child which demand substantial changes in the consultant's usual case examination and evaluation. Opportunities to turn the consultation in a therapeutic direction are minimal but can be achieved by using special measures.

References

American Psychiatric Association. 1982. Child custody consultation: A report of the task force on clinical assessment in child custody. July 1982.

Anthony, J. E. 1974. Children at risk from divorce: A review. In *The child in his family: Children at psychiatric risk,* vol. 3, ed. J. Anthony, and C. Koupernik. New York: Wiley.

Beck v. Beck (1981). 86 New Jersey 480.

Glick, P. C. 1979. Children of divorced parents in demographic perspective. *J. Soc. Issues,* 35(4):170–182.

Levy, A. M. 1978a. Child custody determination—a proposed psychiatric methodology and its resultant case typology. *J. Psych. Law,* summer, pp. 189–214.

Levy, A. M. 1978b. The resolution of child custody cases—the courtroom or the consultation room. *J. Psych. Law,* winter, pp. 499–517.

Levy, A. M. 1980. The meaning of the child's preference in child custody determination. *J. Psych. Law,* summer, pp. 221–234.

Levy, A. M. 1982. Disorders of visitation and child custody cases. *J. of Psych. Law,* 10(4).

Levy, A. M. 1983. Major pitfalls in child custody determinations. Delivered at annual meeting of American Academy of Child Psychiatry, San Francisco, October 1983.

Levy, A. M. (In press, 1984). Father custody, in *Child Psychiatry and the Law,* Vol. II. Ed. D. H. Schetky, & E. P. Benedek. New York: Brunner/Mazel.

Lewis, M. 1974. The latency child in a custody conflict. *J. Am. Acad. Child Psych.,* 13:635–647.

McDermott, J. F., Jr. 1970. Divorce and its psychiatric sequelae in children. *Arch. Gen. Psych.,* 23:421–427.

McDermott, J. F., Tseng, W-S., Char, W. F., and Fukunaga, C. S. 1978. Child custody decision making. *J. Am. Acad. Child Psych.,* 17:104–116.

Olson, D: Marriage-divorce-remarriage: The revolving door. *Contemp. Psychol.,* 22(5):395–396.

Petlicka, M. 1978. Director of Family Counseling Service, Supreme Court, Country of New York. Personal communication.

Sager, C., Kaplan, H., Gundloch, R., Kremer, M., Lenz, P., and Royce, J. 1971. The marriage contract. *Family Process,* 10(3):311–326.

Saxe, D. 1975. Some reflections on the interface of law and psychiatry in child custody cases. *J. Psych. Law,* winter, pp. 501–514.

Sugar, M. 1970. Divorce and children. *South. Med. J.,* 63(12):1458–1461.

Vital Statistics Report, *H.R.A.,* 1977, 26(2):1–3.

Wallerstein, J. S., and Kelley, J. B. 1980. *Surviving the breakup: How children and parents cope with divorce.* New York: Basic Books.

Part II

EVALUATING PROBLEMS: THE DIAGNOSTIC APPROACH

20

The Initial Clinical Evaluation of the Child

RICHARD A. GARDNER

THERE ARE MANY WAYS to approach the initial clinical evaluation of the child. This chapter describes techniques that I have found useful. Needless to say, these techniques can be adapted to each clinician's specific needs. Of course, examiners of other theoretical persuasions will conduct different kinds of evaluations. For example, a cognitive behavior therapist or a classical child psychoanalyst will focus much more on the child's statements and be less concerned with input from the parents. Clearly, a variety of methods can be effective.

Since the full evaluation of the child will include a number of interviews with the child and parents in addition to the initial interview, it should be conducted in a setting in which there are no time constraints. In other medical specialities, examiners do not generally compromise or otherwise restrict their evaluations because of time limitations; other than in emergency situations, they are given free rein to conduct assessments. Because psychiatric evaluations can be quite lengthy, however, time limits are frequently placed on the evaluator. This cannot help but compromise the situation.

Considering the complexity of many (if not most) evaluations, an initial interview of one hour is generally not adequate. Such an interview may provide the evaluator with information about major areas of pathology that warrent further inquiry and possibly some depth of understanding in one or two areas. It cannot, however, provide a diagnosis in the true sense of the Greek origin of the word: to know in depth. Thus, while subsequent interviews of 45–60 minutes are generally adequate, my clinical evaluation generally begins with an initial interview of two hours in which the child and parents are seen in varying combinations. The findings and recommendations are then presented to the family. If warranted, the initial interview is followed by a full, intensive evaluation. Together, the initial interview and the intensive evaluation should provide an in-depth understanding of the child's problems and also establish a good relationship, or at least communication, with the child and family members. Without such a relationship or communication, the likelihood of successful psychotherapy is minimal. Of course, a good relationship does not necessarily predict success for psychotherapy, but it increases the chances for a favorable outcome.

INITIAL TELEPHONE CALL

During the initial telephone call, the examiner should spend a minute or two discussing the child's main problems with the parents so as to be in a better position to deal with the unexpected should it occur later in the consultation room. Psychiatrists or psychologists treating children must be prepared to handle many more "surprises" than with adults—such is the unpredictability of our patients.

From the telephone interview, a number of conclusions may be reached. For instance, one might conclude that an interview is not warranted, or, if the child has symptoms such as headaches or gastrointestinal complaints, that the youngster should first be seen by another medical specialist. Sometimes an evaluation may be premature, as when a child starts to exhibit disruptive behavior in the classroom during the week following a parent's presumably permanent departure from the home. (The authors of *DSM-III* have wisely stipulated a time consideration before many childhood diagnoses can be considered as warranted.)

Often, a question posed to the examiner during this telephone conversation can provide useful information about the parents. For example, a mother may state that she has just discontinued treatment with a therapist because he was "money hungry" (he asked to be paid each month), or because the therapist "started to ask lots of personal questions when I brought my child to see him." A parent may request that the evaluator promise never to tell the child that he or she was adopted. A mother may say that she has no money for treatment, but that the examiner should bill her ex-husband (who does not "believe" in psychiatry and therefore will not be present at the first interview) because her divorce decree states that he should pay all medical bills. Obviously, these are issues that the examiner will want to discuss, even if briefly, on the telephone.

If, after the initial telephone conversation, an interview appears warranted, a two-hour initial interview is scheduled for the child and both parents. The caller is advised that during this time the parents and child will be seen alone and together in varying combinations. This recommendation is made regardless of the parents' marital status. If both parents are involved with the child, their participation in therapy (at some level) is most often warranted. The fact that they are no longer living together does not preclude the need for their cooperation in the child's treatment, and their being together at the initial interview helps establish this precedent. Although on occasion a divorced caller may be surprised at this suggestion, most see the wisdom of it and comply.

The parents should be told that they will be sent a questionnaire to be brought, filled out, to the first interview. The questionnaire should contain questions that will provide basic data about the pregnancy, the delivery, the post-delivery period, the infancy and toddler periods, the developmental milestones, and information about the child's performance in school, at home, and in the neighborhood. The questionnaire should also include questions about the mother and father and might even include a checklist for the presence of the wide variety of symptoms that children can exhibit. (Details of the questionnaire that I devised are to be found elsewhere [Gardner, 1979a, 1982]). The parents are also invited to bring to the initial interview copies of reports from teachers, psychologists, neurologists, social workers, learning disabilities specialists, and other professionals who have been involved with the child.

INITIAL INTERVIEW

It is not expected that an examiner could possibly cover in a two-hour interview all the material that will be presented here. It has been provided to acquaint the reader with the wide variety of possible assessment instruments and techniques that could prove useful in the initial interview.

Parents and Child Together

Seeing the parents and child together in the initial interview, as I do, is not traditional. Traditional practice, when conducting this interview, has been for the therapist to invite the child alone into the consultation room while leaving the parent(s) in the waiting room. One of the arguments for this is that separating the child from the parents at the outset communicates to the child that he or she is to have a special, private relationship—a relationship not shared by the parents. However, one can accomplish this goal without separating the child from the parents at the outset, which is when the child is likely to be most anxious. In fact, pressing for separation at that time may lessen the likelihood that such a relationship will be established since the anxieties that the separation engenders in the child may produce negative reactions to the therapist.

Another reason often given for separating the child from the parents at the outset is that it allows the therapist to observe whether the child has "separation anxiety." It is difficult, however, to imagine any child not being anxious in circumstances where the therapy is an unknown, the therapist is a stranger, and the child has never before been in the clinic or office and has little appreciation of what is going on. It is likely that the youngster has been told something like, "You're going to see a nice lady," "We're taking you to see a nice man who'll be playing lots of games with you," or "We're taking you to see a teacher who will help you learn better." Since such explanations are cover-ups, they may not be believed and may therefore create anxiety. Or the child may be told that he or she is going to see someone who will help with the youngster's "problems." Although the child may not have the faintest idea what the parents mean by the word "problems," he or she is not likely to anticipate that the experience is going to be a pleasant one.

Thus, if a child exhibits anxiety when separating from the parents to go with the therapist, it is likely that this is a normal response. In fact, it is reasonable to say that not being anxious at that point would probably reflect significant psychopathology indicating that the child's capacity to form deep relationships is so impaired that it makes no difference whether he or she is with a parent or a stranger. Or it may reflect such a defect in the parent-child relationship that the child welcomes an opportunity to go off with a stranger. But these are unusual situations. Most often the child is anxious and does not want to be separated from the parents in strange surroundings. One of the worst experiences a child therapist can have is that of trying to force or cajole a screaming, panicky child into accompanying the examiner alone into a private office. As the child desperately implores the parents not to let the stranger take him or her off, the presence of others in the waiting room cannot but increase the child's humiliation. Once in the consultation room, the likelihood of gaining any meaningful information from the child is almost nil.

Another reason many therapists see the parents alone first is because they believe that the child's disruptions and interferences will inhibit the data collection process. In addition, they anticipate that the parents will feel less free to speak when the child is present.

While I recognize the potential drawbacks to my approach of first seeing the parents and child together, I consider that the disadvantages of the traditional approach far outweigh its advantages. First, no matter how accurate the parent's description of the child is, it is very difficult, if not impossible, for the therapist to gain a reasonable appreciation of the kind of person the child is without actually seeing him or her. Furthermore, the aforementioned disruptions and interferences can themselves provide useful information and allow the therapist to observe directly parental interaction with the child—observations that are vital to the evaluation. As for the argument that seeing all three together in the initial interview deprives the evaluator of the opportunity to get information from the parents that they would hesitate to disclose in front of the child, one need not be deprived of this opportunity, which can be obtained when one is alone with the parents during this two-hour interview. In addition, one can also see the child alone and can enjoy the benefits to be derived from that experience, especially in situations where the child might be hesitant to reveal him- or herself in the parents' presence.

Once the parents and child are in the room, I again depart from the traditional approach. In my own training in the 1950s, I was taught that the unstructured interview is best because it allows for free revelations from the universe of information that may come before the evaluator, and that specific questions are likely to be contaminating and restricting. Subsequent experience has led me to conclude that one need not lose the benefits of the open-ended inquiry if one asks specific questions. Both types of inquiry can provide useful information. Thus, during training, I was taught that the best question to begin with was something along the lines of: "Well, why have you come here?" or "So what's the problem?" The rationale for this approach is that since the question is an open one and does not draw the child into specific areas, it therefore does not have any contaminants. Although this position is certainly valid, it does not give proper consideration to the fact that posing open-ended questions to a person who is anxious will not yield helpful information. Accordingly, the initial interview is best begun with general questions that any human being would ask another in a new situation. One might ask whether the parents had trouble finding the office or whether they had difficulty because of the weather. These are innocuous enough questions and are not likely to contaminate anything. They do, however, serve to lessen anxiety and make the examiner (a total stranger) more familiar and "human."

The child is then asked a series of simple questions that will probably be easy to answer, questions about what the youngster's name is and how it is spelled and about his or her address, telephone number, age, school grade, teacher's name, the names and ages of the parents and siblings, and so forth. As the child gets "the right answers," anxiety is alleviated and the child is then in a better position to answer the more open-ended questions about why he or she is there. The specific questions only take a few minutes, do not contaminate, and will provide the examiner with a patient who will generally be in a good position to give accurate answers to the questions that will follow. What is even more important is that the examiner is much more likely to develop a good relationship with the child by starting in this way—with sensitivity to the child's anxiety—rather than by using an approach likely to produce more anxiety and alienation.

At this point, attempts are made to draw the child out, as much as possible, regarding the reasons for coming to the therapist. Occasionally, a child may become involved in a lengthy discussion with the therapist while the parents sit quietly looking on, but this is unusual. If, as most often happens, the child denies having difficulties or mentions only the most innocuous ones, the parents should be invited to give their opinions regarding the presenting problems. The examiner, of course, does not want to be in the position of automatically accepting the parents' versions. Although the parents' recounting of the presenting problems is likely to be far more accurate than the child's, one still does well to hear both sides. This principle should be followed throughout the treatment. It is not being suggested that the therapist strictly refrain from taking the parents' position but rather that conclusions should be made only after hearing both sides and should then support healthy behavior, regardless of who exhibits it—without keeping score, so to speak, as to which party is getting more support. In this way the therapist is more likely to be viewed as impartial.

The examiner would do well to avoid being placed in the position of getting the child to "confess" and admit that he or she has exhibited a particular form of undesirable behavior. If the parents' and the child's renditions are diametrically opposed, and the child insists that the parents (as well as the teachers, baby-sitters, etc.) are lying, the therapist should not be in the position of "nailing down the truth no matter how long it takes." Rather, the therapist might make a statement such as, "Well, you and your parents seem to have different opinions about what's happening here. Let's go on to something else. Perhaps at some other time we'll find out whose opinion is closer to the truth." When a good relationship has been established, the child will be more receptive to revealing deficiencies. A confrontational approach is predictably going to reduce the likelihood that such a relationship will develop.

If during the course of the parents' description of the presenting problems the child interrupts with comments such as, "Don't tell him that," or "I told you never to tell him that," or "You promised me you wouldn't talk about that," one might react with surprise and say something like "What! Keeping secrets from your own psychiatrist? Didn't you know that you're never supposed to keep secrets from a psychiatrist?" One might then reinforce this principle by asking the child to think about television programs he or she has seen in which this fact has been demonstrated.

During the discussion of the presenting complaints it is important to observe the various parties. One should especially observe the child's relationship with each of the parents. Glances and gestures, as well as vocal intonations, provide information about affection, respect, and other forms of involvement. Seat placement, physical contact, and direct statements to one another also give much information about the interpersonal relationships of the parties being interviewed. In fact, this aspect of the interview may be more important than the specific information about presenting problems that is ostensibly the focus.

It is important to concentrate on the child's assets, accomplishments, skills, and hobbies at this time. This serves to counterbalance the ego-debasing material that has been thus far focused upon. By necessity, therapy must concern itself, either directly or indirectly, with the problems that have brought the child to treatment. There is usually little in them that the child can be proud of and much that he or she is ashamed of. In the world beyond the consultation room, the problems may represent only a small percentage of the child's living experiences; in the consultation room, unfortunately, they represent a significant percentage if the therapy is to be meaningful. In order to counterbalance this unfortunate but necessary emphasis, therapists do well to take every opportunity to focus on ego-enhancing material. If warranted, the therapist should compliment the child on a *meaningful* accomplishment. There is no place for gratuitous or feigned praise in therapy. Interest (only if genuine) should be expressed in any activity that is a source of gratification for the child. This, too, can serve to enhance the relationship.

At this point, one can proceed in a number of different ways. If the examiner suspects that there is much useful information that the parents can relate but have been hesitant to reveal in front of the child, the child might be told, "Now I'm going to speak with your parents alone, so I'd appreciate your having a seat in the waiting room. Then, I'll speak with you alone while they sit outside." To some children this might be followed by, "I'll be speaking with them about things that are personal for them. Then, when I'm with you, I'll be speaking about things that you may want to be kept personal." However, it is important for the reader to appreciate that the latter comment is not made very often. I much prefer that the atmosphere reflect an open pool of communication in which all things pertinent to the child are discussed freely with both parents and the child. The examiner may, however, see the child alone at that point, especially if the parents have stated that there is nothing additional that they wish to relate. Or, the interview with all three parties may be continued, if that appears to be the most judicious approach.

Parents Alone

If the situation warrants the parents being seen alone, they should be asked about other problems that they have hesitated to discuss in front of the child. Often such reluctance is ill-advised, and the parents should be encouraged to discuss these issue(s) with the child (who is then brought back into the room). When this is not the case, and the parents are alone, one does well to get some information about the marital relationship. Time does not permit going into great detail at this point, but the therapist wants to get a general idea about its stability and whether significant problems are present. When making inquiries about the parental relationship, each side should be heard; but in the initial interview, it may not be possible to come to any conclusions regarding which party exhibits the greater degree of pathology. The examiner merely wants to obtain a list of the main problems; an in-depth inquiry goes beyond the scope of the initial interview.

On occasion, both parents will claim that they have a good marriage and that they love one another. There are two possibilities here: One is that this is true and the other is, of course, that the parents are denying (either consciously or unconsciously) impairments in their relationship. When presented with the "happy marriage," the examiner might respond with a comment like, "Every marriage has some problems; no marriage is perfect. There are times, I am sure, when the two of you have differences of opinion. Every marriage has its fights from time to time. What are the areas of difference in *your* marriage?" When presented in this way, the parents are generally more comfortable about revealing areas of difficulty. Of course, there are marriages in which the partners never fight, but in such cases one or both generally suffer with a deep-seated anger-inhibition problem, and the "peace" they enjoy is paid for dearly with symptoms and/or character traits resulting from the pent-up hostility that inevitably arises in all human relationships. Sometimes parents who deny marital difficulties in the joint session will provide significant information about their marital problems in individual sessions. Of course, the therapist would then be negligent if he or she did not go into the reasons for the "cover-up" during the joint session.

It is desirable to get some idea about the depth and nature of psychopathology in each of the parents. The interviewer will usually already have some information along these lines from general observations. The level of tension in the initial interview is generally quite high from the outset. Strong emotions are evoked. In such an atmosphere it is likely that many forms of psychopathology will be revealed. This is especially so for such character traits as suspiciousness, dependency, volatility, "low boiling point," strong need to control and dominate, and seductivity. One of the easiest ways to obtain information about the parents' psychopathology is to ask whether either of them has ever been in treatment. If the answer is yes, the therapist has the opportunity to ask about the main problems for which the parent has been or is in therapy. A person who is in relatively good psychological health usually will not hesitate to discuss the major reasons for seeking treatment. Significant secretiveness may, in itself, repressent a problem. One should not, however, expect a person in therapy to reveal every secret or personal problem in the presence of the spouse, although it is reasonable to expect that the major issues will be comfortably discussed. Time only permits an outlining of the major problems for which the parent sought therapy; more detailed information can be gained in subsequent interviews.

Before closing the part of the initial interview in which the parents are seen without the child, they should be invited to talk about anything else they consider important. If a presented issue appears to be significant, some time should be devoted to it—to a superficial degree—reserving detailed elaboration for subsequent sessions.

Child Alone

When the child is brought back into the consultation room, the therapist ought to ask if there is anything he or she wishes to discuss privately. Most often the child has nothing to talk about. One can then direct the child back to the previous conversation and ask if there is anything about it that he or she wishes to comment on. Again, most children have little to say. Sometimes one obtains comments like, "My teacher's a big liar," "The other kids are always picking on me," or "I told my parents there's nothing wrong with me, that I'm not crazy, and that I don't have to see a psychiatrist." With regard to the latter comment, one should try to reassure the child that the overwhelming majority of people who see psychiatrists are not crazy.

Anna Freud (1965) emphasized the importance of the child's gaining insight into the fact that he or she has problems before meaningful psychoanalytic treatment can take place. It is only through such insight, she believed, that the child will be motivated to deal with these problems. It is my experience that the overwheming majority of children are neither interested in nor even capable of gaining insight into the fact that they have psychogenic problems. Denial is a ubiquitous mechanism and it is probably the most common mechanism used by children. Even for those who are capable of such insight, there is a big step from insight to assuming a psychoanalytic stance and attempting to understand underlying psychodynamics in the hope that it will alleviate the psychogenic difficulties. I hold that the child of average intelligence does not attain the capacity for such inquiry until the age of ten or eleven, the age at which a child can understand what Piaget calls *formal operations*. Of course, bright children may be able to do this at a younger age—especially those who have grown up in a home where such inquiry is part of the lifestyle. But whether a formal psychoanalytic approach is desired or a modification of it which involves the child's gaining insight into symptoms, most children are not receptive to this kind of approach. Accordingly, I do not pressure children into providing testimonials regarding an awareness that they have problems, nor are attempts made to get them to profess motivation for change. Therapists who pressure children into such avowals may be teaching duplicity as the children learn to provide the statements they know the examiner wishes to hear. Rather, the therapist should be satisfied if he or she has been successful in luring the child into coming and has been able to make the situation interesting and enjoyable enough to maintain an ongoing therapeutic program. Children are basically hedonistic and the therapist is competing against after-school recreation, television, or just "hanging around and doing nothing." Even the latter is generally preferred to seeing a "shrink."

ENTICING THE VERY RESISTANT CHILD. If the child absolutely refuses to come into the consultation room with the parents, the boy or girl should be allowed to sit outside. For example, if a boy obstinately refuses to leave the waiting room, the examiner might say something along these lines: "Your parents and I will be talking over there in my office. You're invited to come in and join us at any time. If you change your mind, we'll be happy to allow you to join us in the conversation, which, of course, will be about you anyway." If after ten or fifteen minutes he is still outside, the examiner might go out and try to draw the child into a general discussion in the hope of becoming a more familiar figure so that the child will become more receptive. Or the therapist might send a parent out to the waiting room if that approach seems preferable. At the very worst, the child will never come into the examiner's office and will never become a patient. Under such circumstances, therapists should lose no sleep at night but should be satisfied with the knowledge that they have tried their best to engage the child and have therefore "done their duty."

Once in the consultation room, the child may still obstinately refuse to become involved. For such situations, the examiner can try to capture the child's attention through something like magic tricks. In fact, all child psychiatrists might try to master a few of these because they can be valuable in engaging resistant children. Few recalcitrant children can resist the temptation to pull a card from a fan of cards practically under their noses with a dare that the evaluator can guess which card the child picked. Few can resist the challenge to point out under which of the three cups the ball is hidden. The child will usually ask how a particular trick was done. A good reply: "I'll be happy to show you some time. It depends upon how much you cooperate." Such tricks "break the ice," lessen anxiety, and may pave the way for more relaxed involvement in more meaningful diagnostic activities. They also help establish a relationship. (It is not being suggested here that the therapist play the role of a clown or magician; only that some of these stunts, used judiciously, can help facilitate therapeutic involvement.)

Another technique useful in facilitating involvement by extremely resistant children is the Peabody Picture Vocabulary Test—Revised (PPVT-R)(Dunn and Dunn, 1981). Although this test is designed to assess the child's capacity to associate the spoken word with its visual representation (a function that is correlated with verbal intelligence), one can use it quite effectively to engage a resistant child. On each page of the test booklet are four pictures, only one of which is associated with the test word that the examiner verbally presents to the child.

An eight-year-old boy, for example, refuses to talk to me. I introduce the test by telling the child, "This is a test to see how smart you are." I turn to the three-year level pages and ask the child to point to the picture of the *doll*. I might add, "Now I want to see if you're smart enough to tell me which one of these four pictures is a *dolly* [verbalized with childish intonation]." If the child refuses to point or even utter a word, I will dramatically put a cross on the score sheet while mumbling in a disappointed fashion how sad it is that the child doesn't even know what a doll is. I then present the next page and ask the child to point to the man. Again, if there is no response, I will dramatically place another cross on the score sheet with similar murmurings of amazement and disappointment. I might mumble, "Gee, eight years old and doesn't even know what a man is," *or* I might say to the child, "Are you sure you're eight years old?" There are few children who can tolerate more than three or four such responses on my part. (The next two items are a girl and a wheel.) Typically, the child will make a comment like, "What kind of a stupid test is this?" To which I will reply, "As I told you, this is a test to see how smart you are. And I think it's only fair to tell you that you're not doing too well." Again, there are few children who will not respond to such a comment with, "I know what those things are. You don't think I'm stupid, do you?" To which I will reply, "I don't know. The test *does* allow you to change your answer. Do you really know which one of these pictures is the *doll*?" The child will quickly point out the correct pictures, and I will dramatically erase the crosses and replace them with checks. I then proceed with the test and generally the child will complete it. I have then not only learned something about the child's verbal intelligence but, in addition, have broken through the initial resistance and facilitated some early involvement.

I have reservations about using candy or gifts as a way of involving children in therapy. There is too much of a "bribe" quality to this practice, and it may reproduce the pathology of a parent who uses food and gifts as substitutes for love. Games like checkers may be used for short periods to facilitate the child's involvement but, in my opinion, they are of very low efficiency in an ongoing therapeutic process. Elsewhere (Gardner, 1975a) I describe other techniques I have found useful for engaging resistant children.

THE FREELY-DRAWN PICTURE. A good way to start a meaningful interview when alone with a child is to ask the child to draw with crayons a picture of anything he or she wants. I will generally say something like, "I'd like to see how good you are at drawing a picture. Draw anything you want. After you've finished I want to see how good you are at making up a story about the picture that you've drawn. It has to be a completely made-up story, not something that really happened to you or anyone you know, not something that you saw on television or read in a book." By using the phrase "to see how good you are," I hope to enhance the child's motivation. Presumably, if the child draws a "good" picture, I will not only offer praise (which I will), but the child will feel good about him- or herself because of the accomplishment. And the same holds true with regard to the story I hope to elicit. If the child begins to draw something that looks like a design, I will ask what it is. If the child confirms my suspicions, I will say, "It's against the rules to draw a design. The rules of the game are that you have to draw something about which you can tell a story." Of course, the child is under no real compulsion to "follow the rules." Most children, however, will overcome the resistances that contributed to their drawing the design and provide a recognizable drawing.

It is important for the examiner to appreciate that only limited pressure, cajoling, and other forms of "encouragement" should be utilized in this phase of the evaluation. At worst, the child will refuse to draw. The only result of this will be that the examiner would be deprived of some information. In the extreme, the child will absolutely refuse to become involved in any of the diagnostic activities. If such is the case, the child will not become a patient. If the therapist considers this to represent a lack of professional ability, then it is likely that he or she will place undue pressures on the patient. As at other times, the therapist should take the position that he or she did not cause the pathology—it is often generations in the making—and although it is important to *try* to help the patient, it does not behoove the therapist to bring about any kind of alleviation of the presenting problems. Psychopathology is most often complex and we are only at the most primitive levels of our understanding. Considering our ignorance, it is even a bit grandiose of therapists to take the position that help can be given to more than a small fraction of all those who come our way. With this more modest and realistic position, examiners are less likely to place undue pressures on themselves and their patients.

Many books have been written on the analytic meaning of children's pictures. As is true of many aspects of psychodynamic theory, there is little that one can say with certainty. But even within the analytic framework, one must be aware that a psychological interpretation based on the picture itself is very risky business. For example, a boy may draw a picture of a happy scene: a house, a brightly shining sun, and beautiful flowers all around. From the appearance of the picture one is likely to conclude that the boy is a happy child who has an optimistic view of the world. On the other hand, one must consider the possibility that the picture represents a reaction formation against depression, hostility, pessimism, or various other unpleasant feelings. Accordingly, one is in no position to make any statements about a picture in isolation from the child who draws it. The more knowledge the therapist has about the child, the better able he or she is to understand the meaning of the picture. In addition, isolated interpretations are likely to be far less valid than persistent themes that exhibit themselves in many different ways. Thus, if the boy who drew the aforementioned scene was clinically depressed, had a generally "sourpuss" attitude, and had few friends, it is likely that the picture is reaction formation. And this would be supported if he exhibited both clinically and through projective material other manifestations of denial and reaction formation. This caveat about interpretating the child's projections cannot be emphasized too strongly.

The examiner should also appreciate that many age-appropriate, stereotyped pictures may appear to have complex psychodynamic significance when a simpler explanation will suffice and be far more accurate. For example, an eight-year-old boy who draws pictures depicting ships and airplanes in combat should not automatically be considered to have excessive hostility that is being released vicariously through the vehicle of the drawing and its associated war story. All individuals have pent-up anger that they cannot release directly. All of us must utilize various socially acceptable vehicles for vicarious release. Release through space-war fantasy is presently in vogue among children, and the child's utilization of it, to a reasonable degree, is normal and healthy. Accordingly, one should not too quickly impute pathological motives to the child who draws such a picture. It is the *atypical* drawing and story that should command our attention.

What has just been said regarding interpreting the meaning of a picture is also applicable to analyzing the self-created story for its psychodynamic significance. Some children will tell a relatively mundane story depicting events of the day. This is usually a resistance against the expression of more revealing material. Others will tell extremely elaborate stories, sometimes to the point where the examiner will have to interrupt because they appear to go on endlessly. These can also serve the purposes of resistance. However, the therapist may detect one or two themes that are repeated over and over. Such repeated themes may be significant. The repetition may serve the process of working through, in that reiteration and desensitization are central to that process. It is beyond the scope of this chapter to discuss in detail the wide variety of psychodynamic themes that may be revealed in children's stories. The reader who is interested in this area may wish to refer to my work on the Mutual Storytelling Technique (1968, 1969, 1970a, 1970b, 1971a, 1971b, 1972, 1974a).

THE MUTUAL STORYTELLING TECHNIQUE. This technique can be useful in the diagnostic evaluation and as a therapeutic tool. With this method a self-created story is elicited from the child. The examiner then attempts to ascertain which figure(s) in the story represent the child and various facets of his or her personality and which figure(s) represent important individual(s) in the child's life. The therapist then determines whether the child has utilized any pathological modes of adaptation or resolution to the problems with which the protagonists are confronted (usually he has). Ths therapist then creates a story, using the same characters in a similar setting, but introduces healthier modes of adaptation and/or resolution than those revealed in the child's story. In this way, the examiner provides therapeutic messages without subjecting the child to the anxieties associated with attempts to help him or her gain psychodynamic insight, even if the child were capable of such inquiry in a meaningful manner. Because most children (at least those below the age of ten) are unreceptive to and/or incapable of such meaningful inquiry, the method provides an opportunity for the therapist to provide psychotherapeutic messages with a vehicle that is natural for the child.

A vignette from the treatment of a seven-year-old boy, whom I will call Bob, demonstrates the use of the technique. Bob was referred because of generalized apathy, lack of involvement with peers, and disinterest in school in spite of high intelligence. His father was obsessively involved in his work, was away for weeks at a time on business trips, and when home had practically no interest in his son. The mother's father had died before she was two years old, and she was brought up by her mother and two older sisters. She described herself as

> knowing nothing about men. To me they're like strangers from another planet. I just can't relate to them. My daughter, I can understand. We're on the same wave length. But my son, I just can't relate to him. He's just like my husband. As I said, I don't know very much about men, but I do know one thing: I hate them all.

She then went on to describe a series of male therapists whom she had left, and I had the feeling that my name would soon be added to the list. She was basically a bitter, self-indulgent woman with little time for or interest in giving her son affection and attention. Biting sarcasm was her primary mode of relating to men. Near the end of his first two-hour consultation, her son told the following story:

> Once upon a time there was a bear. He was trying to get some honey from a beehive. He got it from the beehive. He went home with it. The bear ate the honey.

Although this story was told during my first meeting with Bob, I believed that I had enough background information to hazard a guess about the meaning of the boy's story. Of course, were he further into treatment I would have been in a much better position to speculate about the story's symbolic meaning. I suspected that the beehive represented the patient's mother. Bees traditionally are associated with stinging and they lend themselves well to symbolizing the mother's hostility. The honey, a sweet food, I suspected, represented whatever affection the mother was capable of providing at times. The combination of bees and honey appeared to be a reasonable statement of the patient's view that acquiring affection from his mother inevitably exposed him to her hostility. In the story Bob revealed his wish to gain his mother's love without being traumatized by her malevolence. Because the mother's psychopathology was deep-seated and because she had absolutely no interest in entering into treatment herself, I considered her prognosis for change very poor. Accordingly, I told the patient the following story:

> Once upon a time there was a bear. This bear loved honey very much. There was a beehive nearby but he knew that the bees were not always willing to let him have some. Sometimes they were friendly and then they would give him a little bit. Other times they were not, and he knew then that it was wise to stay away from them or else he would get stung. When the bees were unfriendly, he would go to another part of the forest where there were maple trees which dripped sweet maple syrup. When the bees were friendly, he would go to them for honey.

In my story I attempted two things. First, I tried to help the patient accept his mother as she really was at that time—someone who could, on occasion, give him some affection but who, at other times, could be punitive and ego-debasing. I advised him to accept this situation and to take her affection when it was available, but not to seek it otherwise. Second, I was suggesting that there were others in the world who could compensate for his mother's deficiencies.

THE DRAW-A-PERSON TEST. During the initial interview many examiners ask the child simply to "draw a person." It is preferable to make this request after the child has drawn the free picture because asking the child to draw a person restricts fantasy significantly. From the universe of possible things a child can draw, selecting a person considerably narrows the child's options. However, there is still a universe of possible drawings and associations (a universe within a universe so to speak), and so the drawing is still fairly useful as a projective instrument. One should not ask the child to draw a person of a specific sex because that may further narrow the possibilities and restrict associations. *After* the child has drawn a figure of a particular sex, one can then ask for one of the opposite sex. Generally, the age and sex of the figure drawn is revealing. If a boy, for example, draws a picture of a girl and, in addition pays significant attention to such details as eyelashes, coiffure, fingernails, jewelry, and other attributes generally of great concern to females in our society, one should consider the possibility that this boy has a sexual identification problem. This would especially be the case if most observers, not knowing the sex of the child, would consider it to have been drawn by a girl. If, however, a boy draws a picture of an older woman, it is likely that the mother or her surrogate is being depicted.

By looking at the picture, the therapist can sometimes learn some important things about the child. However, the reader should be warned that such interpretations are highly speculative and interexaminer reliability is quite low. This drawback notwithstanding, useful information can still be obtained. This is especially the case if speculations from projective material are substantiated by clinical assessment. Placing the feet of a figure flush against the bottom of the paper may connote feelings of instability with a need to anchor or secure the body to a stable place. Children with marked feelings of inferiority are more likely to draw their picture in this way. Significant blackness, especially when drawn frenetically, sometimes symbolizes great anxiety and a view of people as threatening. This kind of picture is more frequently drawn by children who are clinically anxious. Large shoulders and other accentuations of traditionally "macho" features may represent a boy's attempt to compensate for feelings of weakness. This is especially likely in the adolescent with feelings of masculine inadequacy. The way in which the child deals with breast outline may provide information about the child's sexual feelings and attitudes. Family attitudes toward sexuality will often provide clues as to whether the examiner's interpretation in this area is valid. The way in which the child draws the eyes may provide information in a number of areas. Shy children and those prone to use denial mechanisms to a significant degree may draw a figure with the eyes averted. Staring eyes have generally been interpreted to connote suspiciousness and sometimes even paranoia. Again, the examiner does well to make such interpretations cautiously and to use clinical data for support or refutation of these speculations. Machover (1949) has written what may be the most well-known book on the psychological interpretation of children's drawings.

The examiner should try to get the child to tell a story about the picture. One can begin the process by asking for specific information about the person depicted. Some start with the general request that the child tell a story, and then only resort to specific questions if the request is not or cannot be complied with. What has been said about interpreting stories told in association with freely drawn pictures holds for the human-figure drawings as well. The therapist does well to differentiate between age-appropriate stereotyped stories (which are probably normal) and idiosyncratic ones. The latter provide the more meaningful information. But here again there is much speculation.

After drawing the first picture, the child should be asked to draw a picture of the opposite sex. One should take care not to specify whether the picture should be of a child or an adult, lest the universe of possibilities be reduced. One might say, "Now that you've drawn a picture of a male, I want you to draw another picture. This time I want you to draw a female." Or, for the younger child, one might say, "Now that you've drawn a picture of a boy, I want you to draw a picture of either a girl or a woman." After as much information as possible has been extracted from the pictures, the examiner should ask the child to draw a picture of a family. Because of time limitations, it is prudent not to require the child to spend too much time on the details of the various figures. Here, the therapist is primarily interested in the number and sexes of the figures chosen, their relationships with one another, and the story the child tells about the family. Stories elicited from the family picture are generally less revealing than those from the individual pictures. More frequently one obtains stereotyped stories about family excursions or day-to-day activities. These are usually resistance stories and provide little if any psychodynamic information. Of course, at times, one does obtain rich and meaningful stories.

THE MAKE-A-PICTURE STORY TEST. The Make-A-Picture Story test (MAPS) (Shneidman, 1947) is particularly useful for eliciting psychodynamic material from children, especially from those who may not be free enough to reveal themselves through the aforementioned less-structured methods for gaining psychodynamic material, namely, the freely drawn picture, the mutual storytelling technique, and the Draw-A-Person and Draw-A-Family tests. The equipment consists of a series of cards, each of which depicts a scene without human or animal figures, and the child is provided with a collection of figurines (cut from thin cardboard) representing a wide assortment of human and animal figures. The child is simply requested to select one of the cards and one or more of the figurines, put the figurines in the scene, and then make up a story.

Although there is a similarity between the Make-a-Picture Story test and the more commonly used Thematic Apperception Test (TAT)(Murray, 1936), there are definite differences—differences that, in my opinion, make the MAPS a superior diagnostic instrument. First, the scenes depicted in the TAT, although designed to be vague, are still definitely identifiable and have figures with recognizable sex and age. In the TAT these specific figures are placed in specific scenes. In the MAPS the child decides which figure(s) shall be in which scene, thereby increasing almost infinitely the number of possible stimuli for storytelling. In the MAPS the child is much more the creator of the facilitating stimulus. Furthermore, having more of a say in what the picture will be like and playing an active role in determining what picture to create, the child is generally more motivated to associate stories to it.

Another advantage that the MAPS has over the TAT is that the TAT cards are primarily designed for diagnostic work with adults. Although some of the TAT cards do depict children, most depict grown-ups. The adult scenes will certainly elicit fantasies around family life, especially the parents; however, the paucity of children is a definite detriment if one wishes to draw out stories from children. While some of the TAT cards are specifically designated as relevant to boys and girls, the author's experience has been that the child's opportunity to select the figures in the MAPS creates a situation in which more child-type fantasies are likely to be evoked.

Screening for Mild Neurological Impairment

Many, if not most, of the children who come for psychiatric consultation do so with the complaint (it may be one among many) of poor school performance. Sometimes this is in the academic realm, sometimes in the behavioral, and sometimes in both. Of course, in some of these children the school difficulties are related to psychogenic problems. In others, however, there may be a mild neurological impairment. The examiner should consider a neurological factor when evaluating children. He or she should also be familiar with neuropsychological instruments designed to assess for the presence of such impairment. Because these instruments are described elsewhere in this book (see chap. 22), they will not be described here. The reader who is interested in the description of this examiner's assessment battery may wish to refer to his publications in this area (Gardner, 1978, 1979a, 1979b, 1981; Gardner and Broman, 1979a, 1979b; Gardner and Gardner, 1977; Gardner et al., 1979).

Deciding Whether Therapy Is Warranted

There are four areas of inquiry useful in helping the examiner decide whether a child needs treatment. Before elaborating on these, it is important to emphasize that transient symptomatic manifestations are extremely common in children. Practically every child exhibits an occasional tic, short-term phobic reactions, temper outbursts, occasional stealing episodes, lying, bribing, sleep difficulties, and so forth. It is only when atypical, inappropriate, or pathological behavior exhibits itself over a period of time that one should consider therapy. It is difficult, if not impossible, to provide a sharp cutoff point regarding how long symptoms should be present before treatment is warranted, but a few months is certainly reasonable. This important consideration is taken into account in the latest diagnostic and statistical manual—*DSM III* (1980).

The most important area of inquiry, when determining whether a child needs treatment, is school performance. It is the role of parents and society to make every reasonable attempt to change infants into human beings capable of functioning adequately in society. It is in the school that one can ascertain most sensitively whether the first five years of the acculturating process have been successful. It is there that children must constrain their primitive instinctual impulses most consistently. The child with psychiatric problems may not have been properly "civilized" and may therefore manifest behavioral or learning problems in school. There are, however, children with psychiatric difficulties who do extremely well in school (both in behavioral and academic areas). Although they are rigid and overcompliant, they are a joy to their teachers and a source of pride to their parents. But since these children represent a small minority, the basic principle still holds: the child who is doing well in school in the behavioral and academic realms is likely to be well-integrated.

The child's activity in the neighborhood is another important area to explore. Although getting along with peers does not require the degree of integration that successful school performance necessitates, peers will not usually tolerate the degree of uncivilized behavior that parents will accept. In order to maintain friendships, children must have learned to consider the rights of others, wait their turn, adhere to the rules of games, share, and develop a wide variety of other character traits that "win friends and influence people." Accordingly, the therapist should inquire into whether the child seeks friends *and* is sought by them. If both of these occur with reasonable frequency, and if the child and his or her friends are involved in basically healthy endeavors, the child is likely to be relatively healthy. However, if the child seeks and is sought by antisocial individuals, pathology is present. But even this child may be healthier than one who does not make friends.

It is very difficult to determine whether psychopathology is present from the parents' description of the home situation. When a parent presents as a problem the fact that a boy fights often with his brother, the examiner has learned little, if anything. Normal, healthy children fight frequently with their siblings and there is no realistic cutoff point between the normal frequency of such fighting and the pathological. If a child *never,* or hardly ever, fights with a sibling, psychopathology in the areas of inhibition of self-assertion and the expression of hostility may be present. When a parent complains that the child resists cooperating in household chores, dawdles, and is disrespectful of parental authority, the child may be normal. In fact, it is the child who does *not* occasionally exhibit these traits who probably has pathology. Because one cannot differentiate well between the normal and pathological degrees of uncooperative and disrespectful behavior in the home, this is a weak area of inquiry for determining whether a child needs therapy. It is not, however, an area that should be totally ignored. If the child hardly ever cooperates, if fighting with siblings is almost incessant, if conflict and turmoil is the household norm, if power struggles are the rule, then psychopathology is present.

Finally, one wants to assess for the presence of specific symptoms such as obsessions, compulsions, phobias, depression, psychosomatic complaints, and so forth. In my experience, only a small percentage of the patients who come for consultation fall into this category. It is not intrapsychic conflict that plagues the vast majority but interpersonal difficulties. If others were not to complain about them, they would not be in any distress.

By this point, the examiner should have enough information to decide whether treatment is warranted. Although he or she may not know in depth the basic problems that may have caused the psychopathology, enough information should have been obtained to enable the evaluator to come to some conclusion as to whether further work with the family would be useful. At this point, then, the parents should be brought back into the consultation room for a summary and presentation of the examiner's findings and recommendations.

Presenting the Initial Recommendation

A decision has to be made regarding whether the initial findings and recommendations should be made in the child's presence. If what the evaluator is going to tell the parents will be anxiety provoking or otherwise distressful to the child, it is preferable to have the child sit in the waiting room. In my experience, this is most often not the case and so the child remains, even though he or she may not appreciate fully the significance of all that is being discussed. If there is no danger in having the child there, it is better to allow him or her to stay. One reason for this is that sending the child out may contribute to a compromise in the relationship, as the child sits outside knowing that the therapist and the parents are sharing "secrets" about him or her.

At this point, there are three possible courses that the examiner may consider pursuing. The first is that there should be no further sessions scheduled because the examiner has concluded that therapy is not indicated. This has not been a common course in my experience, even though I take a relatively conservative position regarding recommending psychotherapy, because by the time a child is referred for psychiatric treatment, the difficulties have usually reached the point where therapy is warranted.

A second course, the middle road, is one in which the initial interview has not provided enough information to make a definite decision regarding whether or not treatment should be instituted. If, for instance, the child exhibited definite pathology, but there was great resistance during the inquiry, the examiner may be in no position to come to a definitive conclusion. In other cases the two-hour interview may not have garnered enough data to make a decision regarding the nature of the pathology or the type of treatment indicated. It is important for the therapist not to place pressures upon him- or herself, nor to submit to the pressures of others to come to conclusions when the data do not warrant them at a particular point. Submitting to such pressures is likely to compromise one's work. In order to clarify the situation, the therapist might suggest further interviews, further psychological testing, a neurological evaluation, a pediatric evaluation, or request other information. This middle course, fortunately, is unusual.

Most often, I gain enough information in the initial interview to come to some conclusion as to whether or not therapy is required. In some cases, the only recommendation is some form of drug treatment. In others, a combination of medication and psychotherapy appears indicated. Some need only parent counseling, others family therapy, others milieu therapy, and others hospitalization. When the indicated treatment modality involves a form of psychotherapy, I recommend the third course, the intensive evaluation.

In most cases, some form of psychotherapy is the recommendation. In such situations, I outline to the parents what I consider to be the factors that have contributed to the child's difficulties and the kind of therapeutic program that, at that point, I consider warranted. I emphasize that these are *initial* conclusions and that the interpretations as well as the therapeutic program may change as further information is gained. The parents are then advised that the best way to learn more about the child's difficulties is to participate in the full, or intensive, evaluation.

INTENSIVE EVALUATION

The intensive evaluation involves two or three more interviews with the child alone, one or two with each parent alone followed by a joint interview with the parents together, and a family interview if there are siblings who are old and mature enough to make such an interview meaningful. During the course of these clinical interviews, psychological tests are usually administered. If pertinent reports from other examiners have not been brought to the initial interview, the parents are again asked to request them. The parents are then told that following the collection of all the data, the information will be collated and a formal presentation, generally involving two or more hours, will be prepared for them. This will provide them with the opportunity to discuss in detail various aspects of the findings.

Interviews with the Parents Alone

Since the history-taking process will be discussed in detail in other chapters in Part II of this book, the details of the parental inquiry will not be discussed here. During the individual interviews with the parents, one focuses not only on the life history of each parent, but on each parent's involvement with the children. In addition, following the individual interviews, a joint interview is held. This is also part of the data-collection process. Because the therapist may have obtained different information from each parent, it is desirable to see them together in order to attempt to clarify inconsistencies and gain more accurate information. During the joint interview, the examiner does well to focus on the marital relationship and on each parent's methods of dealing with the children, especially the child who has been presented as the patient. Elsewhere (Gardner, 1975a, 1982) I present this aspect of the evaluation in detail.

The Family Interview

Generally, a family interview is conducted in the intensive evaluation phase if there are one or more siblings over the age of ten or thereabouts. Although a family interview with younger children will generally provide some information, the amount is usually not great. Because the intensive evaluation that I conduct is quite extensive, I try to avoid including interviews that would yield a relatively low amount of useful data.

When there are older children, however, especially teen-agers, one does well to routinely conduct a family interview. The parents are advised to tell the youngsters in advance that their assistance is being requested to help the therapist gain a better understanding of the problems of their brother or sister. The parents are asked to encourage the children to be open and honest with regard to what they reveal and to reassure them that they, the parents, will not react punitively to any criticism of them that may be made during the course of the interview. One of the risks of such an interview is that a discussion in which the patient's siblings are asked to identify what they consider to be the youngster's psychiatric difficulties is likely to cause the patient to suffer some ego debasement. However, this drawback can be counterbalanced to some degree by encouraging the siblings to describe the patient's assets as well. In the family interview the therapist wants to observe the various interactions among all the family members and observe how the patient fits into this network.

Individual Interviews with the Child

During the course of the intensive evaluation, I generally conduct two or three more interviews with the child, most often on an individual basis. I may, however, occasionally bring the mother (the parent who most often brings the child—although sometimes it is the father) into the room in order to observe whether or not her presence has an effect on the child. My experience has been that it usually does not squelch the child or otherwise interfere with his or her freedom of revelation. When this is the case, I know that I can utilize the mother more actively in the treatment without fear of her interfering with it and that I am therefore likely to derive the benefits of her active involvement.

It is important for the examiner to appreciate that these two or three interviews are not conducted merely to gain further data, although this is certainly an important aim. Equally, if not more, important is the goal of intensifying the relationship with the child. In the initial interview the child is likely to have been quite anxious, but in subsequent interviews, under more relaxed circumstances, the therapist will have a better chance to achieve a good therapist–patient relationship. He or she will also have the opportunity to determine whether or not a successful relationship is possible with a child who was initially extremely resistive and uncooperative. These sessions allow the therapist the opportunity to try to circumvent and reduce such resistances.

If, during the initial two-hour consultation, no evidence is found for the presence of neurological impairment, the evaluative sessions are devoted to the collection of psychodynamic data—especially information that will assist in understanding the causes of the child's psychogenic symptoms. If, however, a mild neurological problem is present, more tests are administered from the examiner's aforementioned battery, tests that will define more accurately the nature of the deficit(s). A collaborating psychologist will conduct most of these tests so that the examiner will be free to devote these two or three sessions to an evaluation of the secondary psychogenic problems that children with mild neurological impairment often suffer from (Gardner, 1973b, 1973c, 1974b, 1974c, 1975b, 1975c, and 1979c), as well as to the assessment of other psychogenic problems (unrelated to neurological impairment) that may be present. Described here are only those instruments that I have found useful in providing further psychodynamic data, regardless of which of the aforementioned classes of psychogenic impairment may be present.

In the initial interview a few responses to the Make-A-Picture Story cards may have been obtained. In this phase of the evaluation the child is asked to relate more stories from the scenes he or she creates with the test material. Often I will introduce a responding story, in accordance with the principles described in the Mutual Storytelling Technique. When interpreting the child's responses to the MAPS cards, the examiner should not draw any conclusions on the basis of one or two cards. Rather, he or she should look for *themes that are repetitious*. Only these are true reflections of what is going on in the child. Even then, such conclusions must be made with caution.

The child is also presented with variations of the types of verbal projective questions described by Kritzberg (1966). The child is asked: "What animal would you choose to be if you had to be changed into one? You can choose any animal in the whole world." After giving a response, the child is asked why that particular animal was chosen. Second and third choices are elicited and, again, the reasons for the choices are requested. Then the child is asked: "What animal would you *not* want to be?" Following the response, the child is asked why. Again, second and third choices are requested. After getting as much mileage as possible from the original set of responses, a variety of other elaborations of the same question are posed. The child is asked what objects he or she would choose (first, second, and third choices, and why) and *not* choose to be changed into (first, second, and third choice, and why), if such a transformation were required. Older children (above the age of nine or so) are asked what person they would choose to be changed into. Generally, I present the question: "Of all the people in the world, living or dead, past or present, real or from books, famous or not famous, who would you choose to be if you had to be changed into someone?" After obtaining the reasons for wanting to be each person, I ask who the boy or girl would *not* wish to be changed into, and again with reasons why. The child is then asked what animal would *suit* his or her mother's personality if she had to be changed into one. It is important to help the child differentiate between the animal that would suit the mother's personality and the animal that the mother might like to be if she had the choice to choose one. This distinction may be particularly difficult for five and six year olds, but most children of seven and above can make the distinction. Again, the child is asked the first, second, and third choices, and the reasons for each choice. The animals that would *not* suit the mother are also requested. The child is then asked to list a series of objects that would suit (and *not* suit), the mother's personality, and the reasons why. The same series of questions is then requested for the father.

The child is usually asked what things he or she would ask for if three wishes could be granted. In assessing the responses, one should differentiate between age-appropriate, stereotyped responses and those that are unusual and idiosyncratic. A boy, for example, might say that he would wish for "a million dollars" or "all the money in the world." For such a response, one does well to ask the child what he would do with the money. Answers like buying a lot of toys or a big house or a new car are generally in the normal range. If, however, all three wishes are used to purchase material goods, they there may be a problem relating to deprivation or materialism. The examiner should not accept as an answer "as many wishes as I would want." If the child responds with meaningful replies, a fourth or fifth wish might be added. However, I have not generally found this question to be particularly useful because the responses are more often than not stereotyped. Accordingly, I consider it to be among the low-yield questions.

Winnicott's Squiggle's Technique (1968, 1971) can be useful for obtaining psychodynamic information. Like the Mutual Storytelling Technique, it can also be expanded into a psychotherapeutic game. In this game the examiner draws a randomly executed scribbled pattern on a blank piece of paper. No attempt should be made to draw a pattern that has any recognizable shape. Rather, one wants to execute a somewhat amorphous, nonidentifiable scribble. The child is then asked to tell what it looks like and may be invited to add lines if desired. When using the technique for diagnostic purposes, the therapist asks the child to identify the scribble and create a story around it. However, when used therapeutically (more often in the therapeutic sessions than in the intensive diagnostic evaluation), the child is asked to draw the squiggles and the examiner identifies the figures within it and creates his or her own responding stories. In this way, one can combine Winnicott's Squiggle's Technique with the Mutual Storytelling Technique.

It is during the intensive evaluation that I usually introduce The Talking, Feeling, and Doing Game (1973d). Although this game was initially devised for children who were unreceptive to providing self-created stories, it has also proved useful as an additional therapeutic modality for those who are receptive to storytelling and fantasy verbalization. In this game each player in turn throws the dice and moves the playing piece along a path of colored squares. Depending upon which color the playing piece lands, the player takes a talking card, a feeling card, or a doing card. If a player can respond to the questions or directions on the card, a reward chip is given. The talking cards elicit material of a cognitive nature; the feeling cards evoke emotional responses; and the doing cards encourage physical expression. Some typical cards: "Suppose two people were talking about you and they didn't know you were listening. What do you think you would hear them saying?" "A boy has something on his mind that he's afraid to tell his father. What is it that he's scared to talk about?" "Everybody in the class was laughing at a girl. What had happened?" "All the girls in the class were invited to a birthday party except one. Why wasn't she invited?" "If the walls of your house could talk, what would they say about your family?" The questions deal with issues that are relevant to every child, issues that are likely to be at the basis of the child's psychopathology. The responses serve as points of departure for meaningful psychotherapeutic interchanges.

It has been this examiner's experience that the overwhelming majority of children will involve themselves in this game. Even those who are resistant to more traditional approaches, especially those involving direct discussion and/or fantasy elicitation, are usually receptive to playing the game. If the child does play, the therapist can reasonably conclude that meaningful psychotherapeutic involvement is likely. If the child refuses, the course of treatment may be much more difficult. Although the whole decision about therapeutic receptivity cannot be based on the child's response to this single game, it is a very valuable indicator of potential receptivity for the child who is borderline for such involvement. At this phase the examiner is primarily interested in the diagnostic information that the game provides. However, in playing it, the therapist (who also responds similarly to the cards), is given the opportunity to provide some therapeutic input as well.

During this phase the examiner can also utilize traditional play material such as dolls and drawings. As I have said elsewhere (Gardner, 1979d), I consider paints, puppets, clay, water, soldiers, blocks, and sand play to be low-efficiency therapeutic modalities. I do not hold that they are of no value, only that they are of low yield with regard to therapeutic efficacy. Although they may be of higher yield with regard to diagnostic information, they are not as effective in this regard as the instruments discussed previously. Accordingly, I rarely use them in either the diagnostic or therapeutic phases.

Additional Pyschological Tests

On occasion, additional psychological tests are warranted. Chapter 24 deals with the value and choice of different tests that can be used in the initial evaluation phase. It is important for the examiner to appreciate that projective tests provide information about underlying psychodynamics, but that they are of less value for specifically defining the patient's diagnostic category or applicability for therapy. Projections have much in common with dreams. Everyone has dreams and all dreams reveal psychodynamics, but one should not equate psychodynamics with psychopathology. In addition, even if psychopathology is present the tests cannot generally provide much information about motivation for therapy or the capacity of the patient to be involved in treatment. Test findings *must* be combined with clinical observations before one can come to meaningful conclusions about diagnosis and treatment.

FINAL PRESENTATION OF THE FINDINGS

After the interviews have been completed and information from other sources received, all the material is collated and a final presentation for the parents is prepared. An open-ended session is scheduled for the presentation to insure that there will be no pressure of time. The parents are then provided ample opportunity to discuss any issue in as much detail as they wish. These interviews generally take from two to three hours. The child is usually not present at this interview because it often involves discussion of details of marital problems. In addition, most children, especially younger ones, soon become restless and do not absorb much of what is being said.

The therapeutic program is then outlined. This involves setting up a schedule for the therapeutic sessions. It has been this examiner's practice to impress upon the parents that they are his "assistant therapists" and that their active involvement in the treatment is crucial if we are to hope for a positive outcome. I make a strong attempt to impress upon them the point that they should not view the therapy as something that I am doing *to* the child. Rather, it is a cooperative venture in which active participation on the part of all parties is crucial. They are informed that they can rely upon me to *attempt* to help the child, but no promises can be made regarding the duration of treatment or whether or not there will be a positive outcome. Such statements help dispel unrealistic anticipations about what treatment can offer and, it is hoped, will enhance the parents' motivation for involvement and cooperation. The parents are also informed that if therapy reaches a point of nonproductivity, they will be apprised of this and their participation in a discussion of "where do we go from here?" will be invited. This again gets across the point that psychotherapy is a joint endeavor whose success or failure is partly their responsibility and partly the therapist's.

The mother will usually bring the child to the sessions, but the father is informed that he should not feel that he is a stranger. Rather, he is invited to attend any sessions when he is available. The reader should appreciate that such parental participation is not justifiably called family therapy (although on occasion I certainly do use family therapy). Rather, what is described here is best called individual child psychotherapy with parental observation and intermittent participation.

The parents are asked if they would like a full written report prepared. If this is their choice, the report is given to the parents themselves and then *they decide whom they will give it to*—whether it be the school, the child's pediatrician, or anyone else. They then become the ones to decide which material will be divulged and which not. If they decide that they do not want the school to know certain things about their personal lives, they have the freedom to withhold the report entirely or to delete specific material from it. (Of course, they are encouraged to inform the school that they are deleting such material when turning over the report.) In this way, the therapist is protected from the accusation that he or she has provided others with information that the parents did not wish to be revealed. (In this day of mounting malpractice litigation, such a course is most judicious.)

Concluding Comments

I fully recognize that the evaluation described here is more extensive and intensive than that which is traditionally done. I also appreciate that, whether it is conducted in the clinic or private practice situation, it is extremely expensive, which may make it impractical for most therapists. However, to the degree that the therapist can provide such an evaluation, to that degree will the patient be given the optimum service possible.

References

American Psychiatric Association. 1980. *Diagnostic and statistical manual of Mental Disorders (DSM-III)*. Washington, D.C.: APA.

Dunn, L. M. and Dunn, L. M. 1981. *Peabody picture vocabulary test—revised*. Circle Pines, Minn.: American Guidance Service.

Freud, A. 1965. *Normality and pathology in childhood*. New York: International Universities Press.

Gardner, R. A. 1968. The mutual storytelling technique: Use in alleviating childhood oedipal problems. *Contemp. Psychoanal.*, 4:161-177.

———. 1969. Mutual storytelling as a technique in child psychotherapy and psychoanalysis. In *Science and psychoanalysis*, vol. 14, ed. J. Masserman, pp. 123-135. New York: Grune and Stratton.

———. 1970a. Die Technik des wechselseitigen Geschichtenerzählens bei der Behandlung eines Kindes mit psychogenem Husten. In *Fortschritte der Psychoanalyse, Internationales Jahrbuch zur Weiterentwicklung der Psychoanalyse*, vol. 4, ed. C. J. Hogrefe, pp. 159-173. Göttingen: Verlag für Psychologie.

———. 1970b. The mutual storytelling technique: Use in the treatment of a child with post-traumatic neurosis. *Am. J. Psychother.*, 24:419-439.

———. 1971a. *Therapeutic communication with children: The mutual storytelling technique*. New York: Jason Aronson.

———. 1971b. Mutual storytelling: A technique in child psychotherapy. *Acta Paedopsych.*, 38(9):253-262.

———. 1972. The mutual storytelling technique in the treatment of anger inhibition problems. *Int. J. Child Psychother.*, 1(1):34-64.

――. 1973a. *Understanding children: A parents guide to child rearing.* Cresskill, N.J.: Creative Therapeutics.

――. 1973b. Psychotherapy of the psychogenic problems secondary to minimal brain dysfunction. *Int. J. Child Psychother.,* 2(2):224–256.

――. 1973c. *MBD: The family book about minimal brain dysfunction.* New York: Jason Aronson.

――. 1973d. *The talking, feeling, and doing game.* Cresskill, N.J.: Creative Therapeutics.

――. 1974a. La technique de la narration mutuelle d'historettes. *Médecine et Hygiène* (Geneva), 32:1180–1181.

――. 1974b. Psychotherapy of minimal brain dysfunction. In *Current Psychiatric Therapies,* vol. 14, ed. J. Masserman, pp. 15–21. New York: Grune and Stratton.

――. 1974c. The mutual storytelling technique in the treatment of psychogenic problems secondary to minimal brain dysfunction. *J. Learn. Disabil.,* 7:135–143.

――. 1975a. *Psychotherapeutic approaches to the resistant child.* New York: Jason Aronson.

――. 1975b. Psychotherapy in minimal brain dysfunction. In *Current Psychiatric Therapies,* vol. 15, ed. J. Masserman, pp. 25–38. New York: Grune and Stratton.

――. 1975c. Techniques for involving the child with MBD in meaningful psychotherapy. *J. Learn. Disabil.,* 8(5):16–26.

――. 1978. *Reversals frequency test.* Cresskill, N.J.: Creative Therapeutics.

――. 1979a. *The objective diagnosis of minimal brain dysfunction.* Cresskill, N.J.: Creative Therapeutics.

――. 1979b. Throwing balls in a basket as a test of motor coordination: Normative data on 1350 school children. *J. Clin. Child Psychol.,* 8(3):152–155.

――. 1979c. Psychogenic difficulties secondary to MBD. In *Basic handbook of child psychiatry,* vol. 3, ed. J. Noshpitz, pp. 614–628. New York: Basic Books.

――. 1979d. Helping children cooperate in therapy. In *Basic handbook of child psychiatry,* vol. 3, ed. J. Noshpitz, pp. 414–433. New York: Basic Books.

――. 1981. Digits forward and digits backward as two separate tests: Normative data on 1567 school children. *J. Clin. Child Psychol.,* 10(2):131–135.

――. 1982. *Family evaluation in child custody litigation.* Cresskill, N.J.: Creative Therapeutics.

Gardner, R. A., and Broman, M. 1979a. Letter reversals frequency in normal and learning-disabled children. *J. Clin. Child Psychol.,* 8(3):146–152.

――. 1979b. The Purdue pegboard: Normative data on 1334 school children. *J. Clin. Child Psychol.,* 8(3):156–162.

Gardner, R. A., and Gardner, A. K. 1977. *Steadiness tester* (catalog no. 32019). Lafayette, Ind.: Lafayette Instrument Company.

Gardner, A. K., Caemmerer, A., and Broman, M. 1979. An instrument for measuring hyperactivity and other signs of MBD. *J. Clin. Child Psychol.,* 8(3):173–179.

Kritzberg, N. 1966. A new verbal projective test for the expansion of the projective aspects of the clinical interview. *Acta Paedopsych.,* 33(2):48–62.

Machover, K. 1949. *Personality projection in the drawing of the human figure: A method of personality investigation.* Springfield, Ill.: Charles C. Thomas.

Murray, H. 1936. *The thematic apperception test.* New York: Psychological Corp.

Rorschach, H. 1921. *The Rorschach Test.* New York: Psychological Corp.

Shneidman, E. S. 1947. *Make-a-picture story test.* New York: Psychological Corp.

Winnicott, D. W. 1968. The value of the therapeutic consultation. In *Foundations of child psychiatry,* ed. E. Miller, pp. 593–608. London: Pergamon Press.

――. 1971. *Therapeutic consultations in child psychiatry.* New York: Basic Books.

21

Taking a History

IAN A. CANINO

INTRODUCTION

History taking cannot be taken for granted, nor does experience necessarily improve this skill. Clinicians may be influenced by a theoretical orientation which may lead them to focus solely on data they consider relevant, omitting other areas. Just as parents, teachers, siblings, and child patients vary in their capacity to report on past and present events and feelings, so do clinicians vary in their aptitude in eliciting relevant information.

A good history not only provides the basis for decisions about treatment and further investigation, but, in many cases, allows the parents to conceptually organize the events that have affected their children. A historical framework offers cohesion to a series of interacting events, it may serve to explain the presenting symptomatology, and it provides perspectives on the child's strengths, vulnerabilities, and development.

This chapter offers information on the limitations of history taking and provides a summary guide to a history taking protocol.

The Parents' Contribution

Parents may be accurate in reporting some developmental or historical facts and inaccurate in reporting others (Mednick and Shaffer, 1963). Haggard et al. (1966) showed that variables such as weight, height, and health were recalled more accurately by parents than personality variables. Less well-defined problems such as activity levels are not recalled as well as discrete symptoms such as nightmares and stuttering (Laposse and Monk, 1958), enuresis, stealing and temper tantrums (Graham and Rutter, 1968). Parent recall is also less reliable over events of high emotional significance (Wenar and Coulter, 1962), parental attitudes, child rearing practices or feeling states (Evans and Nelson, 1977), and the child's social relationships (Graham and Rutter, 1968). Mothers have been reported to be more reliable informants than fathers (Evans and Nelson, 1977), which underlines the importance of individual parental differences as sources of reliable information.

Robins (1963) studied the accuracy of parental recall for developmental milestones and found considerable inaccuracies on items dealing with toilet training, thumb sucking, demand feeding, and the age of weaning. Reliability was higher for factual questions such as birth weight. She found that inaccuracies tended to follow the recommendations of the popular trends on child rearing. Mothers' recollections were more accurate in this area than the fathers'.

Popular theories about the causes of behavior problems may also produce distortions in parents' accounts of problems (Chess et al., 1966). For example, media stories indicating that children need to have a mother at home may result in a family designating the onset of problem behavior as a time when mother started to work (Mednick and Schaffer, 1968).

Clinicians aware of these nuances can differentially assess the reliability of the data they gather and request more information in potentially unreliable areas.

Patient Variables

There has been less research on the reliability of information provided by children themselves. Some children may deny or minimize their problems out of guilt or fear. Others may feel the examination to be a betrayal of their parents and may fear being punished or abandoned by them as a consequence. Some children are uncooperative or for a variety of reasons displace problem behaviors on others (Cramer, 1975).

Kestenbaum and Bird (1978) present data on the interrater reliability of an interview format with school age children. Helper (1958) compared parental evaluations of eighth and ninth grade children to the children's self-evaluations. He found the correlations between favorability and acceptance (the two variables he studied) to be small but consistently positive. There are a number of child-completed checklists focusing in general on traits such as self-esteem and assertiveness but most lack a situational dimension. Attention to the reliability, validity, and standardization of these child-completed questionnaires is clearly indicated (Mash and Terdal, 1981). Despite these problems, the child's own comments are invaluable for assessing the child's perceptions of his or her parents, teachers, and peers, and for assessing the child's fantasy life.

Interviews with the child's friends or siblings may be useful. Peer evaluation sensitively identifies problem children (Cowen et al., 1973). Information obtained from siblings may be particularly relevant in family situations characterized by high rates of sibling conflict (Leitenberg et al., 1973). Clinicians should also give the child a chance to describe his or her own biography. The child may bring up issues that the parents did not consider to be important or had consciously withheld because they were embarrassed or guilty. If there is a suspicion that the child is exaggerating or distorting past issues, these can be clarified later (with the child's permission and the clinician's good judgment) with the parents. Direct questioning of friends or peers is usually best postponed in order to spare the child from embarrassment. It is best to gather the peers' impressions through the teacher's and parent's own observations. If the child later wants to bring a friend or if, later in the evaluation, a friend's comments or impressions seem important, this issue can be reconsidered and discussed. The views of the child's siblings are in most cases best gathered during a family evaluation, while the child in question is present.

Clinician Variables

Research on the optimal qualities of clinicians who are offering psychotherapy or counseling have been done by Truax and Carkhuff (1967). They stress the importance of empathy, warmth, genuineness, and understanding. Cox, Hopkinson, and Rutter (1981) found that parent informants talked more to interviewers who talked less and who made more use of open questions, at least in an initial interview. Questions asked in a multiple choice style seemed to be more effective and caused less distortion of meaning. Double questions are liable to result in ambiguous replies (Cohen, 1979).

HISTORY TAKING

Special Problems

Taking a history about a child patient differs from taking a history from an adult patient in a number of ways.

First, most of the relevant history on a child will characteristically be supplied by adults (parents, teachers, agency members) who may or may not consider a specific behavior as a symptom. Agreement between what bothers an adult about a child and the clinician's view of salient abnormal child behavior may be quite poor (Ullman and Krasner, 1975).

Second, when interviewing adult patients, symptoms are assessed during a period of slow developmental growth. In children the progression of developmental stages occurs rapidly and expected behaviors change in a relatively short period of time. Adaptive styles and plasticity during these stages are often more marked than well-defined static abnormalities. Children show fewer behaviors that are pathognomonic of disorder than do adults (Achenbach, 1980). This calls for a broader gathering of data, the number of different symptoms being more indicative of a disorder than any single symptom. During childhood, symptoms and tensions are frequently transient and secondary to stressors that are particular to a given developmental stage. These symptoms may take a different form at later stages (Freud, 1962). Knowledge of normal variations in development is thus crucial in order to assess if historical data is indicative of normality or pathology.

Third, many of the presenting behavioral problems in children are intimately linked with intellectual and cognitive difficulties (Evans and Nelson, 1977). Schools are frequent referral agencies, and learning problems often impinge on other developing skills and coping styles of children. Some of these if properly evaluated and treated may still be modifiable. Therefore, a careful school history is critical.

Fourth, children are under much stronger control and are more dependent on their familial and social environment than are adult patients. We often observe that a child may express a series of behaviors under one set of social or familial circumstances and a different set of behaviors under other circumstances. Therefore, the adequate assessment of their present and past environment requires consideration.

General Suggestions

THE PARENTS' ACCOUNT. In terms of the history collected from the parents, we can expect some distortions, biases, and memory lags. It is quite difficult to remember developmental milestones and even harder to be able to relate particular events to particular behavioral responses of children. An attempt to relax the parents as much as possible and allow them, initially, to give recent vignettes of their child's behavior and their family life usually produces further information. It is also of great value, especially if the parents seem uncomfortable and particularly guilty about their child's behavior (seen often when the school has made the referral), to start the interview by asking them what they consider to be their child's strengths and then only later questioning them about their child's problematic behavior. If at all possible, it is recommended that both parents be present during this initial interview. Different points of view and different child-rearing practices, and some ideas regarding the parental interrelationship and nonverbal interactions offer the clinician invaluable information.

It may be important at that time to ask for significant others who may have more accurate information, e.g., the grandmother or baby-sitter who stayed with the child during part of his or her development. If there are special circumstances such as neglect, broken home, previous hospitalizations, physical or sexual abuse, then adults other than the parents may be of primary importance in data collection (Cramer, 1975). Questions and dates regarding major events in the family such as deaths, weddings, moves, financial reversals, and births are usually met with relatively accurate answers. Asking the parents what they remember of their children at those times may offer some significant vignettes about their coping mechanisms, temperaments, developmental strengths, or the situational specificity of their behavior. Evans and Nelson underline the importance of interviewing the parents to assess if they are responsive to behavioral concepts and are serving as adequate mediators to the child. Furthermore, if the interview goes well, not only is some factual information gathered but also a relationship begins to be established with the clinician, and the emotions of the parents can then be elicited (Rutter and Cox, 1981). It is crucial, though, that a good balance between eliciting feelings with empathy and collecting data with discipline be established (Cohen, 1979). Parents should have a clear understanding of the purpose of the interview, and it is often necessary to clarify the relevance of a given question. Of importance for the clinician is not to covertly scapegoat and blame the parents for the behavior of the child.

THE CHILD'S ACCOUNT. In taking a history from the child himself, it is usually better to start the interview by requesting information about the child's immediate field of interest. Questions about a baseball game, a hobby or table game, a favorite movie or television program, are usually met with favorable responses. Gradually the child can be asked to describe his school, teachers, and peers. Questions regarding his family and favorite "grown-ups" or siblings can then be broached. As the child feels more comfortable, questions regarding his dislikes or things he would change about his school, his family, and himself can be asked. If responsive, he can also be asked about his best and most enjoyable memory and then about an incident in the past that he utterly disliked. The clinician should avoid questions like "why" and "how come" and attempt to elicit information by stating: Many children have a favorite person—can you tell me who your favorite person is? During the initial interview it is also convenient to explore the child's view of why he is being evaluated and perhaps clarify what some of the procedures will be—reassuring the child that by understanding what is happening, he may feel better later on. The clinician's demeanor should be non-threatening and non-intrusive. If the child is overly anxious or fearful, it is worthwhile to postpone data gathering and proceed with a reassuring and easy conversation regarding a recent event the child can easily talk about. It is then sometimes helpful to have a family member in the room or limit the interview to a shorter period of time.

A Child's Psychiatric History

With these principles in mind, the clinician then attempts to gather and report his findings in a cohesive and logical manner. It is often true that if the clinician attempts to enforce a particular style of asking for a history and is not flexible, he will find himself with many difficulties. A suggested plan of action—one that cannot always be strictly adhered to—now follows and will serve as a comprehensive approach to history-taking.

Identifying Data and Informants

The first step in reporting a history should be a statement on the identifying data of the child and the informants. The child's age, sex, religion, race, address, and phone number are first registered. A list of names and phone numbers of the child's parents, teachers, and doctors should follow. After this information is gathered, some comments on the source of the referral is helpful. A list of all the important sources of information, including the dates of interviews with each informant, should be given. A brief comment on the reliability of the informants and how this opinion was arrived at is necessary.

Chief Complaints

List and distinguish between the complaints leading to the referral, other prominent complaints, and those complaints from the parents, school, or child. This refers to the immediate reason for the patient's referral and should include the situation specificity of the problem behavior.

Present Illness

The present illness should be evaluated using the following questions: What is the trouble now? What has been going on? Or, Why are you worried about him? Ask the parents what prompted them to bring the child and how recent the behavior is for which the child was brought. The problem behavior should be stated chronologically from the onset of the first symptoms to the present state of affairs; included should be details on the duration as well as the severity and the degree of impairment. At this time, previous psychiatric treatment of the child should be asked about and statements made by the child himself, the referral source, and other informants should also be included. Historical data that may attribute the problem behavior to specific changes in the child's internal or external environment should be elicited.

DEVELOPMENTAL AND PAST HISTORY

There seems to be little doubt that the more time that elapses between the historical event being inquired about and the inquiry, the more are the distortions and the less the reliability. Certainly this seems to be true for attitudinal issues and some child-rearing practices that are or are not in vogue at the time of the history-taking. Since it is our attempt to offer only guidelines, we will include a developmental and past history that will naturally be more reliable the younger the child or the more recent the event. At this stage of the history a review of the child's pediatric chart, a request that the parents bring the baby book, or a photo album that is dated can facilitate memories of the child's developmental stages. Families may be helped by the pictures in recalling the time of their child's first steps, the first spoken phrases, some of their early peer interactions, and other important circumstantial events.

For the clinician, an assessment of the integration, smoothness, timing, and the range of individual variation in behavioral patterns is a basic part of the history. It is generally helpful to ask parents if they have noticed any delay, interruption, or setback in the child's progress as compared to other children or siblings or if there are any areas of precocious development. After asking for a pregnancy, birth, and neonatal history (usually best gathered by asking for a copy of the pregnancy and birth medical records), five major areas of development should be covered: gross motor behavior, fine motor behavior, language behavior, adaptive behavior, and personal social behavior (Knobloch and Pasamanick, 1974).

Some of these developmental facts may be clarified or expanded upon later during the evaluation process. It is always helpful to have available a guideline of normal developmental stages as this history is being asked (see table 21-1).

TABLE 21-1.
Developmental and Past History

I. *Pregnancy and Delivery*
   A. Pregnancy
      Past pregnancies, abortions, miscarriages
      Mother's age and health during prenancy
      Complications of pregnancy
         medications
         bleeding
         accidents
         excessive weight gain, or weight loss
         X rays
         toxemia (high blood pressure, seizures)
         major illness (diabetes, heart disease)
         history of measles, venereal disease, urinary infections, vomiting, or RH negativity
      Addictive habits during pregnancy
         smoking
         drug abuse
         alcohol abuse
      Family attitudes and social stressors
         was the pregnancy planned?
         what sex was preferred?
         how was the name selected?
         what was the family going through at that time?
   B. Delivery
      Type of delivery
         vaginal
         forceps
         breech
         cesarean section
      Length and type of labor
      Complications
      Anesthesia
II. *Birth and Infancy*
   A. Birth
      Apgar scores

TABLE 21-1. (continued)

        Birth weight
        Complications
            need for resuscitation, respiratory distress
            prematurity, blood transfusions
            jaundice, cyanosis
            congenital defects or stigmata
            medications
    B. Infancy
        Undue sleepiness
        Medical problems
        Weak cry, colics
        Did the mother suffer postpartum depression?
        Was child a twin (identical, fraternal)?
        How long did mother and child remain in the hospital?
        Reaction of siblings

III. *Developmental History*
    A. Gross Motor
        When could child keep his head up?
        When did he crawl, sit, stand with support, stand without support, walk, hop, throw a ball, roller skate, ride a bicycle?
        Was child clumsy, or poorly coordinated, or accident-prone?
        Is child overactive or underactive?
    B. Fine Motor
        Pincer grasp, using cup and utensils
        Ability to draw, write, handle small objects, play piano, clap hands, tie shoelaces, use scissors
    C. Language and Communication
        Babbling
        First words
        First phrases
        First sentences, clarity of speech vocabulary, stuttering, lisping
        Delayed speech, echolalia—when?
        How many languages spoken at home?
        Gestures and postural movements in communication; cadence, rhythm of speech
        Language comprehension and expression when following simple commands
        Confusion of garbled speech and thinking
    D. Personal-Social Behavior
        Feeding
            breast- or bottle-fed? reaction to weaning?
            food regurgitation and rumination
            finicky, over- or undereating, vomiting, pica
            food allergies, likes or dislikes
            food habits and dietary intake
            self-feeding
            thumb sucking
            excessive biting or ruminating
        Toilet training
            when, how, and by whom was child toilet trained?
            when was child trained day and night for bladder and bowel control?
            constipation, diarrhea, colics, and enemas
            any bowel movement accidents or bed-wetting? when? how often?
        Sexual attitudes
            sexual abuse or excessive visual sexual exposure

TABLE 21-1. (continued)

    when was child curious about sexual differences? how was this handled?
    is child well identified with his sex? any history of worrisome cross-dressing, effeminacy, or sexual practices—response to opposite sex
    family attitudes and reactions to masturbation
    parental attitudes and practices regarding nudity and sex in the household
    sleeping arrangements
    nature and frequency of sex play
    reactions to sexual body changes in puberty—when did they occur?
    sexual or endocrinological anatomical difficulties
Sleeping
    sleeping habits
    nightmares, sleep talking, sleepwalking, insomnia, early-morning awakening, night terrors
    fear of the dark
    does child sleep alone? if not, with whom and where in the household?
Social interactions
    was child a cuddly infant?
    style and temperament of relating to peers, siblings, teachers, parents, and other family members
    how and with whom does child play—content and quality of sharing? how does he get along with others?
    best friend
    interest in group activities versus individual activities
    aggressive behavior, leadership abilities—is child scapegoated, the clown of the class, shy?
    responses to separations and baby-sitters?
    age of playmates—does he get along better with younger children or with older children and adults?
    overly sensitive, overly competitive, cruel with others, bossy, distant, provocative
    is child gregarious or withdrawn?
    is child moody, appropriate, constricted, labile, explosive?
Habits and fears (when, where, how severe)
    head banging, temper tantrums
    rocking
    thumb sucking
    fire setting
    lying
    stealing
    nail biting
    animal cruelty
    tics
    bruxism
    hair pulling
    phobias, fears
    substance abuse
    how much TV does child watch? what are his favorite programs?
    is child overly concerned about death and dying?
    inappropriate or unusual behavior
Adaptive behaviors
    ability of child to cope with situations of stress
    malleability, frustration tolerance, ability to delay gratification
    ability to adjust to new situations
    ability to use experience in the solution of new problems
    sports, favorite hobbies, and games
    clubs or groups child belongs to

Medical History

The medical history of the child is crucial. We must be able to assess if the presenting symptom is related to a congenital or acquired medical illness presenting with a "psychological" symptomatic picture (see table 21-2). For example, a child's learning problems may be due to his inability to relate to a difficult school teacher or it may be due to a receptive or expressive aphasia, moderate deafness, or a visual motor perceptual disability. Rivinus, Jamison, and Graham (1975) describe twelve children who presented with behavioral symptoms and were treated by mental-health professionals whose final diagnosis was a neurological illness. The clinician must also determine that the behavioral picture is not secondary to substance abuse (e.g., amphetamines presenting a picture of bizarre behavior, paranoia, and/or depression) or medication. For example, steroids may give rise to psychotic symptoms (drugs that cause psychiatric symptoms, 1981) and anticonvulsants to states resembling a dementia. It is usually worthwhile to call the child's pediatrician and/or request a copy of the child's medical records to complement the history taken by the clinician. Other features of the medical enquiry and examination are provided in chapter 22.

TABLE 21-2.
Medical History

1. Contagious diseases
2. Convulsions, fainting spells, seisurelike episodes
3. Operations (ascertain dates)
4. Hospitalizations—reactions, when, how long, for what reason
5. Injuries, accidents, disfigurements
6. Head traumas and sequelae
7. Chronic or acute illnesses
8. Allergies, asthma, hormonal diseases
9. Diseases with consequences on hearing, seeing, or speaking
10. Lead poisoning
11. Impact of illness on school and peer interactions
12. State of immunizations
13. Medications—how much, which
14. Headaches, stomach aches, flatulence, constipation, poor appetite
15. Soiling, bed-wetting
16. Dietary habits—undereating, overeating
17. Mental retardation
18. History of congenital illnesses

Family History

It is important to collect data regarding the family of the child. Not only is it pertinent to identify major historical events but also to gain a sense of the family roles, alliances, and dynamics. A careful family history will nearly always be more relevant (see table 21-3).

There is a reciprocal process between family dynamics and the psychological and social development of the child. Malone (1979) describes the importance of family interviews in relation to diagnosis as enabling us to observe: (a) the child's behavior as it is influenced by and influences the family system, (b) the capacity and motivation against or for change in the family regarding the problematic behavior, (c) nonverbal communication patterns,

TABLE 21-3.
Family History

I. *Family Demographics*
   Age and sex of members
   Places of birth
   Socioeconomic class
   Schooling and type of employment
   Physical aspects of the household and living arrangements

II. *Family Composition*
   Parents
   Siblings
   Other family members
   Other caretakers
   Pets

III. *Family History*
   Families of origin
   Reactions to different developmental stages of children
   Retirement issues
   Marital history
   Who do the children look like, behave like? Who are they named after?
   Medical history
       chronic illnesses
       mental illness
       mental retardation
       suicides
       alcoholism, substance abuse
       antisocial-behavior incarcerations
       learning problems
       hospitalization
       physical or sexual abuse
       disabilities, history of seizures

IV. *Family Events*
   Births
   Marriages
   Vacations, recreational activities
   Shared activities

V. *Family Roles*
   Primary caretaker
   Alliances and coalitions
   Primary disciplinarian
   Sexual roles
   Personalities
   Complementarity (who expresses emotion and who controls it)
   Sibling roles—ordinal position

VI. *Family Function*
   Ability to mourn
   Ability to guide
   Giving autonomy and emancipation
   Giving nurturance and weaning
   Functioning in outside society
   Dealing with crises
   Sharing in activities
   Setting boundaries
   Developing coping styles

TABLE 21-3. (continued)

VII. *Family Communication*
Ability to verbalize
Use of nonverbal styles
Expressing affection and emotion—responsiveness
Ability to be clear
Ability to be intimate and to offer empathy

VIII. *Family Stresses*
Acute or chronic illness in a family member
hospitalizations ⟨ medical / psychiatric ⟩
deaths
divorces
separations
physical and sexual abuse
translocations in neighborhood
economic reversals
incarcerations, legal problems
catastrophic events

(d) the family's patterns in the expression of affect, roles, problem solving, and conflict resolution, and (e) structural imbalances in the family (e.g., splitting, alliances, collusions, and scapegoating). Furthermore, a chance to gather history on the parent's family of origin and to observe sibling interaction is crucial. In the process of taking a history, important adult figures and siblings may be identified who are exacerbating the symptomatology or who may facilitate a cure. Tseng and McDermott (1979) propose a triaxial family classification system. Their first axis considers family dysfunction at different stages of family development, the second axis refers to family-member interaction, and the third axis focuses on the family group as a system and its possible dysfunction as a whole.

There is presently no one ideal approach to family diagnosis and history-taking, and certainly little research exists that can offer guidelines to more reliable information gathering. Furthermore, the amount and depth of family history-taking will depend much on the expressed presenting symptom. In cases of physical and sexual abuse, chronic pediatric illness and psychosomatic illness, divorce and separation, delinquency, and children with separation problems, it seems very important that a more detailed family history be elicited (Tseng and McDermott, 1979). In order both to assess some important relevant history and present interactions, a family interview including the child is helpful. Techinques that have been described as facilitating the collection of material have been summarized by Villeneuve (1979). He gives examples of utilizing sculpting, drawing, puppet play, psychodrama, video playback, and game playing. These techniques will vary according to the developmental stage of the child and the family's ability to participate. It is usually neccessary to determine early what the family likes to do. For example, if the family is particularly creative, a group task to make a large drawing of the family living quarters is suggested. Once they have started, shifts in room allocations, who sleeps with whom, whose room is closest to whom, previous reallocation, and separations can be asked for. Other examples would be to allow the family to produce, direct, or act as in a TV episode regarding something that happened in the family. If the family enjoys sports, ask about what happened at the last ball game they attended. Checking team alliances may relax the family sufficiently, to then enter into a history of family group interactions, alliances, and family dyadic "teams."

SOCIOCULTURAL HISTORY

It is particularly important for those clinicians working in health-delivery systems in large heterogenous communities to be aware of the variety of socioeconomic and cultural differences of the client population. There has been surprisingly little research done to assess the mental-health profiles of minority and/or different ethnic groups. Furthermore, most of the literature describes the problems encountered by clinicians when having to interview these groups but seldom suggests concrete approaches for the assessment, evaluation, and treatment of them. Some authors (Devereux, 1965; Chess et al., 1966) have described approaches and difficulties in the evaluation of children of different groups. While asking questions and eliciting information, the clinician must be aware of child-rearing practices, religious ideology, and differences in communication and language patterns (see table 21-4).

If the child is a migrant member of another society, finding out about the stressors affecting the child on arrival in the present host society will be an important part of the history. Different cultural and socioeconomic groups have different attitudes toward professionals, mental health, and disease, and may consider symptomatic what the clinician may not, or vice versa. A history that includes comments on the families' particular styles, their concepts of socially desirable behavior, and what they consider psychological distress in their children will thus be more contextually relevant. The clinician does better when he assumes a learning position and admits he needs to know more about the culture. He can facilitate this by asking about major holidays, dietary habits, community activities, musical and religious interests, and then gradually entering into the particulars of child rearing and parents' attitudes toward teaching, disciplining, and playing with their children.

This part of the history-taking can be done while doing a family history, and most clinicians will find that the family is usually willing to share their "style of living" more comfortably than more personal or individual areas of conflict.

TABLE 21-4.
Sociocultural History

1. Type of neighborhood
2. Living arrangements
3. Family religion and traditions
4. Family translocations or migration patterns—impact on the child
5. Family festivities, meals, and styles of celebration
6. Languages spoken at home
7. Racial and ethnic membership
8. Level of acculturation and adaptation to their present community
9. Financial and social stressors
10. The family's attitude toward mental health services
11. Familial attitude toward death and illness
12. Familial attitudes of childhood and adolescence
13. Child rearing practices
14. Cultural and social support networks, i.e. church, clubs

School History

Due to the increasing time the child spends in his school as he grows up, it is important to get a good school history from the parents, the teachers, and the child (see table 21-5). It is usually best to wait until the parents' trust has been gained before requesting that a call be made to the teacher. A statement to the effect that the call will just be to gather further information and will not label the child as emotionally ill reassures the parents. It is usual to first contact the guidance counselor, who should initiate communication with the teacher. At that time the home-room teacher can be called and a good sense of the child's cognitive and socialization skills may be acquired.

It is also helpful if the parents have a record of the child's grades for the last couple of years. A request to the parents or child to bring report cards, class pictures, and programs of school activities in which the child has participated can add important data. It is often useful to ask the child who his preferred teacher is and what his favorite subjects are, and to determine which of these he dislikes the most. Recreation and gym time usually evoke many feelings in children regarding socialization skills and difficulties. Questions about the child's participation in school plays and extracurricular activities should be asked as well as the child's school history. This should include his reaction to nursery school, and both growth-enhancing and growth-inhibiting experiences with particular teachers or schools in the past. If the child is going to an inner-city public school plagued by overpopulation, rapid teacher turnover, and underpaid teachers, this should be noted in the history as a potential stressor to the child.

TABLE 21-5.
School History

I. *Parent and Child*
How did the child react to his first day of school? Were there any separation problems?
Is there a history of school phobia or truancy?
Have there been many school changes?
Has the child performed consistently or has he gone through ups and downs in his performance?
What are his grades?
What classes does he enjoy the most? Which does he dislike the most, and why?
Does he like or dislike any particular teacher?
Is the school or present teacher adequate for the patient's particular needs?
What is the attitude of the parents toward the school and the previous history of the parents' own school experiences?
Did he have to repeat any class? Is he in a special class?

II. *Teacher*
Is the child: quarrelsome
submissive
excitable
a daydreamer
squirmy
a smart aleck
easily hurt
a leader, popular
a follower
scapegoated
immature, sensitive

TABLE 21-5. (continued)

          easily frustrated
          uncooperative
          organized
          disorganized
          overactive
          stubborn
          fearful
          clumsy
          moody
Does the child have learning difficulties? In which areas?
How does the child get along with other children?
What are the child's cognitive strengths and weaknesses?
Does the child work well by himself?
In what classes is the child doing well and in which is he doing poorly? Describe the classes the child participates in.
Does he have many teachers? What are the other teachers like?
    Does he have a favorite teacher or a teacher he particularly dislikes?
Does the child enjoy or avoid gym and sports?
Is the child involved in extracurricular activities? Which?
Have there been many changes in the school administration and philosophy?
Is there a high teacher turnover?
Is the school safe? What is the type of neighborhood?
Is the school public or private? Is it coed or not?

CONCLUSION

In taking a history, the clinician will have to consider many factors. He or she should be fully aware of any personal or theoretical biases, and should avoid making any premature decisions and recommendations. The clinician must be careful not to side with the child against the parent or vice versa. He or she must direct the interview with empathy, avoiding ambiguous or leading questions. It is necessary to be structured but flexible, allowing the informants to expand on any given answer and to feel that they can share their own impressions without fear or embarrassment. The data elicited should offer a cohesive framework to a series of interacting events that hopefully will serve as an explanation of the presenting symptomatology.

As has been described, the reliability of some of the historical material varies. Issues that have to do with attitudes and are heavily loaded with feeling, even though crucial for the clinician, usually are least reliable in terms of time of occurrence and veracity of the event. Factual information such as birth weight, and well-defined items such as nightmares, stuttering, and stealing are highly reliable. The importance of the informant and his or her ability to assess and report appropriately problematic behavior also need to be considered. It is the task of the clinician to balance and weigh the importance of all these variables and to develop strategies to elicit if not exact at least sufficiently reliable information that will assist him in making appropriate recommendations.

Finally, the clinician must be sensitive to the particular situation of child patients. They are in a stage of continuous development and growth, and as such, more vulnerable at certain times than at others. They are dependent on adults not only for their physical and psychological sustenance but also depend on adults to serve as their advocates and their intermediaries. A careful assessment of the child's medical and developmental history as well as of his family, sociocultural, and school environment is thus necessary.

The clinician, as a history-taker, will thus serve not only as a detective but as a biographer. He or she will hopefully be the advocate for the child and his family and the initiator of further evaluation and treatment approaches.

REFERENCES

Achenbach, T. 1980. DSM-III in light of empirical research on the classification of child psychopathology. *J. Am. Acad. Child Psych.,* 19(3):395-412.

Chess, S., Thomas, A., and Birch, H. 1966. Distortions in developmental reporting made by parents of behaviorally disturbed children. *J. Am. Acad. of Child Psych.,* 5:226-331.

Cohen, R. 1979. Part A: The approach to assessment. In *Basic handbook of psychiatry. I. Development.* ed. J. Noshpitz, pp. 485-504. New York: Basic Books.

Cowen, E., Pederson, A., Babigian, H., Izzo, L., and Frost, M. 1973. Long term follow up of early detected vulnerable children. *J. Consult. Clin. Psychol.,* 41:438-446.

Cox, A., Hopkinson, K., and Rutter, M. 1981. Psychiatric interviewing techniques. II. Naturalistic study: Eliciting factual information. *Brit. J. Psych.,* 138:283-291.

Cramer, J. 1975. Psychiatric examination of the child. In *The comprehensive textbook of psychiatry,* vol. 2, ed. A. Freedman, H. Kaplan, and B. Sadock, pp. 2055-2060. Baltimore: Williams and Wilkins Co.

Devereux, G. 1965. The voices of children: Psychocultural obstacles to therapeutic communication. *Am. J. Psychother.,* 19:4-19.

Drugs that cause psychiatric symptoms. 1981. *Med. Letter,* 23:9-12.

Evans, I., and Nelson, R. 1977. Assessment of child behavior problems. In *Handbook of behavioral assessment,* ed. A. Ciminero, K. Calhoun, and H. Adams, pp. 603-681. New York: Wiley.

Freud, A. 1962. Assessment of childhood disturbances. In *The psychoanalytic study of the child,* vol. 17, ed. R. Eissler, A. Freud, M. Kris et al., pp. 149-158. New York: International University Press.

Graham, P., and Rutter, M. 1968. The reliability and validity of the psychiatric assessment of the child. II. Interview with the parent. *Brit. J. Psych.,* 114:581-592.

Haggard, E., Brekstad, A., and Skard, A. 1966. On the reliability of the anamnestic interview. *J. Abnorm. Soc. Psychol.,* 61:311-313.

Helper, M. 1958. Parental evaluations of children and children's self-evaluation. *J. Abnorm. Soc. Psychol.,* 56:190-194.

Kestenbaum, C., and Bird, H. 1978. A reliability study of the mental health assessment form for school age children. *J. Am. Acad. Child Psych.,* 17:338-347.

Knobloch, H., and Pasamanick, B. 1974. *Developmental diagnosis.* New York: Harper and Row.

Lapouse, R., and Monk, M. 1958. An epidemiologic study of behavior characteristics in children. *Am. J. Pub. Health,* 48:1134-1144.

Leitenberg, H., Burchard, J., Buchard, S., Fuller, E., and Lysaght, T. 1977. Using positive reinforcement to suppress behavior: Some experimental comparisons with sibling conflict. *Beh. Ther.,* 8:168-182.

Malone, C. 1979. Child psychiatry and family theory: An overview. *J. Am. Acad. Child Psych.,* 18:4-21.

Mash, E., and Terdal, L. 1981. Introduction. In *Behavioral assessment of childhood disorders,* ed. E. Mash, and L. Terdal, pp. 44-53. New York: Guildford Press.

Mednick, S., and Schaffer, J. 1963. Mother's retrospective reports in child rearing research. *Am. J. Orthopsych.,* 33:457-461.

Rivinus, T., Jamison, D., and Graham, P. 1975. Childhood organic neurological disease presenting as psychiatric disorder. *Arch. Dis. Child.,* 50:115-119.

Robins, L. 1963. The accuracy of parental recall of aspects of child development and child rearing practices. *J. Abnorm. Soc. Psychol.,* 66:261-270.

Rutter, M., and Cox, A. 1981. Psychiatric interviewing techniques. I. Methods and measures. *Brit. J. Psych.,* 138:273-282.

Truax, C., and Carkhuff, R. 1967. *Towards effective counselling and psychotherapy: Training and practice.* Chicago: Aldine.

Tseng, W., and McDermott, J. 1979. Triaxial family classification: A proposal. *J. Am. Acad. Child Psych.,* 18:22-43.

Ullman, L., and Krasner, L. 1975. *A psychological approach to abnormal behavior.* Englewood Cliffs, N.J.: Prentice-Hall, p. 475.

Villeneuve, C. 1979. The specific participation of the child in family therapy. *J. Am. Acad. Child Psych.,* 18:44-53.

Wenar, C., and Coulter, J. 1962. A reliability study of developmental histories. *Child Dev.,* 33:453-462.

22

The Physical Examination in Child Psychiatry

LAURENCE L. GREENHILL

THE PHYSICAL EXAMINATION is a much underutilized procedure in child psychiatry. Its unpopularity comes from several sources. Many child psychiatrists have had minimal hands-on experience with child patients in medical school, and few have spent their internship year in pediatrics. Several years of adult psychiatry training engenders a negative attitude toward the stethoscope, black bag, and the white coat, all of which the resident psychiatrist leaves behind as his specialty training advances. Some training programs informally but traditionally maintain that trainees examine colleague's patients, never their own, out of fear that the physical exam may stimulate sexual or aggressive transference emotions or simply ruin the rapport between the child and his "talking doctor." It is as if the psychiatrist's goal of alleviating inner psychological conflict would be diverted by the examination. Physical or neurological examinations rarely are included in the detailed training case work-up, and child psychiatry patients are referred to pediatricians or neurologists for routine examinations.

Several reasons suggest that this subspecializing trend may not be helpful to the patient, the child psychiatrist, or to the future of child psychiatry itself. In theory, the child patient should have the greatest trust in his psychiatrist, and will probably regard a well-done physical examination as a sign of care and attention on the part of his doctor. The child psychiatrist, in doing the evaluation, can become aware of developmental deviations as well as progressive medical disorders masquerading as emotional disturbances. Misdiagnosing a tumor or an anemia as depression can have grave consequences.

The physical examination has more value than the prevention of malpractice. Repeated experience in physical assessment trains the therapist to look at the whole patient. Not only should the child psychiatrist be sensitive to the affective states in his young patients, but he should pick up motor dysfunction, limping, and weight changes. Simple but accurate observation will reveal telltale changes in a child's interest in self-grooming, clothes, or the peer group. The child psychiatrist will then be able to follow the growth and development of the body, development of social functioning, and the child's growing independence as he masters activity of daily living (ADL) skills.

Child psychiatrists should be more comfortable doing physical examinations. After all, the only skill that truly separates child psychiatrists from their nonmedical colleagues is the training in medical diagnosis and treatment. A well-trained child psychiatrist has the potential for utilizing a variety of special techniques, including psychotherapy, family therapy, behavioral management, developmental diagnosis, and physical-examination techniques, and no other professional can duplicate this mix of skills. At present, many other fields are matching or surpassing the child psychiatrist who only does psychotherapy alone.

This chapter will serve as a brief introduction to the examination of the school-age child. No attempt will be made to be comprehensive, since the art of physical diagnosis depends on a thorough understanding of developmental landmarks in the growing child, details of pediatric pathophysiology, and a thorough understanding of anatomy. Each of these topics requires a textbook for adequate coverage and is well beyond the scope of this chapter. But the child psychiatrist can integrate modified physical and neurological examinations into his mental-status evaluation. Key areas of interest will be briefly reviewed here, including the identification and meaning of soft neurological signs, minor physical anomalies, and disorders of growth. Tardive dyskinesia in childhood will also be reviewed.

Approach to the Patient

Some of the child psychiatrist's concerns about disturbing doctor-patient rapport derive from observations of the anxiety exhibited by school-age children due to unpleasant memories of earlier examinations. Much can be done to alleviate this anxiety in a child, and in so doing, actually build better rapport for the psychotherapy sessions. As in many other areas, the correct preparation and approach to the patient will markedly reduce such fears.

One excellent "warm-up" technique is to include the specific developmental testing and evaluation for clumsiness and soft signs just before the physical examination. These tasks have a true "fun-and-games" quality, since they involve playing ball with the examiner and performing tandem gait, running, hopping, skipping, and jumping maneuvers. With the child involved at an early stage, the remainder of the physical assessment can continue this gamelike quality, with the child's cooperation. It also allows the physician to determine how much the child understands simple commands.

This interlude will allow the examiner to make valuable observations on the child's range of affect and facial expressions as well as his attitude toward physical activity. It also gives the physician the opportunity to "lay on the hands" during a nonthreatening game activity. Later on, both hands can be used for examination, one hand carrying out a procedure, and the second hand used as a distracting and comforting force (Hoekelman, 1974).

With experience, the child psychiatrist can develop a given format of observations and physical tests to be used on each child. Generally, a complete child psychiatric evaluation should begin with the history of the present disorder. A past developmental history should follow, with a review of the present level of motor, intellectual, and language function. Next comes the neurological and soft-signs evaluation, followed by the mental status. Finally, the child psychiatrist has the child change to an examining gown for a modified pediatric physical exam, moving from head to foot. Symptomatic body areas can be examined in detail, while other parts of the exam may be shortened, so that the standard approach can be modified to some extent to match the child and his history.

History

The first stage is taking a history to screen for possible physical conditions that might cause emotional difficulties. The parent should be questioned about past family history of learning disabilities, mental retardation, genetic conditions (such as Down's syndrome), and mental illnesses, such as relatives with histories of imprisonment, suicidal behavior, or nervous breakdowns. The reproductive history of the mother should also be reviewed to elicit a history of risk, such as a number of miscarriages or bleeding during the patient's pregnancy, or the need for "hormone shots" such as progesterone to maintain the pregnancy. Mental retardation or genetic syndromes in siblings are other valuable historical details. The labor and delivery history of the patient may also yield valuable historical details, such as prolonged labor, irregularities or cessation of fetal heartbeat, anoxia, withdrawal from maternal drugs, or low Apgar scores. Neonatal sepsis, hypotonia, poor reflexes, irritability, reversal of sleep-wake cycle, and colic at three months are also clues that the child might be at risk for later motor, language, or intellectual developmental delays.

Developmental milestones are important to record. Though most parents have extremely inaccurate recollection for these events, they will recall asking relatives or their pediatrician why their child is delayed. This type of historical detail is more accurate. In addition, it is possible to differentiate among motor, intellectual, sphincter control, and language milestones to pinpoint the area of difficulty. Typical milestones are included in table 22-1.

Other crucial areas can be covered quickly. A record of hospitalizations and operations should be taken, critical for later assessment for child abuse, chronic illnesses, separations, and the general health of the child. Number of days absent from school during the past two years can also reveal a problem of pathological separation anxiety in the child or extreme overprotectiveness in the parent. A history of repeated, severe episodes of otitis media may raise suspicions of a hearing problem, which may be the cause of classroom misbehavior. The presence of a seizure disorder or a history of documented brain injury with loss of consciousness and retrograde amnesia can be associated with an increased incidence of psychiatric disorder. A history of pica should be obtained, since behavior disorders have been linked to subclinical cases of lead intoxication (David, 1978). An allergic history should be inquired

TABLE 22-1.
Developmental Milestones

Motor
- *Sitting* — 5–8 months — *Abnormal* after 10 months
- *Walking* — 13–21 months — *Abnormal* after 24 months

Speech
- Tuneful, repetitive *babble* — 7–8 months — *Abnormal* after 10–11 months
- Spontaneous use of *single words* in correct context — 13–15 months — *Abnormal* after 21 months
- Meaningful *sentences* — 18–22 months — *Abnormal* after 27 months
- Speech *intelligible* to strangers — 3.5 years — *Abnormal* after 4 years

Sphincter Control
- Urine: Day — 5% wetting at age 5
- Night — 15% wetting at age 5
- Feces: Control achieved between 1.5 and 3 years

after, and a detailed record of psychotropic medication usage should be taken. If a child has been on such medications, questions concerning beneficial responses, side effects, toxic reactions, and evidence of tolerance should be asked. A good history of drug response can save much unnecessary trial-and-error medication adjustment.

OBSERVATION

Much can be learned about a child simply by his or her appearance, movements, and spontaneous speech. Are gross handicaps present, such as blindness or deafness (child is using sign language with parents), or does the child need a minor or major appliance to ambulate, such as a wheelchair or walker? Body size itself is revealing, for the tiny-for-age child may suffer from chronic renal disease, severe maternal deprivation, and abuse (Goodwin, 1978), or Cushing's syndrome from excessive cortisol (Blodgett et al., 1956; Falliers et al., 1963; Loeb, 1976), while the unusually tall child may have hyperthyroidism. Gait should be examined carefully for subtle signs of mild hemiparesis (lack of normal arm swing on one side, dragging one foot) or a limp secondary to a joint abnormality or a congenitally short tibia. Motor coordination can be quickly assessed, with the examiner being vigilant for signs of spasticity (as seen in children with cerebral palsy secondary to neonatal hyperbilirubinemia), tremor, or choreoathetoid movements.

Minor physical anomalies are often revealed by inspection alone and will often lend the child a peculiar appearance. These signs include such findings as low-set ears; congenitally wide-set eyes with broad intercanthal distance (hypertelorism); epicanthal folds; high, arched hard palate (cathedral palate); bilateral single, transverse palmar creases (simian lines); short, incurving fifth fingers; and large space between a short big toe and longer second toe. These are often seen in profusion in children with genetic problems such as Down's syndrome, a disorder that can often be reliably diagnosed by appearance alone. Some evidence exists associating a high minor physical anomaly score with levels of gross motor activity in children in general (Waldrop and Halverson, 1971) and with attention deficit disorder with hyperactivity (ADDH) in particular (Waldrop and Goering, 1971; Rapoport and Quinn, 1974). An attempted replication of these studies failed to find a significant correlation between the presence of ADDH and a high score on minor physical anomalies (Mattes et al., 1984). Even so, a child with a large number of these minor findings should be examined for a possible genetic syndrome.

EXAMINATION FOR SOFT NEUROLOGICAL SIGNS

An examination for soft neurological signs fits in well as a warm-up procedure prior to the actual physical, since it involves ballcatching, running, and hopping. It is utilized to measure the number and severity of nonlocalizing, subtle signs of clumsiness or dysfunction in the neuromusculature system. A number of studies have suggested an increased incidence of these signs appearing in groups of children with behavior or learning difficulties (Shaffer, 1978). Carefully done epidemiological studies attest to the fact that they can be readily and reliably elicited (Rutter et al., 1970; Rieder and Nichols, 1979) with the use of instruments such as the NIMH-developed physical and neurological examination for soft signs (PANESS) (Guy, 1976). Yet other more recent studies have questioned the sensitivity and ease of administration of the PANESS (Camp et al., 1978; Porrino et al., 1983; Sarma, 1983). Sarma has successfully tested a new procedure, the EXAMINS, which includes 18 items, scored as pass or fail, including digit span, visual tracking, speech, nystagmus, eye symmetry, hand dominance, crossed dominance of arm and leg, identifying right-left on self, right-left on examiner, bilateral hand stimulation, face-hand test, finger localization, graphesthesia, stereognosis, synkinesis, finger-to-nose test, diadokokinesis, and passive head turning. There appears to be a significant correlation with "cross-situational" hyperactivity, which is defined as the sum of hyperactive factors from Conner's parent and teacher questionnaire.

Problems have existed with the interpretation of soft-sign findings, as pointed out by Shaffer. The base rate of these signs is as high as 14% in populations of children with no disorders (Rutter et al., 1970). When age and IQ are covaried for, the soft-sign variables fail to distinguish between normals and children with problems. Yet two types of studies suggest that the presence of soft signs in childhood may have prognostic significance at predicting later psychopathology. Quitkin and his colleagues (1976) found significantly higher rates of these signs (dysdiadokokinesias, dysgraphesthesias, mirror movements, finger apraxia, poor gait, and poor speech) in adult schizophrenics with premorbid histories of childhood asociality than in psychiatrically disturbed controls. A recent epidemiological study selected 110 seventeen-year-old subjects from the Columbia sample frame of the NIH Collaborative Perinatal Project, each of whom had shown positive evidence of having soft signs at age seven. Analysis of the data showed significant evidence that the soft signs persisted, and thus had no developmental course, and predicted later psychopathology in late adolescence (Shaffer et al., 1981; Shaffer et al., 1982). In general, there appears to be value in the assessment of soft neurological signs in the physical examination of the child psychiatric patient.

The actual examination for soft neurological signs may be conducted in three main phases, those while the subject is *sitting,* those while the subject is *standing,* and those with the patient *walking or running.* These procedures are reviewed in detail in several sources, each of which utilizes particular techniques for eliciting neurological soft signs (Touwen and Prechtl, 1970; Bialer et al., 1974; Guy, 1976, pp. 394–406; Sarma, 1983).

It may prove more feasible to begin with the child seated opposite the examiner, and then proceed stepwise to the next two phases. All procedures must be demonstrated by the examiner and rehearsed with the patient until the examiner is satisfied the patient completely understands what he is to do. Otherwise, the failure of the patient to accomplish these simple motor tasks is a cognitive problem, and not a soft neurological motor sign. It is also essential for the examiner to identify the patient's dominant hand by asking him to hold up his writing hand, his dominant foot by asking for the foot he kicks with, and the dominant eye, by asking him to sight a target with an imaginary gun. These dominant sides can be rechecked during the course of the test.

The procedures will be presented first, and the interpretation and thresholds for abnormality will be covered in table 22–2 below.

Procedures while Patient Is Seated

RIGHT-LEFT ORIENTATION. Right-left orientation can be questioned facing the patient. By combining several instructions, one can also test the number of commission commands the child can process. Then the patient should be asked to identify the right and left parts of the examiner. If the child becomes confused at this point, reach across with your

TABLE 22-2.
Age Thresholds for Soft Signs

Test	Abnormal Findings	Cutoff Age
1. Tongue extension	Motor impersistence	> 8 years
2. Finger-to-nose	Tremor, past pointing	> 8 years
3. Left-right, orient	Inaccurate on self	> 8 years
	Inaccurate on examiner	> 9 years
4. Mouth open, eyes closed	Fingers spread	> 8 years
5. Rapid alternating	Mirroring, overflow	> 10 years
6. Finger opposition	Mirroring, overflow	> 10 years
7. Stereognosis	Dysgraphesthesia	> 10 years
8. Squeeze clip	Motor impersistence	> 8 years
9. Mod. Romberg	Involuntary movements	> 10 years
10. Localize sound	Cannot point to sound	> 5 years
11. Tandem gait	Falls from line 2 times	> 8 years

right hand, grab his right hand, and prove they are on the right side by turning your body to face in the same direction as his. Several examples of this type of instruction can teach normal eight-year-old children quickly.

HEAD OR FACE TESTS. Tests directed at parts of the head or face may elicit clumsy, awkward, and irregular movements in those children with multiple soft signs. In particular, one looks for either *choreiform* (small, jerky, twitchlike movements) or *athetoid* (writhing, snakelike, slow movements of fingers or tongue) movements. Instruct the patient to open and close the mouth rapidly; those with soft signs develop an irregular pace with many associated movements. Ask the individual to stick out the tongue as far as possible and move it from side to side quickly. Irregularity of motion will be evident in the attempts of those children with soft signs. Then the child is asked to protrude the tongue as far as possible while holding it still. Examine for an inability to maintain the tongue in extension, and watch the surface of the tongue for fine, vermicular, writhing motions.

FINGER-TO-NOSE TEST. Instruct the patient to alternately touch the index finger of his dominant hand to the tip of his nose and then to the tip of your index finger. At first, move your finger to the extremes of the patient's visual field and then stop. Watch the patient's finger: does a tremor develop just as he is about to touch your stationary finger? Then move your finger just as the patient is about to touch yours: does the patient "past point," missing your finger, or develop a tremor? Ask the patient to use his nondominant hand as well: does a tremor develop now?

HAND TESTS. Rapid alternation—ask the patient to hold up both hands at face level. Taking one hand at a time, suggest that the patient rapidly supinate and pronate the wrist. Look for smoothness and regularity of this motion as the patient is asked to speed up. Irregularity and clumsiness are signs of dysdiadokokinesis. Also look for mirror movements (synkinesis), which can overflow into the other hand and appear as damped alternations at the wrist. Associated movements, such as facial grimacing, tongue protrusion, or head movements are also scored as soft signs.

Stereognosis—one may test for cortical parietal lobe function by placing objects (coins of various denominations) in the hand or drawing numbers on the palm, and asking the patient to identify them with the eyes covered. Inability to recognize numbers drawn is termed *dysgraphesthesia.* It is critical to trace the numbers so they are right-side up for the patient.

Opposition test—the patient is instructed to rest both hands on the knees, with the palms facing upward. The thumb is then touched to each finger in a serial fashion, as rapidly as possible, but only for one hand at a time. Look for mirror movements in the opposite hand.

Squeeze-clip test—with the hands in the same position as the opposition test, ask the patient to squeeze a bulldog clip. Look for mirror movements in the opposite hand and for associated movements in the face.

DEEP-TENDON REFLEXES. Deep-tendon reflexes should be evaluated. Use a reflex hammer and concentrate on the upper and lower extremities. Besides looking for "hard" findings, such as ankle clonus or extensor plantar responses, try to determine if reflex asymmetry exists.

EVALUATE MUSCLE STRENGTH. Moving from the head and neck down to the lower extremities, evaluate the patient's major muscle groups on both sides of the body. For example, ask the patient to turn his head to each side with your hand blocking the motion at the chin. For the upper and lower extremities, try to move a limb at each major joint after the patient has fixed the posture, stating, "Keep your arm flexed and don't let me move it," for example. Look for serious asymmetries in muscle strength between one side of the body and the other, suggestive of a subclinical hemiparesis. Also be on the lookout for generalized weakness, or *hypotonia,* now being reported in children with atypical psychosis or pervasive developmental disorder, childhood onset (Cantor, 1980).

Procedures while the Patient Is Standing

CATCHING A BALL. A child of eight should be able both to throw a tennis ball overhand across a ten foot distance and catch it two out of three tries.

THE MODIFIED ROMBERG. The standard Romberg exam involves the patient standing with feet together, arms raised and pointed forward, and eyes closed. The patient must hold that posture for ten seconds without falling; this indicates intact vestibular functioning. In modified form the patient is asked in addition to open his mouth as wide as possible, protrude his tongue as far as possible, and spread his fingers, holding this posture for twenty seconds. Shine a flashlight on the tongue to observe fine athetoid writhing movements. Look for drift downward of one arm, indicating possible weakness. Small, jerky, arrhythmic movements at the wrist, fingers, or shoulder suggest a choreiform movement disorder, while writhing athetoid movements may be seen in the tongue or fingers. These movements have been called Prechtl movements (Touwen and Prechtl, 1970, pp. 38-40). They are also observed in cases of tardive dyskinesia (Gualtieri, 1983).

MOUTH-OPENING FINGER-SPREADING PHENOMENON. While the child is standing, the examiner supports the child's extended arms so the hands and wrists are not under tension. The child is asked to close his eyes and open his mouth as wide as possible. Maximal spreading and extension of fingers, in an involuntary manner, is significant in a child over eight, and is a positive soft sign (Touwen and Prechtl, 1970).

STANDING ON ONE FOOT. Ask the patient to stand on the dominant foot for ten seconds. Repeat for the other foot. Observe for problems in balance and strength on both sides.

Procedures while Patient Is Walking or Running

These procedures are often carried out on linoleum-tiled floors that have a natural grid built in from the pattern of square tiles. Otherwise, it is useful to lay out a one-foot square using tape. In addition, put down a six-foot stretch of tape in a straight line for the tandem gait tests.

HOPPING TEST. Ask the child to hop on one foot at least ten times, while remaining inside the square of tape. As earlier, the test should be carried out with the dominant foot and then the nondominant one. Clumsy, uncoordinated children over eight years of age with soft signs have trouble remaining inside the square and hopping on one foot without putting down the other foot for balance.

TIPTOE WALKING. Most children over the age of three can walk the entire six-foot tape line on tiptoe without having their heels touch the floor. Certain children with the pervasive developmental disorder will be able to carry out this test before the age of three because of the predominance of toe walking in that syndrome.

TANDEM GAIT. The examiner needs to exhibit this test by walking heel to toe down the tape, like a high-wire performer in a circus. The child above eight should be able to carry out tandem gait for a six-foot distance without falling away from the line once or using the walls for support. If this is completed successfully, ask the child to walk the tape in tandem gait, first on the heels, then on the toes. Walking backward in tandem gait takes more practice.

RUNNING. Ask the child to run down a hallway and return. Is the motion graceful or clumsy? Is arm swing identical on both sides or is one arm hanging limp, suggesting a mild hemiparesis? Does the child run on the balls of his feet or flat-footed?

OTHER TESTS. These tests are related to speech production, hearing, and strabismus.
Speech—rate the child's speech in terms of its intelligibility. Can it be understood without a knowledge of the context? Are there prominent articulation problems, such as slurring or consonant omission, that require the examiner to ask the child to repeat words or phrases? Does the child stutter?
Strabismus—using the Hirschberg test (see later), ask the child to fixate on a distant object. If the uncovered eye moves just as the other eye is covered up, the child may have a latent strabismus.
Auditory sensitivity—the child's basic hearing can be tested if the examiner sits from 8 to 18 feet behind the patient and whispers or talks in a low voice, uttering a series of numbers and letters and asking the child to repeat each.
Ability to localize sound—most children over five years old should be able to point to the direction of a noise behind them. Tap with the reflex hammer directly behind the child and ask him to point in the direction of the noise.

This series of tests will generally provide the child psychiatrist with a comprehensive picture of the general central nervous system functioning of the patient. In particular, repeated examinations of a number of children will increase the practitioner's acumen in spotting deviancy. Table 22-2 lists some of the soft-sign tests, the abnormal signs, and the age thresholds for each test.

MENTAL STATUS EXAMINATION

The mental-status examination is often thought to be the special province of the child psychiatrist. Yet the examination actually exists as part of any specialized evaluation of the child done by a number of professionals, including child psychologists, pediatricians, speech therapists, and others. In this chapter the mental-status examination becomes part of the sequence of the general physical examination rather than the main routine of the practitioner. As such, it will contain bits and pieces of other specialist's tests, such as the activity of daily living (ADL) questions taken from the Denver developmental or the Vineland social maturity index (Doll, 1965), and certain questions from the child psychology intelligence-test batteries, such as the Stanford-Binet or the Wechsler intelligence scale for children—revised (Anastasi, 1976). Borrowing from these fields, the child psychiatrist can screen his patients for developmental delays and mental retardation in a limited fashion, but enough to know whether more formalized testing need be done. The child psychiatrist then can assume more of the role of a generalist and act as the child's advocate in the health-care and academic systems, coordinating special evaluations and following through on obtaining special class or school placements, tutoring programs, or even specialized medical evaluations or treatments.

The mental-status examination can be structured to increase rapport, much like the ancillary warm-up function of the soft-signs neurological examination. Starting with the Goodenough-Harris drawing test (Harris, 1963) and the house-tree-person drawings (Hammer, 1960), the mental status can then move into the more intimidating question-and-answer process of the actual mental-status assessment. As with the actual physical, the more intrusive segments of the mental status are saved for last.

ADL Assessment

This segment of the examination involves the child's mother. Questions cover the child's basic skills in self-care, such as his ability to dress himself, buckle belts, tie shoelaces, and button shirt fronts. These skills should be present by primary-school age, between six and seven years. The level of feeding can also be evaluated, since most eight year olds feed themselves, cut their own meat with a knife, and can use a fork. Mobility skills will depend upon the parent's assessment of the child's age and judgment, but many ten year olds are allowed to ride the bus alone and find their own way to and from their local school. By age seven most children should know their own address and phone number, and have enough telephone skills to call a parent at home if they are stranded. The child psychiatrist can determine if missing skills are due to poor training at home or to developmental delays or retardation.

Observation of the Child

Although observation was mentioned in a previous section, it is worthwhile to reconsider the child's behavior at this time. Can the child separate from his parent for the examination?

Children with separation anxiety may be hesitant to leave their mothers behind in the waiting room, become tearful, or even cling to her and totally resist coming into the office. Does the child look his stated age? Younger-appearing children may be emotionally immature or retarded, and this physical trait can be reinforced by adults and peers who treat them as they would a younger, less apt child.

Is the child dressed neatly and is he clean? Unkempt children may have received less-than-optimal parental care, or have attention deficit disorder with hyperactivity (ADDH), a condition in which children's high level of physical activity and inattention to detail produces a picture of dirty faces and hands, untied shoelaces, scuffed, worn-out shoes, unzipped zippers, and shirttails hanging out. What is the child's activity level? The ADDH child will leave no room for doubt during the first few minutes of the evaluation. He will constantly fidget in his seat, walk around the room, and in severe cases, jump on chairs, desks, or tables and run out of the room.

Can the child make eye contact with ease? Even when children are shy, they will make eye contact with the examiner during the warm-up procedures listed earlier. Those who are reluctant to look at the examiner throughout the interview may be very depressed or, in rare cases, may have a form of pervasive developmental disorder.

What is the child's primary affect and does he show a sufficient range of emotional expression? This observation comes from the examiner's natural response to the child and the feelings that arise in the interaction. It is sometimes helpful to consider what feelings are stimulated within the examiner by the child. Is there a sense of sadness and depression? Does the child act reserved and somehow invoke a tense, anxious feeling in the examiner? Occasionally this reaction can arise with a highly anxious child or even one who is belligerent and whose primary affect is sullen rage. Watch the child's face for signs of pleasure as he becomes involved in the physical activity of the soft-signs examination—does he smile or laugh? Other reactions seen include the promiscuous fast attachment of the deprived youngster who ends the interview with a request that the examiner take him home with him.

Be certain to observe for the presence of an involuntary movement disorder. Although benign tics may occur around the age of four, if there is a history of chronic tics, subvocalizations, and vocal tics with a waxing and waning course, the possibility of Gilles de la Tourette's disorder should be investigated. If a child has been taking neuroleptics and shows signs of generalized choreiform movements or buccal-lingual-masticatory tics, the child must be thought to have a drug-related dyskinesia until proven otherwise (Polizoes and Engelhardt, 1978; Gualtieri et al., 1980; Gualtieri, 1983). If the dyskinesia lasts longer than three months after the cessation of neuroleptic drug therapy, tardive dyskinesia may be suspected. Children as young as six years of age have been shown to suffer from the disorder (Gualtieri, 1983).

Goodenough-Harris Drawing Test

This test screens for signs of mental retardation but cannot be used to make a diagnosis. The original test asks a child to make three drawings (a man, a woman, and self), but one drawing will suffice. Hand the child a pencil and a blank piece of typing paper, and instruct him to make a drawing of a person large enough to fill the page. Although the quality of the artwork will help, the actual scoring depends upon the detail in the drawing. A count of specific features such as eyelashes, lips, teeth, earlobes, the correct number of fingers, and details of clothing can be summed. A loose approximation would rate the child as normal if the sum of details drawn is equal to or greater than twice his age. Eight-year-old retarded children will often produce the typical disembodied, fingerless drawing done by a four year old, with a few strands of hair and oversized eyes that flow outside of the simple circle of the head. Details of clothing are lacking and the lower extremities, if present, do not touch the ground.

When the child completes the drawing, ask him to sign his name in script and date the drawing with today's date, stating "I'd like to keep this picture and know who did it and on what day it was done." This will yield a sample of handwriting, which can be evaluated for fine motor skills in producing either smooth, relatively quick penmanship or a slow, laborious, messy scrawl. In some cases the fine motor control for script, which should be present by age eight, is so lacking that the child tells you he has been allowed to print by his teachers. The dating procedure requested here is a typical classroom orientation measure and should be in place by the third grade, or by age eight.

House-Tree-Person Test

This can be the second drawing requested of the child, and although the formal test asks the child to draw three pictures, for purposes of this examination, only one drawing need be done. The typical second grader often draws such scenes, with the ground as a line, the sun as a circle, and the house and tree in the foreground. Projective interpretations of the tree, house, and person are possible, but the picture itself serves as a conversation piece for the examiner to ask questions about the child's house, family, and play area. Some find it useful at this point to inquire about other projective questions, such as asking the child to list three wishes.

General Fund of Information

Here the examiner attempts to get an impression of the child's general knowledge about the world. Indirectly, it can be a measure of vocabulary as well, which gives the psychiatrist a rough estimate of the child's intelligence. One question that should be assessed is the child's understanding concerning his reasons for coming for the evaluation. Brighter children will grasp the reasons by the age of eight and be able to give a version of their parent's chief complaint (but only if the parent has been truthful with them!). Typical inquiries include questions about the name of the president, the mayor's name, and details about some current event that appeared in the newspaper or on the television news. Boys can be asked about the names of baseball and football teams as well. These questions should be continued, each requesting more detailed factual information until the child begins to make mistakes. By age ten most children should have a wide range of general information for immediate retrieval.

Short-term Auditory Memory

Short-term recall of spoken commands and instructions is critical for success in school beyond third grade. Many assignments are given orally, and the child with ADDH or receptive language difficulties typically misinterprets oral assignments. One test entails giving the child a number of unrelated commands. For example, the examiner might ask the child to "pick up the pencil; move the book to the other desk; push the green chair over to the door." Performing these tasks without reminders entails carrying out a triple-commission command, a feat every normal six year old should be able to accomplish. Children with retardation or receptive language problems find it difficult to master such requests.

Number of digits recalled forward provides an excellent test of rote storage and retrieval, and should be at least six digits by the age of eight. Number of digits recalled backward is a trickier task, since the entire set must be held as a visual representation in memory to be reversed; therefore it tests visual memory as well. Serial sevens or serial threes involve the child counting backward from one hundred by subtracting either seven or three in a sequential fashion. This task is taxing and should be saved for the end of the memory section, since it involves the repetition of a subtraction operation multiple times, without losing one's place. It tests goal directedness, ability to pay attention, and memory, and as such is an excellent procedure for evaluating the child with attention deficit disorder. Normal children of age eight should do quite well on the serial three test, whereas twelve year olds will manage the serial sevens with proficiency.

Ability to Abstract: Proverbs and Similarities

Many proverbs and analogies used in the adult mental-status examination can be used successfully with children from the age of eight on. Similarities are also useful, such as asking the child to identify the common element linking an apple and an orange (they are both fruit) or a table and a chair (both furniture). Middle school-age children do quite well explaining proverbs such as, "Look before you leap" and "People who live in glass houses shouldn't throw stones." Concreteness may be seen in the learning disabled and the retarded.

Simple Calculations

Most first graders can perform simple calculations without paper and pencil, though some will use their fingers. By the end of the third grade, many eight year olds can make simple change calculations in their head. The serial three sequences will also serve as an evaluation of numerical skills on a screening basis.

Hallucinations

Hallucinations must be differentiated from *hypnogogic* (seen upon falling asleep) and *hypnopompic* (seen upon awakening) images, which are normal. Auditory hallucinations reported during daytime hours take on more clinical significance, but are not specific to psychotic states in childhood, since they may be reported by children with severe conduct disorders or major depressive disorders. In some cases they arise because so many other professionals ask the child about voices that the child finds an accepted reason for his troublesome behavior, e. g., "the voices told me to hit my brother." Mood congruent hallucinations may be seen in cases of prepubertal major depressive disorder, in which the voices tell the young patient he is bad and should be punished.

Suicidal Ideation

In general, children will respond to questions about suicidal ideation if it has been present. A particularly nonthreatening manner of investigation is to link the question to a specific feeling, such as "Have you ever been so disappointed or has something made you so angry that you have wanted to hurt yourself?"

If one gets a positive response to a suicidal probe like this, it is important to follow up with specific questions related to major depressive illness. Ask the child about prolonged sadness (exceeding two weeks in which the child felt sad more than 50% of the time). Inquire about initial, middle, and terminal insomnia; diurnal mood shifts; anhedonia, or lack of pleasure, in any pursuit (lasting more than two weeks); anorexia and weight loss. For a more detailed interview schedule, consult the K-SADS (Puig-Antich and Chambers 1978).

MODIFIED PHYSICAL EXAMINIATION

First of all, school-age children tend to be modest. Because an examination of the trunk and extremities is essential for determining sexual development, evidence of child abuse, and various rashes and neurological and genetic conditions, it is best to ask the patients to disrobe and change into gowns. Examiners who are the opposite sex of the late preadolescent/ early adolescent patient should leave the room while the child undresses; some children will prefer to have parents and siblings of the opposite sex step outside as well. Underpants should be left on in both sexes, and girls as young as seven should be supplied with gowns.

Growth-Rate Evaluation

Height and weight measures can be recorded by the child psychiatrist, particularly if the examiner plans to administer medications that might affect weight or height. Growth suppression has been reported for ADDH males taking the stimulant drugs, including d-amphetamine (Safer and Allen, 1973), as well as for magnesium pemoline (Dickinson et al., 1979) and methylphenidate (Greenhill, 1981; Mattes and Gittelman, 1983). Reviews of the literature (Roche et al., 1979; Greenhill, 1981) suggest that the weight velocity reduction is more often seen than is the height velocity slowdown. While negative studies on the effects of stimulant-related growth inhibition have also been reported, the bulk of the data, especially at higher drug doses, indicates that a degree of growth retardation can occur in susceptible children who take stimulants regularly (Greenhill et al., 1984). Major neuroleptics also increase children's weight velocity, leading to weight gain when these drugs are used chronically (McAndrew et al., 1972; Simeon et al., 1977).

Height and weight should be included as a standard part of the initial evaluation, and should be checked every three months for those patients on maintenance stimulant or neuroleptic medication. Standardization of measurement technique will produce meaningful data and is only slightly more involved than casual methods. Children should be weighed after urinating, in their examining gowns, and with shoes off, ideally at the same time of day. The most reliable height measures are taken in a recumbent position (nullifying the effects of gravity and poor posture) using a Harbington stadiometer (Sobel, 1975; Greenhill et al., 1981). Other authors suggest a vertical stadiometer or ruler placed against a wall, since children will even out their posture if they can press against a wall (Hoekelman, 1974).

Various age-corrected growth charts have been created that can be used to estimate the height and weight percentile a particular child's growth pattern matches. These charts have been assembled from cross-sectional measurements of many children of different ages, and joined together with computer-generated curve-smoothing techniques to produce smooth regular growth curves. As a result, these charts can only be rough approximations of curves generated by longitudinal follow-up of a large group of children measured at different ages. The largest database of growth information was collected by the National Center for Health Statistics (NCHS), with hundreds of individual children's measures collected for each six months of age represented (Malina, 1974; Hamill, 1976). Ross laboratories supplies charts based on the NCHS data, as shown in figure 22-1a and 22-1b.

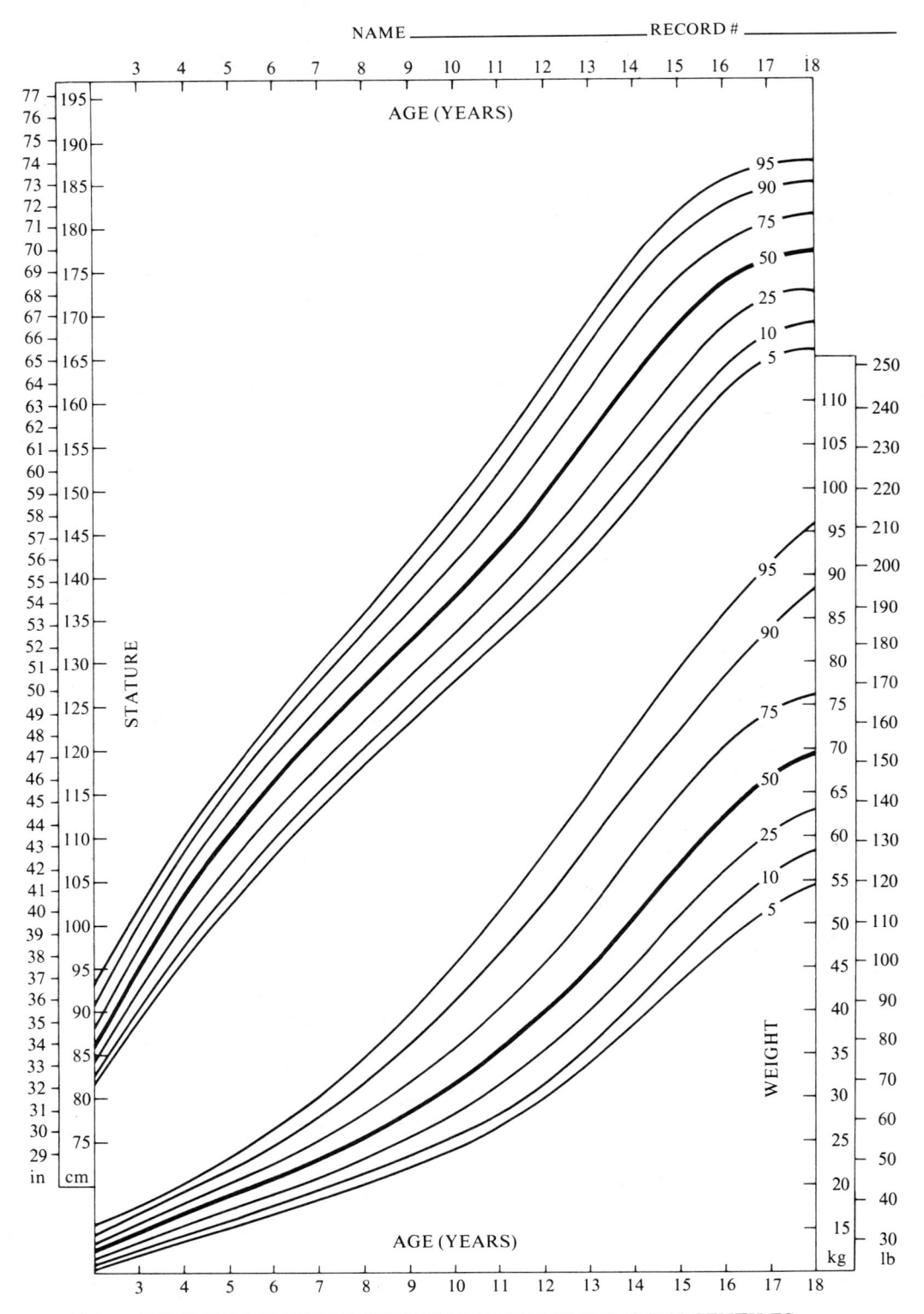

Fig. 22-1a. BOYS: 2 TO 18 YEARS PHYSICAL GROWTH NCHS PERCENTILES

Adapted from: National Center for Health Statistics: NCHS Growth Charts, 1976. Monthly Vital Statistics Report, Vol. 25, No. 3, Supp. (HRA) 76-1120, Health Resources Administration, Rockville, Maryland, June 1976. Data from the National Center for Health Statistics. © 1976 ROSS LABORATORIES. Reproduced with permission of Ross Laboratories, Columbus, Ohio.

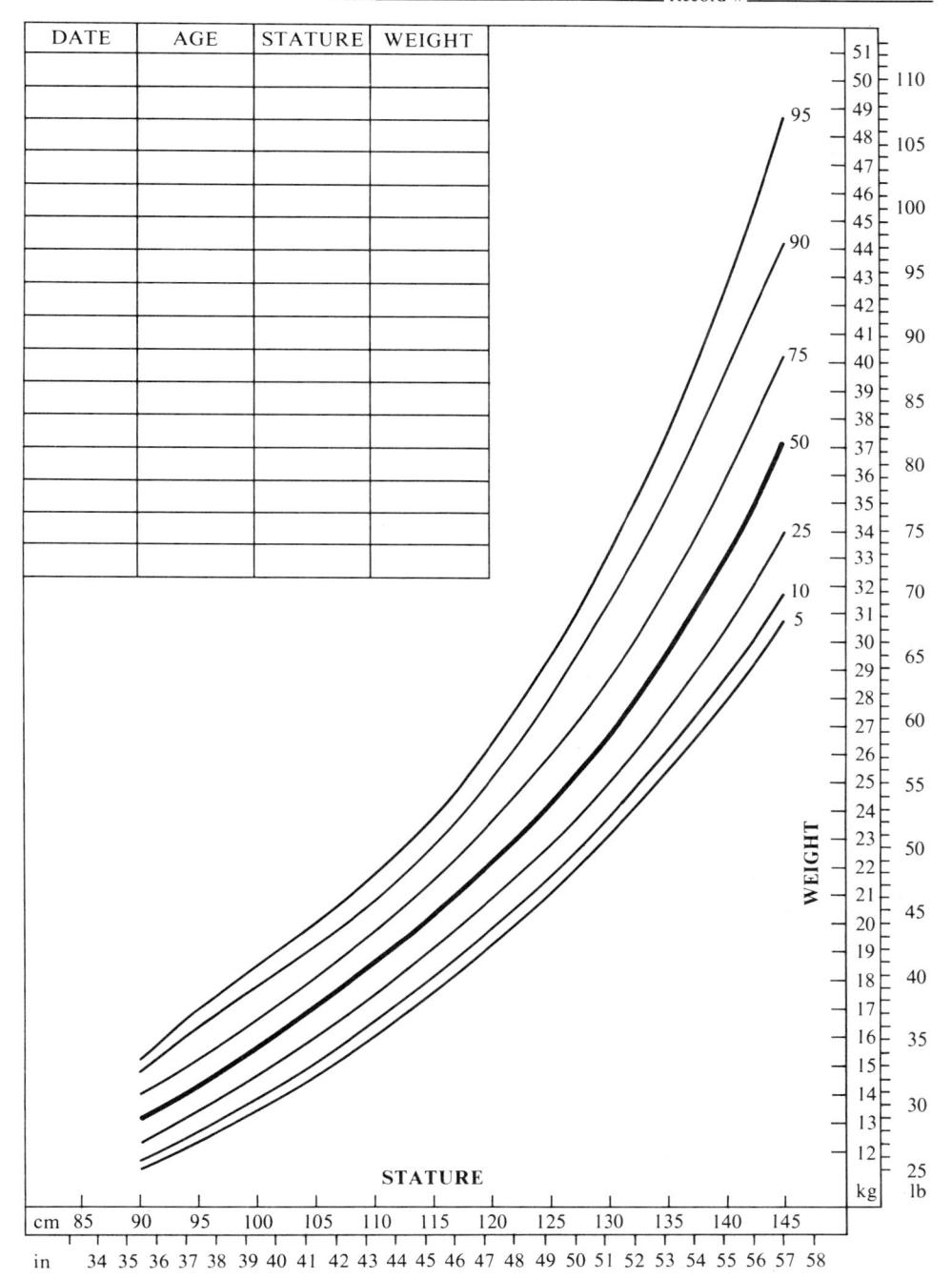

Fig. 22-1b. BOYS: PREPUBESCENT PHYSICAL GROWTH NCHS PERCENTILES*

Adapted from: National Center for Health Statistics: NCHS Growth Charts, 1976. Monthly Vital Statistics Report. Vol. 25, No. 3, Supp. (HRA) 76-1120. Health Resources Administration, Rockville, Maryland, June, 1976. Data from the National Center for Health Statistics. © 1976 ROSS LABORATORIES. Reproduced with permission of Ross Laboratories, Columbus, Ohio.

Using these growth charts, a child psychiatrist can monitor the growth curves of a child on stimulant medication. If an ADDH child shows more than a 25 percentile drop on drug, a drug holiday is indicated. After two to four months, "catch-up" growth occurs (Safer et al., 1975); then the child can be restarted on another stimulant. Measurements of height and weight that are greater than 97 or less than 3 percentile points may indicate a growth disturbance and require investigation.

Measurement of Head Circumference

Head circumference should be measured using a cloth or soft, plastic centimeter tape wrapped around the skull and over the occipital, parietal, and frontal prominences to obtain the greatest circumference. The measurement should be conducted every two years. In the neonate and toddler, rapid growth may be indicative of subdural hematoma, brain tumor, or hydrocephalus. Microcephaly is often associated with mental retardation. Figure 22-2a and 22-2b show the normative, age-corrected curves for head circumference for boys and girls separately, from a convenient chart supplied by the Mead-Johnson Company.

Vital Signs

Vital-sign measures may show increases due to anxiety. Temperature is most accurately determined by rectal thermometer in children under ten, and it should be noted that temperatures as high as 101 degrees Fahrenheit (38.3 degrees C) will occur in an active, school-age child after several hours of gross motor activity. Between six and fourteen years, pulses average 95 ± 30 (two standard deviations) normally. For blood pressures, the cuff size is all-important; too small a cuff (using a toddler cuff on a big ten year old) will produce a falsely high reading, while too big a cuff will produce low numbers. The cuff width should be ½ to ⅔ the width of the upper arm. Although muffling of the heart sounds signals the diastolic blood pressure (BP), this change may not be heard in younger children. Use the disappearance of the heart sound as the diastolic reading. When hypertension is found in children, its causes are not mysterious. Increased BP in children may be attributed to renal disease in 78% of cases, to renal artery disease in another 12%, to coarctation of the aorta in 2%, and to pheochromocytoma in 0.5% of cases.

Skull and Neck Examination

As suggested in the foregoing, the examiner should be on the lookout for characteristic facies that reflect chromosomal abnormalities (Down's syndrome), endocrine defects (hypothyroidism shown by large, protruding tongue), perennial allergic rhinitis, or battered-child syndrome. It is wise to listen for bruits over the skull with a stethoscope, for such sounds in nonanemic school-age children may indicate increased intercranial pressure from a tumor, an arteriovenous malformation or shunt, or an aneurysm. Nuchal rigidity may also indicate intercranial problems, in particular meningitis, and is best tested by having the child sit up with legs extended on the examining table and touch his chin to his chest without pain. The neck should also be examined for large nodes (adenopathy) secondary to otitis media or tonsillitis and for the presence of an enlarged thyroid gland.

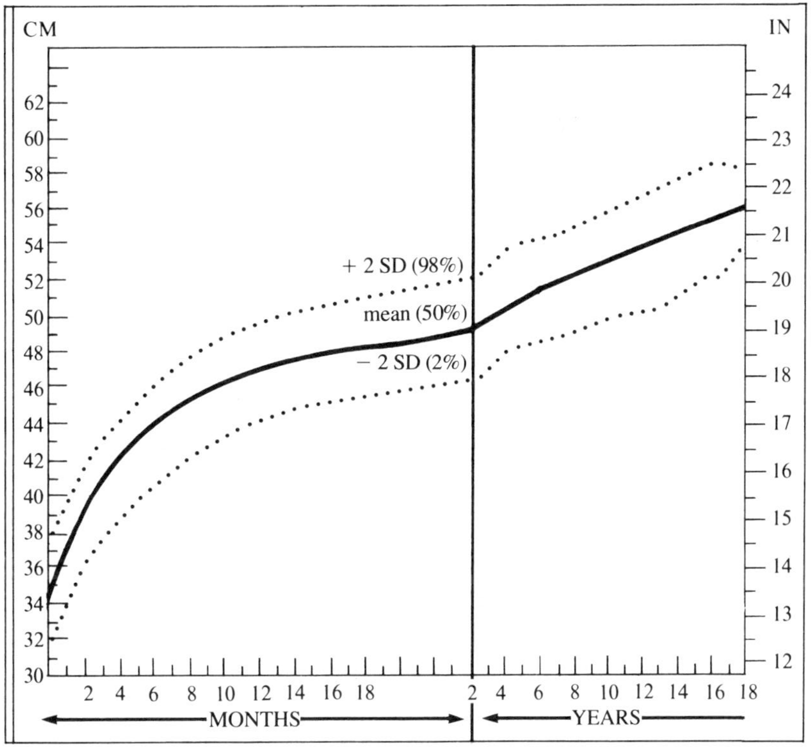

Fig. 22-2a. HEAD CIRCUMFERENCE—BOYS. G. Nellhaus, Composite International and Interracial Graphs. PEDIATRICS, 41:106, 1968. Reproduced with permission of Mead Johnson Laboratories.

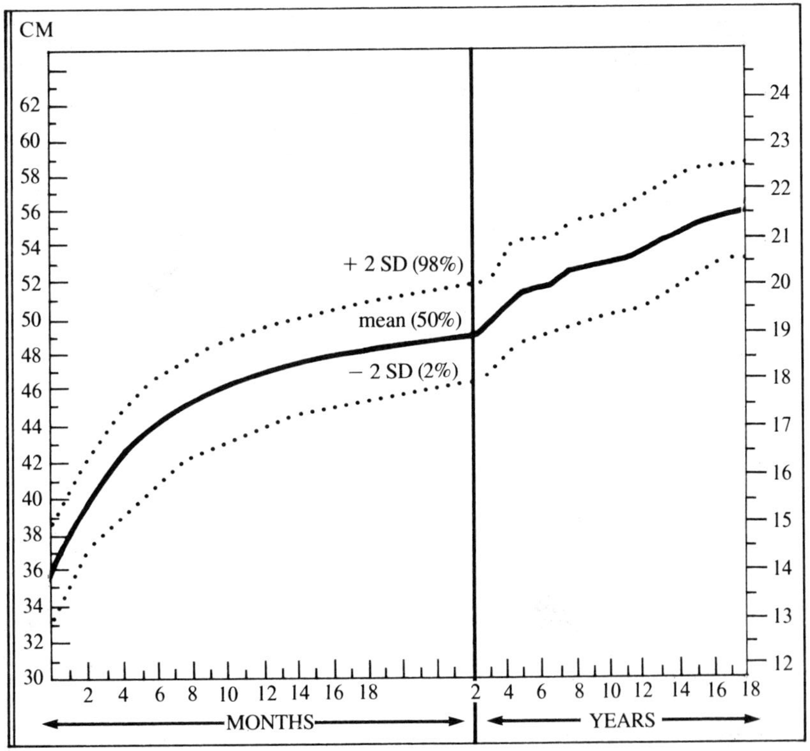

Fig. 22-2b. HEAD CIRCUMFERENCE—GIRLS. G. Nellhaus, Composite International and Interracial Graphs. PEDIATRICS, 41:106, 1968. Reproduced with permission of Mead Johnson Laboratories.

Eye Examination

Three ocular examinations can be done by the child psychiatrist. First, check the extraocular muscles. Using the Hirschberg Test, determine the presence of strabismus or squint due to weakness in eye musculature causing misalignment of the two eyes. The Hirschberg test is performed by having the examiner hold a small flashlight at his own midforehead, allowing him to see its reflection in both corneas of the patient. Reaching out, the examiner then turns the patient's head up and down and from side to side, having told the patient to watch the light at all times. Should the reflection disappear from one of the eyes, strabismus should be suspected. Strabismus, and anisometropia (one eye having a refractive index of more than 1.5 diopters greater than the other eye) are the leading causes of amblyopia exanopsia, a condition in which the occipital cortex switches off the visual input from one eye (because of its confusing, misaligned information), leading to disuse atrophy of that eye.

Next, the examiner should check visual acuity for both eyes separately using a small Snellen E chart for children who cannot read, or a near-vision test card (available from Low Vision Lens Service, New York Association for the Blind, 111 East 59th Street, New York, NY 10022.) Poor vision may be a cause of classroom misbehavior.

A funduscopic examination of both eyes should also be done. Using the ophthalmoscope, the examiner asks the child to look carefully at a spot on the wall in a darkened room. Both retinal disks should be seen and should be flat with clear demarcations of the borders and no papilledema.

Auditory Acuity

Hearing should always be checked by the child psychiatrist in this modified physical examination. Poor hearing can cause academic underachievement, depression, paranoia, and problems in discipline. Although some ADDH children seem to tune out requests from parents and other authority figures, the child with hearing problems may not be showing passive-aggressive behavior when he does not cooperate. A history of repeated ear infections should raise one's suspicions that poor hearing may be at the root of the problem.

As indicated previously, the examiner can stand from eight to eighteen feet behind the patient, asking questions and giving commands in a low voice or a whisper. Care should be taken that the patient not see the examiner's lips when this procedure is carried out. Tuning forks can be used to screen for hearing problems with the examiner using his own auditory acuity as a check.

Chest, Heart, and Lungs Examination

The exterior of the thorax should be examined first. Scars, burns, and other sign of trauma may be found. Certain congenital conditions, such as neurofibromatosis, will leave characteristic cafe-au-lait markings on the back. Breast development may start early in preadolescence and is usually asymmetrical. Subaxillary hair and breast development will allow the clinician to stage the extent of the pubertal process using Tanner criteria.

Lung fields should be examined over the back and upper thorax to map the extent of breath sounds. Percussion of the back is useful, and, of course, the stethoscope can be used to pick up wheezing and rales in the chronic asthmatic patient.

Heart sounds should also be auscultated. In young children the apical impulse, or point of maximum impact (PMI), can be felt at the fourth intercostal space. After seven years of age, the PMI moves to the fifth intercostal space. It is wise to check for the presence of regular sinus rhythm, and for murmurs. Loud murmurs, irregular heart rate, or extremely prominent PMI may suggest cardiac disease, which may be a cause of what appears to be depression. Tricyclics are the treatment of choice for depression, and yet if the problem is cardiac in nature, these drugs may be contraindicated.

Abdominal Examination

One should examine the abdomen for signs of former surgical procedures. Using the stethoscope, the psychiatrist should listen for normal bowel sounds and should press down on the abdomen to determine tenderness and examine for the presence of abdominal masses. Neither the liver, kidney, or spleen should be palpable.

Genital and Rectal Examination

This part of the examination involves the most embarrassment for the patient and potentially the most discomfort, so it should be saved for last. The genital examination also serves to stage the pubertal process, for the presence of pubertal hair may occur as easily as the eighth year. Small male genitalia in early childhood and in prepubescence is of no significance. Abnormalities, such as enlarged female clitoris and nondescended testicles in the male require referrals to a specialist in endocrinology or urology. The rectal examination may be facilitated if the child is asked to breathe in and out quickly "like a puppy dog" (Hoekelman, 1974).

Musculoskeletal System

Joint and skeletal difficulties can best be detected in the school-age child by observing him in various postures. Looking from the front and rear, the examiner can watch the child standing straight with the feet together and then touching the toes or the shins while standing. Hip abnormalities become evident when the child is seen from behind as weight is shifted from one leg to another; the pelvis tilts toward the diseased hip when weight is put on that leg but remains level when weight is put on the other leg. This is Trendelenburg's sign.

Another examination should be done. The child should be observed rising from the floor when he starts from a position laying on his back. Those children with proximal muscle weakness of muscular dystrophy have pelvic girdle weakness, and literally climb up on their legs with their hands (Gower's sign).

SUMMARY

There are many important reasons for conducting a physical examination on the child psychiatric patient. First and foremost is to rule out physical causes of poor social and emotional adjustment. Second, one wants to be certain that physical child abuse is not going on with a child who is sullen and withdrawn in school. For those children who benefit from chronic treatment with psychotropic medication, one must monitor growth and development. Since soft neurological signs may predict later psychopathology, their documentation is essential. The physical examination trains the physician to look at the child systematically and carefully. Finally, the physical examination can provide comprehensive care for the child and increase rapport through the caring physical contact of a child psychiatrist.

REFERENCES

Anastasi, A. 1976. *Psychological testing.* 4th ed. New York: Macmillan.

Bialer, I., Doll, L., and Winsberg, B. 1974. A modified Lincoln-Oseretsky motor development scale: Provisional standardization. *Percep. Motor Skills,* 38:599-614. A copy of the manual can be obtained on request from the first author at 524 Clarkson Avenue, Brooklyn, NY 11203.

Blodgett, F., Burgin, L., Iezzoni, D., Gribetz, D., and Talbot, N. 1956. Effects of prolonged cortisone therapy on the statural growth, skeletal maturation, and metabolic status of children. *N. Eng. J. Med.,* 254:636-641.

Camp, J., Bialer, I., Sverd, J., and Winsberg, B. 1978. Clinical usefulness of the NIMH physical and neurological examination for soft signs. *Am. J. Psych.,* 135:362-364.

Cantor, S., Trevenen, C., Postuma, R., Dveck, R., and Fjeldsted, B. 1980. Is childhood schizophrenia a cholinergic disease? I. Muscle morphology. *Arch. Gen. Psych.,* 37:658-667.

Close, J. 1976. Manual for the neurological examination for soft signs, the PANESS. In: *ECDEU assessment manual for psychopharmacology.* Rev., ed. W.Guy, pp. 394-406. Dept of Health, Education, and Welfare, DHEW pub. no. (ADM) 76-338.

David, O. 1978. Central effects of minimally elevated lead levels. In: *Proceedings of the National Institute of Mental Health on the hyperkinetic behavior syndrome, June 1978.* ed. N. Reatig, pp. 14-18. Doc. no. PB-297804 (code A12). National Technical Information Service.

Dickinson, L., Lee, J., and Ringdahl, I. 1979. Impaired growth in hyperkinetic children receiving pemoline. *J. Ped.,* 94:538-541.

Doll, E. 1965. *The Vineland social maturity scale.* Circle Pines, Minn.: American Guidance Service.

Falliers, C., Tan, L., Szentivanyi, J., Jurgensen, J., and Bukantz, S. 1963. Childhood asthma and steroid therapy as influences on growth. *Am. J. Dis. Child.,* 105:41-51.

Goodwin, D. 1978. GCRC research teams study link between psychosocial dwarfism and child abuse. U.S. Dept. of Health, Education, and Welfare, 2(7):1-16.

Greenhill, L. 1981. Stimulant-related growth inhibition in children: A review. In: *Strategic interventions for hyperactive children,* ed. M. Gittelman, Armonk, N.Y.: M. E. Sharpe.

Greenhill, L., Puig-Antich, J., Chambers, W., Rubinstein, B., Halpern, F., and Sachar, E. 1981. Growth hormone, prolactin, and growth responses in hyperkinetic males treated with d-amphetamine. *J. Am. Acad. Child Psych.,* 20:71-84.

Greenhill, L., Puig-Antich, J., Novacenko, H., Solomon, M., Anghern, C., Florea, J., Goetz, R., Fiscina, B., and Sachar, E. 1984. Prolactin, growth hormone, and growth responses in boys with attention deficit disorder with hyperactivity treated with methylphenidate. *J. Am. Acad. Child Psych.,* 23:24-34.

Gualtieri, C. 1983. Tardive dyskinesia. Report on 30th Annual Meeting of the American Academy of Child Psychiatry, October 27, 1983, San Francisco, Calif.

Gualtieri, C., Barnhill, J., McGimsey, J., and Schell, D. 1980. Tardive dyskinesia and other movement disorders in children treated with psychotropic drugs. *J. Am. Acad. Child Psych.,* 19:491-510.

Guy, W. 1976. ECDEU assessment manual for psychopharmacology. Revised. U.S. Department of Health, Education, and Welfare, DHEW publication no. (ADM) 76-338:287-299; 383-394.

Hamill, P., Drizd, T., Johnson, C., and Lemeshow, S. 1976. *NCHS growth charts,* Monthly vital statistics report, examination survey data, National Center for Health Statistics (HRA) 76-1120, 25 (Suppl. 3):1-22.

Hammer, E. 1960. The house-tree-person (H-T-P) drawings as a projective technique with children. In: *Projective techniques with children,* ed. A. I. Rabin and M. A. Haworth. New York: Grune and Stratton.

Harris, D. 1963. *Children's drawings as measures of intellectual maturity.* New York: Hartcourt, Bracer, Jovanovich.

Hoekelman, R. 1974. The pediatric physical examination. In: *A guide to physical examination,* 2nd ed., ed. B. Bates, and R. Hoekelman, pp. 367-427. Philadelphia: J. B. Lippincott Co.

Loeb, J. 1976. Corticosteroids and growth. *N. Eng. J. Med.,* 295:547-552.

Malina, R. 1974. *Body dimensions and proportions, white and negro children, 6-11 Years (United States).* National Center for Health Statistics. Vital and health statistics, series 11, National Health Survey, no. 143, DHEW publication no. (HRA) 75-1625. Washington, D.C.: U. S. Gov. Printing Office, pp. 22-23.

Mattes, J. and Gittelman, R. 1983. Growth of hyperactive children on maintenance regimen of methylphenidate. *Arch. Gen. Psych.,* 40:317-321.

Mattes, J., Gittelman, R., and Levitt, M. 1984. Subclassification of hyperactive children on the basis of minor physical anomalies and plasma dopamine-beta-hydroxylase activity: An attempted replication. In: *Psychobiology of childhood,* ed. L. Greenhill, and B. Shopsin, pp. 159-182. New York: Spectrum Publications.

McAndrew, J., Case, O., and Triffint, D. 1972. Effects of prolonged phenothiazine intake on psychotic and other hospitalized children. *J. Aut. Child Schizo.,* 2:75-91.

Polizoes, P., and Engelhardt, D. 1978. Dyskinetic phenomena in children treated with psychotropic medications. *Psychopharm. Bull.,* 14:65-68.

Porrino, L., Rapoport, J., Behar, D., Sceery, W., Ismad, D., and Bunney, W. 1983. A naturalistic assessment of the motor activity of hyperactive boys. I. Comparison with normal controls. *Arch. Gen. Psych.,* 40:681-687.

Puig-Antich, J., and Chambers, W. 1978. The schedule for affective disorders and schizophrenia for school-age children (6-16 years): Kiddie-SADS (K-SADS). For copies of this instrument, contact Drs. Puig-Antich and Chambers at the Department of Child and Adolescent Psychiatry, New York State Psychiatric Institute, 722 West 168th Street, New York, NY 10032.

Quitkin, F., Rifkin, A., and Klein, D. 1976. Neurologic soft signs in schizophrenia and character disorder. *Arch. Gen. Psych.,* 33:845-853.

Rapoport, J., Pandon, C., Renfield, M., Lake, R., and Ziegler, M. 1977. Newborn dopamine-beta-hydroxylase, minor physical anomalies and infant temperament. *Am. J. Psych.,* 134:676-679.

Rapoport, J., and Quinn, P. 1975. Minor physical anomalies (stigmata) and early developmental deviation: A major biologic subgroup of "hyperactive children." *Int. J. Men. Health,* 4:29-44.

Rieder, R., and Nichols, P. 1979. Offspring of schizophrenics. III. Hyperactivity and neurological soft signs. *Arch. Gen. Psych.,* 36:665-674.

Roche, A., Lipman, R., Overall, J., and Hung, W. 1979. The effects of stimulant medication on the growth of hyperactive children. *Ped.,* 63:847-849.

Rutter, M., Graham, P., and Yule, W. 1970. *A neuropsychiatric study in childhood.* Clin. in Dev. Med., no. 35/36. London: Heinemann/SIMP.

Safer, D., and Allen, R. 1973. Factors influencing the suppressant effects of two stimulant drugs on the growth of hyperactive children. *Ped.,* 51:660-667.

Safer, D., Allen, R., and Barr, E. 1975. Growth rebound after termination of stimulant drugs. *J. Ped.,* 86:113-116.

Sarma, P. S. B. 1983. A new examination for minor neurological signs in children (EXAMINS). Presented at the Annual Meeting of the American Academy of Child Psychiatry, 1983, San Francisco, Calif. A copy of the procedure for scoring and administration is obtainable upon request from Dr. Sarma, associate professor of child psychiatry, University of Health Sciences, Chicago Medical School, 3333 Green Bay Road, Chicago, IL 60064.

Shaffer, D. 1978. Annotation: "Soft" neurological signs and later psychiatric disorder—a review. *J. Child Psychol. and Psych.,* 19:63-66.

Shaffer, D., O'Connor, P., Shafer, S., and Feldman, R. 1981. The neurological soft signs and antisocial behavior. Presented at the Annual Meeting of the American Academy of Child Psychiatry, October, 16, 1981, Dallas, Texas.

Shaffer, D., Schoenfield, I., O'Connor, P., and Shafer, S. 1982. Possible mechanisms in the development of psychiatric disorders in minimal brain dysfunction. Presented at the Annual Meeting of the American Academy of Child Psychiatry, October 22, 1982, Washington, D.C.

Simeon, J., Gross, M., and Mueller, J. 1977. Neuroleptic drug effects on children's body weight and height. *Psychopharm. Bull.,* 13:50-53.

Sobel, E. 1975. Abnormal growth patterns in infancy and childhood. In: *Endocrine and genetic diseases of childhood and adolescence,* ed. L. Gardner. pp. 64-84. Philadelphia: Saunders.

Touwen, B., and Prechtl, H. 1970. *The neurological examination of the child with minor nervous dysfunction.* Clin. in Dev. Med., no. 38. Spastics International Medical Publications. Philadelphia: J. B. Lippincott Co.

Waldrop, M. and Goering, J. 1971. Hyperactivity and minor physical anomalies in elementary school children. *Am. J. Orthopsych.,* 41:602-607.

Waldrop, M., and Halverson, C. 1971. Minor physical anomalies and hyperactive behavior in young children. In: *The exceptional infant.* New York: Brunner and Mazel.

23

Functional Analysis of Children's Behavior

RICHARD S. FELDMAN

BEHAVIOR ANALYSIS IS COMPRISED of a set of discovery procedures for specifying the functional relationships between behavior and its determinants. It originated in the experimental psychology laboratory, in particular the early operant conditioning studies. As the principles derived from those studies have been applied to an increasingly broad and complex array of behaviors and eventually to nearly the whole range of clinical problems, the techniques of behavior analysis itself have enormously expanded. As Mash and Terdal (1981a) note in their review, behavioral assessment and behavioral interventions have developed jointly in the closest possible relationship. This is not surprising, since it is one of the defining characteristics of behavior analysis in the clinical context that it should have direct implications for designing and monitoring treatment.

As the field of behavioral assessment has grown to include a host of tools and procedures other than direct observation, it is important to stress that the idea of a *functional* analysis remains central. Mash and Terdal speak of behavioral assessment in terms of a "problem-solving strategy based upon ongoing functional analysis" (p. 7); Marholin and Bijou (1978) discuss behavioral assessment in terms of an "interactional model of human behavior which is based on a functional analysis of behavior" (p. 14); and Nelson and Hayes (1979) seek to "identify meaningful response units and their controlling variables" (p. 1).

The extent to which clinical decision-making is actually based on such a functional analysis of behavior will no doubt depend largely on the extent to which the clinician views a behavioral model as comprehensive. The choice of assessment techniques, the manner in which those techniques are employed, and the selection of therapeutic goals all follow to an important degree from the various theoretical frameworks in which clinicians operate and the intervention strategies they are prepared to employ. (Other factors, such as administrative requirements for diagnostic labeling, for example, may also play their part.) Observation of a child during projective testing may indeed furnish a useful (if hardly sufficient) sample of behavior in such areas as, say, cooperativeness and attention span, but a psychodynamically oriented clinician will employ such testing in the first place because of an interest in eliciting signs of underlying personality dynamics, while a behaviorist interested in assessing cooperativeness and attention will not be likely to choose a setting primarily structured with so little intrinsic relevance to behavioral formulations. It is not the purpose of this chapter to review and compare the various approaches to assessment of children's behavior (see, for example, Mischel, 1968; Kanfer and Saslow, 1969; Mash and Terdal, 1981b). Rather, the content has been selectively guided by a consideration of those procedures most directly relevant to the formulation of therapeutic goals and interventions in behavioral terms.

How is the clinician to proceed? This chapter will consider the following principal issues: (1) the unit of analysis; (2) scope of the inquiry; (3) methods of data collection; and (4) selection of target behaviors.

UNIT OF ANALYSIS

Fundamental to a functional behavioral analysis is the *reinforcement contingency,* which consists of a behavior (response), its antecedents (discriminative stimuli), and its consequences (reinforcing stimuli). The terms "reinforcement contingency" and "contingency analysis" sometimes have the unfortunate effect of focusing attention too exclusively on the behavior-reinforcer connection; we continually speak of some reinforcing consequence being contingent on the child's behavior, but much less frequently of the behavior being contingent on some particular antecedent or concurrent circumstance. Partly this is because reinforcing stimuli are often more obvious and easier to manipulate; for example, we instruct parents or teachers to give or withhold attention (praise, points, or whatever) for a behavior we want to change, without adequately investigating the ways in which the child's environment might be rearranged, at least temporarily, to improve things. The teacher who moves a child to the front of the room "so he'll work instead of fooling around" is attempting to use this idea. However, the teacher might not have the right program, for a behavioral analysis might show that while the child does indeed "fool around" less when he sits closer to the teacher, he also gets less attention than before and in fact does not do more work. Changing the discriminative stimuli for the child has reduced behavior hypothesized to be incompatible with working, and thus our analysis has taught us something about the conditions under which it might be easier to increase the amount of schoolwork the child does. At the same time, we may note that the child's closer proximity has apparently not served as a discriminative stimulus for the teacher to deliver more positive reinforcers either in general for acceptable classroom behavior or in particular for whatever amount of work the child actually does. This will have to be dealt with if the teacher in this case is to play a significant role as mediator (Tharp and Wetzel, 1969) in the intervention program designed for the child.

Behavior, of course, occurs as part of an ongoing stream of events, and our unitization will depend on our purpose. A parent's reprimand may be both the consequence of a child's sloppily done homework and the antecedent of a spouse's criticism for being too demanding of the child. If it is determined that the quality of the child's homework should indeed be the target of intervention, and if the data show that both the reprimands and the subsequent criticism are frequent or severe enough to cause concern, then both will have to be examined for their possible functional relationship to the child's behavior. The parental reprimand may be functioning as an inadvertent positive reinforcer because of the attention the child thereby receives (particularly if a lengthy argument ensues), while the spouses' disagreement, expressed as criticism in response to such reprimands, will, for obvious reasons, make it more difficult for the parents to work effectively to change the child's behavior. To be successful, the therapist may have to spend as much time in determining what maintains the parental reprimands in spite of the fact that they have not led to improvement in the child's behavior as in determining what maintains the child's behavior itself. However, in both instances, the functional principle and the unit of analysis will be the same.

Precise quantitative measures of reinforcement contingencies are difficult to obtain without direct observation. When, in interviewing parents, we ask such questions as "Where or with whom is that behavior most likely to occur?" and "How do you usually respond to the child when that behavior occurs?" we are asking about contingencies. Some widely used instruments—behavior problem checklists, for example—tell us nothing directly about contingencies. The essential point is that the reinforcement contingency is of conceptual as well as methodological significance. It reminds us that few behaviors are equally probable and equally appropriate (or inappropriate) under all circumstances and that a successful therapeutic intervention will require knowledge of at least some of the functional connections between the child's behavior and the context in which it occurs.

Scope of the Inquiry

The "S-O-R-K-C" model, in which Kanfer and Saslow (1969) expanded Lindsley's (1964) behavioral-analysis format to include the biological condition of the organism, is among the most comprehensive and widely cited guides to behavioral assessment. Although not devised specifically for children, it incorporates many features of particular relevance to them (including reference to developmental norms), and it seems eminently useful in child-behavior assessment (Ollendick and Cerny, 1981). The S refers to antecedent stimulus events, O to organismic (i.e., biological) variables, R to behaviors (responses), K to contingency-related factors (e.g., reinforcement schedules), and C to the consequent events following R. Kanfer and Saslow provide a detailed outline of the kinds of information required to fill out the S-O-R-K-C schema. In brief, they are as follows.

Initial analysis of the problem situation must take place, in which complaints are given behavioral definition and are at least tentatively classed as excesses or deficits in terms of their frequency, appropriateness to the occasions of occurrence, etc. The distinction is not always easy—for example, physical assaults in response to minimal provocation might be viewed as either excessive aggression or deficient social skill. However, the emphasis of the intervention strategy would most likely differ depending on how additional information leads us to classify the behavior. If the child in this case frequently gets along well with peers (i.e., typically uses the social skills necessary for appropriate interaction), then training the child to recognize the particular cues that sometimes lead to inappropriate aggression, perhaps along with some contingent punishment such as loss of a privilege when it does occur, might be a major treatment component. But if the child does not in general have such skills, the emphasis would be on teaching them in a broad range of contexts and then reinforcing their appropriate use; penalizing the unacceptable behavior could only lead to further misfortune if acceptable alternatives are not readily available in the child's behavioral repertoire.

Also part of the initial analysis is an assessment of the child's behavioral assets. Parents and others are sometimes at a loss for words when asked for such information, and, if pressed, tend to search for outstanding skills or talents. However, it is also important to identify what are simply areas of exceptionally good functioning within the range of that child's behavior, such as helpfulness with siblings. Such assets or strengths suggest natural starting points or "staging areas" from which new behaviors can be shaped or social relationships altered; they also suggest classes of discriminative and reinforcing stimuli already of functional importance for the child's behavior and therefore of potential usefulness in programming for behavior change.

Clarification of the problem situation should include assessment of who finds the behavior objectionable and why. One issue in this regard is whether any particular behavior in question is truly maladaptive for the child or whether the parent or other informant who finds it objectionable is applying an unwarranted criterion—e.g., complaints about bedwetting in a child too young to be fully trained or complaints about fighting in a child who lives in a rough neighborhood where fights are frequent. The latter case is not straightforward: Is the child also concerned about the behavior? Does he fight more than his peers, and even if he does so only to defend himself, why is he in that position so often? Or is the behavior really not a problem at all except for the parent's concern? Such possibilities point to another major consideration in this phase of assessment: the conditions or circumstances associated with occurrence of the behavior.

Also a major focus at this stage is the likely impact on the child and others (especially the family) if the problem behavior were significantly altered. For example, if a withdrawn child's social skills are improved to the point where he or she wants to stay out with friends after school instead of coming right home, will there be someone else to take over that child's task of caring for the younger sibling until their mother or father gets home from work?

Motivational analysis is primarily an assessment of current and potential positively reinforcing and aversive events (including fears). Also to be considered here is the possible change in reinforcer availability if a problem behavior is successfully altered—e.g., will the child still be able to get a half hour of her father's undivided attention every evening if she begins to do her homework by herself?

Developmental analysis should include the determination of relevant biological limitations such as perceptual handicaps or chronic illnesses. Medical or other special consultations may be required if the condition seems to be functionally related to a behavior targeted for change (e.g., megacolon in an encopretic child or hearing loss in a socially withdrawn child).

Also assessed here are sociological changes, such as new demands or norms resulting from a change of school, and behavioral changes, such as an increase or decrease in the kinds of situations in which the target behavior occurs.

Analysis of self-control includes assessment of control strategies the child appears to use (e.g., avoiding situations where the problem behavior is especially likely to occur) and the conditions that appear closely related to the degree of self-control exhibited (e.g., verbal abuse directed toward peers during classroom activities but not on the playground).

Analysis of social relationships should take into consideration the characteristic ways in which the child's behavior varies with different people, their mutual expectations, and the potential therapeutic role of individuals in the child's environment. This last point is critical, because so many interventions depend on the active participation of parents or others.

Analysis of the social-cultural-physical environment encompasses such factors as economic constraints (which, to cite only one aspect, may limit the availability of material reinforcers or even social ones, such as privacy in an overcrowded apartment or time with a parent who is trying to hold down two jobs); lack of congruence between the family's and the neighbors' values or standards as they impinge on the child's behavior (the downstairs tenants who threaten to take some sort of action if the children do not make less noise in the evening); and disparities in norms among the various settings in which the child has to function (e.g., a strict school and a permissive home, or vice versa).

If anyone is still surprised by the range of data sought in the Kanfer and Saslow or some similar framework in the name of behavior analysis, they should be reminded that significant functional relationships are not necessarily to be found in the most obvious places and that the search for them is guided by empirical considerations. Kanfer and Saslow state that "A behavioral analysis excludes no data relating to a patient's past or present experiences as irrelevant" (p. 438). The criterion is a *significant functional relationship to any current behavior targeted for change,* and the goal is therapeutic decision making, not diagnostic categorization and not all-inclusive description for its own sake.

It is certainly true that sometimes the whole process is simple, relatively speaking: the problem is easily targeted, the adequate assessment quite narrow, and the intervention straightforward, with child and family living happily ever after or for the duration of the follow-up period, whichever is shorter. But not always; not even very frequently. In this connection, the earliest behavior-modification studies may inadvertently have fostered an expectation of simplicity not necessarily common in clinical experience. Kanfer and Saslow, in encompassing organismic variables and a broad behavioral and social perspective, are neither attempting to make their approach more appealing to traditionalists nor submitting grudgingly to practical exigencies. Just as the three-part reinforcement contingency looks at behavior in the context of its functionally related antecedents and consequences, beginning with the most immediate ones, similarly does the assessment approach described earlier place the reinforcement contingency in the broader context of relevant biological and ecological factors.

Unfortunately, recognition of the breadth of the data base which may be necessary for planning and monitoring sound interventions has not been matched by the development of adequately detailed and well-researched guidelines for deciding exactly how to collect the data and how to know when one has collected enough. It is therefore doubly helpful that behavioral interventions are in a sense self-correcting; when they do not work as intended (and we will know if they are not working because the behaviors are clearly defined and assessment is ongoing), a likely cause is an incorrect or incomplete behavioral analysis leading to an unworkable or inadequate program, and so we go back and try again. An assessment approach such as the one by Kanfer and Saslow can at least tell us what we might have omitted from consideration.

Methods of Data Collection

Mash and Terdal (1981a) have provided a wide-ranging discussion of the many kinds of procedures and instruments used for behavioral assessment of children, and the contributors to their book furnish many examples of the ingenuity and care with which data-collection methods have been created or adapted for specialized assessment needs in particular clinical areas (Mash and Terdal, 1981b). Most conspicuously in conjunction with behavioral interventions, there has been such a proliferation of paper-and-pencil instruments, observation codes, laboratory analogue situations, etc., that Evans and Nelson (1974) were led to observe, "Behavior therapists seem to be in the awkward position of coming to depend on tests that are less psychometrically sophisticated than those they have spurned" (p. 602). Mash and Terdal (1981a) argue for the development of behavioral assessment methods that are more standardized and population specific, but they also point out that "when assessments focus on identifying relevant behavior and controlling variables for the individual child, in order to design effective treatments, the need for standardization seems less evident" (p. 42). The issues here serve to highlight the fact that traditional methods often fail to provide just those aids to highly individualized assessment and treatment design that the more behavioral approaches are intended to supply.

In fact, virtually all the familiar methods can yield information relevant to a functional analysis. Even behavior checklists and rating scales, for example, can suggest broad classes of discriminative or reinforcing stimuli worthy of more detailed examination—as in the case of reliable but discrepant ratings by a teacher and by a parent. Thus, there is often the temptation to use as many avenues of assessment as time and resources permit. Time and resources typically being limited, there is perhaps some degree of paradoxical comfort to be drawn from Mash and Terdal's observation that "the hypothesis that using as many different methods as possible will result in a truer or more useful description of the child has not been tested" (p. 41).

Nevertheless, adequate assessment typically requires more than one mode of data collection. The classes of methods to be discussed here are interviews, rating scales and checklists—which are in many respects interview equivalents, observations, and standardized tests.

Interviews, for all of their endlessly debated difficulties, are indispensable, as writers repeatedly note. Indeed, although some discussions of assessment appear to take it for granted that clinicians always have ready access to any mode of data collection, many—especially private practitioners—do not. For better or worse, the interview is undoubtedly the mainstay.

Even when the principal complaint about the child originates with the school or with some other agency or individual outside the home, the first person interviewed in detail about the child is often a parent, usually the mother. Regardless of who the informant is, the primary purposes of the behavioral interview are (1) to clarify the nature of the complaint in terms of specific behaviors that the adult is concerned about and that appear to be maladaptive for the child, (2) to identify the contextual variables functionally related to those behaviors, (3) to identify resources in the child's environment available to mediate change, and (4) to communicate to the informant, through the form, content, and timing of comments and questions, the kinds of data the interviewer thinks are necessary to obtain and the nature of the framework in which the child's behavior is to be discussed. This last point is an often unstated factor, not always systematically thought out but fundamental to the achievement of the other goals. Often, for example, extensive questioning about the child's early development may, contrary to an interviewer's intention, strengthen parents' frequent tendency to explain current behavior primarily by historical factors. At the same time, repeated insistence on specific behavioral examples of vague or global attributions (such as "stubborn," "unhappy," "aggressive," and so on), and the delivery of suitable reinforcement by the interviewer when they are provided, can further the interviewer's aim of increasing the behavioral precision of the informant's replies and descriptions. The extensive literature on verbal conditioning in interviews and similar situations (e.g., Salzinger, 1978) points the way to more effective shaping of functional behavioral statements by informants, but too seldom is sufficient attention paid to the notion of systematically applying behavioral principles to the assessment interview itself. There are occasional happy exceptions; Rekers (1981), for example, suggests that in interviewing a child, the use of positive reinforcement for any speech at all, and the temporary avoidance of direct, leading questions, is a useful technique for obtaining an extended baseline sample of the child's verbal behavior which can then be analyzed for content or other characteristics of interest.

Kanfer and Saslow, as discussed earlier, provide a detailed account of the areas to be covered in a behavioral interview, and Holland (1970) has published a useful guide for behavioral interviews with parents. All such guides leave a good deal unspecified. For instance, it is not clear whether reviewing a list of situations and asking the informant if they are associated with any problem behaviors (Atkeson and Forehand, 1981) is any better or worse than reviewing a list of problem behaviors and asking if there are any situations in which they occur (Patterson, et al., 1975). One possible disadvantage of the latter approach is that it concentrates on undesirable or maladaptive behaviors, whereas an inquiry initially organized by situation allows quite naturally for questions about both good and poor aspects of the child's functioning in each case. It must be said that there is little hard evidence on which is the better way to go about it. However, especially in interviewing someone who finds the child very aversive, there would seem to be a number of potential advantages to a format that calls the child's healthier and more desirable behavior to frequent attention. In addition, when a child has a pervasive disorder (such as autism or a perceptual handicap) or shows serious deviance over a considerable range of behaviors or situations, it becomes critical to emphasize close scrutiny of the child's areas of best functioning for clues to the design of intervention programs. Whatever the format, the most important consideration is that it be comprehensive and that, when an area of apparent significance is touched on, the interviewer obtain a clear picture of exactly what the behavior is, how concerned the informant or anyone else is about it, the best possible estimate of its frequency or intensity, the situations in which it is most likely and least likely to occur, the response of others to the child's behavior, and the child's subsequent response to whatever the other person does.

One very helpful strategy is to review a complete typical weekday and weekend, including all the household routines, who is with the child at each point, characteristics of the child's interactions with others in each situation, what problems arise, and how the problems are handled. If the informant is a teacher or someone else not a regular member of the household, the inquiry will obviously be modified accordingly. It is then often highly informative to do the same thing for "yesterday," because there are likely to be differences from what has been described as the typical day; detailed examination of these differences will not only reflect on the informant's apparent degree of reliability but will most likely also clarify important aspects of the relevant reinforcement contingencies for the child by identifying circumstances under which the child's behavior departs from the typical.

Issues of reliability and validity are reviewed in most discussions of assessment and will not be repeated again here. However, it seems worth emphasizing in the present context that reliability and validity are likely to increase, the more recent and the more precisely behavioral is the information being reported (Ciminero and Drabman, 1977), and that functional analysis and subsequent behavioral interventions depend heavily on just such information.

Interviews with children have not always received much attention in discussions of functional analysis of behavior, but that is changing somewhat for a number of reasons, including increased interest in the role of private events (which, from a behavioral point of view, are largely what cognitive formulations are all about). While it is surely essential to have observable behavioral validation criteria when, say, fears or problem-solving strategies are at issue, the child's reports of feelings, thoughts, or self-instructions are of obvious value and in fact are sometimes themselves the targets of intervention. Similarly useful, though again not necessarily sufficient, are children's reports of what they do and do not find reinforcing, and even their perceptions of those persons whom the therapist may wish to consider for roles as mediators in the intervention. Tharp and Wetzel (1969) developed a thirty-four-item incomplete-sentence instrument, the Mediator-Reinforcer Incomplete Blank, which can be used to provide the framework for that part of the interview dealing with the child's reinforcers and the persons who mediate their delivery. It contains such items as "My favorite grown-up is _____," "If I had ten dollars I'd _____," and "I will do almost anything to avoid _____." Follow-up questions are used when necessary to get clear specification of reinforcing and punishing events (including behaviors of people the child mentions) and of the ranking of reinforcers.

Taking the child's age and general level of functioning into account, questions about activities, interactions with family members and peers, worries and fears, likes and dislikes, etc., can produce useful clues about discriminative and reinforcing stimuli. The reinforcement-contingency unit should be kept in mind here, too, as in interviewing an adult informant; in discussions about any particular behavior, the interviewer should make an attempt to elicit contextual information.

There is some evidence that parents' and children's reports of behavior show substantial agreement (Herjanic et al., 1975). That in itself says nothing about either's accuracy, but at least it is encouraging, and in any case not only the children's reports, but the adult informants' as well, are subject to checks on internal consistency and validation from other data sources. The earlier comments about the application of reinforcement procedures to the interview with informants apply here as well. Not only can the child's speech output and general cooperativeness be increased by the use of reinforcement, as noted previously (see also, S. Salzinger et al., 1962), but where the interviewer already has some information as a basis, there is no reason why more accurate reporting by the child cannot be shaped as has sometimes been done in studies of children's self-monitoring. The possibilities here seem worthy of more detailed investigation.

Rating scales, behavior checklists, and similar compilations have limited utility for functional behavior analysis for several reasons: typically lacking information on positive or adaptive behaviors (the Achenbach Behavior Profiles are an exception—Achenbach and Edelbrock, 1981), they tell little about the child's strengths or assets which can be taken advantage of in designing a program; lacking contextual information, they have few specific treatment implications beyond the indication of possible target behaviors; and while they are usually designed to require a fairly low level of inference on the part of the rater, not all of the items refer to specific behaviors. Mash and Terdal (1981a) suggest that situational content would add to the value of such instruments. While that is certainly true, it must be noted that the brevity and simplicity of their current formats, designed primarily for paper-and-pencil administration with minimal instruction of the informants, account for a significant measure of their popularity, as does the ease with which they can be scored.

For the present purpose, these instruments are noteworthy primarily for their use as adjuncts to the interview or other data-gathering methods, suggesting possible target behaviors, problem situations, or other significant items that might otherwise be overlooked. Atkeson and Forehand (1981) refer to them as "structured paper and pencil interview[s]."

Similarly structured instruments designed to identify current or potential reinforcers have, not surprisingly, received considerable attention in the context of functional analysis.

Homme (1970), for example, describes a "reinforcement menu" wherein the names or pictures of possible reinforcers appear, making it suitable for use with even quite young children. Clinically the concept of reinforcement has been of particular interest in behavioral models of depression, and in that context Costello (1981) discusses the various other instruments that have been used or that might be adapted from their adult versions for the identification of a child's reinforcers, with either the child or someone else as the informant.

It should be noted that reinforcers assessed in this way do not necessarily have any more functional significance than do behaviors targeted from checklists. A reinforcer must ultimately be defined in its functional context by its ability to maintain or increase the strength of some behavior on which it is contingent. Nevertheless, reinforcement survey instruments are valuable for much the same reason as behavior checklists: as reminders of possibilities that we or the informant might otherwise overlook and that should be assessed more thoroughly.

Direct observation of the child's behavior, particularly in so-called natural settings, has been a distinguishing feature of behavior analysis and modification from the outset, and the development of observational techniques, along with the systematic study of their difficulties and sources of potential error (Lipinski and Nelson, 1974), is a major contribution to the field of behavioral assessment. Obviously and unavoidably, there is a sense in which observational data have always played their part: as a basis for descriptions by parents and teachers of the presenting complaints about children's behavior; in clinicians' impressions of children's behavior with them or with parents during interviews or even in the waiting room; in judgments of children's cooperativeness and attentiveness when the validity of psychometric test results is at issue; and so on. However, our concern here is with the collection of observational data as a principal, systematically employed assessment modality.

The most common reasons for collecting observational data are well-known—first, to obtain a current sample rather than some form of retrospective report of the child's behavior and the reinforcement contingencies of which it is a part, and second, to provide an objective baseline for the behavior(s) targeted for change, against which therapeutic effectiveness can later be measured. Such data are especially valuable when the informant (adult or child) is having difficulty supplying clear verbal descriptions, and the observations can, in fact, serve to furnish examples that are then used to instruct the informant on the kinds of reports the clinician wishes to obtain.

The technical and practical considerations vary enormously with the particular nature of the behavior being assessed. In the case of bed-wetting, for example, the response definition should be a matter of little dispute. It is impossible to conceive of a reasonable program that would not include a frequency tally of wet and dry nights; the observer/reporter is clearly going to be a member of the household, possibly even the child, but not the clinician; and there is virtually no choice of situations in which the behavior is to be observed. Toward the other extreme, consider "uncooperative" behavior, where the response definition, the schedule of sampling, the most reliable observer, and the sites of observation all require decisions based on the best interview or other data available. Still more troublesome are behaviors with significant private target components—self-instructions, for instance—although even here a bit of ingenuity can often lead to the collection of the necessary data, as when a mother switches on an unobtrusive recorder at her son's bedtime to obtain a tape of his use of the self-instructions he was being taught for coping with fear of the dark (Karoly, 1981). Very low frequency behaviors also present an obstacle to direct observation, especially when practical or ethical considerations prevent their deliberate elicitation (the purpose of which would, of course, not be to obtain a measure of frequency but to observe the nature of the behavior and how it could be elicited). Here, it might be possible to identify a higher-frequency, functionally related correlate of the behavior which might later be targeted for intervention; physical assaults, for example, might be rather rare but might always be preceded by intense arguments or verbal abuse which themselves might be of sufficient frequency to make the collection of observational data feasible and useful.

The literature provides a number of examples of detailed, carefully constructed, and extensively studied observation systems, of which Patterson's (Patterson et al., 1969) and Wahler's (Wahler et al., 1976) are particularly well-known. However, it seems unlikely that any such scheme will soon serve the needs of routine assessment, if only because of the extensive training the observers must have to achieve an acceptable level of reliability.

A small number of objectively defined behaviors, typically selected and defined on an ad hoc basis to serve the immediate assessment needs of the case at hand, was the hallmark of the early behavior-modification studies and continues to be the most practicable clinical strategy in any setting where the services of trained observers—or of students or research assistants who can be trained at other than the client's expense—are not readily available. As previously discussed, the objective specification of behaviors to be targeted for change, requiring the translation of vague or global characterizations of the child's problems into more precise, less inferential terms, is a major component of functional analysis. To the extent that this can be accomplished by means of behavioral interviews or other reports, the most basic requirement of a simple, clinically practical observation schedule will already have been met.

Technical and methodological problems aside, two main strategies are available for circumventing the cost of sending trained observers into the field: using parents, teachers, or others in the child's natural environment to collect observational data, and carrying out systematic observations in the clinic as part of the regular assessment battery. The first of these is of particular importance, for in addition to its clear practical advantages, we should remember that parents and others often play a significant role in carrying out the actual therapeutic interventions, and if these mediators are to do their job properly, they must necessarily learn to observe the targeted behavior and surrounding events with some accuracy in the settings where the behaviors are likely to occur.

There is evidence that parents, for example, for all the potential sources of serious bias and error, can indeed learn to provide accurate observational records of their children's behavior (Wahler et al., 1976). Salzinger, Feldman, and Portnoy (1970) reported that the real problem was to get some of the parents to keep the records in the first place; those that did so learned without much difficulty to record in behavioral terms, and in addition, home observations by trained observers not only tended to confirm the accuracy of the parents' observations but added little useful information to them. As with all other kinds of assessment data, the clinician will use whatever cross-checks on reliability and validity are available.

While it is no longer tenable to assume that observations in natural settings will always be more useful and error-free than other assessment procedures, it seems that such data can be obtained in a relatively efficient manner, and it is probably fair to say that most assessments, as well as most interventions, will profit from having parents or other significant individuals in the children's environment, or the children themselves, keep track of at least one or two behaviors of chief concern, along with the appropriate contextual information. Some parents or other informants will be able to manage only the simplest formats—e.g., a chart already set up for them, with the day broken into hourly or even longer intervals, requiring only a check mark if the targeted behavior occurs at all during a given interval. Although neither a precise measure of the behavior (its frequency, intensity, or duration) nor any contextual information beyond the approximate time of occurrence is obtained, the record will nevertheless provide a useful indication of response strength, and by at least locating the behavior as to day and time, it can serve as a structured memory aid to the informant when more detailed information is sought by the clinician in an interview. In addition, such record keeping imposes minimal demands on the informant while at the same time establishing a pattern of regular homework. Once this takes place and the informant has been duly praised for providing the records and, it is hoped, has been convinced of their usefulness, it may become easier to obtain more functionally oriented records in which the observer notes not only the date and time of the behavior's occurrence, but also the circumstances (including place and people present), specific antecedent events, the behavior itself, others' responses to the behavior, and the child's response to whatever consequences ensued. It will be helpful to obtain as well notations of any special circumstances bearing on the representativeness of the record, such as an illness of the child or of someone else in the household, or a change in some aspect of the regular household schedule or routine.

It should be kept in mind that observational records are valuable not only for purposes of initial behavioral assessment but also for monitoring the course of the subsequent intervention and follow-up. Therefore, however much the clinician would like to have all the potentially useful details, the most important thing is to settle on a recording format that the informant is likely to maintain reliably over a substantial period of time. At the opposite pole from informants who will keep only the most skeletal records are the occasional ones who write what amounts to a series of short stories documenting the child's and their own difficulties. Impressive and informative as these accounts may be, such industry on the part of informants is unlikely to continue indefinitely, and furthermore, a good deal of discussion is typically necessary to translate these narratives into functional terms. Just as it is essential during assessment interviews to establish at the outset the terms in which the child's behavior is to be discussed, it is essential to establish a useful and manageable observation format as soon as possible.

Systematic behavioral observations in the clinic or laboratory, sometimes in relatively free but often in structured situations, have been widely employed as a convenient and economical alternative to field observations, although they present their own difficulties along with their virtues (Hughes and Haynes, 1978). Even the briefest and simplest of these procedures typically require more training in observation and coding than many clinicians are likely to have had. In view of the time psychometricians invest in learning to administer and interpret a variety of tests which often turn out to have little value in making treatment decisions and none in monitoring behavior change, perhaps some of that time would be better spent in learning basic observation skills, particularly with reference to parent-child interactions, a frequent focus of interest in clinic observations; observations could then more easily be incorporated into the assessment process.

Forehand (see Forehand and Peed, 1979; Atkeson and Forehand, 1981), in assessing conduct-disordered children, observes the mother-child interaction for only approximately ten minutes, and the observer codes the behavior directly through a one-way window. (Some more complex systems require videotaping for later analysis, another barrier to routine use.) Three child behaviors (compliance to parents' commands, noncompliance, and inappropriate behavior) and six parent behaviors (including verbal or physical rewards, and commands) are coded. The brevity and simplicity of the system make it suitable for use during every clinic visit and in other settings as well.

Barkley (1981), who presents a detailed discussion of the way he handles clinic observations of hyperactive children, notes that the typical playroom situation becomes inappropriate for children older than about twelve. With younger children, following a free-play period for mother and child, the mother is instructed to give a variety of commands (e.g., "Give me one of those toys," "Do all the math problems"). A television set is left on as a deliberate distraction, further decreasing the likelihood, as Barkley reports, that behavior-problem children will complete all the commands in the maximum of twenty minutes allowed. With adolescents, parents are instructed to engage in a discussion of such topics as "completing chores when requested," "bedtime on school nights," and "the type of music your son/daughter likes to listen to," and to attempt to resolve disagreements when they arise.

In discussing the observations with parents immediately afterward, Barkley attempts to determine whether the behavior observed is typical. It is interesting that this point is raised less often in connection with home and school observations, where it is frequently assumed, with little confirmation, that a brief sample of observed behavior is more or less typical of the child simply because the setting is familiar. Also, while it is easy to focus almost exclusively on the problem of obtaining a representative sample of the child's behavior, a proper functional analysis will usually require that we also obtain a representative sample of the behavior of the parent, teacher, or anyone else whose interactions with the child are of interest. Indeed, to the extent that the child's behavior is functionally related to the behavior, or even the mere presence, of these other persons, the representativeness of all aspects of the observation context must be considered.

Formal test administration has a useful role to play in behavioral analysis where it permits an important aspect of the child's behavior—e.g., problem-solving strategy—to be sampled, where there are suitable norms against which to determine the presence of significant deficits or assets (as, for example, with some developmental scales and achievement tests), and especially where the behavior actually required by the test is very much like the behavior of immediate clinical interest (as in some tests of expressive and receptive language functioning). Among the reasons for the administration of formal tests, Mash and Terdal (1981a) note "institutional or legislative requirements, situational expectancies, ease of administration, habit, and perceived usefulness" (p. 60). It is a familiar and not very reassuring list. Intelligence tests furnish an instructive example. Widely administered and widely reported as the tests are, it is frequently impossible to discern on clinical grounds why they were given or how, if at all, the results figured in the intervention strategy. Where the child is suspected of suffering from a significant degree of either retardation or genius, that is another matter—although even here, it is not immediately obvious in what ways the intervention for, say, tantrums would necessarily differ in the two cases, other factors (such as reinforcing stimuli) being equal. The time is perhaps approaching when the routine administration of lengthy test batteries will no longer constitute a kind of semi-autonomous enterprise. Instead, in behavioral assessment anyway, there is an increasing emphasis on developing instruments and procedures to serve the needs of assessment in particular clinical problem areas—fears, learning disabilities, social-skill deficits, etc.—and to consider formal testing as not always the first or most productive means of assessment, but simply one possible avenue to be used only when specifically appropriate.

Discussions of standardized testing in relation to the assessment of children's behavior can be found in Ollendick and Cerny (1981) and Evans and Nelson (1977), among others, and the contributors to Mash and Terdal's (1981b) assessment volume discuss the use of tests addressed to a variety of circumscribed clinical problems.

SELECTION OF TARGET BEHAVIORS

The decision process by which a behavior is singled out for treatment is often not specified beyond noting that a parent or teacher complained about the behavior, or that the problem was "obvious." Such complaints are certainly to be taken seriously, though not necessarily accepted at face value, and sometimes the problem *is* obvious. Nevertheless, the selection of target behaviors, either positive or negative, has become increasingly recognized as problematic and in need of careful study and systematization.

Furman and Drabman (1981), in discussing methodological issues in behavior-therapy research with children, list four major ones: target-behavior selection, measurement of the behavior, treatment design, and assessment of treatment effectiveness. The order is interesting, implying as it does what surely is often the case in clinical practice—that the target behavior is already selected, probably according to one or more of the conceptual and empirical criteria summarized by Mash and Terdal (1981a), before systematic measurement procedures are employed. In other words, the target behaviors may not actually be derived from careful functional analysis of a broad range of the child's behavior (although subsequent observational or other data may lead to alterations in the choice or definition of targets), but, rather, measurement procedures are likely to be selected on the basis of their suitability for assessing the type of behavior already targeted, with one possible consequence being that other, even more significant, targets are precluded.

It is easy to state the problem in a way that makes it appear unsolvable, since clearly there must be limits to the range of possibilities that can be thoroughly explored before treatment decisions are made (including the most basic decision of whether to intervene at all), and those possibilities include not only the full spectrum of the child's behavior but also the behavior of significant others in the child's environment and nonsocial aspects as well. The point is that some such comprehensive assessment scheme as Kanfer and Saslow's (1969), discussed earlier, is absolutely essential to minimize the chances of overlooking a significant intervention target. Kanfer and Grimm (1977) have formulated guidelines specifically for selecting target behaviors based on information obtained in interviews. They based their outline on work with adults, and thus there is no consideration of developmental and other factors of particular relevance to children. However, the five major target categories that they discuss—behavior deficiencies, behavior excesses, inappropriate external stimulus control, inappropriate self-generated stimulus control, and problematic reinforcement contingencies—are all conceived in functional terms and are as relevant to children's as to adults' behavior. The use of these categories, along with a comprehensive interview guide, should help assure that no important potential targets are overlooked and that the ones chosen have true functional significance for the child.

REFERENCES

Achenbach, T. M., and Edelbrock, C. S. 1981. *Behavioral problems and competencies reported by parents of normal and disturbed children aged four through sixteen.* Monograph of the Society for Research in Child Development, no. 388.

Atkeson, B. M., and Forehand, R. 1981. Conduct disorders. In *Behavioral assessment of childhood disorders,* ed. E. J. Mash, and L. G. Terdal. New York: Guilford Press.

Barkley, R. A. 1981. *Hyperactive children: A handbook for diagnosis and treatment.* New York: Guilford Press.

Ciminero, A. R., and Drabman, R. S. 1977. Current developments in the behavioral assessment of children. In *Advances in clinical child psychology,* vol. 1, ed. B. B. Lahey, and A. E. Kazdin. New York: Plenum Press.

Costello, C. G. 1981. Childhood depression. In *Behavioral assessment of childhood disorders,* ed. E. J. Mash, and L. G. Terdal. New York: Guilford Press.

Evans, I. M., and Nelson, R. O. 1974. A curriculum for the teaching of behavior assessment. *Am. Psychologist,* 29:598-606.

———. 1977. Assessment of child behavior problems. In *Handbook of behavioral assessment,* ed. A. R. Ciminero, K. S. Calhoun, and H. E. Adams. New York: Wiley.

Forehand, R., and Peed, S. 1979. Training parents to modify noncompliant behavior of their children. In *Treatment and research in child psychopathology,* ed. A. J. Finch, Jr., and P. C. Kendall. New York: Spectrum.

Furman, W., and Drabman, R. S. 1981. Methodological issues in child behavior therapy. In *Progress in behavior modification,* vol. 2, ed. M. Hersen, R. M. Eisler, and P. M. Miller. New York: Academic Press.

Herjanic, B., Herjanic, M., Brown, F., and Wheatt, T. 1975. Are children reliable reporters? *J. Abnorm. Child Psych.,* 3:41-48.

Holland, C. J. 1970. An interview guide for behavioural counseling with parents. *Beh. Ther.,* 1:70-79.

Homme, L. E. 1970. *How to use contingency contracting in the classroom.* Champaign, Ill.: Research Press.

Hughes, H. M., and Haynes, S. N. 1978. Structured laboratory observation in the behavioral assessment of parent-child interactions: A methodological critique. *Beh. Ther.,* 9:428-447.

Kanfer, F. H., and Grimm, L. G. 1977. Behavioral analysis: Selecting target behaviors in the interview. *Beh. Modif.,* 1:7-28.

Kanfer, F. H., and Saslow, G. 1969. Behavioral diagnosis. In *Behavior therapy: Appraisal and status,* ed. C. M. Franks. New York: McGraw-Hill.

Karoly, P. 1981. Self-management problems in children. In *Behavioral assessment of childhood disorders,* ed. E. J. Mash, and L. G. Terdal. New York: Guilford Press.

Lindsley, O. R. 1964. Direct measurement and prosthesis of retarded behavior. *J. Ed.,* 147:62-81.

Lipinski, D., and Nelson, R. 1974. Problems in the use of naturalistic observation as a means of behavioral assessment. *Beh. Ther.,* 5:341-351.

Marholin, D., and Bijou, S. W. 1978. Behavioral assessment: Listen when the data speak. In *Child behavior therapy,* ed. D. Marholin II. New York: Gardner Press.

Mash, E. J., and Terdal, L. G. 1981a. Behavioral assessment of childhood disturbance. In *Behavioral assessment of childhood disorders,* ed. E. J. Mash, and L. G. Terdal. New York: Guilford Press.

Mash, E. J., and Terdal, L. G., eds. 1981b. *Behavioral assessment of childhood disorders.* New York: Guilford Press.

Mischel, W. 1968. *Personality and assessment.* New York: Wiley.

Nelson, R. O., and Hayes, S. C. 1979. Some current dimensions of behavioral assessment. *Beh. Assess.,* 1:1-16.

Ollendick, T. H., and Cerny, J. A. 1981. *Clinical behavior therapy with children.* New York: Plenum Press.

Patterson, G. R., Ray, R. S., Shaw, D. A., and Cobb, J. A. 1969. *Manual for coding of interactions.* Rev. New York: Microfiche.

Patterson, G. R., Reid, J. B., Jones, R. R., and Conger, R. E. 1975. *A social learning approach to family intervention: Families with aggressive children.* Vol. 1. Eugene, Oreg.: Castalia Publishing Co.

Rekers, G. A. 1981. Psychosexual and gender problems. In *Behavioral assessment of childhood disorders,* ed. E. J. Mash, and L. G. Terdal. New York: Guilford Press.

Salzinger, K. 1978. Language behavior. In *Handbook of applied behavior analysis.* ed. A. C. Catania, and T. A. Brigham. New York: Irvington Press/Halstead Press.

Salzinger, K., Feldman, R. S., and Portnoy, S. 1970. Training parents of brain-injured children in the use of operant conditioning procedures. *Beh. Ther.,* 1:4–32.

Salzinger, S., Salzinger, K., Portnoy, S., Eckman, J., Bacon, P. M., Deutsch, M., and Zubin, J. 1962. Operant conditioning of continuous speech in young children. *Child Dev.,* 33:683–695.

Tharp, R. G., and Wetzel, R. J. 1969. *Behavior modification in the natural environment.* New York: Academic Press.

Wahler, R. G., House, A. E., and Stambaugh, E. E. 1976. *Ecological assessment of child problem behavior.* New York: Pergamon Press.

24

The Use of Psychological Tests in Clinical Practice with Children

Rachel Gittelman

Psychological testing is an important professional resource to clinicians involved in the diagnosis and treatment of children with psychiatric problems. Yet its role is puzzling since there are, literally, hundreds of psychological tests, many with titles that promise much.

It would be impossible to acquaint the reader with all, or even a sizable proportion, of the marketed tests. Rather, we will discuss the tests for functions most commonly assessed in pediatric psychiatry settings, and address issues such as when to refer a child for testing and what can be reasonably expected from psychological testing. The tests mentioned in the text are listed in the Appendix.

There are some important conceptual and technical issues that influence the usefulness of psychological tests. They include concepts of standardization, reliability, validity, sensitivity and specificity. These are touched upon briefly at the beginning of the chapter; the clinical aspects of psychological testing follow.

General Issues

Standardization

It is very difficult to evaluate the significance of a test score in the absence of standards regarding how others perform on the test. The establishment of standards, or norms, permits a comparison of the child's performance to others and allows for interpretation of discrepancies for an individual on diverse measures.

For example, a reading disorder is defined by discrepant scores on IQ and reading tests. This is possible because norms are available for each test, permitting us to determine the child's relative rank on each measure compared to his peers.

I am indebted to Donald F. Klein, M.D., for the tables. His very helpful comments regarding the discussion of test sensitivity and specificity are most gratefully acknowledged.

Since age ordinarily has a tremendous influence on what children do, norms are needed for various ages. In addition, IQ also affects performance on many other measures, and a requirement for standardization is that a broad range of IQ values should be represented in the sample used to standardize a test.

It is important to remember that a test purported to have been standardized does not necessarily provide norms that are useful for all purposes. A key consideration is whether the standardization sample is adequately representative of the children to whom we compare the tested child. An arbitrary example is used to illustrate the point. A widely used reading test is the Gray Oral Reading Test. It provides norms for first to twelfth graders. Because boys and girls differed in performance, separate norms were given for each sex. However, the entire standardization sample, for a single age group of either sex, numbers as little as seventeen, and at most twenty-four. One can question the adequacy of norms based on such small groups. In addition, the children's IQs in the standardization sample were well above average. The practical consequence is that the test scores of children with low and average IQ levels are difficult to interpret, because the standardization sample failed to include them. Even with higher IQ children, the test presents problems because there were so few of them in the standardization sample. Thus, the mere fact of standardization does not automatically provide standards adequately representative of the general population.

The essential point is that there are varying standards of quality in standardization; and it cannot be assumed invariably that these have been met.

Another factor influencing the utility of norms is their recency. Those developed many years ago may no longer be valid due to cultural changes such as the advent of television, preschool programs, a greater degree of education in the general population, and so on. In general, newly standardized tests are better than old ones.

It is possible to norm a test for any type of group, such as individuals with schizophrenia, affective disorders, or people in lower-class or upper-class standing. In psychological testing, one major concern is to evaluate a child relative to other children of the same age and, sometimes, sex. Other characteristics may also be important. For example, if an intelligence test has been standardized on English-speaking children only, its use with bilingual youngsters is limited, since a clear interpretation of test results is impeded by a lack of norms in bilingual groups. The use of the test is not unjustified if one wishes to compare the ability of the bilingual child to English-speaking youngsters, but if no standards are available for bilingual children, it is not possible to determine the deviance of test results for these children.

In summary, for norms to provide good guides of performance, the standardization sample must be well representative of the children tested. The use of tests in groups not included in the standards renders interpretation of results most difficult.

Reliability

For the most part, clinicians are concerned with relatively enduring characteristics, not with transient, ephemeral phenomena. Therefore, it is essential that the information generated by a test be stable. If children's IQ scores differed markedly from one hour or day or month to the next, we would loose all interest in IQ measures, since they are intended to evaluate functions that are relatively consistent.

Most commonly, clinicians will be concerned with the test-retest reliability of psychological tests. It reflects the stability of children's performance over various time intervals. For a test to have any usefulness in the usual clinical setting, it must have adequate short-term or immediate reliability. The clinician will be interested in stability of performance over extended periods of time only if the characteristic tested is expected to remain relatively constant. This is usually the case in the evaluation of personality traits and overall intellectual ability. It is not the case in the assessment of a mood disorder or any other symptom or characteristic that should change over time.

There are many ways of computing reliability. They are usually expressed by a correlation coefficient. Unfortunately, there is no specific coefficient value that can be identified as reflecting adequate short-term reliability since its significance will depend in part, on the size of the group from which it was obtained and whether the same level of reliability is obtained across the whole range of scores. Some tests may be more reliable at one level of performance than at another. An arbitrary rule of thumb is that tests whose immediate reliability falls at or above coefficient values of 0.80 can be considered to reflect satisfactory consistency of performance. Those with reliability coefficients below 0.60 can be considered to have poor reliability. Above 0.60 but below 0.80 indicates a moderate, but not unacceptable, level of stability. (This is assuming that reliability values are precise.)

Individual versus Group Testing

Tests can be devised for many purposes, but in the clinical setting we are always assessing an *individual* child and making decisions about that child, not about a group of children. Group testing can be used for selection purposes. An example is the achievement testing necessary for entry into universities. By using test scores to eliminate very large groups of applicants, admission offices can concentrate their selection procedures on smaller groups. Similarly, during WW II, psychologists devised tests to select pilots, navigators, and other special personel. Though the tests will miss many outstanding individuals, they will, as a whole, generate a much more accurate group definition than would be accomplished if they were not applied. Furthermore, the cost of excluding other competent individuals is of little concern.

If the goal of psychological testing is to identify the extreme of the distribution of a clinical characteristic, our standards for the quality of the tests can be more lax than they need to be in the individualized clinical situation. Evaluation procedures may be only slightly better than chance or random selection, and yet still produce a considerable advantage in the selection of very deviant individuals. Thus group testing could be used for clinicial purposes to cull out a small subgroup from a very large pool of children. For example, one might want to select, from an entire school population, those children most likely to develop psychiatric problems, in order to implement a preventative therapeutic program, such as in case-finding procedures.

However, in clinical evaluations group-selection process is never relevant; as a result, much more rigorous demands are placed upon the tests. They have to be extremely accurate to generate confidence in the assignments made for a specific child. Consequently, for the clinician it is useless to know that scores on a test differentiate significantly between children who have a disorder, or a trait, and those who do not. Significant differences between groups can be obtained in spite of very poor discrimination. Even if a test correlates significantly with the presence of a disorder, it may yield a very substantial number of claims that a disorder or characteristic is present when it is not (false-positive errors), and that a disorder is absent when it is in fact present (false-negative errors). This is clearly an intolerable situation in the clinical setting. Therefore, to be useful to clinicians, psychological tests must be very good, to be any good at all. What is meant by good? In psychological assessment, goodness refers to validity. The type of validity we are most concerned about in psychological testing is construct validity. Do the tests really measure what we want them to? For example, if we are trying to detect defects in attentional ability, are the tests truly capable of assessing attentional ability? If we are evaluating a child's anxiety level, do the tests measure anxiety accurately?

Types of Diagnostic Decisions

There are essentially two types of diagnostic test usage. In one, the child fits within a category by virtue of the test score, and the test score defines the diagnosis. In the other, the psychologist must infer the presence of a disorder. The diagnosis of mental retardation is an example of a test-defined diagnosis. If the diagnosis is based on IQ alone, any child with an IQ score below 70 is, by definition, in the mental retardation class, and vice versa. One can debate the merits of the definition in terms of its predictive validity (i.e., whether it is associated with various future life events); or one can be concerned with other important issues regarding the diagnosis, but the diagnostic process itself is completely straightforward. It requires no inferential judgment—only a test score. The same is true for the diagnosis of a specific reading or arithmetic disorder, where a set of scores are required: IQ and achievement scores. Here again, the diagnostician's clinical judgment is not called upon, merely his testing and scoring skills. The major concerns in the individual assessment of children for mental retardation or for learning disorders are the reliability and construct validity of the tests. Indeed, we want to be sure that the reading tests are good estimates of the child's reading ability, and so on.

The preceding two examples are exhaustive of the cases where test scores constitute definitional diagnostic criteria. In the rest of psychological test diagnosis, the judgment of the psychologist is called upon to arrive at a diagnostic formulation. Examples abound: children are tested to assess their "potential," to determine whether brain damage or schizophrenia or a personality disorder or minimal brain dysfunction is present. In no instance is there a clear-cut test definition for any condition, other than for mental retardation and specific reading or arithmetic disorders.

We now face serious problems because we find that children with identical scores may belong to different diagnostic classes, since there is overlap in test scores between different clinical conditions. Not all children with poor scores on attentional tests have an attention-deficit disorder; not all youngsters who show *no* sign of thought disturbance on test measures are free of schizophrenia, and vice versa. Affecting the accuracy of the diagnostic decision when discrete groups share test characteristics, will be the overall sensitivity and specificity of the test.

Sensitivity and Specificity

Two types of mistakes can occur in the diagnosis process, false-positive and false-negative errors. The terms *sensitivity* and *specificity* are now used. They are related to the concepts of false-positive and false-negative errors but are not synonymous with them. Sensitivity values refer to the rate of detection of true positives, that is, finding that something is present when it is truly present. Specificity values denote the rate of true negatives, i.e., saying that something is absent when it is truly absent.

This discussion may seem a bit too technical for clinicians mostly interested in the basic principles of testing. Nonetheless, clarification of these issues will help immensely to understand that, in many cases, diagnostic assignment based on psychological test performance is a very tricky procedure.

When tests are being developed, for example, for a type of brain damage, patients with the damage are compared with others without it. Let us assume, as is often the case, that the groups are roughly equivalent in size; half the patients examined have the disorder and half do not (this ratio represents a base rate of 50% for the disorder). The test is found to select the affected patients well beyond chance. The test is now touted as a good measure for that type of brain damage. (The use of brain damage as an example is purely arbitrary. We could also speak of personality type.) As a result, clinicians will use the test with the expectation that it is useful for that particular diagnosis. Are the clinical patients distributed in a fashion similar to the 50% base rate of the original study? Most likely not. Does it matter? Yes, definitely. Because a very different rate of success will be found in clinical situations where the prevalence, or base rate, of a diagnosis or other characteristic deviates from the rate in the validation sample. This phenomenon can be demonstrated graphically without resorting to the relevant mathematical formulas that prove it.

In tables 24-1, 24-2, 24-3, the rate of accurate diagnosis is presented for tests with identical sensitivity and specificity; in all instances the tests have 60, 70, 80, 90, and 95% accuracy in ruling in, and ruling out, a disorder. Only the base rate of the disorder has been varied. In table 24-1 the base rate of a diagnosis in the clinic is 5%; in table 24-2 it is 20%, and in table 24-3 it is 50%. The entries in the tables represent what percentage of those diagnosed will be correctly identified by the diagnostician in each respective setting. Note that where only 5% of the clinic patients have a condition, there is extremely poor accuracy, even

TABLE 24-1.
Percentages of Accurately Identified Cases with Varying Sensitivities and Specificities in Settings with a 5 Percent Prevalence of Affected Cases

Test Specificity (Percent)	Test Sensitivity (Percent)				
	60	70	80	90	95
60	7	8	10	11	11
70	10	11	12	14	14
80	14	16	17	19	20
90	24	27	30	32	33
95	39	42	46	49	50

TABLE 24-2.
Percentages of Accurately Identified Cases with Varying Sensitivities and Specificities in Settings with a 20 Percent Prevalence of Affected Cases

Test Specificity (Percent)	Test Sensitivity (Percent)				
	60	70	80	90	95
60	27	30	33	36	37
70	33	37	40	43	44
80	43	47	50	53	54
90	60	64	67	69	70
95	75	78	80	82	83

TABLE 24-3.
Percentages of Accurately Identified Cases with Varying Sensitivities and Specificities in Settings with a 50 Percent Prevalence of Affected Cases

TEST SPECIFICITY (PERCENT)	TEST SENSITIVITY (PERCENT)				
	60	70	80	90	95
60	50	54	57	60	61
70	57	61	64	67	68
80	67	70	73	75	76
90	80	82	84	86	86
95	89	90	91	92	93

when both sensitivity and specificity are excellent. For example, if a test has 90% accuracy for establishing the diagnosis when it is present, as well as for dismissing it when it is absent, among those diagnosed as having it, only 32% will actually have the disorder. In contrast, if the test were not used, but all patients were declared not to have the disorder, a 95% rate of accuracy would be achieved.

Given similarly high sensitivity and specificity (90%) in clinics with a base rate of 20% for the disorder, the percentage correctly diagnosed will improve markedly. We now reach a 69% accuracy among those diagnosed. Still not as good as the 80% rate of accuracy we would obtain if we again said that no one had it.

The picture changes when the base rate is 50%. Now, with the same test that has the optimistically high (90%) sensitivity and specificity, the accuracy rate reaches 86%. A very respectable level, and one far better than if the test had not been used.

In almost all clinical situations, each condition for which a diagnosis is sought has a very low base rate. It seems fair to state that, in general, any one disorder does not much exceed the 20% frequency, with many being far less prevalent; therefore, we must conclude it unlikely that impressively accurate diagnostic statements can be derived from tests.

A few more observations from these tables are in order. Note that improving *sensitivity* does not matter much. For instance, for a test with a specificity of 60% (i.e., the test has been found to identify correctly 60% of those who do *not* have the disorder), improving the sensitivity from 60% to 90% only improves the diagnostic accuracy from 7 to 11% if the base rate is 5% (table 24-1), and from 50 to 60% if the base rate is 50% (table 24-3). A different pattern occurs if *specificity* is increased for a test with a 60% sensitivity (i.e., 60% of those with the disorder are identified). A change in the specificity (the true negative rate) will have a remarkable influence on the accuracy of the diagnosis. In table 24-1, for example, with a 5% base rate, the hit rate goes from 7 to 24% when the specificity changes from 60 to 90%; in table 24-3, where the base rate for the disorder is 50%, the diagnostic accuracy will go from 50 to 80%, with changes to specificity from 60 to 90%. This means that it is not sufficient to attend to the adequacy of a test in *identifying affected cases,* but it is essential to know how good the test is in *ruling out,* or confirming the absence of, a condition.

The discussion concerning the poor diagnostic showing of tests when the base rate is low and the specificity is poor may seem counterintuitive, or even dubious. It is unfortunate that many important issues such as this concerning clinical assessment require expert critical review. The well-intentioned clinician does not have the background necessary to judge the diagnostic adequacy of the myriad of tests available. Nor is test popularity an index of excellence.

Practical Issues

Referrals for Psychological Testing

Psychological testing is not called for in all cases, but certain presenting clinical symptoms regularly require that such testing be done.

ACADEMIC DIFFICULTIES. Reports of poor school performance always require an evaluation of intellectual ability to clarify the possible presence of limited intelligence. Some may feel that it is possible to assess IQ with confidence through clinical interviewing. However, the likelihood of error from clinical impressions is too great to forego formal evaluation. In addition to intellectual ability, the child's scholastic achievement requires objective assessment. Here again, a cursory impressionistic approach often can be misleading.

BEHAVIOR PROBLEMS IN SCHOOL. Many children who are referred because of disruptive behavior may not be reported to be performing poorly academically, yet their intellectual resources and their academic skill development may be limited. The detection of impaired cognitive ability in children with disruptive behavior will influence treatment plans. Clinicians will most likely want to address the treatment of both behavioral and academic problems in those who present not only complaints of conduct, but who also have failed to acquire appropriate skills. Therefore, children with conduct problems in school should be referred for psychological testing. Other school problems, such as school phobia for example, do not automatically necessitate psychological testing. The latter may be advisable in individual cases but is not a necessary routine procedure.

DEVELOPMENT LAG. Some children may have unusual language construction, seemingly poor comprehension, or may be slow in getting work done, and yet have no conduct problem. These difficulties are frequently subtle manifestations whose presence is often noted by teachers or parents who may contrast the affected child to his peers. An assessment of intellectual and specific cognitive abilities is necessary for proper diagnosis of these youngsters.

ANXIETY ABOUT SCHOOL PERFORMANCE. Children who overvalue high grades may become seriously distraught when they receive average or less than top grades, and may come to professional attention because of anxiety, depression, poor sleep, somatic complaints, and other more general problems. Some of these children may be overzealous students who spend long hours at schoolwork but may lack intellectual ability or have different difficulties. It is helpful to assess these children's cognitive skills to determine whether they have specific skill deficiency or inefficient work habits. For example, a student with excellent intellectual ability may have a mild reading problem. The child may have excelled while scholastic demands remained relatively simple, but with more academic complexity, the youngster may encounter failure with consequent bitter disappointment.

Psychological testing will also provide useful information if the results rule out the presence of cognitive impairment, since attention will then focus on the emotional factors that interfere with smooth functioning.

CHANGE IN FUNCTIONAL LEVEL. Testing is regularly indicated when children show a marked deterioration in functional capacity, such as worsening in school performance or in social interest. We are not referring to temporary or mild fluctuations in behavior, which are very common in children, but to significant shifts in social and intellectual performance. Test results will provide a baseline measure that can be used to compare the child's performance as time goes on. Testing can thus help to evaluate whether the deterioration is a progressive one and may also give clues regarding the causes for the change in functioning.

ASSESSMENT OF INTERVENTION EFFECTS. Some children are so impaired that it may seem superfluous to use tests to document their disability. For example, a twelve year old who is clearly not mentally retarded and is practically a nonreader very likely does not require costly individual educational assessment to verify the presence of a reading disorder. However, the tests should be performed if an intervention is planned, in order to establish an objective assessment of level of ability so as to enable monitoring of treatment effects. The same is true for any type of disability to which therapy is geared, assuming there exists a means for objective assessment.

How to Refer for Testing

Psychological testing in children is regularly conducted within the context of a multidisciplinary evaluation; therefore, the psychologist must address questions raised by other professionals and tailor the assessment accordingly. The value of testing will be affected by the relevance and appropriateness of the questions, and by the quality of the information provided to the psychologist concerning the observations that have led to a request for psychological testing.

By making very explicit the goals of assessment, the referring professional will facilitate the selection of appropriate psychological tests and will render the assessment more meaningful as well as more efficient. If the clinical problem is presented in vague fashion, much testing will be done in search of the problem, rather than the answer, with consequent loss of time.

It is not sufficient to state that an assessment of the child's capacity is requested; the reasons for the request, and if possible the purpose of testing, should be stated. Ideally the referral should indicate the overall concern, as well as specific questions. As an example:

> The child is doing poorly in school. He is reported to be behind his classmates in all academic subjects. Assessment of his intellectual functioning and academic abilities is requested to rule out low intellectual ability and document level of academic skills.

This type of referral requests objective information regarding two important aspects of cognitive performance, IQ and academic achievement. It does not request a full examination of possible factors that might contribute to poor school performance in this child. No demand is made to provide assistance in the disposition of the case, or in treatment plans, or in understanding the possible influences that may be at the origin of the difficulties.

This referral should lead the psychologist to administer an IQ test and achievement tests of relevant school subjects. There need not be further testing.

In other instances the referring clinician may want assistance in planning a child's treatment program. The referral should then state:

> The child is doing poorly in school. He is reported to be behind his classmates in all academic subjects. Psychological testing is requested to assist in the treatment plan.

With such a referral, the psychologist will not only assess intellectual ability and academic ability but also relevant developmental cognitive functions. These might include language development, attentional ability, and specific difficulties in decoding (reading) and encoding (writing). The avenues pursued will depend on the nature of the dysfunctions observed as testing progresses. The psychological test report should then include specific recommendations regarding class placement, the advisability of remediation, the types of assistance, and the reasons for such help.

Cognitive development is not the only pertinent issue for children having school difficulties; psychosocial influences within and outside the family affect academic performance. If the psychiatrist desires assistance in elucidating the nature of the interpersonal emotional factors that may contribute to a child's academic problems, it should be stated in the referral.

Need for Individual Testing

Some children may have been evaluated in school; clinicians can then obtain IQ and academic achievement scores that have resulted from the child's participation in group testing.

Group IQ tests are really achievement tests, since they rely heavily on reading ability. Children with adequate intellectual ability but poor reading skills are penalized on group tests. Poor performance may also result from lack of self-application rather than skill deficiency. Therefore, group IQ tests can be helpful only to rule out intellectual impairment when a child receives a good score.

Inadequate motivation can also affect performance on individually administered tests, but it is less likely to occur since psychologists are trained to obtain good cooperation from children. If, however, the psychologist fails to enlist the child's interest, a note can be made of it and testing rescheduled, or the results can be interpreted accordingly. This information is not lost, as it is in the case of group testing.

Need for Retesting

We have discussed the clinical circumstances that call for psychological testing. There are some situations that should alert the clinician to request retesting of a child. A good rule of thumb is that very peculiar, unexpectected test outcomes should be a signal to reevaluate a child. There are many factors that may lead to clearly deviant patterns of results when no abnormality is present. Therefore, if psychological testing produces conclusions that are inconsistent with a host of other observations, such as the child's history, school behavior, or careful clinical observations, it is judicious to request a repeat testing. This procedure is akin to repeating medical laboratory tests that yield unsuspected deviant findings. It is best to insure that measurement error, or some other source of error, is not responsible for making important decisions about a child.

CLINICAL APPLICATIONS: PROJECTIVE TESTS

Broadly speaking, there are two types of tests, projective and objective. Projective tests are used for the evaluation of personality and for psychodiagnosis. All other assessments rely on objective tests consisting of specific tasks.

It is not unusual for psychologists to be asked to assess personality characteristics, such as self-image and esteem, aggressive fantasies and the propensity for their expression, sexual identification, the nature of the child's intrapsychic conflicts, and many more. In order to address those important clinical questions, psychologists use several projective tests. They differ from objective tests in that they do not call for a correct answer from the child, but allow free rein. Their use is rooted in psychoanalytic theory. More specifically, it is predicated on the projective hypothesis, which posits that the interpretation of all experiences is colored by unconscious, repressed mental content. Reliance on intrapsychic material is greater when interpreting experiences that are ambiguous, rather than well-defined in content. Consequently, when responding to test materials that do not have clear intrinsic structure, the child will expose aspects of psychic content not otherwise accessible. In this way, a glimpse is offered of the child's unconscious drives and the nature of the defenses against these drives. The projective tests can be viewed as a controlled form of dream production, or projective play, and the analytic interpretation process of the test responses can proceed in the same vein.

The most commonly used projective tests are described briefly:

The Rorschach Test

The Rorschach test, a series of ten inkblots, is the least structured test available since it is nonrepresentational. The child is told to state what the card looks like; responses are recorded without interruption and verbatim. After the ten cards have been responded to, inquiry follows to determine the location and nature of the percepts on the card. Features such as the content, form, color, shading, and other determining characteristics of the responses can be scored. Response latencies, consisting of the time lag between card presentation and the child's response to the card, can also be noted. Long latencies may be interpreted as evidence of an active defensive process against the anxiety experienced upon immediate viewing of the card. The anxiety might be due to the activation of important unconscious conflicts by the content of the card.

The test responses can be subjected to two types of analysis. One is an interpretation of the response scores, the other is an informal clinical interpretation of the test responses. There are age norms available for the quantitative scores (Levitt and Truumaa, 1972).

Thematic Apperception Test (TAT)

In this test a number of cards are selected from thirty black and white cards depicting a wide variety of scenes, some with ambiguous content. One card is blank. The child is asked to tell a complete story for each card. Scoring procedures have been devised, but these are not usually used by clinicians. Rather, a qualitative analysis of the story content is conducted.

Children's Apperception Test (CAT)

This test was designed to be a child version of the TAT (though the TAT is used with children); it provides pictures of animals, cartoon-style, instead of the TAT's photographs and stylized drawings. The animals are situated in scenes specifically designed to evoke associations concerning eating and toilet behavior (oral and anal-phase conflict), sibling rivalry, and parent-child interaction.

Drawings

Among projective drawings there are the figure drawings, or Draw-A-Person Test where the child is asked to draw a person. The House-Tree-Person calls for a drawing of a house and a tree, as well. Some ask children to draw a family. Inquiry follows regarding various aspects of the drawing, such as the age and sex of the person, and the child may be asked to talk about the picture. Characteristics such as body image, gender typing, self-esteem, sexual anxiety, capacity for warmth, aggression, and many other personality constructs are inferred from the drawings.

Personality Testing

Personality testing is often requested when there is doubt regarding the significance of the child's symptoms. For example, a child is reported to be aggressive, but the diagnostician wants confirmation of the characterological nature of the aggressive behavior. If the child produces aggressive responses on projective tests, the clinician will be confident that the child's aggression is an important aspect of his personality. If no aggressive themes are present, the significance of the child's overt aggression may be minimized. Conversely, a child who is not aggressive but who produces aggressive themes on the projective testing may be viewed as having great propensity for aggression, or as having a conflict about the expression of hostile feelings. In turn, this trait would be viewed as playing a role in the child's emotional adjustment.

The foregoing assumptions are not rooted in empirical evidence. In fact, there is very little evidence to document the belief that children's personality characteristics are well estimated by projective testing. For example, in a study of the TAT, only one of five ratings of aggression differentiated aggressive and nonaggressive children. In the one discriminant measure, the difference in frequency of response between the two types of children was only one (Kagan, 1956). This magnitude of difference is too small to be applied in a diagnostic fashion. In a study of disturbed children, the Draw-A-Person Test was not found to predict levels of current or future aggression (Breidenbaugh et al., 1974). Similarly disappointing results were reported with the Bender-Gestalt. The clinical criteria believed to indicate symbolic representation of aggression—heavy drawing over, progressively larger figures—were unrelated to levels of expressed aggression (Trahan and Stricklin, 1979).

Attempts to identify differences in various aspects of emotional well-being among children whose fathers had died (Lifshitz, 1975), whose parents had divorced (Kelly and Berg, 1978), or who had been placed in foster care (North and Keiffer, 1966) also have failed. (For a more comprehensive discussion of these issues see Gittleman-Klein, 1978; Gittleman, 1980; Lachar and LaCombe, 1983.)

The empirical literature dealing with personality assessment in children is surprisingly scant. Therefore, it is not possible to draw definite conclusions concerning the accuracy of personality testing in children. Among the tests, the DAP emerges as an invalid personality test—the indicators of emotional disturbance have not been shown to be reliable (Hammer and Kaplan, 1966).

The TAT has also failed to show satisfactory validity (Reddy, 1960). Too little work has been done with the Rorschach to assess its validity. Certainly, given the state of our knowledge, it is unjustified to rely on the test results to rule out the presence of disorders when symptoms are evident; or to assume from the tests that personality deviance is present when it is not evident in the child's behavior.

In addition to describing the current personality pattern, some use projective tests to reconstruct the child's early dynamic genetic process. Statements regarding oral or anal conflicts may be advanced to account for the present clinical picture. This practice is of very dubious merit. Schafer (1978), a leading psychoanalyst, believes that it should be avoided. He states,

> Since at present there seems to be no evidence in Rorschach test records to support or refute genetic relationships, and since current representations of the remote past are historically unreliable even though revealing of current pathology, interpretation can and should pertain only to the present personality structure and dynamics of the patient, or to changes in these and in the relatively recent past (p. 563).

Though this statement was made about the Rorschach test as it pertains to adults, it is equally relevant to all forms of projective testing and for all ages.

Just as questionable is the practice of predicting what is likely to happen to a child on the basis of projective testing. Some report the likelihood of future decompensation into a psychotic state or suicide or sexual maladjustment. Since there is a total absence of support for the merit of this practice, it must be viewed, unfortunately, as being totally deceptive.

To illustrate concretely the type of unwarranted reconstructions and predictions that are made from projective testing, a few excerpts from psychological test reports are quoted:

> The potential for ideas of reference, feelings of depersonalization are indicated. The groundwork for suicidal ideation has been laid in the desire to retreat back to the maternal womb.

> During childhood the patient tried to maintain a phallic, assertive concept of herself, but intense sibling rivalry brought such gross feelings of rage to the surface that it threatened her dependent adjustment. Projection of the rage left her guilt-laden and fearful of impending destruction.

> He had achieved a dependent attachment to a mother figure whom he couldn't grasp or understand, but he experienced her as cold and demanding.

> Along with her repression has come a loss of awareness of the sexual differences in objects, indicating that sexual relationships could occur with both males and females, with little emotional impact.

> A tendency, related perhaps to homosexual strivings, toward severe repression, leading to suicide and imagined rebirth, is evidenced and suicide precautions are indicated.

Statements such as these are extremely seductive, since clinicians often believe that heretofore unknown events have been revealed. These interesting reconstructions and predictions have not fared well when put to the test.

Diagnosis

The practice of classifying patients on the basis of projective tests has a long history. Over the years many claims have been made regarding the characteristics of schizophrenia, psychopathy, neurosis, and other disorders on psychological tests. As an example, the presence of "primary-process" responses on projective tests has been used to make a diagnosis of schizophrenia.

The detailed evidence regarding the use of psychological tests for diagnostic purposes is beyond the scope of this summary. It has been presented elsewhere (Gittelman-Klein, 1978; Gittelman, 1980). The unequivocal conclusion drawn from critical reviews of the literature is that there is no evidence whatever to support the use of such testing for diagnostic purposes, except in two instances: mental retardation and specific developmental disorders.

As an example of what cannot be done, a recent observation is reported. The testing of a school-phobic child reportedly indicated psychosis. Because of the test results, the youngster was treated with neuroleptics (in this instance, totally without success).

In this anecdote the use of antipsychotic medication follows logically from the report of schizophrenia. However, the diagnosis is based on the erroneous presumption that psychological tests are diagnostically informative. It is a grave error to make diagnostic or pharmacotherapeutic decisions on the basis of projective testing. This is not to say that the conclusions from the tests should have been ignored completely. They might have raised concern regarding the possible evidence of psychosis and called for a clinical review of the diagnosis. If no evidence for a history of psychosis had been elicited from further interviewing, the test results should have been ignored.

There is a common view that the skill of the psychologist makes up for the inadequacy of the diagnostic tests and that, therefore, in the hands of a talented clinician, projective tests can produce accurate information concerning children's personality and diagnosis. There is no support for this view whatsoever, if one is referring to the interpretation of tests results. As a matter of fact, the evidence points in the opposite direction. When one can make accurate diagnostic interpretations, it is because the deviance is so obvious most can discern it even in the absence of special training. Subtle inferences by expert clinicians have never been shown to be useful. It is important to keep in mind that I am referring to projective test result interpretations, and not to the observations that can be made from a child's behavior, either during testing or interview. In these situations it is very likely that talented clinicians come to valuable conclusions and that their judgment is better than that of less capable clinicians.

To conclude, it cannot be emphasized sufficiently that psychiatric diagnosis cannot be made, or even advanced, on the basis of projective test results. This view is echoed even by some with unambivalent enthusiasm for insights derived from projective tests. For example, Kline (1976) states, "At present, with current interpretive scoring methods, projective tests should not be used to make important decisions about people" (p. 56).

It is most regrettable that other professionals continue to recommend the use of psychological tests to establish a diagnosis, without providing any supporting evidence (Weiss, 1978).

Clinical Applications: Assessment of Intellectual Ability

Unlike testing for personality traits or diagnosis, the goal of intellectual assessment is to determine a child's capacity compared to other children of the same age. To do so properly requires the availability of standards established in large groups representative of the population to which the tested children belong. The issue of standardization has been discussed in the "General Issues" section of the chapter.

Tests that have been standardized and yield age norms are the most useful. The many tests of ability or skill development that have not been standardized cannot provide an accurate evaluation of how tested children compare to their peers, and hence, have much more limited clinical utility; the conclusions so generated are much more tentative than when standardized instruments are used.

Several measures yield IQ scores. None is applicable to children below the age of two. However, clinicians may in some instances be interested in evaluations of the developmental level of children during the first two years of life.

Testing of Infants

The Bayley Scales of Infant Development is the best measure for evaluating infants. It was standardized on a large sample representative of the United States population, and provides norms from two months to two and a half years. By necessity, the evaluation of infants consists mostly of sensory-motor tests.

Initially, it was hoped that the assessment of these functions during the first two years would provide information related to intellectual ability later on. This has not turned out to be the case (e.g., Honzig et al., 1948). Therefore, infant testing should be viewed as providing a picture of the child's developmental status at the time, with the understanding that it bears little relationship to intelligence as measured by IQ tests in older children.

In spite of the overall lack of relationship between scores on infant tests and later IQ, infants who receive scores in the extreme bottom of the distribution are more likely to be intellectually handicapped eventually. In grossly impaired infants, the appearance of deviance is readily apparent to the naked eye. Yet, the availability of test scores to document retardation in development may be helpful. It often facilitates communication to parents and other professionals. Nevertheless, even in the case of severely developmentally retarded youngsters, early test results are not good predictors of the *degree* of impairment later on. Much more important to this prediction is the cause of the retardation. If it is due to social factors, the eventual outcome may be benign depending on future events. If the early retardation is due to biological factors, the nature of these may be more informative than the early test scores. Therefore, even in the case of retarded infants, the test scores are not sufficient for individual case disposition.

Conversely, eventual intellectual retardation cannot be ruled out in infancy. Though, here as well, children who obtain normal or superior test scores are much less likely to have later IQs in the retarded range than other infants. It would be unfortunate if great hopes for intellectual superiority were communicated to parents when their infants obtained high developmental scores. In many cases, disappointment would ensue.

Testing of Preschool Children

The age group referred to as pre-school falls between the ages of two and six years. A number of well-standardized tests are available for IQ testing. The Stanford-Binet Intelligence Scale, the first carefully constructed individual intelligence test was redesigned and restandardized in 1972. It is suitable for children from the age of two. For the preschool ages it includes verbal tasks such as object naming, storytelling, and nonverbal tasks such as bead stringing. The tests are organized by age. Because very marked changes in ability occur over short time spans, different tasks are provided for each at half-year intervals until the age of five, but at yearly intervals thereafter.

The McCarthy Scales of Children's Abilities are applicable to children of two and a half to eight years of age. Unlike the Stanford-Binet, it organizes tasks by function, rather than by age. The test includes verbal, perceptual, performance, quantitative, general cognitive, memory, and motor scales. The potential difficulty in this practice is that the functions may not be as discrete as the labels imply; the test items may reflect a number of abilities, not only the name they are assigned. Therefore, it is important not to assume that these scales represent discrete developmental skills. An overall score, general cognitive index (GCI), is obtained which is based on fifteen of the eighteen test items. Standardized scores are provided for three-month intervals.

The Wechsler Preschool and Primary Scale of Intelligence, the WPPSI (pronounced wipsy), is applicable to ages four and a half to six and a half years. It is organized by test, not by age level. The eleven tests are divided into a Verbal and a Performance scale, each providing separate IQs which are combined to generate an overall IQ. This test was modeled after the earlier Wechsler tests for adults and school-age children. The verbal scale includes: information, vocabulary, arithmetic, similarities, and comprehension. The performance scale consists of animal house (the child picks the appropriate house for different animals), picture completion, mazes, geometric designs (a copying task), and block design. Norms are provided for half-year intervals.

All these tests, the Stanford-Binet, McCarthy scales and WPPSI are well-standardized instruments with very good reliability. The WPPSI is not useful for children below four. Its advantage is that it provides verbal and performance IQs, whereas the others do not.

The possible advantage of the Stanford-Binet over the McCarthy scales is that it is much more widely known, has been extensively studied, and is familiar to most professionals, while the McCarthy Scales are not. It also provides norms from two years on, the McCarthy from two and a half years.

The three instruments all take about one hour to administer. Most children enjoy the procedures due to the ingenious use of colorful materials and rapid shifting from one type of task to another.

The use of IQ tests in children between the ages of two and four is limited by the same considerations that affect infant testing. Early IQ scores are not good predictors of later IQ. It is only by the age of five or so that IQ scores become very stable in groups of children.

There are probably two major reasons why early and later status are not strongly associated. For one, different behaviors are assessed at different ages. On the Stanford-Binet, for example, the vocabularly test requiring a child to explain the meaning of words does not appear before the age of six. The disparity in test items at various ages is striking when one considers that among preverbal infants and young children, there is no opportunity for assessing language, and one is inferring overall intelligence mostly from nonverbal tasks. It is apparent that the skills necessary to master many of the complex motor and perceptual developmental milestones are not the same as those that underlie overall intellectual capacity in older children.

In addition to the fact that very different functional domains are assessed early and later on, the uneven *rate* of children's development limits the stability of IQ. Skill development does not proceed in smooth, gradual progression, nor at the same rate in all children. There are discrete periods of sudden increments, and these may occur relatively early or late. Their timing has little bearing on ultimate ability. Compared to the norm, if a child develops a skill early in life, we consider the youngster precocious. However, precocity is not a reliable index of superior ability. An example in point is the development of walking. Those who have observed infants appreciate how complex and difficult walking is when it first begins. Some do it early, by the age of ten months for example, others not until three months later. Both milestones are within the norm, but the age difference is very large; it represents almost one-third of the life span of the early walker. Yet, there is no reason to expect that the two types of children will ultimately differ in walking ability. Thus, precocity does not always indicate true superiority, and vice versa. There is enough similarity in eventual skill between slow and rapid developers as to render early assesment an inaccurate predictor of end-point ability.

In summary, two principles of development prevent satisfactory early assessment of later ability. One is the fact that important aspects of later function cannot be tested early in life. And two is that although the timing, or initial appearance, of ability varies, this early variation is often unrelated to eventual capacity.

Testing of School-Age Children

The Stanford-Binet is standardized on groups up to age eighteen, and therefore can be used for school-age children. The nature of the tasks changes with the age level; they are heavily weighted for verbal ability.

The Wechsler Intelligence Scale for Children—Revised (WISC-R) is appropriate for ages six through sixteen years. It includes eleven subtests. The verbal scale includes: information, similarities, arithmetic, vocabulary, comprehension, and digit span. The performance scale includes picture comprehension, picture arrangement, block design, object assembly, and coding. Both scales are very well standardized and have been shown to be reliable.

As noted earlier, the advantages of the Wechsler test over the Stanford-Binet test is that the Wechsler provides separate IQs for verbal and performance scales. Furthermore, the subtests are organized by type of task and thereby provide a quantitative estimate of a child's ability in various areas of knowledge and competence.

However, this aspect of the Wechsler test has some disadvantages. The fact that two IQ scores are generated has created the erroneous notion that there are separate types of intelligence, one verbal and the other nonverbal. Yet, the two IQ scores are highly correlated and do not represent independent abilities. The same thing is true for the subtests that comprise the verbal and performance scales. Each test has been reified, by some, as representing discrete abilities; yet, there is great overlap in the functions assessed by each subtest.

Another unfortunate practice is to view all the component aspects of mental development as proceeding at the same rate. Consequently, differences in subtest scores, called test scatter, are interpreted as reflecting pathology, either of emotional or organic origin. As a consequence it is not uncommon for clinicians to interpret differences in verbal and performance scale scores, as well as among subtest scores, as having diagnostic significance. There is ample evidence that score inconsistency is the rule, not the exception (Kaufman, 1979). Therefore, scatter on the WISC tests is not an index of psychopathology or brain damage. However, it can reflect differences in various abilities and may permit a description of children's strengths and weaknesses. When very large differences occur, they are a signal to look further, but, in themselves they have no precise diagnostic meaning.

To document this point, it is helpful to review the data from the standardization of the test. Among the 2,200 children who comprised the normative sample, the *average* difference between the lowest and highest scores on two subtests was 7 points (the scores can range from 1 to 20, 10 being average). Similarly, a difference somewhat greater than 7 was found in 50% of the children (Kaufman, 1976a). The average difference between the verbal and performance IQ was 8. It can be expected that 50% of nonclinic children will have verbal-performance discrepancies of 7 to 8 points (Kaufman, 1976b). Because the differences between subtest scores are unstable, score differences should be calculated between the scale score and the *average* of the subtests (either verbal, performance, or all) to obtain a more accurate measure of interest scatter. This approach also requires caution, since 30% of normal children will have discrepancies of at least 3 points from their own average score on three subtests (Kaufman, 1976b).

The advantage of the Wechsler scale is that it gives the opportunity for signaling that a child may have specific difficulties. For example, test results indicating a high performance IQ but a very low verbal IQ would legitimately raise the possibility of a language disorder. Future evaluation would be necessary to elucidate this question, since the IQ test alone would not suffice for a definitive diagnostic statement. Score discrepancies, when large, are signals to look further. (There may seem to be an inconsistency in the juxtaposition of the two arguments that (1) the verbal and performance IQs do not reflect totally different types of intelligence, and (2) that score discrepancies between the two IQs are very common. There are differences between the tasks in each scale that may influence performance, but these are not clearly related to differences in reasoning ability or overall intelligence. The tests of the performance scale are almost all timed and may require motor ability; this is not true of the tests on the verbal scale. These no-intellectual factors may affect performance.)

A rapid screening measure of IQ is the Peabody Vocabulary Test. The child is told a word and has to point to the picture that represents it. Because no verbal expression is called for, the test is not adequate for diagnostic purposes, and adequate performance cannot be construed as ruling out the presence of specific intellectual deficits that require expressive language and comprehension of more complex verbal materials.

Misconceptions Regarding IQ Testing

There are many misconceptions regarding IQ. Those encountered frequently are discussed briefly. The comments apply to IQ scores obtained from individually administered tests and not to group IQ tests that present their own special problems.

Johnny has an IQ of 125. An IQ score is not a characteristic that one possesses, as eye color. It is a score obtained on a test. Different IQ tests will yield different scores. A more accurate restatement of the foregoing is: Johnny obtained an IQ score of 125 on the WISC-R. His actual score on the test probably falls between 120 and 130. The statement as originally phrased communicates an unwarranted degree of exactness regarding IQ scores. This practice often leads to attributing undue importance to differences of 5-10 points at different times.

IQ scores mean nothing because they can change radically from one testing to another. Over short time spans, IQ scores are very stable. The correlation between individual scores and true scores is about 0.90. It is possible for IQ scores to be affected by environmental factors such as the race and skill of the examiner, the temporary mood state of the child (fatigue, anger, poor motivation), but, in general, only to a slight degree—not to the point where children will show large drops or increases in IQ. IQ scores are among the most robust test measures. By that, we mean that they are not vulnerable to capricious vagaries of circumstances surrounding the testing procedure or to changes in the child's mental health.

Since IQ scores are stable, they do not change over time. Reports of stability of IQ are expressed in correlational terms. These refer to *groups* of individuals. It is true that, in groups, those with high scores at one time will be overrepresented among those with high scores at a future time. However, this important observation is misinterpreted as indicating that IQ is an unmodifiable individual characteristic. It is not only possible, but very frequent, for the IQs of individuals to change to a remarkable degree over long periods of time (e.g., Honzik et al., 1948; Pinneau, 1961).

When very large differences occur at two time points, they generally reflect gradual shifts, not sudden fluctuations. Therefore, when we report that an individual's IQ may differ by 50 points over time, the conclusion should not be that the first time the IQ was 80, the second 130, and the third time it was 30. The discrepancies are not random but follow a pattern, which is probably related to the timing of skill development and environmental factors. Decrements in IQ are often associated with impoverishment of environmental opportunities for intellectual development, and increments with intellectual stimulation. For example, if a six year old is a slow maturer but has grown up in a richly stimulating environment, the child's early IQ may seriously underestimate later scores. The converse situation could also occur.

Large discrepancies between verbal and performance IQs are common among children with high IQ. The erroneous notion has gained credence that large verbal-performance IQ discrepancies (of 15 points or more) are not unusual if they occur among children of high IQ, as compared to those with average low IQs. This is not the case. IQ scale differences are unrelated to children's IQ levels, or to their age, social class, or race.

Children from socially disadvantaged homes have lower verbal than performance IQ. It is often assumed that an unstimulating environment penalizes the development of verbal skills but not manipulative, nonverbal reasoning. Social disadvantage is a nonselective handicap; it affects all aspects of mental development. It is important for professionals to appreciate that there is no component of mental ability that is spared the deleterious effects of an intellectually limiting milieu.

The child's potential ability is higher than the IQ score indicates. It is very commonplace for psychologists to state that a child's IQ score underestimates the youngster's true ability. (Claims that the IQ score has overestimated ability are conspicuously nonexistent.) Psychologists often come to this optimistic conclusion because they assume that psychopathology depresses IQ scores. Therefore, performance is necessarily reduced if a child is seen in times of difficulty; the expectation is that when well, the child will obtain higher scores on IQ tests. As a rule, psychological disturbance does not have a deleterious effect on IQ, though in some children it may. This possibility should be considered if the IQ score is clearly inconsistent with a youngster's premorbid performance. In such cases, a plan to reevaluate the child is essential.

In another instance, a child might indeed have better intellectual ability than the overall test result indicates if the IQ score is depressed by low scores on parts of the test that involve little reasoning, such as the repetition of numbers (digit span) or the mechanical writing task (coding).

The circumstances are very limited for conjecturing better intellectual ability than provided by the test. One can only conclude that the extremely frequent reporting of better potential intelligence in children than indicated by IQ scores is, for the most part, unjustified, perhaps motivated by well-wishing goals.

Since intelligence is inherited, IQ is unchangeable. Puzzlingly, some retain the notion that characteristics that are influenced by heredity are immutable. There is excellent evidence demonstrating the positive influence of education on IQ, and the detrimental effects of inadequate environments. These findings do not challenge the notion that genetic influences exist.

Jane is an overachiever, her academic achievement is too good for her IQ. It is often ignored that IQ tests estimate ability and are not precise instruments of it. They tap only some of the skills that are necessary for school achievement. If a child's grades and school placement seem better than one would anticipate given her IQ scores, consideration should be given to the possibility that the test has failed to assess some of the factors that go into being a good student.

At times, children who are excelling in school are discouraged from pursuing academic goals because their IQ score is felt to be inadequate. The child is viewed as an overachiever. Overachievement is a term often used but whose validity is without empirical basis. We do not know enough about its meaning to permit us to counsel children to abandon specific goals. It is illuminating to note that, among professionals, a wide range of IQ is represented. For example, among a group of lawyers enlisted in the Air Force, scores obtained on a group test ranged from 94 to 157 (Brody and Brody, 1976). Though the average IQ score of the lawyers was high (127.6), it seems that superior IQ scores are not a necessary condition for obtaining an advanced degree. It is also noteworthy that among these professionals subnormal IQ scores were nonexistent. Therefore, a minimum level of performance is necessary, but that minimum is not very high. It follows that in any one individual it is not necessary to rule out higher education in the absence of a superior IQ score.

IQ tests are discriminatory because ethnic groups differ in test scores. Many well-intentioned, but uninformed, objections to IQ testing would be avoided if it were understood that IQ tests do not measure innate ability. Whatever capacities psychologists assess, these are always the result of interactions between biological and environmental events. There is no way of identifying how much of a child's intelligence is the result of felicitous or poor genetic material, and how much is due to experiential factors. If it were generally appreciated that in individual cases the two processes cannot be extricated, and that an IQ score cannot estimate the person's true potential, much resentment of IQ testing might be eliminated.

This issue bears on the concerns regarding the testing of children from minority groups. In the United States these youngsters obtain lower IQ scores than white children. As a result, some have demanded that IQ tests be banned in minority groups. This view would have merit if it were shown that IQ scores have less predictive validity among various ethnic and racial groups. However, similar predictive value and similar patterns of performance have been found to exist in various groups.

High IQ is associated with better academic achievement regardless of the group's racial composition, and the factors derived from IQ tests do not differ between whites and blacks (Reynolds, 1982). (It has been suggested that intelligence tests may not reflect the same intellectual processes in white advantaged and black disadvantaged children. However, this possibility has not been well studied.)

Since we know that social disadvantage limits intellectual development, it would seem more sensible to indict the social conditions that have contributed to limiting the cognitive development of minority children, rather than to indict the tests that document the tremendous price our society pays for its pervasive discriminatory practices.

The issue of racial difference in IQ continues to arouse much interest and passion on both sides of the controversy. It is unlikely that either side will be able to provide irrefutable arguments as long as social inequities continue. As clinicians involved in educational planning for children, we should be aware of the practical implications of the debate regarding the claim that certain racial ethnic groups have lower intelligence due to constitutional factors.

As mentioned, IQ differences between white and black children are factual. What is in doubt is the origin of these differences (for a review of these issues, see Richardson et al., 1972). Of crucial importance is the very large overlap in IQ distributions between the racial groups. Therefore, knowing the race of a child does not provide useful information regarding intellectual resources. As a consequence, racial identification cannot serve any purpose for educational placement or diagnostic assessment, and racial differences should not influence practice whether it be educational or clinical. Academic assessment and clinical evaluations should proceed regardless of a child's race, and race can never explain deficits identified through formal testing.

Academic Skills

Clinicians are concerned mostly about a child's ability to read, spell, and perform arithmetic. For all these, performance must be interpreted in the light of IQ. Discrepancies between ability and IQ signal the possible presence of a disorder. Therefore, academic test results are interpretable only when one knows overall intellectual ability.

READING. The most important skill for academic performance is reading. To that end, the recognition of words is necessary, but clearly not sufficient. In addition, language construction and comprehension are essential.

There are many very well standardized tests of reading. As with all clinical evaluations, reading must be tested on an individual basis; results from group testing should not be relied upon to make important decisions about a child.

The Wide Range Achievement Test of reading is widely used because it requires little time and is very well standardized. However, it has the important limitation of being a measure of word recognition exclusively. Many children perform adequately on this reading task, but are deficient when presented with meaningful text. Word-recognition tests may be useful to spot some reading handicaps; however, they are not satisfactory for ruling out difficulties in reading.

There are a number of reading tests that consist of prose and include an assessment of comprehension. Some well-standardized oral tests include the Gilmore and the Durell. The Gilmore generates three reading scores: accuracy, comprehension, and rate. Its limitation is that it cannot be used for children beyond the eighth grade. The Durell is applicable to children through the sixth grade only and does not have norms for comprehension.

The Gray Oral Reading Test is one of the widely used tests for paragraph reading and reading comprehension. Its advantage is that it has reading material up to twelfth-grade level. Unfortunately, the group of children on whom it was normed was small, and their average IQ was above average. Another detriment is that no norms are provided for the comprehension test.

These are all oral tests. Their advantage is that the examiner can observe the type of errors a child makes while reading, and may thereby identify sources of difficulty that might lead to specific therapeutic recommendations. However, much of the reading done in and out of school after the very first years is silent. There are some children who perform satisfactorily on oral reading tests, and yet their teachers report poor language skills. In some instances the use of paper-and-pencil reading tests is appropriate. There are many very well standardized measures for all grades that were devised as group tests, such as the SRA Achievement Series which includes very early reading skills, the Iowa Silent Reading tests, and the Stanford Achievement Tests.

All these silent tests have been standardized using very large groups (up to 70,000 in some cases) with great care to obtain truly representative samples of the U.S. population. Furthermore, these tests all have considerable validity in predicting children's school performance. They can be used for clinical purposes, provided the child is supervised during the task in order to be certain that he or she has expended appropriate effort to perform the task. Some of the tests are time-consuming (from twenty minutes to one hour for the reading and language tests), and that may be why they are not more frequently used in clinical settings. They should be viewed as screening procedures and not as diagnostic instruments, since they rely heavily on verbal ability.

The Peabody Individual Achievement Test (PIAT) is the only individual test of achievement that includes a range of academic content. Both reading recognition and comprehension are included. It is easy to administer and includes norms from kindergarten to twelfth grade, making it widely applicable. The reliability of the reading recognition test is good, but that of the reading comprehension is relatively low. On the whole, this test is less reliable than the group achievement tests. However, it is a useful screening device. The types of difficulty encountered by children with disorders of reading can be assessed. For this purpose there is little need for norms obtained from the general population. Rather, the issue is whether the child is able to perform various important aspects of reading such as syllabification, decoding of beginning, middle, and end sounds, blending of sounds, etc. (This type of testing is known as criterion-referenced, since the goal is to ascertain whether a criterion of performance is met by the child.) Several other measures are available for this purpose: the Roswell-Chall tests, the Woodcock Reading Mastery Test, the Durell Analysis of Reading Difficulty Test, the Bryant (Bryant, 1983), and the Standard Reading Tests (Daniels and Diack, 1973). All have the goal of identifying the deficient aspects of decoding in a child diagnosed as having a disorder of reading.

Clinicians often look for possible language impairment in children with reading dysfunction, since reading is a symbolic language task not the mere recognition of printed forms. A growing body of data indicates that reading impairment is associated with deficits in language development.

Besides impaired language development, other types of disturbances have been reported in disorders of reading, such as poor visual and auditory perception leading to misinterpretations of reading matter, and poor sequencing ability leading to a deficit in organization of words into meaningful structure. Attentional defects have also been reported in children with reading disabilities.

As a result, a typology of reading has emerged: some types characterized by verbal/language deficits, others by graphomotor difficulties, as well as other types, all based on the pattern of a child's performance on various psychological tests (e.g., Mattis et al., 1975; Rourke, 1978). The diagnostic subclassification of reading disorders is potentially important. However, so far there is no evidence that the patterns of test scores used to classify children are reliable, that children with different syndromes differ in the types of reading failure, that the various types respond differently to treatment, or that their outcomes differ. Therefore, we must conclude that, at present, psychological testing of children for purposes of diagnosing different types of reading disorders has no established validity. Whether it will eventually emerge as useful is unknown. Therefore, at this time it cannot be recommended that children with reading deficits routinely receive costly extensive testing of cognitive development.

ARITHMETIC. The WISC-R includes an arithmetic test. It is a timed, oral test that relies exclusively on mental computation and, therefore, is insufficient to assess mathematical skill. The ability to perform mental arithmetic problems is not identical to the demands required to do written problems where one has a graphic display of one's work and computation can be done in writing. Consequently, the testing of arithmetic ability cannot be limited to the test on the IQ test.

Tests of arithmetic include those on the Wide-Range Achievement Test, where no contextual reading is required, the Peabody Individual Achievement Test, and the mathematics tests of any of the group achievement tests noted. All are well standardized. It is important to note that performance on the mathematics tests is influenced greatly by the curriculum a child has been exposed to. It is important to ascertain that the capacities tested have been taught to the child before inferring an arithmetical disorder.

SPELLING. Poor reading is associated with poor spelling. But many poor spellers are fine readers. Children are not brought to professional attention because of poor spelling. The assessment of this skill is performed to provide a comprehensive assessment of a child's strengths and weaknesses. It is not an essential diagnostic procedure.

The best measures are those that demand writing from dictation (encoding) rather than the recognition of spelling errors from printed words. The Wide Range Achievement Test (WRAT) contains such a test and is very well standardized.

ADDITIONAL SKILLS. It is possible to assess children's academic skills other than reading and arithmetic—for example, science and social studies. However, this is rarely done for clinical purposes. Tests that provide norms for performance in a variety of academic areas include all the group achievement tests noted under the section dealing with reading.

Other Assessments

There is a new and growing branch of psychological assessment that specializes in the evaluation of specific mental abilities, such as language development, and, by extension, brain damage and dysfunction. Historically, it had its beginning in the work of those involved in the study of brain-damaged individuals. Because one of the major concerns of this field is the relationship of brain function to behavior, it has become known as neuropsychology.

It is a specialized, empirical discipline whose practices are changing relatively quickly based on evolving research findings. Therefore, it would be misleading to discuss the use of various assessments as if they were established. A complicating factor in presenting current practices is the idiosyncratic manner in which psychologists proceed in their clinical assessment of children. Unlike the field of intelligence testing that has very well established procedures, there is no standard means for testing component aspects of cognitive ability in children. The application of neuropsychology to the clinical assessment of children is a new field, and many changes are likely forthcoming.

A very schematic summary of assessment of language and brain damage is presented to acquaint the reader with some of the approaches used. However, it should not be construed as a comprehensive survey of currently available measures. Unfortunately, there is no text available that summarizes this branch of testing in children.

LANGUAGE DYSFUNCTION. The diagnostic concern in evaluating a cognitive ability such as language is whether the development of specific functions is impaired *relative to overall ability*. The performance of a child on cognitive measures is interpretable only in the context of intellectual ability. If two children perform identically on language tests, but one has retarded overall intellectual functioning and the other does not, the scores will have very different implications. Therefore, it is essential to obtain IQ scores in order to interpret properly a child's performance on measures of language function.

Most of the tests used to evaluate language, as well as other specific aspects of mental development, do not have well-established norms. This shortcoming makes it difficult to pinpoint the magnitude of dysfunction or delay, except in clearly abnormal cases. Consequently, it is ill-advised to reach important diagnostic conclusions on the basis of a single measure. If abnormality is suspected, assessment on several measures of language is called for to provide a confluence of information on which to base a decision.

One approach to the assessment of language disorders has been to distinguish between phonological, structural, and syntactic components of language. Phonological content refers to the sounds of language. These are measures that enable the detecting of difficulty in a child's decoding ability (they are mentioned in the section on reading). The structural aspect of language refers to its grammatical structure, the syntactic to its content. There is a great deal of overlap among these three constructs, but it is helpful to distinguish them to identify areas of deficiency.

Perhaps the best known test of language skills is the Illinois Test of Psycholinguistic Abilities (ITPA). It has the appealing characteristic of including twelve subscales, thereby giving the impression that it provides a comprehensive assessment of language. Its practical disadvantage is that the norms are only for children up to the age of ten. Therefore, only gross deficiencies can be detected in older adolescents. Of greater concern is the failure to demonstrate diagnostic validity for the test. Furthermore, ITPA scores are strongly influenced by IQ. As noted earlier, this is a detriment in a measure of cognitive skill, since we are interested in knowing if a child has a specific deficiency, not one that is mostly a function of IQ. The ITPA does not meet this goal.

Many of the other instruments used in the assessment of language disorders have been adapted from those developed for adult aphasia (Spreen and Benton, 1969). They focus on language comprehension, repetition, and naming tasks. A well-known test of simple comprehension is the Token Test (De Renzi and Vignolo, 1962). It evaluates the child's ability to comprehend simple verbal instructions. Commands are given, using various colored circles and rectangles. The easiest is "touch the red circle," the most difficult is "before touching the yellow circle, pick up the red rectangle."

Tests of sentence repetition include the Stanford-Binet Memory Test for Sentences and the Spreen-Benton Memory for Sentences Test. Naming tests consist of the presentation of pictures which have to be named by the child, such as the Rapid Automatized Naming Test; other tests require the child to find words spontaneously.

In naming tests, clinicians look for deficits in word retrieval, a form of anomia which may vary in severity from mild to severe. Mild-word retrieval problems may be characterized by accurate but slow performance. More severe word-retrieval problems would be suspected in those who, instead of labeling the object, give a description of its function. Other types of misses, or paraphasias, consist of distortions so that a noun close to the correct one is given (milophone for xylophone, for example), substitutions for similar sounding nouns (telescope for stethoscope), or substitutions for nouns with similar functions (glass for cup).

BRAIN DAMAGE AND DYSFUNCTION. Only a highly condensed and limited coverage of this topic is attempted. The limited goal is to introduce some of the approaches used in the assessment of brain damage in children. One of the most unfortunate traditions in psychology is the testing for "organicity" or "brain damage." This concept has carried the implicit notion that brain damage is a unitary concept that can be detected with specific tests designed to elicit organicity. The belief that there are tests of organicity, or that there is a battery of tests that will unerringly reveal the presence of brain damage, needs to be dispelled. Testing for brain damage has not yet reached this level of precision.

There are two types of assessment for brain damage. One, where there has been a known insult or trauma, the other where no definite positive history exists, but the presence of brain dysfunction or damage is suspected.

For children with documented brain injury, testing is done to provide objective information regarding the child's mental abilities and handicaps. Cognitive impairments may be subtle, though clinically important, and may be missed in the absence of systematic evaluation. Evaluations should be performed at regular intervals to determine the course of identified difficulties and to check on the possibility of delayed appearance of other dysfunctions. Specific intervals for assessment will depend on the age of the child, the nature of the insults, and the magnitude of the impairment obtained initially.

The testing for brain damage in children without known trauma has a different goal. Assessment is often conducted to establish a diagnosis, as well as to evaluate current disabilities. The diagnostic procedures for determining brain damage have greater validity than the ones for other so-called functional psychiatric disorders but they are not without problems.

The general approach is to assess functions that are known to be affected in individuals with frank brain lesions, and to infer the presence of central nervous system dysfunction based upon a confluence of findings. A number of developmental abilities are assessed to make the diagnosis of brain dysfunction. Disorders of language are preeminent in this assessment. Visual perceptual development is often examined when assessing a child for possible brain dysfunction. To this end, the Children's Embedded Figures Test may be used. It requires the child to find the "hidden," embedded, design in a picture.

In addition, visual-motor development is of concern. The tests commonly used are the Bender-Gestalt test, for which scores with norms are available for children from five to ten (Koppitz, 1964, 1975), and the Developmental Test of Visual-Motor Integration, which also has age norms, from two to fifteen years. Both tests require the copying of printed geometric figures. These tests have a graphomotor component.

Because the motor system is often affected by brain damage, other motor abnormality may be looked for. The Purdue Pegboard is a motor test that requires the child to place pegs in spaces on a board. Performance with each hand and with both hands is recorded.

Vigilance, or the ability to sustain attention, may be examined when the integrity of the central nervous system is in question. Unfortunately, there is no measure of vigilance or attention that has demonstrated validity. Several measures exist, such as: The Porteus Maze Test, where a child must draw a line from the center of printed mazes to the exit; the Matching Familiar Figures Test, requiring the identification of one of several pictures as being identical to the model presented; and cancellation tests, where the child must cross out a specific symbol (letters, numbers, or geometric pictures) from an array in which the critical symbol appears randomly. None of these measures has been shown to be satisfactory for determining the presence of attentional disorders or to be better than clinical observations.

Visual-spatial constructional abilities may also be tested, via the use of tests of block design assembly such as the Block Design Test of the WISC-R. If impairment is found, it remains to be determined whether the difficulties lie in the visual-spatial perceptual system or in the constructional demands of the task.

Other forms of perceptual impairment can be assessed—the recognition of facial expressions for example—where photographs of adults expressing common emotions such as anger, sadness, and fear have to be identified; or spatial orientation, which includes right-left orientation, and the ability to perceive objects in space such as on the Block Counting Task of the Stanford-Binet where the task requires the child to infer, on a design, the presence of blocks that are not visible on the card but are hidden by other blocks.

Finally, various aspects of memory may be impaired, such as visual memory. The Benton Visual Retention Test requires children to reproduce geometric designs they have been shown. Tests of auditory memory, which involve repetition or recall of verbal materials, have been mentioned in the discussion on language.

By integrating findings from the preceding assessments, as well as a number of other developmental functions, inferences may be drawn about the likelihood of the presence of brain dysfunction. However, it is important to note that information obtained from tests can only be interpreted properly in the context of the child's IQ, history, and current clinical status.

Conclusions

Psychological testing of children has much to offer in documenting overall intellectual development, scholastic progress, and other abilities. It is best viewed as a means of assessing cognitive assets and limitations, and not as a means of classification or diagnosis. Psychological test results provide important information about current status, but they are not tools for predicting future status, especially in young children.

Too much is generally expected from psychological testing. An objective examination of its usefulness should not lead to the proverbial discarding of the baby with the bathwater. A baby exists, if conclusions are restricted to observations derived from well-standardized instruments with demonstrated reliability. Psychological testing is in an unusually advantageous position in behavioral science since it has such measures. The unfortunate history of these tests lies in the unwarranted claims that have been advanced for them. The statement made by Meehl in 1956 is still most appropriate.

> A great deal of skilled psychological effort is probably being wasted in going through complex, skill demanding, time consuming test procedures of moderate to low validity, in order to arrive at conclusions about the patient which could often be made with high confidence without the test, and which in other cases ought not to be made (because they still tend to be wrong).

References

Breidenbaugh, B., Brozovich, R., and Matheson, L. 1974. The Hand test and other aggressive indicators in emotionally disturbed children. *J. Pers. Assess.*, 38:332-334.

Brody, E. B., and Brody, N. 1976. *Intelligence: Nature determinants and consequences.* New York: Academic Press.

Bryant, N. D. 1983. *Diagnostic test of basic reading decoding skills.* New York: Teacher's College Press.

Daniels, J. C., and Diack, H. 1973. *The standard reading tests.* London: Chatto and Windus.

De Renzi, E., and Vignolo, L. A. 1962. A token test for the measurement of dysphasia. *Brain,* 85:665–678.

Gittelman, R. 1980. The role of psychological tests for differential diagnosis in child psychiatry. *J. Am. Acad. Child Psych.,* 19:413–437.

Gittelman-Klein, R. 1978. Validity of projective tests for psychodiagnosis in children. In *Critical issues in psychiatric diagnosis,* ed. R. L. Spitzer and D. F. Klein, pp. 141–166. New York: Raven Press.

Hammer, M., and Kaplan, A. M. 1966. The reliability of children's human figure drawings. *J. Clin. Psychol.,* 22:316–319.

Honzig, M. P., MacFarlane, J. W., and Allen, L. 1948. The stability of mental test performance between two and eighteen years. *J. Exper. Ed.,* 17:309–324.

Kagan, J. 1956. The measurement of overt aggression from fantasy. *J. Abnorm. Soc. Psychol.,* 52:390–393.

Kaufman, A. S. 1976. Verbal performance IQ discrepancies on the WISC-R. *J. Consult. Clin. Psychol.,* 44:739–744.

———. 1976b. A new approach to the interpretation of test scatter on the WISC-R. *J. Learn. Disabil.,* 9:160–68.

———. 1979. *Intelligent testing with the WISC-R.* New York: Wiley.

Kelly, R., and Berg, B. 1978. Measuring children's reactions to divorce. *J. Clin. Psychol.,* 34:215–222.

Kline, P. 1976. *Psychological testing.* London: Malaby Press.

Koppitz, E. M. 1963. *The Bender Gestalt test for young children.* New York: Grune and Stratton.

Koppitz, E. M. 1975. *The Bender Gestalt test for young children: Research and application, 1963–1973.* New York: Grune and Stratton.

Lachar, D., and LaCombe, J. A. 1983. An introduction to the personality inventory for children: Applications in the school setting. *School Psychol. Rev.,* 12:399–406.

Levitt, E. E., and Truumaa, A. 1972. *The Rorschach technique with children and adolescents: Application and norms.* New York: Grune and Stratton.

Lifschitz, M. 1975. Social differentiation and organization of the Rorschach in fatherless and two-parented children. *J. Clin. Psychol.,* 31:126–130.

Mattis, S., French, J., and Rapin, I. 1975. Dyslexia in children and young adults: Three independent neuropsychological syndromes. *Dev. Med. Child Neurol.,* 17:150–163.

Meehl, P. E. 1956. Wanted—a good cookbook. *Am. Psychologist,* 11:263–272.

North, G. E., and Keiffer, R. S. 1966. Thematic productions of children in foster homes. *Psychol. Rep.,* 19:43–46.

Pinneau, S. R. 1961. *Changes in intelligence quotient from infancy to maturity.* Boston: Houghton Mifflin.

Reddy, P. V. 1960. A study of the reliability and validity of the children's apperception test. *Brit. J. Ed. Psychol.,* 30:182–184.

Reynolds, C. 1982. The problem of bias in psychological assessment. In *The handbook of school psychology,* ed. C. R. Reynolds, and T. B. Gutkin, pp. 178–208. New York: Wiley.

Richardson, K., Spears, D., and Richards, M., (eds.) 1972. *Race and intelligence: The fallacies behind the race-IQ controversy.* Baltimore, Md.

Rourke, B. P. 1978. Reading, spelling, arithmetic disabilities: A neuropsychological perspective. In *Progress in learning disabilities,* ed. H. H. Myklebust, pp. 97–120. New York: Grune and Stratton.

Schafer, R. 1978. Criteria for judging the adequacy of interpretations. In *Problems of human assessment,* ed. D. N. Jackson, and S. Messick, pp. 559-574. Huntington, N.Y.: R. E. Krieger Co.

Spreen, O., and Benton, A. L. 1969. *Neurosensory center comprehensive examination for aphasia.* Neuropsychology Laboratory, University of Victoria, Victoria, B.C., Canada.

Trahan, D., and Stricklin, A. 1979. Bender-Gestalt emotional indicators and acting-out behavior in young children. *J. Pers. Assess.,* 43:365-375.

Weiss, J. L. 1978. The clinical use of psychological tests. In *Harvard guide to modern psychiatry,* ed. A. M. Nichol, pp. 41-55. Cambridge, Mass.: Belknap Press.

APPENDIX

The following is a list of the psychological tests mentioned in the text. The age range to which the tests are applicable is indicated in parentheses.

Bayley Scales of Infant Development
(2-30 mo.)
The Psychological Corporation
757 Third Avenue
New York, NY 10017

Bender-Gestalt Test (4 yr. and above)
Western Psychological Services
12031 Wilshire Boulevard
Los Angeles, CA 90025

Benton Visual Retention Test
(8 yr. and above)
The Psychological Corporation
757 Third Avenue
New York, NY 10017

Children's Apperception Test (CAT)
(3-10 yr.)
Human Sciences Press
72 Fifth Avenue
New York, NY 10011

Children's Embedded Figures Test
(5-12 yr.)
Consulting Psychologists Press
577 College Avenue
Palo Alto, CA 94306

Developmental Test of Visual Motor Integration (2-15 yr.)
Follett Publishing Company
1010 West Washington
Chicago, IL 60607

Durell Analysis of Reading Difficulty (grades 1-6)
The Psychological Corporation
757 Third Avenue
New York, NY 10017

Durrel-Sullivan Reading Capacity and Achievement Tests (grades 2-6)
World Book Company
Merchandise Mart Plaza
Rm. 510
Chicago, IL 60654

Gilmore Oral Reading Test (grades 1-8)
The Psychological Corporation
757 Third Avenue
New York, NY 10017

Gray Oral Reading Tests (grades 1-16)
Bobbs-Merrill Company, Inc.
4300 West 62nd Street
Indianapolis, IN 46206

Illinois Test of Psycholinguistic Abilities (2-10 yr.)
University of Illinois Press
Urbana, IL 61801

Matching Familiar Figures Test (6 + years)
Jerome Kagan, Ph.D.
Harvard University
33 Kirkland St., 1510 William James Hill
Cambridge, MA 02138

McCarthy Scales of Children's Abilities
(2.5–8.5 yr.)
The Psychological Corporation
757 Third Avenue
New York, NY 10017

Peabody Individual Achievement Test
(grades kgn.–12)
American Guidance Service
Circle Pines, MN 55014

Peabody Picture Vocabulary Test
(2.5–18 yr.)
American Guidance Service
Circle Pine, MN 55014

Porteus Maze Test (3 + yr.)
The Psychological Corporation
757 Third Avenue
New York, NY 10017

Purdue Pegboard (5 yr. +)
Science Research Associates
259 East Erie Street
Chicago, IL 60611

Rapid Automatized Naming (3–11 yr.)
Rita Rudel. Ph.D.
Box 29, Neurological Institute
710 West 168th Street
New York, NY 10032

Rorschach (3 yr. and above)
Grune and Stratton, Inc.
111 Fifth Avenue
New York, NY 10003

Roswell-Chall Auditory Blending Tests
(6 yr. +)
Essay Press
P.O. Box 5, Planetarium Station
New York, NY 10024

Roswell-Chall Diagnostic Reading Test
(6 yr. +)
(see above)

SRA Achivement Series (grades 1–9)
Science Research Associates, Inc.
155 North Wacker Drive
Chicago, IL 60606

The Standard Reading Tests, 1973 (5–9 yr.)
Chatto and Windus
3 Upper James Street
London W1R 4BT, England

Stanford Achievement Test, 1982
(grades 1.5–9.5)
The Psychological Corporation
757 Third Avenue
New York, NY 10017

Stanford-Binet Intelligence Scale, Form L-M, 1972 (2 yr.-adult)
Riverside Publishing Company
1919 South Highland Avenue
Lombard, IL 60148

Thematic Apperception Test (TAT)
(4 yr. and above)
Harvard University Press
79 Garden Street
Cambridge, MA 02138

Weschsler Intelligence Scale for Children—Revised, 1974 (6–17 yr.)
The Psychological Corporation
757 Third Avenue
New York, NY 10017

Wechsler Preschool and Primary Scale of Intelligence, 1967 (4–6.5 yr.)
The Psychological Corporation
(see above)

Wide Range Achievement Test (5 yr.-adult)
Jastak Associates, Inc.
1526 Gilpin Avenue
Wilmington, DE 19806

Woodcock Reading Mastery Test
(kgn.–12th grade)
American Guidance Service
Circle Pines, MN 55014

25

Organization and Use of *DSM-III*

Dennis P. Cantwell

It will be the purpose of this chapter to describe the principles of classification of psychiatric disorders of childhood; to describe the organization of the *Diagnostic and Statistical Manual of Mental Disorders (DSM-III)* including its unique features; to describe multiaxial system and how to use it; and to give a detailed description of the section in *DSM-III* describing psychiatric disorders of infancy, childhood, and adolescence. In addition, this chapter will address the use of *DSM-III* in the diagnostic process in child psychiatry and areas of contention and controversy surrounding its publication. A fuller discussion of some of the issues to be examined here can be found in the introduction to *DSM-III* and in several previous essays (Cantwell, 1980; Spitzer and Cantwell, 1980; Rutter and Shaffer, 1980; Achenbach, 1980; Gittelman, 1980).

Why Diagnose?

The diagnostic process in child psychiatry has been conceptualized in previous publications as geared toward answering a number of questions (Cohen, 1976; Cantwell, 1980). These questions will be briefly reviewed. The instruments available to the clinician in going through the diagnostic process and the role that *DSM-III* can play in the diagnostic process will then be discussed.

The questions that the diagnostic process is geared toward answering in child psychiatry include the following: (1) Does the child who is being presented for evaluation have any type of psychiatric disorder whatsoever? (2) If the child does have a psychiatric disorder, does the clinical picture of the disorder fit a known recognized clinical syndrome as described in *DSM-III*? (3) In this individual child, what are the intrapsychic, familial, social, and biological roots of the disorder, and what are the relative strengths of each of these roots? (4) What forces in this child are maintaining the problem? (5) What forces are facilitating the child's normal development? (6) What are this child's individual strengths and competencies? (7) What is the likely untreated natural history of this child's disorder? (8) Is intervention necessary in this particular case? (9) What types of intervention are most likely to be effective?

In order to respond properly to the last three questions, it is necessary to rely heavily on *DSM-III*. The answer to question 7 depends partly on the natural history of the clinical syndrome described in the answer to number 2. Thus, it is helpful if the child's clinical picture does meet that of a known and recognizable syndrome, since there is likely to be a body of knowledge recorded in the literature about untreated natural history. However, the answer to this question also depends partly on the answers to questions 3 through 6. The natural history of the child's disorder also determines how urgent we should be with our interventions and at what level we should intervene. It is obvious that a disorder (such as an anxiety disorder), which tends to pass with time and leaves little or no residual effects, requires much less urgent and much less intense intervention than a disorder (like infantile autism), which is likely to be significantly disabling without treatment.

The natural history of a child's disorder offers a test of the efficacy of our treatment modalities. For any single treatment or any combination of treatments to be considered efficacious with a particular problem, the outcome for that problem with treatment must be better than that which is obtained with no treatment at all.

The answers to questions 8 and 9 are facilitated if the child meets a definitive *DSM-III* diagnosis. In those cases there should be a body of literature reporting on different types of intervention techniques used with different types of disorders. However, it must be said that currently for many of the disorders this is not true. While many areas of child psychiatric research are weak, the areas of treatment intervention and assessment of treatment outcome are probably the weakest.

Treatment planning depends not only on the answer to question number 2 (what *DSM-III* diagnosis the child has) but also on the answers to questions 3 through 9. In fact, there are individual practitioners who feel that making a specific psychiatric diagnosis is not useful or important. For example, some who use a systems-oriented approach to diagnosis and treatment may feel that the individual child, although he may be presented for psychiatric evaluation, is really not the patient. Rather, a disordered family system is the true patient, and a categorical, behavioral-descriptive system like *DSM-III* does not allow for classification of pathological family systems. While this is true in some sense, many feel that the state of the art has not reached the point where a valid and reliable classification of family systems that has utility for clinical purposes and/or research purposes has yet been developed. Moreover, the making of an individual diagnosis in a child and/or in a parent does not preclude the use of any therapeutic orientation or the use of any therapeutic modality.

Likewise, there are those who say that the process of making a psychiatric diagnosis is merely a form of labeling a child and is a meaningless exercise for clinical purposes. As is emphasized elsewhere in this chapter, making a diagnosis does result in applying a label to the psychiatric disorder a child presents with. It does not result in applying a label to a child. A child may have measles at one age of his life and pneumonia at another age. He may present with one psychiatric disorder at one age and another disorder at a different age. For clinical purposes no one would state that it is a meaningless exercise to distinguish between measles and pneumonia. Therefore, it is difficult to fathom why it should be a meaningless exercise to distinguish similarly between two psychiatric disorders.

A third objection is often stated in a way that emphasizes the fact that the focus on a child's disorder may minimize the importance of the individual patient. The making of a psychiatric categorical diagnosis, such as a *DSM-III* diagnosis, does imply in many respects that the focus of scientific inquiry will be an individual disorder A or disorder B rather than the patient with disorder A or disorder B. This focus of scientific inquiry, however, in no way diminishes the importance of the child as an individual patient. Every child patient is a unique human being, and obviously this uniqueness must be taken into account in any doctor-patient relationship. This consideration is part of the art of medicine. However, excess emphasis on unique aspects of each patient and a lack of recognition of common factors shared by patients who present with a particular disorder will impede scientific study. For if patients share no common factors, then training and experience are valueless, and dealing with each new patient becomes a research project in itself.

For research purposes a valid diagnostic classification scheme is a vital necessity. If findings from various centers are to be compared, investigators with different theoretical backgrounds must have a common language with which they can communicate. A proper classification serves this purpose. A classification system emphasizes what a particular patient has in common with other patients. It is not to be confused with a diagnostic formulation which emphasizes what a particular patient has that is different from other patients. Both are necessary. One cannot do the work of another.

Principles of Classification of Childhood Psychiatric Disorders

The basic principles of classification in child psychiatry have been discussed fully elsewhere (Rutter, 1978; Cantwell, 1980). The important points will be reviewed briefly here.

Categorical and Dimensional Systems

Previous classification systems, including *DSM-I* and *DSM-II*, Group for Advancement of Psychiatry (GAP), and *DSM-III*, have been categorical in nature. The categorical approach to classification emphasizes the use of clinically obtained knowledge to set up specific diagnostic criteria for each psychiatric disorder. Thus, one either meets the criteria for one psychiatric disorder or another or may meet the criteria for more than one. A second approach, the dimensional approach, emphasizes statistical and mathematical methods to define specific syndromes. Mathematical techniques can then be applied to ascertain whether a given patient fits into a dimensionally defined syndrome.

These two approaches, although often thought of as mutually exclusive, may in fact be considered to be complementary to each other. Achenbach (1980) reviewed the evidence for the validity and stability of such mathematically defined syndromes of behavior. These are generally produced by factor, pattern, and cluster analyses of rating scales completed by parents, teachers, and significant others. Only some of these empirically derived syndromes have counterparts in *DSM-III*, although there does tend to be a large degree of overlap. There are mathematically derived syndromes that have no apparent counterpart in *DSM-III*, and likewise there are *DSM-III* diagnostic categories that apparently have no counterpart among mathematically derived syndromes of behavior as described by Achenbach.

Categorical Diagnoses

In other areas of medicine, etiology has often been assumed to be the best basis for classification. However, this is only true in those conditions in which known agents can be isolated and specific treatments can be applied from this knowledge. This is not necessarily so in all of general medicine. A phenomenological-descriptive approach to fractures (simple versus compound) offers much more information than an etiological one which would tell whether the fracture was due to an auto accident or being hit by a falling object. At the time of writing, it must be said that there is no absolutely "right way" or "natural way" to classify psychiatric disorders of childhood.

In child psychiatry there is a relative lack of hard facts regarding the natural history, family pattern, clinical features, etc., of various psychiatric disorders. We know much less than we do about the more traditional well-defined syndromes in adult psychiatry such as schizophrenia and major depressive disorder. In child psychiatry one man's fact is often still considered to be another man's fantasy, and yet for any classification system to be successful, it must be based as much as possible on known facts and not on theoretical concepts.

RELIABILITY. To structure a classification system effectively, the categories described must be reliable. Of course the categories must have validity as well, but a category cannot be valid if it is not reliable. It can be reliable, however, and not be valid. In diagnostic classification of psychiatric disorders, reliability means that when one patient is evaluated at a given time in a certain fashion by one clinician, that clinician will come up with the same diagnosis as another clinician who evaluated the same patient at the same time in a similar fashion. There are multiple sources of unreliability in psychiatric diagnosis: information variance, observation and interpretation variance, and criterion variance.

Information variance can be minimized by the use of standardized evaluation instruments such as interviews with the parents, interviews with the child, and behavior rating scales. Observation and interpretation variance can be reduced by training in rules of interpretation of clinical evidence. Criterion variance can be minimized by the use of operational diagnostic criteria. Probably the most ambitious effort to do so was that by Feighner and his colleagues from the Washington University School of Medicine in 1972 (Feighner et al., 1972). This was further elaborated by Spitzer et al. in the Research Diagnostic Criteria in 1975 (Spitzer et al., 1975). The *DSM-III* classification makes use of operational diagnostic criteria for psychiatric disorders in both childhood and in adults. Thus, only criterion variance can be minimized or eliminated by use of a diagnostic classification system itself, and then only if the diagnostic system utilizes operational diagnostic criteria to describe each psychiatric disorder.

VALIDITY. For a classification system to be effective for either clinical use or research use, the diagnostic categories in the system must have validity. The types of validity to be considered include: face validity, descriptive validity, and predictive validity. Face validity begins by obtaining descriptions from experienced clinicians about what they think the essential features of a particular psychiatric disorder of childhood are. Many of the categories in the childhood section of *DSM-III* currently have only face validity. Some also have descriptive validity. When a category has descriptive validity, it is characterized by symptoms that are not commonly seen in persons with other types of mental disorders or in individuals with no mental disorder, and it justifies the assumption that the psychiatric disorder represents a distinct behavioral syndrome rather than a random collection of clinical features.

From the standpoint of the clinician and the researcher, the most important type of validity is probably predictive validity. A classification system like *DSM-III* differentiates psychiatric disorders from each other on the basis of their clinical picture; predictive validity refers to ways in which these disorders differ *other* than in their clinical picture with respect to natural history, and response to treatment. In child psychiatry as compared to adult psychiatry, there is a relative lack of this type of knowledge leading to a lack of knowledge about predictive validity of the various types of psychiatric disorders described in *DSM-III* for children and adolescents.

DIFFERENTIATION AND COVERAGE. *DSM-III*, like all classification systems, must strive to provide adequate coverage. Thus, ideally we would like to see every child who presents for evaluation present with only one disorder and present with a disorder that is described somewhere within the classification system. This is unlikely to happen since we know from studies of adult psychiatric patients that 25% receive a diagnosis of undiagnosed mental disorder (Goodwin and Guze, 1979). In addition to providing adequate coverage, a useful system must also provide adequate differential between the syndromes. One of the weaknesses of *DSM-II* was that certain diagnoses, such as adjustment reaction of childhood, may be overused to cover nearly every patient who comes through the door of a psychiatric clinic. While providing tremendous coverage, it is often useless for differentiating between syndromes that require different types of intervention or have different natural histories without treatment.

DEVELOPMENTAL FRAMEWORK. Psychiatric classification systems attempting to categorize psychiatric disorders of infancy, childhood, and adolescence must have a developmental framework. Child psychiatrists see many children presenting with conditions that are considered normal at one time of life but may be pathological at another (i.e., bed-wetting at age two versus bed-wetting at age fourteen). All psychiatrists must contend with the question of distinguishing normality from abnormality. However, the child psychiatrist has the added problem of defining normality for different ages and different developmental levels.

PRACTICAL UTILITY. Most importantly, *DSM-III*, if it is to be a useful diagnostic classification system, must be practical and clinically useful in everyday clinical practice. All diagnostic classification systems have multiple purposes. They will be a necessary basis for communication, for information retrieval, for research, and possibly for forensic, legal, and other issues. However, their most important purpose is clinical usefulness. If a system is so complicated and so difficult to deal with that mental-health practitioners will avoid using it in everyday clinical practice, it will not turn out to be an effective system.

WHAT IS *DSM-III*?

The third edition of the American Psychiatric Association's *Diagnostic and Statistical Manual of Mental Disorders* (*DSM-III*) became the official psychiatric nomenclature in the United States in January of 1980. The publication of *DSM-III* was the end product of many years of work by the Task Force on Nomenclature and Statistics of the American Psychiatric Association. This task force was appointed in June 1974 under the chairmanship of Robert L. Spitzer. The charge given to the task force was to develop the new diagnostic and statistical manual. It was to be a classification system that would closely reflect the current state of knowledge regarding mental disorders, be useful for both those in clinical practice and those in research, and be as compatible with the *International Classification of Diseases*—Ninth Edition (*ICD-9*) as possible.

The task force had primary responsibility for overseeing the ongoing work of advisory committees and consultants and was heavily involved in formulating the basic principles that underlie *DSM-III*. There were advisory committees, composed of individuals with recognized expertise in a particular field, for each of twelve major areas of classification, as well as for the multiaxial system and for the glossary of technical terms.

This "multiple-committee" approach assured inputs from a wide variety of professionals with different theoretical orientations and widely divergent views on the existence and nature of certain psychiatric disorders. However, this same approach is likely to ensure that no single individual will be perfectly happy with the final document. In some cases final decisions were made by a close vote of the task force.

Basic Features

There are certain basic features of *DSM-III* that make it rather unique as an official classification system. These include the nonetiological descriptive approach, the comprehensive systematic description of each psychiatric disorder, the use of operational diagnostic criteria for the diagnosis of each disorder, the overall inclusiveness of the system, the fact that it was field tested in several ways prior to its publication, the many useful appendices that appear at the end of the manual, and the multiaxial approach to psychiatric diagnosis. Brief comments will be made about each of these particular features.

NONETIOLOGICAL DESCRIPTIVE APPROACH. *DSM-III* has taken an atheoretical approach to psychiatric classification. The task force thought that there were only a few psychiatric disorders in which the etiology or pathophysiological process was known. These include the organic mental disorders and some of the drug-induced psychiatric disorders. Thus, *DSM-III* attempts to describe very comprehensively and systematically *what* is wrong with the patient. However, it only rarely attempts to describe *how* the disturbance came about.

COMPREHENSIVE SYSTEMATIC DESCRIPTIONS. The text of *DSM-III* systematically describes each disorder in terms of the current knowledge available at the time the classification system was developed. A description of each disorder is outlined under the following headings: Essential Features, Associated Features, Age of Onset, Course, Impairment, Complications, Predisposing Factors, Prevalence, Sex Ratio, Familial Pattern, and Differential Diagnosis. Obviously, for some disorders (such as schizophrenic disorders) a substantial amount of information is under each heading. For other disorders, including many in the childhood section, there is either one line or a statement that no knowledge is available.

OPERATIONAL DIAGNOSTIC CRITERIA. *DSM-I*, *DSM-II*, and *ICD-9* only provide general descriptions of the psychiatric disorders in their classification systems. With the one exception of schizo-affective disorder, *DSM-III* outlines specific diagnostic criteria for the diagnosis of each of the psychiatric disorders listed in the classification.

OVERALL INCLUSIVENESS. As mentioned previously, many of the psychiatric disorders in the childhood section of *DSM-III* only have face validity. That is, the description of the disorder on the face of it seems to describe accurately the characteristic features of individuals with that disorder at least as agreed upon by experienced clinicians. The approach taken in *DSM-III* was that it was best to include conditions for which only face validity had been demonstrated because clinicians need to be able to communicate with each other about the types of problems they see. It is more difficult to demonstrate more powerful types of validity—descriptive and predictive—for childhood psychiatric disorders.

However, the task force recognized that it was incumbent upon the psychiatric profession to assess the existence of other types of validity for those disorders in *DSM-III* that at that time had only face validity. If over time other types of validity cannot be demonstrated, despite thorough investigation, then there is serious question whether these conditions should continue to be included in a psychiatric classification of mental disorders.

FIELD TESTING. Only rarely were reliability and validity studies done on disorders described in *DSM-I* and *DSM-II*, even after the classification system had been established. During the course of development of *DSM-III*, once preliminary diagnostic criteria had been drafted, field tests were carried out prior to the document being finalized. Repeated use by several clinicians in different areas led to revisions of diagnostic criteria and attempts to make the wording less ambiguous than it had been originally. Formal reliability trials were conducted and are described in an appendix of the manual.

APPENDICES. *DSM-III* contains many appendices including the description of the field trials and interrater reliability for various diagnostic categories. Some of the more useful ones are decision trees for differential diagnosis, an updated glossary for technical terms, and an annotated comparative listing of *DSM-II* and *DSM-III* which contains explanations for the major changes made and for new categories added, with references justifying the changes. The decision-tree approach to differential diagnosis will be described subsequently in more detail.

MULTIAXIAL SYSTEM. A complete *DSM-III* diagnosis will require codings on five separate axes. On axis I, all clinical psychiatric syndromes will be coded with the exception of two, the specific developmental disorders and the personality disorders. On axis II, the specific developmental disorders and the personality disorders will be coded. There is no theoretical reason for coding both of these on the same axis, nor is there a theoretical reason for separating them from a coding on axis I. The reasons are very practical. Both of these types of disorders tend to be overlooked and not coded if an individual presents with a more acute condition such as a conduct disorder in children or an acute episode of alcoholism in adults. Coding them on a separate axis has been found in systematic studies to insure their coding more reliably (Cantwell et al., 1979).

On axis III will be coded all *physical* disorders and conditions that are current, exist outside of the mental-disorder section of *ICD-9CM,* and are potentially relevant to either the understanding or management of an axis I or axis II disorder. For example, in a child with a conduct disorder who has juvenile diabetes, it is important for the management of the disorder to know that the juvenile diabetes is present, although it may have nothing to do with the etiology of the disorder. On the other hand, a child with acting-out impulsive behavior who has a temporal lobe seizure disorder may be a child in whom the temporal lobe seizure disorder does in fact have an etiologic role in an axis I condition.

On axis IV is coded the overall severity of psychosocial stressors. A seven-point rating scale is used for coding the *overall severity* of stress that is considered to be a significant contributor to either the etiology or the exacerbation of the axis I or axis II condition. The manual provides anchor points for each scale level with examples for adults as well as for children and adolescents.

Axis V requires the clinician to code the highest level of adaptive functioning that the patient has experienced in the past year for at least a few months duration of time. Again, a seven-point rating scale is provided and anchor points are given with examples for children as well as for adolescents and adults. Adaptive functioning is conceptualized as consisting of a composite of three major areas: social relationships, the use of leisure time, and occupational functioning. The latter is considered school functioning for children and adolescents.

Two examples will suffice to give an example of how the multiaxial system is used. In the first case we have an eight-year-old boy who presents with a long-standing history of difficulty in relating to others, ritualistic and compulsive behavior, and early and severe problems with receptive language. He meets the operational diagnostic criteria for axis I diagnosis of infantile autism. In addition, at the time of presentation he has a significant degree of reading disability not explainable on the basis of his IQ which is in the normal range. On axis II, then, one would code a developmental reading disorder. The patient also presents with a temporal lobe seizure disorder which would be coded on axis III. It is well known that autistic children have high rates of seizure disorders. It is not clear whether or not the seizure disorder is an etiologic factor in the autism, but is is clearly something that is important for the management of the child. The eight-year-old boy also happens to come from a home in which the mother has a current severe episode of depression, and there is a good deal of marital strife. The appropriate severity codings on axis IV would be rated for psychosocial stressors. Finally, prior to the current episode of presentation, it was noted that the child was functioning reasonably well in a special school program and had fairly good peer relationships until about a month before the hospitalization for the current episode. In this case an appropriate coding on axis V, highest level of adaptive functioning, would be in the fair to good range.

Take another case of a twelve-year-old boy who presents with a long-standing history of attention deficit disorder with hyperactivity. In addition, he has had significant problems with reading, math, and spelling in school all throughout his academic years. But his current presentation is for a two-month-long episode of depression manifested by dysphoric mood, anhedonia, and many vegetative symptoms. A suicide attempt precipitated the current evaluation. It is found that both parents have a history of unipolar affective disorder, and there is a good deal of marital strife in the family. There is no current biological condition that is thought to play a role either in the recognition, development, or management of the disorder coded on axis I or axis II. Prior to the episode of depression, the child had done very poorly in school academically and had done so for a number of years. He had very few friends and in general was functioning very poorly.

For this case, on axis I the primary diagnosis would be single episode of depression. Another diagnosis on axis I would be attention deficit disorder. Even though attention deficit disorder with hyperactivity was present for the longest time and was present prior to the episode of depression, it was the episode of depression that led to the current evaluation. Thus, it goes first on axis I. On axis II the patient clearly has a mixed specific developmental disorder. This is because there are problems in multiple academic areas, none of which predominate. There is no axis III diagnosis because the patient does not have any physical disorder or condition that currently plays a role in etiology or the management of the disorder. On axis IV again a proper severity rating would be made for psychosocial stressors considering the impact of two mentally ill parents and significant marital strife on the child. Finally, prior to the current episode of depression, the patient had multiple problems of peer relationships and was doing very poorly throughout all of his schooling. Thus, the highest level of adaptive functioning would be rated as very poor because of marked impairment in both school functioning and social relationships.

Thus, it can be seen that in these cases the use of a multiaxial system gives a much fuller description of the patient's current problems than would be possible without its use. In both cases using the *DSM-II* scheme, the developmental disorder may have been overlooked in face of the more significant axis I impairment. There would have been no clear way of relating the presence of the temporal lobe seizures in the first patient using a uniaxial system. And *DSM-I* and *DSM-II* would not have allowed the axis IV and axis V evaluations which tell us a significant amount about the patient's psychosocial environment and also about how well he has been functioning prior to the current episode of illness.

The Infancy, Childhood, and Adolescence Section

While in many ways *DSM-III* represents a radical departure from *DSM-II* and *DSM-I*, its immediate predecessors, it is in the childhood section that there has been the greatest change. *DSM-II* had 146 specific diagnostic categories. There are 176 when *DSM-III* axis I and axis II are considered together. Thus, there is not that great a change in the overall number of diagnostic categories. However, in *DSM-II* there was one category for children's disorders (Behavior Disorders of Childhood and Adolescence) which included six specific conditions. *DSM-I* did not have a separate section for disorders of childhood and adolescents. The diagnostic class in *DSM-III* titled "Disorders Usually First Evident in Infancy, Childhood, and Adolescence" contains more than four times as many categories as there were for children in *DSM-II*. A detailed description of each of these disorders can be read in *DSM-III* itself or in previous publications (Spitzer and Cantwell, 1980).

Some important general points will be discussed here. First, it should be recognized that there are many children who present for child psychiatric evaluation who have problems in development that are not contained within any of the specific *DSM-III* diagnostic categories. Studies of adults and adolescents, for example, have shown that as many as 25% of patients presenting for evaluation will have an "undiagnosed mental disorder" if one uses specific diagnostic criteria to make a specific diagnosis. It is not surprising that the figure will be at least as high in children.

Often children with severe aggressive behavior, precocious sexual activity, or other symptoms may be presented for evaluation to a child psychiatrist. Yet these symptoms may not be part of a diagnosable psychiatric disorder using *DSM-III* criteria. In these cases one can use a diagnosis of "unspecified mental disorder" and describe the predominant features.

Moreover, there may be children presenting to a child psychiatrist with conditions that do not warrant the diagnosis of a mental disorder at all. In these cases a V code such as "parent-child problem" or "other specified family circumstances" can be used.

Second, it is to be emphasized that this section of *DSM-III* contains those conditions that usually *arise* and are *first manifested* in infancy, childhood, and adolescence. This does not mean that children and adolescents can only be given diagnoses from this section of the manual. For example, obsessive-compulsive disorder is not in this section, yet there are children who present with such behavior. The reason for its absence is that it *usually* does not arise and first manifest itself in childhood. The same is true with certain types of phobic disorders. Thus, a child who presents with a phobic disorder should be given the appropriate diagnosis from other areas of the manual. The introduction to the childhood section of

DSM-III names the diagnostic categories that although listed elsewhere in the manual may be appropriate for children or adolescents.

There are several special situations that have been handled in different ways. For example, in the case of affective disorders and schizophrenic disorders, it was thought that the *essential* features of both of these conditions were the same in children and adults. Thus, there are no special categories corresponding to these disorders in the infancy, childhood, and adolescent section of *DSM-III*. That means that if a child or an adolescent has a condition that meets the criteria for one of the affective disorders or for a schizophrenic disorder, these diagnoses should be given, regardless of the age of the individual. The rationale behind this was that we do not have an infantile pneumonia, a child pneumonia, and an adult pneumonia. Pneumonia is pneumonia regardless of the age of the individual. However, it is also recognized that in many cases, especially in the case of the affective disorders, there are *age-specific associated features*. These features have been written up for infants, children, and adolescents in the text of the disorder. However, they do not affect the diagnostic criteria nor do they affect where in the classification scheme the disorder is placed.

A second type of problem arises when a condition in childhood has a very strong relationship to a condition in adult life but not a one-to-one relationship. The most concrete example of this is conduct disorder in childhood and antisocial personality disorder in adult life. It is quite clear that very rarely, if ever, does one develop an antisocial personality disorder in adult life without having manifestations of a conduct disorder in childhood and adolescence. It is also true that many children with conduct disorders do in fact have antisocial disorders when they are adults. However, there is not a one-to-one relationship going from one to the other. That is, some 40 to 50% of those with diagnosable conduct disorder will be diagnosed as antisocial personality in adult life—the others will not. Since there is no way of predicting which conduct-disordered child will in fact become an antisocial personality disorder, one overall category was not used for children and adults. That is, children who meet the criteria for a conduct disorder are not given the diagnosis of antisocial personality disorder until after the age of eighteen. A separate condition—conduct disorder—with various subtypes having different diagnostic criteria, was written up and placed in the infancy, childhood, and adolescent section. There are other conditions like this, such as overanxious and avoidant disorders in childhood. These may have some relationship to the adult diagnoses of generalized anxiety disorder and avoidant personality disorder. However, the evidence is less clear in these conditions than it is with conduct disorder and antisocial personality disorder.

A third situation arises when a condition that manifests itself first in infancy, childhood, and adolescence does persist into adult life, but in a somewhat modified form. This quite commonly happens with autism and with attention deficit disorder. In these cases a residual category is written up for those individuals who had the disorder in childhood and met the specific criteria. They continue to have problems in adult life related to their original diagnosis but no longer meet the original criteria. It is for these conditions that the residual categories of attention deficit disorder and pervasive developmental disorder are used.

How to Use *DSM-III*

What tools are available to the clinician in the diagnostic process? In general they can be divided up into six types: an interview with the parents about the child (this may include family interviews); an interview with the child himself or herself; behavior rating scales completed by parents, teachers, and significant others in the child's life; a physical exam; a neurological exam; and laboratory studies, including psychological testing. Only in rare cases do the physical and neurological exams or the laboratory studies contribute to making a specific diagnosis. This does not mean that they do not play an important part in many cases in providing *other* information regarding the diagnostic formulation and the patient's history and management. With the exception of chromosomal studies in certain cases of mental retardation and specific psychometric testing for confirmation of the diagnosis of some specific developmental disorders, laboratory studies do not exist for the diagnosis of specific psychiatric disorders in childhood. Thus, the making of a *DSM-III* diagnosis—that is, the defining of a clinical syndrome in childhood—most likely will be done on the basis of the interviews with the parents, the interviews with the child, and the behavior rating scales. The astute clinician will look for as much information from as many areas as possible and will arrive at a diagnostic formulation of an individual child's problem in terms of a specific *DSM-III* diagnosis.

The multiaxial scheme of *DSM-III* makes a nice framework upon which to anchor the diagnostic process. Thus, the question of diagnosis is answered if the child meets one or more of the conditions on axis I or axis II. This includes the diagnosis of "unspecified mental disorder." Again, only rarely will the physical exam, neurological exam, or laboratory studies be helpful in this area. Axis III allows the clinician to look at the physical and neurological findings and laboratory findings to confirm the diagnosis of some specific physical disorder. Interviews and observations of the parents and of the child will generally be used to assess the impact of psychosocial stressors as coded on axis IV, and along with parent and teacher rating scales will be used to make an assessment about the level of adaptive functioning to be coded on axis V. The author also feels that axis V can be used in a *clinical sense* to rate the current level of impairment produced by the axis I and/or axis II conditions. This can be done by rating it as none, mild, moderate, or severe impairment in the three areas mentioned before (use of leisure time, school functioning, and peer relationships).

DECISION-TREE APPROACH TO DIAGNOSIS

One of the more helpful appendices, in the author's opinion, in DSM-III is the appendix containing decision trees for differential diagnosis. These decision trees outline a branching-tree approach to differential diagnosis for ruling in or ruling out appropriate axis I or axis II diagnoses. Two of these will be illustrated for common presenting problems in childhood.

The first decision tree to be illustrated will be that used for the differential diagnosis of children who present with *antisocial aggressive, defiant, or oppositional behavior*. The first question to be answered is: Does the child have a known organic etiology for this condition? If the answer to that is yes, one must then consider an organic mental disorder such as substance intoxication or organic personality disorder. Also to be considered is intermittent explosive disorder which can be diagnosed when it is symptomatic of an organic mental disorder. If the answer to the question of whether there is a known organic etiology is no, the next question to be answered is whether or not the child has subaverage general intellectual and adaptive functioning. A yes answer requires a diagnosis of mental retardation. A no answer allows one to proceed to ask the next question: Are there any psychotic features, including bizarre behavior? A yes to this question refers the clinician to the differential diagnosis of psychotic features, which is a different decision tree. A no answer leads one to ask the next question: Are there isolated discrete episodes of sudden loss of control of aggressive impulses resulting in assault, violence, or other destructive acts? If the answer is yes, the diagnosis is intermittent or isolated explosive disorder. If the answer is no, the next question is: Is there a personality pattern of continual antisocial behavior in which the rights of others are violated with onset in childhood and persistence into adult life? If the answer to that is yes, the diagnosis is antisocial personality disorder, which is only made after the age of eighteen. If the answer is no, a related question is then asked: Is there a repetitive and persistent pattern of behavior in which either the rights of others or major age-appropriate societal norms or rules are violated? If the answer to that question is yes in the child, the diagnosis is conduct disorder. If the answer is no the next question posed is: Is there a pattern of disobedient, negativistic, and provocative opposition to authority figures? If yes, the diagnosis is oppositional disorder. If no, the next question is: Is there a maladaptive reaction to a psychosocial stressor in the child's environment? If the answer is yes, the diagnosis is adjustment disorder with disturbance of conduct. If the answer is no, the diagnosis is a V-code diagnosis of child, adolescent, or adult antisocial behavior.

Many children present with *academic or learning difficulties* as the major or predominant disturbance. The first question to be asked in such cases is: Are there demonstrable signs of focal central nervous system disease? If the answer is yes, one must consider a neurological disorder which would be coded on axis III and which may or may not be associated with other disorders to be uncovered by answers to the later questions. If there is no demonstrable sign of focal central nervous system disease, the next question is: Is there subaverage general intellectual and adaptive functioning? If yes, the diagnosis of mental retardation should be considered, which again can be concurrent with other diagnoses occurring later down the line of the decision tree. The third question: Is there a specific delay in development, not symptomatic of the other disorder? A yes answer requires a diagnosis on axis II of specific developmental disorder, which again may coexist with other diagnoses along the decision tree. A no answer allows one to continue to the next question: Is there a developmentally inappropriate short attention span and poor concentration? If yes, a diagnosis of attention deficit disorder should be considered. A no answer leads one to ask the next question: Is there a repetitive and persistent pattern of behavior in which either the rights of others or major age-appropriate societal norms or rules are violated? A yes answer gives a diagnosis of conduct disorder. A no causes one to ask: Is there a pattern of disobedient, negativistic, and provocative opposition to authority figures? A yes answer would lead one to consider a diagnosis of oppositional disorder. A no answer leads to the following: Is there one or more of the preceding disorders present to account for academic or learning difficulty. A yes answer would then stop the decision tree. Thus, either mental retardation, a neurological disorder, attention deficit disorder, conduct disorder, oppositional disorder, or specific developmental disorder may exist separately or concomitantly to explain the academic learning difficulties which are the major physical disturbance. If the answer to the previous question is no, the next question arises: Is the academic or learning difficulty symptomatic of another mental disorder? A yes answer would lead one to consider such things as an adjustment disorder with academic inhibition. A no answer would lead to consideration of a V code such as academic problem or borderline intellectual functioning.

Advantages and Disadvantages of *DSM-III*

There have been multiple critiques written about *DSM-III* both before and after its publication (Schacht and Nathan, 1977; Zubin, 1977; Garmezy, 1978; Rutter and Shaffer, 1980).

Some of the major critiques will be reviewed here and the rationale for the approach taken in *DSM-III* will be outlined. First a major criticism is that there is no overall definition of mental disorder in *DSM-III* and the guidelines of what constitutes a disorder as listed in the introduction are problematical. Second, there are multiple critiques about the multiaxial system (the number and types of axes that were created, the failure to have mental retardation as a separate axis, and the codings on axis IV and on axis V). A third criticism has to do with what is perceived as excessive subdivision of the psychiatric disorders in the infancy, childhood, and adolescence subsection. A fourth related criticism has to do with presenting operational diagnostic criteria with insufficient evidence. A fifth and final criticism relates to why *DSM-III* had to be created in the first place in lieu of the use of *ICD-9* in the United States. Each of these will be discussed in turn.

Definition of Mental Disorder

Neither *DSM-I*, *DSM-II*, nor *ICD-9* contain an overall definition of mental disorder. On theoretical grounds this is a serious defect, for if there is a *classification* of mental disorders, there should be an overall *definition* of mental disorder so that one can decide the criteria by which a particular disorder either does or does not get into the classification system. For a variety of reasons it was decided (Klein, 1978; Spitzer and Endicott, 1978) that no generally accepted satisfactory definition could be formulated. There is a statement, however, in the introduction to *DSM-III* advising that each of the mental disorders described in the document is conceptualized first as a clinically significant behavioral or psychological syndrome—that is, a pattern that occurs in an individual—and that moreover, this pattern of behavior is specifically associated with either distress (such as a painful symptom) or disability (impairment in one or more areas of functioning). Finally, there is an inference that a dysfunction exists in the individual which may be behavioral, psychological, or biological, and that the disturbance is not *solely* in the relationship between the individual and society. Thus, *DSM-III* does not have an official definition of mental disorder but does have guidelines in the introduction that allow each individual disorder to be assessed as to whether or not it should have been included in the manual. Some objections have been raised to these guidelines as they are published. These have been discussed fully by Rutter and Shaffer (1980).

Multiaxial Classification Issues

MENTAL RETARDATION AS A SEPARATE AXIS. As Rutter and Shaffer point out, field studies both by the World Health Organization (WHO) and by Cantwell et al. (1979) do support the idea that mental retardation is more often diagnosed when it is a separate axis. In actual fact, this author agrees that mental retardation should have been a separate axis. The major reason for it not being included separately was the desire to keep the number of axes to a minimum to insure their use by clinicians who might feel a proliferation of axes would be too difficult. As a point of interest, the American Association on Mental Deficiency, in its new classification scheme includes a multiaxial approach to the classification of mental retardation itself—one axis being for the classification of level of IQ, another axis for the classification of level of adaptive behavior. It is only logical, then, that some coding should be available for the severity level of each of these two dimensions of mental retardation. Up till now all systems have allowed a severity coding only on level of IQ and not on the level of adaptive behavior. In individual cases the severity level of IQ and adaptive behavior are not necessarily congruent.

AXIS IV CODING. The coding on axis IV is an overall coding of the severity of stress produced by any psychosocial stressor. It does not consider the *type* of psychosocial stressor nor does it consider the *severity* of the stressor as it applies to the individual. Rather, the severity that an average person would be expected to receive from such a stress is coded. Obviously, in coding psychosocial stressors, one might code the type of stressor, the severity of the stressor, or both. And in considering the severity of the stressor, one could consider the idiosyncratic reaction of an individual to the stress, recognizing the fact that the same stressor (such as death of a mother-in-law) might in fact have very different impacts on different individuals. The other approach is to take the view that a certain stressor has a rather uniform impact on the average individual. Rutter and Shaffer (1980) have rightly criticized the approach taken in *DSM-III* on the grounds that some important advances in methodology of stress research have been neglected. The present author also believes it would have been useful to have been able to code both type and severity and to take into account idiosyncratic reaction of the individual when assessing the stress. Needless to say, there would have been more methodological problems with this approach than with the current approach, but probably more useful data would have been collected with each patient.

AXIS V CODING. The author believes that axis V should have been a dual coding: one for impairment level produced by the current episode of illness, and one for highest level of adaptive functioning attained by the individual. Thus there would have been a coding on one axis to compare current level of impairment with a previous level of adaptive functioning. Again, Rutter and Shaffer have criticized the idea of restricting the level of adaptive functioning to a period within a year from the time that the individual is seen for the axis I or axis II condition. This means that in all cases we are not considering premorbid functioning but rather functioning in an arbitrary time limit. Setting such a time limit means this coding will be different for individuals whose disorder lasts for longer than a year versus those who had the disorder for a shorter period of time.

Excessive Subdivision of Categories

It has been shown in many studies, both with the *ICD-9* classification system and with the *DSM-III* classification system, that there generally tends to be agreement on broad categories of disturbance, such as conduct disorder and emotional disorder, between individual clinicians. However, when finer subdivisions are made, the agreement is less. Yet *DSM-III* did take a "splitter" rather than a "lumper" approach. That is, if certain types of conditions could be described with essential features and associated features, that condition was included. As noted earlier, this meant the inclusion of many categories in the childhood section for which no validity other than face validity had been demonstrated. Rutter and Shaffer feel that the opposite approach should have been taken, that is, restricting the categories to the more broad categories of conduct disorder, emotional disorder, etc., without the finer subdivisions, unless there is justification in the literature for such a subdivision. They also feel that the inclusion of mixed types, such as mixed disturbance of conduct and emotions, would have been more practical and more fruitful than the use of separate diagnostic categories that need to be diagnosed together to get the same picture (e.g., overanxious disorder and conduct disorder—both diagnoses must be made rather than choosing a single diagnosis of mixed disturbance of conduct and emotion).

Use of Inconclusive Operational Diagnostic Criteria

The criticism as to the use of operational diagnostic criteria without the support of sufficient evidence is related to the preceding criticism. That is, if there is little evidence for the predictive validity of finer subdivisions in categories, there is even less evidence for the use of specific operational diagnostic criteria for these disorders. The counterargument is that without these specific diagnostic criteria, one could lump together conditions that might appear similar on the face of overall clinical symptomatology but actually do have some finer distinctions that may turn out to have some predictive validity. The argument here being that if they do not exist in the classification system, they cannot be studied to assess other types of validity.

Need for DSM-III

Rutter and Shaffer point out that the *International Classification of Diseases*—Ninth Edition, has a solid research background behind it. The classification system for psychiatric disorders of childhood was well studied prior to being developed and codified in *ICD-9*. They question why a separate diagnostic system needed to be made for use in the United States. The counterargument to that is, of course, that American clinicians who reviewed the drafts of *ICD-9* did not feel that it met their needs in many areas. Only systematic research can answer which of the systems is better. In fact, there is a great deal of overlap between them.

SUMMARY

This chapter has attempted to review the background and the development of *DSM-III*, the principles of classification upon which *DSM-III* was based, the organization and use of the manual, how it can be used in the diagnostic process, and the areas of controversy and contention. It is likely that over the years the categories in *DSM-III* will be studied from many points of view and that some will be found to be very valuable and very valid. Others will be found not to have solid reasons for their subdivision or indeed for their inclusion in *DSM-IV*. However, overall it can be said that *DSM-III* does mark an improvement for both the clinician and the researcher in the often neglected but important area of nosology and classification of the psychiatric disorders of childhood.

REFERENCES

Achenbach, T. M. 1980. DSM-III in light of empirical research on the classification of child psychopathology. *J. Am. Acad. Child Psych.,* 19:395–412.

American Psychiatric Association. 1980. *Diagnostic and statistical manual of mental disorders (DSM-III)*. Washington, D.C.: APA.

Cantwell, D. P. 1980. The diagnostic process and diagnostic classification in child psychiatry—DSM-III. *J. Am. Acad. Child Psych.,* 19:345–355.

Cantwell, D. P., Russell, A. T., Mattison, R., and Will, L. 1979. A comparison of DSM-II and DSM-III in the diagnosis of childhood psychiatric disorders. *Arch. Gen. Psych.,* 36:1208–1228.

Cohen, D. J. 1976. The diagnostic process in child psychiatry. *Psychiat. Ann.,* 6:29–56.

Feighner, J. P., Robins, E., Guze, S. B., Woodruff, R. A., Winokur, G., and Munoz, R. 1972. Diagnostic criteria for use in psychiatric research. *Arch. Gen. Psych.,* 26:57–63.

Garmezy, N. 1978. DSM-III. Never mind the psychologists: Is it good for the children? *Clin. Psychologist,* 31 (3).

Gittelman, R. 1980. The role of psychological tests for differential diagnosis in child psychiatry. *J. Am. Acad. Child Psych.,* 19:413-438.

Goodwin, D. W., and Guze, S. B. 1979. *Psychiatric diagnosis.* New York: Oxford University Press.

Klein, D. F. 1978. A proposed definition of mental illness. In *Critical issues in psychiatric diagnosis,* ed. R. L. Spitzer, and D. F. Klein, pp. 41-55. New York: Raven Press.

Rutter, M. 1978. Classification. In *Child psychiatry,* ed. M. Rutter, and L. Hersov, pp. 359-384. London: Blackwell Scientific Publications.

Rutter, M., and Shaffer, D. 1980. DSM-III: A step forward or back in terms of the classification of child psychiatric disorders? *J. Am. Acad. Child Psych.,* 19:371-394.

Schacht, T., and Nathan, P. E. 1977. But is it good for the psychologists? *Am. Psychologist,* 32:1017-1025.

Spitzer, R. L., and Cantwell, D. P. 1980. The DSM-III classification of the psychiatric disorders of infancy, childhood, and adolescence. *J. Am. Acad. Child Psych.,* 19:356-370.

Spitzer, R. L., and Endicott, J. 1978. Medical and mental disorder. In *Critical issues in psychiatric disorders,* ed. R. L. Spitzer, and D. F. Klein, pp. 15-39. New York: Raven Press.

Spitzer, R. L., Endicott, J., Robins, E., Kuriansky, J., and Gurland, B. 1975. Preliminary report of the reliability of Research Diagnostic Criteria applied to psychiatric case records. In *Predictability in psychopharmacology: Preclinical and clinical correlations,* ed. A. Sudilovsky, S. Gershon, and P. Beer, pp. 1-47. New York: Raven Press.

Zubin, J. 1977. But is it good for science? *Clin. Psychologist,* 32:5-7.

Part III
GENERAL NOTES ON TREATMENT APPROACHES

26

Pediatric Psychopharmacology

LAURENCE L. GREENHILL

HISTORY

The development and widespread application of neuroleptics and tricyclic antidepressants twenty years ago changed the entire structure of American psychiatry, leading to shorter hospital stays for schizophrenic and depressed patients, and to a reduction in state hospital inpatient populations. The field has moved forward in a series of stages, beginning with the serendipitous discovery of the antipsychotic chlorpromazine, through a period of clinical empiricism involving drug trials correlated with plasma level measures, and on to the use of these agents as pharmacological tools to dissect receptor function and neurotransmitter chemistry and pathophysiology. Phenothiazines have been shown to prevent deterioration in the majority of hospitalized schizophrenics, and continued drug treatment after discharge greatly lessens the rate of relapse. Other studies have shown that these neuroleptics have more than a sedating anxiolytic effect, for they truly ameliorate the "core" schizophrenic defect of abnormal thought processes in the anxious-agitated patient as well as in the apathetic patient, both acute and chronic.

Building on these psychopharmacological findings, a series of imaginative investigations have explored the various activities of drugs with different structures. The relationship of dopamine receptor blockade to antipsychotic activity has been elucidated, and neuroendocrine responses have been utilized to determine the role of neurotransmitters in mental disease states (Sachar, 1978).

The treatment effectiveness of clinical adult psychopharmacology eventually led to the development of neurochemical and neurophysiological theories of schizophrenia and depression. The correlation of therapeutic response with plasma levels of psychoactive medications has shed light on the perplexing absence of response to tricyclic treatment (Glassman et al., 1975) and to phenothiazines (Davis et al., 1978) in certain patients. These patients had unusually low plasma concentrations of unbound drug due to a genetically determined, high metabolic elimination rate for the drug (Sjoquist, 1979) or to increased binding because of elevated serum protein levels (Shand, 1979).

The success of psychopharmacological treatments has revived the field's interest in the disease model which links specific pathological states, as defined by Research Diagnostic Criteria (Spitzer and Robins, 1978) or *DSM-III* (American Psychiatric Association, 1980) classifications, to improvement with specific drug treatments. Structured interview questionnaries have allowed the clinician to correlate changes in drug plasma level concentrations with change scores in key diagnostic variables (Puig-Antich et al., 1979). These forms include the Schedule for Affective Disorders and Schizophrenia (SADS) (Spitzer and Endicott, 1978), the Kiddie-SADS (K-SADS) version for children ages six to twelve years (Puig-Antich and Chambers, 1978), and Diagnostic Interview Schedule (DIS).

Child psychopharmacology has generally lagged behind the impressive accomplishments of adult drug research. Besides Bradley's serendipitous discovery of Benzedrine's calming effects in childhood behavior disorders (Bradley, 1937), most early work involved the empirical application of research drugs from adult psychiatry to severely impaired child inpatients. As Werry (1982) points out, these adult-derived drugs were given to children in conspicuously different ways than they had been used in adults. Until recently, drugs were used to ameliorate childhood target behavioral signs which were not syndromally linked, quite different from studies employing adult self-reported disease symptoms. Hyperkinetic and conduct-disordered children often have no complaints themselves, but their misbehavior produces intense discomfort in their caretakers, who, in turn, request the drug treatment. Werry (1982) states that it is usually others, not the child, who require that the child's behavior be changed. In addition, the unsettled nature of childhood nosology, complicated as it is by issues of developmental change, prevents a precise match of drug type to childhood disorder.

Drug Review

A review of pediatric psychopharmacology may be approached from a variety of directions: by drug category, by diagnostic condition, or by patient-oriented indications/contraindications. Because childhood psychiatric nosology remains controversial and in flux, and indications/contraindications must be addressed to the needs of the individual patient, these approaches can be subsumed within a drug classification. A list of general clinical guidelines will be given before the specific drug categories are reviewed. In addition, guidelines for clinical usage will be mentioned for each drug category.

Drug Management Issues

The murky, ill-defined state of prepubertal psychiatric nosology has prevented the establishment of a stable diagnostic classification system for child psychiatry. Attention deficit disorder overlaps and merges with conduct disorder, childhood schizophrenia is a rare, undefined phenomenon frequently argued over, and childhood affective disorder exists at a much lower prevalence than seen in older age groups. The child's rapid emotional, social, and cognitive development in this time period make it difficult for the clinician to establish a stable treatment baseline to track the efficacy of his or her intervention.

The natural history of a psychiatric disorder is one of the most powerful validation measures because it gives a sense of "caseness" and defines the presenting problem as a medical entity. Yet very few child psychiatric disorders except hyperactivity fit the medical model making them suitable for drug treatments. In fact, Werry (1982) has correctly identified the symptomatic treatment approach of much of child psychopharmacology as a process of suppressing target symptoms, rather than curing well-defined syndromes. Thus, neuroleptics are used to calm unmanageable behaviors across a wide variety of childhood disorders, including the self-abuse observed in pervasive developmental disorder, the violent temper and aggressivity associated with undersocialized conduct disorder with aggressivity, the screaming behavior found in the institutionalized child with moderate mental retardation, and the classroom disruptiveness associated with severe attention deficit disorder with hyperactivity. Furthermore, the phenomenology of these conditions often changes in appearance and in manageability as the child becomes older, making it difficult to know whether the child is responding to the drug or to development.

Thus, treatment success in child psychopharmacology is measured by symptom suppression. These symptoms and their functional disabilities reappear immediately as the drug wears off. Enuretic children wet as soon as the imipramine stops, and hyperactive children become more hyperactive than ever as their medication wears off. Their hyperactivity rebounds at the end of a day on stimulants.

The parents form the key to success in the treatment of the child with psychoactive drugs. They supervise all drug administration and must coax the child to swallow the pills or capsules. Their expectations of symptom improvement and fears about socially stigmatizing side effects must be assessed before treatment is to begin. Many adults worry about the child's chemical dependency on the pills, and whether he must take the drug for the rest of his life (Grinspoon and Singer, 1973). Will treatment produce physical dependence, or tolerance with increasing amounts of drug needed to get the same effect? Will pill taking lead to adult drug abuse? Can a child form an emotional dependency on this treatment and then manipulatively blame the medicine if he gets into trouble?

Parents also fear that the child's cooperation has been obtained at the expense of a loss of spontaneity or creativity. Children who are taking phenothiazines look sleepy or "glazed," and seem zombified. This glassy-eyed appearance suggests that the children are mindlessly under the control of their psychotropic medications. Behavior-controlling drugs are commonly thought to prevent ethical development, and it is feared that the treated child may fail to develop an independent sense of moral responsibility and social judgment (Schrag and Divoky, 1975).

Many of these concerns and questions can be managed by a sensitive clinical interview, allowing the parents to ventilate their fears and have their questions answered in a careful, thoughtful manner. Direct answers to questions convey much more sincerity than vague generalizations. Many parents find reading material helpful and appreciate the clearly written booklets available from the drug companies describing the medication's therapeutic actions and side effects. Other parents delve into the current medical literature and ask detailed, penetrating questions about current psychopharmacological controversies. Physicians may find themselves threatened if a parent seems knowledgeable about a particular drug. Other therapists may become uncomfortable if they are unable to answer a question. Although it is reassuring to know the answer, parental anxieties respond best to a concerned, tolerant, caring approach. Since pediatric psychopharmacology continues to be an empirical exercise rather than an exacting science, it is generally better to share uncertainty than to hide it, only to have to deal with the parent's disappointment when several medications fail. An overenthusiastic therapist can unwittingly support unrealistic parental expectations that the therapist has a perfect "silver bullet" to cure their child's global behavioral problems.

Many parental worries can be assuaged if the clinician includes a long-term management plan with drug holidays and off-drug assessment periods. Most children can be titrated off maintenance pharmacotherapy during the summer. The drug vacation allows family and physician to observe the results of therapy and normal development. Many children will cope surprisingly well. In the fall, the child should be allowed to return to school off medication. Regular teacher reports should be collected. The longer the child can attend class without the support of drugs, the more progress can be shown to parents and child. If he must return to pharmacotherapy, it may be at a lower dose. Even so, the parents should be supported through this period. Remedication is not a sign of failure, but the end of one cycle off drug.

Placebo trials provide the therapist with another modality for checking the progress of treatment. Many pediatric patients are maintained on medications without the assurance that they are being helped by them. Inconsistent teacher reports or severe disparity between teacher and parental rating forms is an indication for a placebo trial. This technique can be most easily managed with stimulants. The ten-item Conners Questionnaire (Guy, 1976) allows for rapid scoring and assessment. A simple design, using four four-day periods, can be set up with a placebo-active-placebo-active format (ABAB design). The teacher is asked to fill out four ten-item forms for the sixteen-day trial. Both therapist and parent should be ignorant about the exact timing of the four phases, and individual day's medications can be prepared in separate envelopes by a nurse or other professional who will keep the code. If the child shows no major changes throughout the trial, or becomes worse on active drug, a drug vacation is strongly warranted. On the other hand, a display of the child's characteristic pre-drug behavior problems while on placebo can end doubts about the medication's benefits.

What about the child's concerns? Children characteristically report few subjective changes during treatment. Sedating side effects from neuroleptics, constipation, dizziness, and weakness from tricyclics, and upset stomach from lithium give the characteristic somatic orientation of most of the pediatric self-reports. It is the social impact of the drugs that concern many school-age children. As Whitehouse and his coworkers (1980) noted, taking pills makes the child vulnerable to peer ridicule. One report (Sprague and Sleator, 1975) indicated that many children, left to their own devices in school, avoid going to the nurse to obtain their noontime doses of medication. Perhaps some of the drug-unresponsive academic and social problems found in treated ADDH children is a result of the failure to take the in-school medication. Long-acting sustained release medication preparations, including Ritalin-SR, slow-release Dexedrine capsules, and magnesium pemoline offer an alternative for the child concerned with peer disfavor.

Minde (1980) points to another intrapsychic level of dysfunction resulting from pediatric psychopharmacology. Children who come to believe that they themselves are incapable of functioning and succeeding without the intervention of medication may suffer a form of iatrogenic disability. It is preventative to introduce the medication as a tool or crutch that can be discarded as soon as the child can cope successfully by himself. Even when he succeeds on the drug, accomplishing and achieving in school as never before, it is the child, not a pill, who makes the grade.

Ages-Associated Differences in Psychopharmacology

Adolescent psychiatric disorders show very different patterns of prevalence than do their childhood equivalents. Schizophrenic hallucinations, delusions, and loosening of associations or incoherence begin to be found in adolescents referred for admission to hospitals, comprising up to 20% of incoming patients. Unlike the children with pervasive developmental disorder, these disturbed adolescents show a clear deterioration from a better-functioning premorbid personality. This symptom picture only begins to occur around age fourteen, in much greater frequency than the extremely rare cases of childhood onset pervasive developmental disorder or schizophrenia occurring in childhood.

This is also true of major endogenous depressive disorder. Rutter et al. (1970) reported that 3 of 2,199 prepubertal children on the Isle of Wight were depressed. He went on to report a tenfold increase in the frequency of depression from childhood to adolescence from the same population. Kashani and coworkers (1983) assessed 641 children from the New Zealand general-population longitudinal study—at nine years of age. They found, after administering the K-SADS-E (epidemiology version) to a screened sample of 94 children, that the current point prevalences of major and minor depressive disorder could be estimated at 1.8% and 2.5%, respectively. These measures escalate during adolescence into adulthood, with the prevalence rates of depression going up as much as ten times, as they did when adolescents were interviewed in the Isle of Wight study. For adults, Weissman and Myers (1978) have reported a 4.3% prevalence for major depression and 2.5% prevalence for minor depression. In addition, Kashani et al. found an equal representation of male and female children in the depressed sample, whereas more adolescent girls become depressed than boys.

Another indicator of the increased prevalence rates of psychiatric disorder in adolescents can be found in the rates of completed suicides. Shaffer and Fisher (1981) have shown a remarkable difference in suicide rates for the two age groups. During the seven-year period studied in his British Isles survey, Shaffer could find not even a single record of a completed suicide for a child under twelve years of age. The age-specific mortality rate for prepubertal suicide is 0.81 per 100,000; it is almost ten times greater for the fifteen to nineteen year olds, being 7.64 per 100,000.

Furthermore, during the period 1964-77, there was a large increase in suicide rate for fifteen to eighteen year olds (125% for males, 70% for females), while the ten to fourteen year olds maintained a stable rate (Shaffer and Fisher, 1981). The increased prevalence of depression and suicide make these disorders a key issue for the practice of adolescent psychiatry.

One particular type of anxiety disorder that shows a marked age trend is that linked with refusal to go to school. School phobia appears to be most common at three different periods during the child's school life—at and soon after entry at five years, at eleven years, and at fourteen years. The first two peaks may be related to developmental phases wherein anxiety levels are high to start with, but the third peak is linked to the onset of a more widespread disorder such as depression or schizophrenia (Graham, 1979).

Several other disorders are extremely rare in the preadolescent period. The occurrence of conversion reactions, that is, a disturbance of physical function, including seizures, paralysis, aphonia, and blindness, strongly suggests an organic etiology in the child, but may be psychological in origin in the adolescent. In rare cases, conversion disorders may be an associated finding in childhood depression and may have been treated successfully with tricyclic antidepressants (TCAs) (Weller and Weller, 1983). With suspected conversion disorders, Weller and Weller suggest the use of 250 mg of amobarbital following the method of Perry (Perry et al., 1981), taking caution to avoid this technique in paranoid children or those who are sensitive to barbiturates or with a history of porphyria.

Manic depressive disorder was reported by Kraeplin (1921) to occur at a prevalence of less than 0.01% in preadolescence, and is extraordinarily rare. The last case at the New York

State Psychiatric Institute was seen three years ago, and the ten-year-old girl in question actually turned out to have multiple sclerosis. Using New York Hospital data, the modal age for first break in bipolar disease is close to twenty years of age.

Adolescent psychiatry, therefore, shifts from the softer nosological definitions of childhood disorder to adolescent syndromes which are more stable over time. Severe endogenous depression, schizophrenia, or manic-depressive psychosis will predominate, leading to proportionally more adolescents treated as inpatients. Secondary psychosis and secondary bipolar syndromes emerge as adolescents abuse cannabis, alcohol, and amphetamines. Many of those treatments will be somatic ones, involving psychopharmacological agents.

Working with Disturbed Adolescents

Disturbed adolescents have traditionally been the toughest patients. This is partially due to the fact that the reason for treatment comes from both the patient and the parent, so it is both "other" and "child" based. In addition, the use of psychotropic medicine in adolescents is split between the need to control the adolescent's disturbing behavior and to treat the adolescent's disease. At times the two goals can be contradictory; for example, the parents may be upset by their son throwing a chair through the living-room window during an argument, while the boy may complain that the parents generated his anger, hurting his feelings. Although the therapist may want to start medication to reduce the adolescent's irritability and projection, drugs may be viewed by the patient as punishment.

Other problems revolve around the adolescent's continual demand for and sensitivity to independence from parental control. This arises immediately over the issue of medication control. Should the parents keep track of the drug and give the pills? To some adolescents, this is an insult to their intelligence. But for the highly suicidal, impulsive adolescent depressive, the urge to swallow the entire bottle of tricyclic antidepressant may be overpowering.

Unfortunately, tricyclic antidepressants have a narrow therapeutic to toxic ratio. TCAs are creating a significant public-health problem because of accidental poisoning of young children (FDA Drug Bulletin, 1980) who ingest medicine intended for their parents or older sibs. These compounds are highly lethal, causing death in 1% of children taking overdoses accidentally, compared to the 0.3% death rate from other drugs. Doses over 10 mg/kg may be dangerous, and death in children has occurred from doses as low as 15 mg/kg (Saraf et al., 1974). The prudent clinician instructs the parents to lock up TCA medication, particularly if the youngster being treated is impulsive. One medical center treated two such overdoses in the same month several years ago. Although both acts were impulsive gestures carried out in front of the parents, one of the adolescents died within thirty minutes from cardiac arrhythmia while receiving good medical care at the university hospital emergency room. Tricyclic antidepressants should be dispensed directly to parents when the adolescent, treated as an outpatient, has a history of impulsiveness or has actually overdosed.

Compliance is the most critical component of clinical psychopharmacology, and everything should be done to encourage the adolescent patient to follow the drug regimen. Those adolescents taking less lethal drugs than lithium or antidepressants should be given the opportunity to control their medications. This will emphasize that their own inner comforts, not just their parent's complaints, are being addressed. With greater involvement, the adolescent patient will be a better reporter of side effects. In my experience, adolescents do not overreport or drown the therapist with imagined somatic complaints. Certain tricyclics, like imipramine, reliably produce many side effects in adolescents and adults, but there is no greater preponderance of side effects reported by either group.

Stimulants

Stimulant medications represent the best studied, safest, and most utilized class of drugs for outpatient children in the United States. There have been extensive reviews published (Gittelman-Klein, 1975; Klein et al., 1980; Conners and Werry, 1980), and a complete discussion of their clinical use is given in chapter 14. Several pharmacological issues have emerged from the clinical use of these compounds and will be highlighted.

Do Stimulants Work Best Only in Certain Groups?

Theories that the beneficial response to stimulant medication was limited to one age range (school-age children) or to one diagnostic group (children with cross-situational attention deficit disorder with hyperactivity [ADDH]) have not been supported. Shaffer and coworkers (1974) demonstrated that medication response on a variety of activity and attentional measures differentiated poorly among groups of hyperactive, brain-damaged, and ADDH children. Rapoport et al. (1978) carried out a d-amphetamine study comparing the response of normals with that of ADDH children. The calming response to stimulant medications occurred in ADDH children, as well as in other groups. Both hyperactive and normal boys treated with acute single doses of 0.5 mg/kg amphetamine showed significant drug responsiveness on tests of language, memory, and attention, with striking decreases in motor activity (Rapoport et al., 1978). The reputed "paradoxical" stimulant calming effect in ADDH children was not found in a study of seven males given 10 mg d-amphetamine long-acting capsules at bedtime; instead true stimulant enhancement of the lighter sleep stages, arousal, and wakefulness was produced, but with improved cooperativeness upon rising (Chatoor et al., 1983). In addition, studies of the sleep patterns of methylphenidate-treated ADDH boys revealed no particular pattern of restlessness during sleep, regardless of drug state (Greenhill et al., 1983b).

Children with ADDH who are younger than the usual school-age group are now being treated in clinical research protocols. Preschoolers, once thought to be unresponsive to stimulant medication, have been shown to display significant reductions in hyperactive behavior in two controlled studies. Schleifer and his colleagues (1975) treated twenty-six nursery-school students (mean age 4.1 years, range 3 to 5 years) with an average methylphenidate dose of 10 mg and found significant decreases in hyperactivity in a fourteen- to twenty-one-day placebo-controlled crossover trial. Conners (1975) found similar significant improvements in 95% of methylphenidate-treated, physician-selected nursery-school children (mean age 4.8, range 3 to 6 years) in a double-blind, parallel-design study at two, four, and six weeks, when compared to a group of hyperactives on placebo (response rate 10%).

Do Adolescents Respond to Stimulants?

Psychiatric lore has perpetuated the idea that ADDH diminishes with age and vanishes during adolescence. Clinicians have traditionally discontinued stimulants at age twelve for a variety of reasons, including: the anticipated loss at puberty of the unique paradoxical calming response to stimulants; possible growth suppression because long bone growth stops during adolescence when the epiphyses close (Greenhill, 1981); and because of possible dependence upon or abuse of these medications (Goyer et al., 1979).

In general, there is little empirical evidence to support any notions that the adolescent's response to stimulant medications differs greatly from that found in children. They respond to d-amphetamine by releasing catecholamines from the presynaptic neuron (Scheel-Kruger, 1972), just as children and adults do.

Several studies show positive treatment results in adolescents. Three studies of male delinquents treated with stimulants (Korey, 1944; Eisenberg et al., 1963; Maletzky, 1974) report significant drug response with improvement in social and behavioral areas. An open-label study by Lerer and Lerer (1977) of twenty-seven adolescents meeting criteria for ADDH found improvements on the Conners ten-item brief questionnaire scored by the teacher. Varly's 1983 study of twenty-two adolescents utilized a double-blind, Latin-square design to compare three drug treatments: placebo given at 8:00 A.M. and noon; 0.15 mg/kg of methylphenidate given at 8:00 A.M. and noon; or 0.30 mg/kg of methylphenidate administered at 8:00 A.M. and at noon. When the children took methylphenidate, they reported mild side effects, some complained of mild sleep disturbances, some had appetite disturbances. The blood pressure of the methylphenidate-treated subjects showed a mean diastolic elevation of 7 mm Hg, and an increase in heart rate of 10 beats/min. There was a significant drug effect ($p < 0.05$) and a significant positive correlation between teachers' and parents' ratings. The stimulant medication response was an improvement of attention and decrease in impulsivity, quite similar to the drug-related changes found in childhood. There was no evidence that the adolescents showed excitement or euphoria on the methylphenidate, and no evidence of a reversal of positive drug effect.

These studies suggest that the prudent clinician may consider continuing treatment on patients as they grow into adolescence. Routine drug holidays should be given each summer, with stimulant medication restarted during the school year only as needed, to clarify the persistence of the signs of hyperactivity in the teenager. If there is doubt about the efficacy of the stimulants, a placebo trial can be most revealing.

Dose-Response Studies

There has been a strong interest in stimulant dose-response studies in children. Sprague and Sleator (1977) have suggested that there is a dose-related dissociation of the cognitive and social response to stimulant medication. A 0.3 mg/kg dose was reported to induce optimal matching-to-sample task performance (fewest errors and shortest latency of response) for an immediate-memory picture-recognition task in twenty hyperactive subjects. Increasing the dose to 1 mg/kg resulted in a return to baseline (or worse) for performance error rates, but classroom social performance improved. Methylphenidate has been shown to produce a limited type of state-dependent learning (Swanson and Kinsbourne, 1976). Both Swanson et al.'s dose-response work (1977) on a similar paired-associates learning (PAL) task and Gan and Cantwell's more recent study (1982) tend to support the lower dosage—0.3 mg/kg methylphenidate dose level—as being more effective in this one immediate-memory laboratory task than higher stimulant dose levels. By examining the children's performance under no-drug, placebo, and drug conditions, Gan discovered that a number of ADDH children do worse (more errors of omission) on placebo than on no-drug, and show improved PAL task performance on both 0.3 and 1 mg/kg. Gan found no evidence for state-dependent learning during relearning of the task twenty-four hours later. She suggested that expectation effects of taking a pill (even placebo) could affect performance. Such expectation effects show interactions with drug effects during direct behavioral observations in experimental classrooms (Whalen et al., 1978). These expectation effects can also show their presence in the type of interaction, directive or supporting, adults have with ADDH children (Barkley and Cunningham, 1979).

The complexities of this data do little to support the dissociation of dose-response curves for stimulants. Werry and Aman (1975) have produced other evidence that linear dose-cognitive response curves are far more common in children, even across drug types. Still, the "lowest dose is best for learning" point of view has been very influential. There has been a widespread acceptance of the dissociation hypothesis, even though the original study has yet to be replicated in an independent lab. A *de facto* 0.3-0.6 mg/kg dosage guideline has emerged, even though no independent evidence for a therapeutic methylphenidate window has been published. Recent research papers no longer use the clinically based titration method of dosage adjustment over a 20-60 mg/day range (Sprague and Sleator, 1975).

Pharmacokinetic studies have recently been carried out for methylphenidate in hyperactive children. These projects had to await the development of reliable assay (Iden and Hungund, 1979). Most groups report a large degree of variability in peak methylphenidate plasma levels for the same oral dose, both between individuals and within the same individual on different days (Hungund et al., 1979, Gualtieri et al., 1981; Gualtieri et al., 1982). In spite of this variability, Kupietz and coworkers (1982) reported a significant negative correlation between learning errors on a PAL task and peak methylphenidate levels in five ADDH males. Blood sampling was carried out at baseline and five times over the next seven hours following oral ingestion. Other studies demonstrated an inverse relationship between the increase in plasma level of methylphenidate (MEP) and the decrease in error rate on a test of motor persistence (Gardner et al., 1979; Greenhill et al., 1983a). Achieving this significant dose-response correlation was a result of the high resolution time-tracking pharmacokinetic MEP analysis used.

Pharmacokinetic MEP studies in children have been primarily same-day acute-dosing studies. The longest period of observation was utilized by Winsberg's group (1982), who carried out a six-week, placebo-controlled study of varying mg/kg MEP dosages between 0.25 and 1 mg/kg in twenty-five ADDH boys. Weekly plasma levels correlated with teacher and parent responses in a linear dose-response fashion. Maintenance treatment of ADDH often last months or years, not weeks. With the trend in the methylphenidate literature showing successful short-term effects, but long-term drug tolerance (Greenhill, 1977) and persistent academic failure (Weiss et al., 1975; Charles et al., 1979), this question is not trivial. Could long-term changes in metabolism, in volume of distribution, or in timing of peak MEP plasma levels explain the drug's lack of efficacy in those cases who show tolerance and require ever increasing doses over the long haul? One study examined pharmacokinetic parameters at baseline and after six months on maintenance MEP in eight ADDH males and found no significant changes in MEP time to peak, MEP peak values, MEP half-life, or volume of distribution (Greenhill et al., 1983a).

Prognosis

What does happen to the hyperactive syndrome in adolescence? In many cases the predictive validity of the diagnosis of ADDH is very weak, with no characteristic treatment response holding over time and no characteristic outcome emerging from many follow-up studies (Shaffer and Greenhill, 1979). There has been a tendency to include active males without other functional deficits, particularly when inappropriately low cutting scores, based on small samples, are used on global teachers' questionnaires (Trites et al., 1979).

Some data have developed from recent studies that have been well controlled and show a low attrition rate. The hyperactive boy who shows out-of-seat motor hyperactivity in the classroom, impulsiveness, and distractibility as a prepubertal child will probably continue to have these features as an adolescent, according to Gittelman's follow-up study (1982) that retrieved 98% of the original sample at age eighteen. In addition, as Weiss and Hechtman (1979) report from their Toronto sample, hyperactive adolescents openly express their frustration and disappointment over school failure. Studies of Weiss and coworkers (1975, 1979) as well as the two-year follow-up of seventy-two ADDH children by Riddle and Rapoport (1976) indicate that over half the ADDH children continue to exhibit signs of impulsivity, motor restlessness, and short attention span well into adolescence.

Long-term treatment with stimulants, with a follow-up of from two to twelve years from first identification, has failed to show any stable benefit to academic performance or to social outcome (Weiss et al., 1971) for adolescents in school. Charles et al. (1979) found no significant differences in outcome between a group of thirteen children who discontinued their methylphenidate and those who remained on the drug during a three-year follow-up study. Satterfield and colleagues (1980) reported substantial maintenance of early drug improvements in academic performance, delinquent behavior, and emotional adjustment for a group of sixty-one children with ADDH followed for two years in a multimodality program of carefully adjusted medicine and psychotherapy. This study was not controlled, and it suffered a 48% attrition rate, so interpretation of the results must be cautious.

What Effects Do Stimulants Have on ADDH Children?

In contrast to Weiss and Laites's notion (1962) that amphetamines could "increase cognitive capacity," there has been no empirically derived evidence to prove that the stimulants can increase intellectual abilities above baseline measures. A detailed controlled investigation of behaviorally normal children with reading disability showed no significant drug effect on the acquisition of reading skills (Gittelman-Klein, 1976). Barmack (1979) noted that performance changes from stimulants were not a direct result of biochemical alterations alone, but were probably mediated by psychological processes such as pacing and task acceptability. He believed stimulants did not show more than small percentage improvements over starting baseline measures, whereas major percentage differences between placebo and active drug were seen due to early performance decrements when the individual was treated with placebo.

Both hyperactive and normal children show significant performance changes on certain laboratory-based tests. Amphetamines have been shown to produce mood state-dependent enhancement of memory retrieval and storage when given to depressed adults (Weingartner et al., 1978). Controlled continuous performance test (CPT) amphetamine studies involving hyperactive children, normal children, and young adults show that amphetamines significantly increase perceptual sensitivity (d') and reponse bias (B), with younger children showing a much larger effect (Sostek et al., 1981). Recent work on electrophysiological tests of the late positive complex (LPC) and event-related potentials (ERP) associated with cognitive processing during CPT exercises shows significant reductions of placebo levels of errors and reaction time on two different dosage levels of methylphenidate in twenty-seven cross-situational hyperactive children and a maximal enhancement of the LPC at the 0.3 mg/kg oral dose level (Klorman et al., 1983). How these performance enhancements on laboratory measures translate to the social ecology of the classroom is not yet clear.

Naturalistic studies utilizing portable activity monitors with solid-state memories have revealed that a 15 mg amphetamine dose, compared to placebo in a double-blind ABAB design, significantly reduced the motor activity of twelve hyperactive boys for eight hours after ingestion across a wide variety of situations and different tasks (Porrino et al., 1983). The half-life of d-amphetamine in ADDH children has been shown to range from ten to nineteen hours (Ebert et al., 1976; Brown et al., 1978), and studies of continuously treated hyperactive males under steady-state drug conditions (Ebert and Perel, personal communication) show plasma amphetamine concentrations as high as 40 ng/ml eighteen hours after oral dosing.

The dopamine-deficiency hypothesis (Wender, 1971; Wender, 1975) of ADDH, which proposed a putative central neurotransmitter disorder underlying the clinical symptoms, was generally not supported by a number of controlled studies using the dopamine (DA) agonist Sinemet (60 mg/day carbidopa, and 600 mg/day L-dopa) (Langer et al., 1982) and piribedil, a relatively specific DA agonist (Brown et al, 1979). Clinical effects on the signs of ADDH were either weak (Sinemet) or nonexistent (piribedil). Side effects of the dopamine agonists were far greater and the clinical effects less beneficial than the regular stimulant, d-amphetamine. The investigators concluded that central noradrenergic systems were more likely to be involved in the mechanism of stimulant drug action in ADDH (Langer et al., 1982).

Some investigators have utilized animal models of ADDH to understand the effects of stimulants on specific brain receptors. Rat brain membranes have demonstrated the presence of high affinity, saturable, and stereospecific binding sites for $[H^3]$ threo-($\pm$)-methylphenidate (Skolnick et al., 1984, in press). Data on the relative motor stimulant activation potencies of a group of ritalinic acid esters correlated at a highly significant level with their ability to displace $[H^3]$ threo-($\pm$)-methylphenidate from these striatal membranes, which appear to be presynaptic dopamine receptor sites. The MEP receptor involved in the stimulant treatment of childhood ADDH may have a specific brain locus in the striatum, which may turn out to be the actual site of drug action in the ADDH child.

Interaction with Other Therapies

The interaction between stimulants and nonpharmacological treatments has not received the attention it might. Two types of studies exist. One category compared behavioral-modification techniques with methylphenidate pharmacotherapy (Gittelman-Klein et al., 1980) and found the medication showed the strongest and quickest benefits, although both modalities were effective. The second showed improved outcome when stimulant treatment was combined with a program of educational remediation and parental counseling (Satterfield et al., 1980). Rarely have interactions between stimulants and other drugs been studied, although methylphenidate and thioridazine appear to be useful when used together (Gittelman-Klein et al., 1976).

Long-Acting Preparations

A longer-acting, enteric-coated, sustained-release methylphenidate preparation has received FDA approval and is now available. Drug administration can be limited to a once-per-day schedule, allowing for parental administration and avoiding the in-school midday dose and its attendant peer ridicule thought to be a major source of poor patient compliance. Dosage has been set at 20 mg to approximate a total daily drug intake (at 0.6 mg/kg) for the typical 33 kg child. Controlled clinical studies have been limited to one published report (Whitehouse et al., 1980), and the new drug is currently under investigation to determine its true dosage equivalency and actual efficacy when compared to the well-proven shorter-acting Ritalin formulation. A series of papers reporting on sustained-release d-amphetamine found few pharmacokinetic differences between the two formulations (Brown et al., 1978, 1980).

These authors showed that the maximal clinical response to d-amphetamine occurred within the first three hours after ingestion, which is called the absorption phase, regardless of whether the short-acting tablet or the long-acting capsule was used. A similar plasma concentration time course may be present for both short- and long-acting MEP, and only a time-tracked dose-response pharmacokinetic study of Ritalin-SR in ADDH children will tell.

Long-term Side Effects

Although stimulant medication constitutes one of the safest forms of pharmacotherapy, concern with potential long-term growth inhibition has existed since the first report of this side effect by Safer, Allen, and Barr (1972). Review articles (Roche et al., 1979; Greenhill, 1981) suggested that weight velocity losses occurred more often than height velocity decrements, and that methylphenidate was less apt to cause this side effect than d-amphetamine. Prospective studies of children receiving continuous, long-term d-amphetamine (Puig-Antich et al., 1978) and methylphenidate (Mattes and Gittelman, 1983) suggested that the growth slowdown was dose related. Loney and coworkers (1982) reported that complaints of stimulant side effects were far more predictive than oral dose in a sample of eighty-five boys (mean age at follow-up = 14.5 years) treated a mean period of thirty-six months on a mean dose of 33.1 mg/day. Treatment-related variables such as initial nausea and vomiting explained 7% of the variance in adolescent height and 17% of the variance in weight, even though the majority of adolescents reported that all stimulant-related appetite-suppressant effects disappeared by the end of the first month of treatment. While the mechanism of growth suppression remains obscure, a simultaneous suppression of mean sleep-related plasma prolactin concentrations has been reported (Greenhill et al., 1981; Greenhill et al., 1984) from the dopamine agonist action of the stimulants. Kilgore and colleagues (1979) have suggested, from their tissue culture *in vitro* work, that stimulants suppress somatomedins, a group of peripherally synthesized peptides necessary for bone growth.

ANTIDEPRESSANTS

The tricyclic antidepressants have been applied to the treatment of childhood depressive states, school phobia, and ADDH. Their actual clinical application has been limited to the short-term treatment of enuresis (Werry, 1982). Even though a large body of controlled drug literature exists showing TCAs effective in suppressing the symptoms of enuresis (Rapoport et al., 1980), there are only a scattering of controlled studies in other conditions.

Use of Tricyclics for Enuresis

The treatment of enuresis constitutes the best studied pharmacological therapeutic application of TCAs in pediatric medicine and child psychiatry, with over forty controlled studies published showing imipramine's clear benefit over placebo in suppressing nighttime wetting (Rapoport et al., 1980). The mechanism of action remains unknown, but recent work shows that the drug's antienuretic effect is not a simple matter of either central or peripheral anticholinergic influence on bladder tone. Given by themselves, powerful anticholinergic drugs fail to suppress the symptoms of enuresis. Rapoport and coworkers (1980) reported significant correlations between plasma concentration of TCA and clinical response (r = 0.59, p < 0.01), with no evidence of a therapeutic "window," for all responders with TCA plasma concentrations of 150 ng/ml or greater showed dryness. A plasma concentration at this level was no guarantee of clinical response, since several subjects exhibited either transient dryness or no response at that blood level. Total bedtime dose was 75 mg of either imipramine or desipramine, except for nonresponders and transient responders, who were given more drug (up to 125 mg at bedtime).

Even though most controlled TCA studies of enuretics report response rates approaching 60%, these medications have a limited application in the treatment of this disorder. TCAs suppress enuresis in good responders, who still wet as soon as the drug is stopped. Transient responses, symptom breakthrough, and tolerance effects occur regularly in those children treated for enuresis. As shown in chapter 2, there is good evidence that bell-and-pad conditioning is a more effective and long-lasting treatment. TCAs are useful for short-term suppression of enuretic episodes, as when a child is going for a sleep-over visit with a friend.

Treatment for ADDH

The use of antidepressants in the treatment of ADDH is of considerable pharmacological interest. Rapoport and coworkers (1974) have indicated that TCAs can be effective in the treatment of ADDH, although there tend to be more side effects than with stimulants. Drug tolerance develops in many after several months, even though plasma levels of TCAs remain unchanged. The clinical benefits occur within days of starting the TCAs in ADDH children, in contrast to the four- to six-week period required for antidepressant action to develop. This suggests that the TCA's mechanism of clinically beneficial action differs in the two disorders. Comparisons of stimulants to TCAs in a controlled, Latin-square design drug study showed that antidepressants produced less dramatic results, but worked controlling behavior into the evening hours without causing insomnia (Garfinkel et al., 1983). Work with other classes of antidepressants also appears promising, and early studies show that monoamine oxidase (MAO) inhibitors may show some benefit in cases of ADDH (Rapoport, personal communication).

Use of Tricyclics for Depression

Puig-Antich and coworkers (1978) have identified a group of depressed prepubertal children whose symptoms meet the Research Diagnostic Criteria for major endogenous depression. With antidepressant medication response serving as a validating criterion for this disorder, these investigators have shown a significant correlation between plasma level concentrations of total TCAs exceeding 200 ng/ml and clinical response on the mood-change scores of the K-SADS (Puig-Antich et al., 1979). Other studies have shown similar results in this age group but at slightly lower plasma concentrations of TCAs (Weller et al., 1983).

The response to TCAs in major depressive illness may vary according to age group, for some preliminary work has shown that placebo response rates equal those of active drug in adolescents with major depression (Kramer and Feiguine, 1981). More studies need to be done in this area to show the long-term efficacy of the TCA treatment for childhood depression, as well as the long-term side effects in the developing child.

Treatment for Adolescents with Mood Disorders

Adolescence is a time of increased suicide rates, depression, and the emergence of bipolar disorders. Prepubertal major depressive disorder has a lower prevalence than depression in adolescence. Typically, depressed teenagers are female, report frequent mood swings, boredom, extreme rejection sensitivity from peers, and display outbursts of rage toward their parents. When clinically depressed, they experience a persistent depressive mood and anhedonia for a two-week duration and have a number of vegetative signs—anorexia, insomnia, and diurnal mood variations. Overdoses are common. Antidepressants would seem to be indicated for treating adolescents. But do they work?

There has been a paucity of controlled studies of adolescents treated with tricyclic antidepressants. Kramer and Feiguine's 1981 double-blind, placebo-controlled study of twenty adolescents treated with amitriptyline is one of the few published. They found no significant difference between amitriptyline and placebo, since both groups showed a 75% improvement rate.

Puig-Antich and colleagues at the New York State Psychiatric Institute extended the Kramer and Feiguine study with an open-label trial of imipramine in thirty-eight children over a five-week period (Puig-Antich et al., 1983). All subjects were Tanner stage 3, and 18% were inpatients. For a positive clinical response, criteria were set so that the K-SADS ratings had to be less than or equal to 3 (mild) at five weeks on two items—mood and anhedonia. Again there was a high placebo response rate (68%), which did not differ from the active drug response (58%). Whereas plasma level of imipramine plus desipramine best predicted response in Puig-Antich's group of prepubertal major endogenous depressive disordered children, there was no significant relationship between plasma level and positive clinical response in the adolescents. The only clinical predictive factor was the symptom of separation anxiety, which predicted nonresponse.

Two possible variables in these adolescents might explain the findings. The relative resistance to TCA treatment in adolescence may be related to a biological change, i.e., both males and females show the highest plasma estrogen levels at that time. Estrogen may competitively inhibit receptors critical for the action of the TCAs. In addition, the adolescent's clinical picture most closely resembles adult atypical depressives described by Quitkin (in press). These patients differ from typical depressives by a reversal of vegetative signs—too much sleep, overeating, no response to imipramine, and good response to MAO inhibitors.

Future research will be conducted with depressed adolescent patients treated with MAO inhibitors. But that raises the concern about diet, since tyramine-rich foods can cause dangerous elevations in blood pressure and teenagers are notorious violators of dietary limits. Although the Food and Drug Administration and the pharmaceutical companies warn that combining a tricyclic and an MAO inhibitor may lead to serious side effects, many therapists use the combination because it is believed to be safer and, perhaps, more efficacious for patients unresponsive to single agents. A recent controlled study of sixty adult depressives by Simpson's group (Ranzani et al., 1983) randomly assigned patients to combined treatment (an MAO inhibitor plus a tricyclic antidepressant), to a single tricyclic, and to a single MAO inhibitor. The investigators carefully followed certain guidelines to insure a minimum of side effects. Both types of drug were started on the same day at low dosages, and then gradually increased to a maximum point that was exactly half those used with each single drug. A typical schedule might include Parnate at 30 mg in the morning and amitriptyline 150 mg at night. The outcome suggests that when MAO inhibitors are begun simultaneously with small doses of TCAs, there are no increases in hypertensive crisis or other cardiovascular side effects. Therefore, a few investigators have begun treating adolescents with combined antidepressant medication schedules. Anecdotal reports to date are encouraging.

Other clinicians favor the use of nortriptyline for adolescents. Kragh-Sorensen's early work (Kragh-Sorensen et al., 1976) indicated a therapeutic window in plasma levels, and most treating physicians attempt to set the plasma levels between 150 and 180 ng/ml. Typically, this is achieved with a daily oral intake of 50 to 250 mg of nortriptyline.

The observation of Klein et al. (1980) that adult agoraphobic patients had past childhood histories of separation anxiety led them to utilize imipramine, a drug that relieved panic anxiety, in the school-phobic children with pathological separation anxiety. They launched a six-week, placebo-controlled study of thirty-five children between the ages of seven and fifteen who had been absent from school for at least two weeks, and a two-week attempt was made to get them back to school before entering the study. Then approximately half the group was placed on imipramine, and half on placebo, 81% of the imipramine group returned to school, and 100% felt better. In contrast, only 47% of the placebo-treated group returned to school and only 21% felt better. Analysis showed that alleviation of the separation anxiety does not guarantee a return to school (Gittelman-Klein and Klein, 1973). Although anecdotal reports have indicated d-amphetamine and chlordiazepoxide may help in school phobia, there is no firm evidence. The only controlled study involving another drug was carried out by Abe (1975) using sulpride, an antidepressant and antipsychotic. It helped thirteen of twenty-one school phobics, who ranged in age from nine to seventeen years, to go back to school within a few days.

Subtypes of other clinical disorders in child and adolescent populations may respond to the action of antidepressants. Puig-Antich et al. (1983) described a subgroup of prepubertal males with primary depression and secondary conduct disorder who responded to imipramine with mood elevation and the cessation of antisocial acts. Eight depressed children with cancer responded to low doses (1–2 mg/kg/day) of imipramine or amitriptyline (Pfefferbaum-Levine et al., 1983). Bulimia, the syndrome of compulsive binge eating sometimes starting in adolescence, has responded to treatment with imipramine in a controlled study of twenty-two females (Pope et al., 1983). The reported efficacy of clomipramine (CMI) in adults with obsessive-compulsive disorder has been as convincing for children. A controlled study of CMI in children and adolescents with severe obsessive-compulsive disturbance showed significant differences between placebo and active drug (Rapoport, personal communication). The positive reports cited here require replication before they can be applied to everyday practice.

NEUROLEPTICS

Despite their widespread use in child and adolescent psychiatry, neuroleptics do not have a specific target disorder for treatment in the majority of school-age children. There are a small number of first-break schizophrenics who become symptomatic before their sixteenth birthday and may benefit from the antipsychotic action of these drugs, although their prognosis is poorer when treated with these agents (Werry, 1982). Haloperidol has been used in the management of children with pervasive developmental disorder for limited, symptomatic control of stereotypies, fidgetiness, hyperactivity, and abnormal object relations (Campbell et al., 1983). Most of the neuroleptics prescribed in child psychiatry settings are used for sedation in the institutionalized retarded (Lipman et al., 1978).

The situation is different in adolescent psychiatry, where neuroleptics of all types receive a good deal of use. The emergence of schizophrenic and bipolar syndromes at this developmental stage establishes a first-line indication for the use of the major tranquilizers. With the increased amount of drug abuse and the toxic psychoses from marijuana, PCP, LSD, mescaline, cocaine, and heroin that can occur in this age group, staffs in psychiatric emergency rooms dispense neuroleptics on an acute basis. As with childhood disorders, major tranquilizers are often used for extreme aggressivity, extreme hyperactivity, Tourette's syndrome, and psychotic states.

One frequent application of these drugs is for the long-term management of adolescents and young adults with retardation who reside in institutions and in community foster care. Lipman et al. (1978) and Breuning et al. (1983), in separate surveys, have discovered that 55% of these patients are treated with major tranquilizers for behavioral management to limit aggressivity and screaming. The drug of choice in these situations appears to be thioridazine, or Mellaril. Unfortunately, this population, because of cognitive deficits, tendency to become obese, meager behavioral gains, and an inability to question the use of these drugs, is particularly ill-suited for the use of such medication.

There is no doubt that neuroleptics are of value in the treatment of the agitated, psychotic adolescent patient. Depending on the patient's pharmacokinetics, metabolism, and the drug's bioavailability, the agitated psychotic adolescent may be treated with rather sizable amounts of these drugs. Werry (1982) has pointed out that juvenile schizophrenics do respond to neuroleptics, but somewhat less well than do adult-onset cases. For the older adolescent patient with manic phase bipolar illness, doses of haloperidol can be titrated against his agitation with good results, particularly when waiting for the lithium to exert control.

The problem with neuroleptics more and more is the cost of their use. Many neuroleptics produce weight gain, which seems to be a direct stimulatory action of these drugs on hypothalamic nuclei. Only molindone hydrochloride, or Moban, an indole amine-like compound, seems to promote weight loss (Gardos and Cole, 1977), making it a good choice for an already overweight patient. Another action of all neuroleptics is an acute elevation of serum prolactin in both sexes. Prolactin release is tonically inhibited by dopamine and released in abundance by agents that block the postsynaptic dopamine receptor, which is true of all major tranquilizers (Gruen et al., 1978). Prolactin is thus released, and its effects on the developing adolescent are unknown at this time. Although one report attributed granulocytopenia in children to taking phenothiazines (Shabry and Wolk, 1980), the reported blood dyscrasia seemed mild and was not convincingly linked to the medication.

Neuroleptics also appear to interact negatively in laboratory tests of cognitive functioning (Aman, 1978). This feature raises serious questions about their use in mentally retarded populations. Bruening and coworkers (1983) conducted a controlled study showing that sustained use of thioridazine, 3-6 mg/kg, blocked the normal increase in IQ test scores found when retarded adolescents were rewarded with sodas and other treats for correct answers. These particular adolescents had demonstrated an 80% diminution of objectionable social behaviors when treated with the drug, so were considered clear-cut responders. The controls, who were nonresponders, also failed to show the reinforcement-cued performance improvement on the tests, but showed an improvement in social behavior when taken off the drug. Bruening likened these effects to the differential, dissociative dose-response curves for methylphenidate described by Sprague and Sleator (1977). As dose is increased, two peaks appear—one for best cognitive performance (at a low dose) and one for best social performance (at the higher doses). Most clinicians titrate on the basis of social responses and have no practical outcome variable for cognitive performance. Adjusting the adolescent's thioridazine dose to give the minimal social difficulties may produce problems, for the patient may no longer be as responsive to social praise from the teacher. In addition, Bruening's study raises serious questions about the treatment of adolescent patients simultaneously with neuroleptics and behavioral modification, since the neuroleptics appear to block the response to reinforcement.

Finally, there is the question of tardive dyskinesia (TD). This persistent dyskinetic movement disorder was first reported in elderly inpatients who had been treated with large doses of neuroleptics over many years (Medical Letter, 1979). Gualtieri and colleagues (1980) have estimated that all adolescents and young adults who have a total lifetime exposure to major tranquilizers that exceeds 375 *grams* are at serious risk for TD. Although the most common presentation involves choreiform, jerky movements of the oral-buccal-masticatory musculatory (BLM syndrome), other areas can be involved. Severe akathisia may accompany the facial movements, as we saw in a fourteen-year-old psychotic girl who developed severe tongue protrusion and paced constantly after treatment with chlorpromazine, 400 mg/day. Technically, patients must have a movement disorder that lasts three or more months for it to qualify as TD. Ferguson and Breuning (1982) have shown that drug-related movement disorders significantly interfere with the performance of retarded children and adolescents on structured workshop tasks.

TD can strike children and adolescents, somewhat going against the clinical lore that younger patients are protected from the disorder (Gualtieri et al., 1980). A consortium has been formed to collect cases of adolescents, young adults, and children with the disorder (Gualtieri et al., 1983). Children as young as age six, as well as many adolescents, with classic BLM syndrome, Bon-Bon signs, dystonias, and tongue protrusion have begun to appear in referral centers. Also worrisome are the growing number of lawsuits against the treating psychiatrist over young adults with TD. Gualtieri (1983) recommends that neuroleptics be used sparingly in children and adolescents because of this risk.

Fenfluramine, an anorectic agent that inhibits serotonin release, has been used in the treatment of pervasive developmental disorder. One double-blind but essentially uncontrolled study reported significant gains on a ward behavior checklist and Catell intelligence test scores in two autistic preschool children treated for six weeks with the drug (40 mg/day) in a placebo-fenfluramine-placebo design (Geller et al., 1982). An interinstitutional collaborative group has been established, and they recently reported weight loss, decreased plasma serotonin levels, but little clinical improvement in the group of autistic children treated with the drug (Klykylo and Realmuto, 1983).

LITHIUM

Lithium prophylaxis against mania has been shown to have a most reliable and predictable action. Most episodes of bipolar affective disorder make their appearance in the late teens or early part of the twenties, so few adolescents will be found on maintenance lithium treatment.

Lithium has proven helpful in some areas of child psychiatry, such as the treatment of very aggressive children, regardless of *DSM-III* diagnosis (Campbell et al., 1982b). Some promising early work had been done by Sheard (1971) and Tupin (1978) on prison populations using lithium for limiting violent outbursts. Campbell's work with lithium includes controlled studies of a number of drug types in the treatment of autistic children, ADDH children with severe aggressivity, and undersocialized conduct disorder, aggressive type (Campbell et al., 1978; Campbell et al., 1982a). Lithium appears to be as clinically efficacious as haloperidol in curtailing aggressivity when compared to placebo, but with fewer sedating side effects (Campbell et al., 1983). The two drugs differentially interfered with cognitive functioning, haloperidol producing slower and more variable reaction times and lithium causing a deterioration in qualitative performance on the Porteus maze test (Platt et al. 1981).

These findings suggest that both lithium and the neuroleptics reduce aggressivity and lead to mild cognitive impairment as assessed in the laboratory. The major advantage of lithium treatment is the reduced vulnerability to the development of tardive dyskinesia. Treatment of aggressive children with phenothiazines would lead to lengthy treatments and a great risk for TD. Further work with lithium should be done.

Although some clinicians have combined lithium with phenothiazines in the treatment of very violent children and adolescents, there are no controlled studies to date describing the efficacy or risks of such a combination in child or adolescent populations. Lithium has not proven helpful in the treatment of hyperactivity (Greenhill et al., 1973).

The drug is a weak antidepressant (Klein et al., 1980), although recent reports suggest it may potentiate the actions of first-line antidepressants such as nortriptyline in cases unresponsive to conventional drug therapy. This suggests another combination that may prove useful in treating adolescent major depressive disorder.

Rifkin et al. (1972) conducted a study on a series of twenty-one adolescent female patients he believed to have an atypical mood disorder. He called them emotionally unstable character disorders because of chronic maladaptive behavior patterns, short-lived depressive and hypomanic mood swings lasting a few hours or days, which were not triggered by external events. A six-week, double-blind crossover study comparing lithium to placebo showed that lithium significantly stabilized mood swings, and did not produce the sedation that neuroleptics had. Today, these cases might be called rapid-cycling manic depressives, borderlines, or schizo-affectives.

Propranolol

This beta adrenergic blocking agent has been used effectively in controlling explosive rage outbursts in adults otherwise unresponsive to other drugs, including anticonvulsants and major tranquilizers. Several investigators (Elliot, 1977; Yudofsky et al., 1981; Williams et al., 1982) have treated episodic belligerence in young adults and adolescents with propranolol, in divided doses, in doses ranging from 320 to 520 mg/day. Schreier (1979) found that lower doses, namely 100 mg/day, controlled rage in a twelve-year-old child. Many of these cases had positive neurological histories and many of the patients successfully treated could be diagnosed in *DSM-III* as either conduct disorder, undersocialized, aggressive type, or as intermittent explosive disorder. Williams and coworkers (1982) treated thirty patients, including fifteen adolescents. The optimal dosage yielding maximal therapeutic effects with least side effects ranged from 50 to 960 mg/day, with a median dose of 160 mg/day. Seventy-five percent of the patients showed either moderate or marked improvement in apparent response to this drug. Side effects included somnolence and lethargy, four cases of hypotension, and one case of bradycardia. One adolescent patient became clinically depressed on 960 mg/day and one other patient developed asthma. All side effects were reported to be transient and easily reversible with dosage adjustment. This drug should be considered for the management of episodic, violent, uncontrolled behavior, since stimulants, anticonvulsants, and neuroleptics are mostly ineffective.

CLONIDINE

Clonidine is an alpha$_2$ adrenergic agonist originally marketed for the central control of hypertension. It appears to act mainly in the locus ceruleus, a pontine area rich in adrenergic neuron bodies. The drug stimulates adrenergic presynaptic receptors, thus decreasing the neuron's output of norepinephrine by means of inhibitory feedback pathways. Using clonidine to decrease adrenergic responsivity, Gold and coworkers (1978) have been able to withdraw heroin addicts without the hypersensitive adrenergic "cold-turkey" response.

Clonidine has been applied by Leckman et al. (1983) of the Yale group in a novel fashion to an entirely different population, children and adolescents suffering from Tourette's syndrome (TS). The syndrome is a severe, familial neuropsychiatric disorder characterized by childhood onset and lifelong duration of simple and complex motor and phonic symptoms that wax and wane in severity. Clonidine has proven helpful in the treatment of TS. Leckman et al. studied six cases with TS before and after twelve weeks of clonidine treatment. Two of these were adolescents and three were eleven years of age. Doses were set at 2–3 μg/kg, and a mean reduction in symptoms of 38% occurred ($P < 0.005$). Patients continued to maintain improvement over a twelve-month period, and three out of four patients put in a double-blind discontinuation study relapsed. Clonidine appears to be an effective treatment of TS.

CARBAMAZEPINE

Carbamazepine (Tegretol) is an iminodibenzyl derivative. It has a multitude of therapeutic uses (Ballenger and Post, 1980). It is the drug of choice for the control of temporal lobe epilepsy, but has also been used for pain syndromes, trigeminal neuralgia, diabetes insipidus, and dystonic disorders. It has been noted that half of the 2,500 seizure patients in forty studies of carbamazepine showed improvement in psychiatric functioning. Seven of these studies were controlled and showed a positive psychotropic effect from the drug. Patients report feeling brighter, more alert, and have fewer symptoms of anxiety, depression, and irritability. A number of studies on patients with episodic violent and psychopathological difficulties, abnormal EEG, but no documented seizures, improved on carbamazepine.

Ballenger and Post studied nine bipolar young adult patients in a double-blind, placebo-controlled trial. Antimanic effects were observed in seven patients throughout the trial, while the antidepressant effects required two weeks to appear. Therapeutic effects were achieved with 600–1,600 mg/day at blood levels of 8–12 μg/ml. Side effects included dizziness in one-third of the patients, pruritus in one patient, and dropping white count (from 8,000 to 6,000) in most patients. Carbamazepine is an alternative to lithium because it produces no tremor and no thyroid problems, and it will not induce mania as do the TCAs when they are used to treat depression in bipolars. It may prove to be an effective drug for treating depression in adolescents with major depressive disorders refractory to tricyclics.

Conclusions

Pediatric psychopharmacology has a few impressive accomplishments, which justify it as an effective treatment modality. Certainly, the short-term treatment of ADDH with stimulants has chalked up an impressive record of benefits with a minimum of risks. Yet the field remains burdened with a number of primitive asumptions, difficult to modify, e.g., that sedating a retarded patient is therapeutic management. Other therapists undertreat patients, convincing the parents that poor response to one underutilized drug means that their child is unresponsive. Unfortunately, there are no sensitivity tests, as with antibiotics, that can serve to pinpoint the optimal therapeutic agent. As Werry (1982) has pointed out, pediatric psychopharmacology has provided many heuristic observations and few clinically meaningful guidelines. The therapist must be willing to be an optimistic empiricist, always hoping to find a moderate degree of improvement, not a miraculous cure.

References

Abe, K. 1975. Sulpride in school phobia. *Psychiat. Clin.,* 8:95–98.

Aman, M. 1978. Drugs, learning, and the psychotherapies. In *Pediatric psychopharmacology: The use of behavior modifiying drugs in children,* ed. J.S. Werry, pp. 79–108. New York: Brunner/Mazel.

American Psychiatric Association. 1980. *Diagnostic and statistical manual of mental disorders—third edition (DSM-III).* Washington, D.C.: American Psychiatric Association.

Ballenger, J., and Post, R. 1980. Carbamazepine in manic-depressive illness: A new treatment. *Am. J. Psych.,* 137:782–790.

Barkley, R., and Cunningham, C. 1979. The effects of methylphenidate on the mother-child interactions of hyperactive children. *Arch. Gen. Psych.,* 36:201–208.

Barmack, J. 1979. Letter to Judith L. Rapoport.

Bradley, C. 1937. The behavior of children receiving Benzedrine. *Am. J. Psych.,* 94:578–584.

Breuning, S., Ferguson, D., Davidson, N., and Poling, A. 1983. Effects of thioridazine on the intellectual performance of mentally retarded drug responders and nonresponders. *Arch. Gen. Psych.,* 40:309–313.

Brown, G., Ebert, M., and Hunt, R. 1978. Plasma d-amphetamine absorption and elimination in hyperactive children. *Psychopharm. Bull.,* 14:33–35.

Brown, G., Ebert, M., Mikkelsen, E., Buchsbaum, M., and Bunney, W. 1979. Dopamine agonist piribedil in hyperactive children. Presented at the annual meeting of the American Psychiatric Association, Chicago, Illinois.

Brown, G., Ebert, M., Mikkelsen, E., and Hunt, R. 1980. Behavior and motor activity response in hyperactive children and plasma amphetamine levels following a sustained release preparation. *J. Am. Acad. Child Psych.,* 19:225–239.

Campbell, M., Cohen, I., and Small, A. 1982a. Drugs in aggressive behavior. *J. Am. Acad. Child Psych.,* 21:107–117.

Campbell, M., Perry, R., Bennett, W., Small, A., Green, W., Grega, D., Schwartz, V., and Anderson, L. 1983. Long-term efficacy and drug-related movements: A prospective study of haloperidol in autistic children. *Psychopharm. Bull.,* 19:80–83.

Campbell, M., Schulman, D., and Rapoport, J. 1978. The current status of lithium therapy in child and adolescent psychiatry. A report of the Committee on Biological Aspects of Child Psychiatry of the American Academy of Child Psychiatry. *J. Am. Acad. Child Psych.,* 17:717–721.

Campbell, M., Small, A., Green, W., Jennings, S., Perry, R., Bennett, W., Padron-Gayol, M., and Anderson, L. 1982b. Lithium and haloperidol in hospitalized aggressive children. *Psychopharm. Bull.*, 18(3):126–129.

Charles, L., Schain, R., and Gutherie, D. 1979. Long-term use and discontinuation of methylphenidate with hyperactive children. *Dev. Med. Child Neurol.*, 21:758–764.

Chatoor, I., Wells, K., Conners, C., Seidel, W., and Shaw, D. 1983. The effects of nocturnally administered stimulant medication on EEG sleep and behavior in hyperactive children. *J. Am. Acad. Child Psych.*, 22:337–342.

Conners, C. 1975. Controlled trial of methylphenidate in preschool children with minimal brain dysfunction. In *Recent advances in child psychopharmacology,* ed. R. Gittelman-Klein. New York: Human Sciences Press.

Conners, C., and Werry, J. 1980. Pharmacotherapy. In *Psychopathological disorders of children,* ed. H. Quay, and J. Werry, pp. 336–386. New York: Wiley.

Davis, J., Erickson, S., and Dekirmenjian, H. 1978. Plasma levels of antipsychotic drugs and clinical response. In *Psychopharmacology: A generation of progress,* ed. M. Lipton, A. DiMascio, and K. Killiam, pp. 905–915. New York: Raven Press.

Dayton, P., Perel, J., Israili, Z., Faraj, B., Rodewig, K., Black, N., and Goldberg, L. 1975. Studies with methylphenidate: Drug interactions and metabolism. In *Clinical pharmacology of psychoactive drugs,* ed. E.M. Sellers, pp. 183–202. Toronto: Alcoholism and Drug Addiction Foundation.

Ebert, M., van Kammen, D., and Murphy, D. 1976. Plasma levels of amphetamine and behavioral response. In *Pharmacokinetics, psychoactive drug blood levels, and clinical response,* ed. L. Gottschak, and L. Merlis, pp. 157–169. New York: Spectrum Publications.

Eisenberg, L., Lackman, R., Molling, P., Lockner, A., Mizell, J., and Conners, C. 1963. A psychopharmacologic experiment in a training setting for delinquent boys: Methods, problems, findings. *Am. J. Orthopsych.*, 33:431–437.

Elliot, F. 1977. Propranolol for the control of the belligerent behavior following acute brain damage. *Ann. Neurol.*, 1:489–491.

Ferguson, D., and Breuning, S. 1982. Antipsychotic and antianxiety drugs. In *Drugs and mental retardation,* ed. S. Breuning, and A. Poling, pp. 168–214. Springfield, Ill.: Charles C. Thomas.

Food and Drug Administration Drug Bulletin. 1980. Tricyclic antidepressant poisoning in children. 10:22–23. Available from the Dept. of Health and Human Services, Public Health Service, Food and Drug Administration, Rockville, Maryland, 20857.

Gan, J., and Cantwell, D. 1982. Dosage effects of methylphenidate on paired associate learning: Positive/negative placebo responders. *J. Am. Acad. Child Psych.*, 21:237–242.

Gardner, R., Gardner, A., Caemmerer, A., and Broman, M. 1979. An instrument for measuring hyperactivity and other signs of MBD. *J. Clin. Child Psych.*, Fall, pp. 173–179.

Gardos, G., and Cole, J. 1977. Weight reduction in schizophrenics by molindone. *Am. J. Psych.* 134:302–304.

Garfinkel, B., Wender, P., Sloman, L., and O'Neill, I. 1983. Tricyclic antidepressant and methylphenidate treatment of attention deficit disorder in children. *J. Am. Acad. Child Psych.*, 22:343–348.

Geller, E., Ritvo, E., Freeman, E., and Yuwiler, A. 1982. Preliminary observations on the effect of fenfluramine on blood serotonin and symptoms in three autistic boys. *New Eng. J. Med.*, 307(3):165–169.

Gittelman, R. 1982. Follow-up study of 100 children with attention deficit disorder with hyperactivity into adolescence. Presented at the 29th Annual Meeting of the American Academy of Child Psychiatry, Friday, October 26, Washington, D.C.

Gittelman-Klein, R. 1975. Review of clinical psychopharmacological treatment of hyperkinesis. In

Progress in psychiatric drug treatement, ed. D. Klein, and R. Gittelman-Klein, pp. 661-674. New York: Brunner/Mazel.

Gittelman-Klein, R., Abikoff, H., Pollack, E., Klein, D., Katz, S., and Matter, J. 1980. A controlled trial of behavior modification and methylphenidate in hyperactive children. In *Hyperactive children: The social ecology of identification and treatment,* ed. C. Whalen, and B. Henker. New York: Academic Press.

Gittelman-Klein, R., and Klein, D. 1973. School phobia: Diagnostic consideration in the light of imipramine effects. *J. Nerv. Ment. Dis.,* 156:199-205.

Gittelman-Klein, R., and Klein, D. 1976. Methylphenidate effects in learning disabilities. *Arch. Gen. Psych.,* 33:655-664.

Gittelman-Klein, R., Klein, D., Katz, S., Saraf, K., and Pollack, E. 1976. Comparative effects of methylphenidate and thioridazine in hyperactive children. *Arch. Gen. Psych.,* 33:1217-1231.

Glassman, A., Kantor, S., and Shostack, M. 1975. Depressions, delusions, and drug response, *Am. J. Psych.,* 132:7-12.

Gold, M., Redmond, D., and Kleber, H. 1978. Clonidine blocks acute opiate withdrawal symptoms. *Lancet,* 2:599-602.

Goyer, P., Davis, G., and Rapoport, J. 1979. Abuse of prescribed stimulant medication by a 13 year old hyperactive boy. *J. Am. Acad. Child Psych.,* 18:170-175.

Graham, P. 1979. *Psychophatological disorders of childhood.* ed. H. Quay, and J. Werry, pp: 185-209. New York: Wiley.

Greenhill, L. 1977. Methylphenidate (Ritalin) and other drugs for treatment of hyperactive children. *Med. Letter,* 19(482):53-55.

Greenhill, L. 1981. Stimulant-related growth inhibition in children: A review. In *Strategic intervention for hyperactive children,* ed. M. Gittelman. Armonk, N.Y.: M.E. Sharpe.

Greenhill, L., Perel, J., Curran, S., and Gardner, R. 1983a. Attentional measures and plasma level correlations in methylphenidate treated males. Presented at the 30th Annual Meeting of the American Academy of Child Psychiatry, October 28, San Francisco, California.

Greenhill, L., Puig-Antich, J., Chambers, W., Rubinstein, B., Halpern, F., and Sachar, E. 1981. Growth hormone, prolactin and growth responses in hyperkinetic males treated with d-amphetamine. *J. Am. Acad. Child Psych.* 20:71-84.

Greenhill, L. Puig-Antich, J., Goetz, J., Goetz, R., Hanlon, C., and Davies, M. 1983b. Sleep architecture and REM sleep measures in prepubertal children with attention deficit disorder with hyperactivity. *Sleep,* 6:91-101.

Greenhill, L., Puig-Antich, J., Novacenko, H., Solomon, M., Anghern, C., Florea, J., Goetz, R., Fiscina, B., and Sachar, E. 1984. Prolactin, growth hormone, and growth responses in boys with attention deficit disorder with hyperactivity treated with methylphenidate. *J. Am. Acad. Child Psych.* 23, 1:58-67.

Greenhill, L., Rider, R., Wender, P., Buchsbaum, M., and Zahn, T. 1973. Lithium carbonate in the treatment of hyperactive children. *Arch. Gen. Psych.,* 28:636-640.

Grinspoon, L., and Singer, S. 1973. Amphetamines in the treatment of hyperkinetic children. *Harv. Ed. Rev.,* 43:515-555.

Gruen, P., Sachar, E., and Langer, G. 1978. Prolactin responses to neuroleptics in normal and schizophrenic subjects. *Arch. Gen. Psych.,* 35:108-116.

Gualtieri, C. 1983. Tardive dyskinesia litigation. Presented at the 30th Annual Meeting of the American Academy of Child Psychiatry, October 27, San Francisco, California.

Gualtieri, C., Barnhill, J., McGimsey, J., and Schell, D. 1980. Tardive dyskinesia and other movement disorders in children treated with psychotropic drugs. *J. Am. Acad. Child Psych.,* 19:491-510.

Gualtieri, C., Kanoy, R., Hawk, B., Koriath, U., Schroeder, S., Youngblood, W., Breese, G., and

Prange, A. 1981. Growth hormone and prolactin secretion in adults and hyperactive children: Relation to methylphenidate serum levels. *Psychoneuroendocrin.,* 6:331-339.

Gualtieri, C., Wargin, W., Kanoy, R., Patrick, K., Shen, D., Youngblood, W., Mueller, R., and Breese, G. 1982. Clinical studies of methylphenidate serum levels in children and adults. *J. Am. Acad. Child Psych.,* 21:19-26.

Guy, W. 1976. *ECDEU Assessment manual for psychopharmacology.* Rev. ed. U.S. Dept. of Health, Education, and Welfare. DHEW pub. no. (ADM) 76-338.

Hungund, G., Perel, J., Hurwic, M., Sverd, J., and Winsberg, B. 1979. Pharmacokinetics of methylphenidate in hyperactive children. *Brit. J. Clin. Pharmacol.,* 8:571-576.

Iden, C., and Hungund, B. 1979. A chemical ionization selected ion monitoring assay for methylphenidate and ritalinic acid. *Biomed. Mass Spectrometry,* 6:422-426.

Kashani, J., McGee, R., Clarkson, S., Anderson, J., Walton, L., Williams, S., Silva, P., Robins, A., Cytryn, L., and Mcknew, D. 1983. Depression in a sample of 9-year-old children. *Arch. Gen. Psych.,* 40:1228-1235.

Kilgore, B., Dickinson, L., Burnett, C., Lee, J., Schwedie, H., and Elders, M. 1979. Alterations in cartilage metabolism by neurostimulant drugs. *J. Ped.,* 94:542-545.

Klein, D., Gittelman, R., Quitkin, F., and Rifkin, A. 1980. *Diagnosis and drug treatment of psychiatric disorders—second edition.* Baltimore: Williams and Wilkins, pp. 590-696.

Klorman, R., Salzman, L., Bauer, L., Coons, H., Borgstedt, A., and Halpern, W. 1984 (in press). Effects of two doses of methylphenidate on cross-situational and borderline hyperactive children's evoked potentials. *Electroenceph. Clin. Neurol.*

Klykylo, W., and Realmuto, G. 1983. A multicenter study on the effects of fenfluramine in autism: A preliminary report. Presented at the 30th Annual Meeting of the American Academy of Child Psychiatry, October 27, San Francisco, California.

Korey, S. 1944. The effects of benzedrine sulfate on the behavior of psychopathic and neurotic juvenile delinquents. *Psychiat. Quart.,* 18:127-137.

Kragh-Sorensen, P., Hansen, P., Gaastrup, T., and Huidberg, E. 1976. Self-inhibiting action of nortriptyline to antidepressant action at high plasma levels: A randomized double-blind study controlled by plasma concentration in patients with endogenous depression. *Psychopharm.* 45:305-312.

Kramer, A., and Feiguine, R. 1981. Clinical effects of amitriptyline in adolescent depression: A pilot study. *J. Am. Acad. Child Psych.,* 20:626-644.

Kraepelin, E. 1921, *Manic-depressive insanity and paranoia,* Edinburgh: E. & S. Livingston Ltd.

Kupietz, S., Winsberg, B., and Sverd, J. 1982. Learning ability and methylphenidate (Ritalin(R)) plasma concentration in hyperkinetic children. *J. Am. Acad. Child Psych.* 21:27-30.

Langer, D., Rapoport, J., Brown, G., Ebert, M., and Bunney, W. 1982. Behavioral effects of carbidopa/levodopa in hyperactive boys. *J. Am. Acad. Child Psych.,* 21:10-18.

Leckman, J., Detlor, J., Harcherik, D., Young, J., Anderson, G., Shaywitz, B., and Cohen, D. 1983. Acute and chronic clonidine treatment in Tourette's syndrome: A preliminary report on clinical responses and effect on plasma and urinary catecholamine metabolites, growth hormone, and blood pressure. *J. Am. Acad. Child Psych.,* 22:433-440.

Lerer, R., and Lerer, M. 1977. Responses of adolescents with minimal brain dysfunction to methylphenidate. *J. Learn. Disabil.,* 10:223-228.

Lipman, R., DiMascio, A., Reatig, N., and Kirson, T. 1978. Psychotropic drugs in mentally retarded children. In *Psychopharmacology: A generation of progress,* ed. M. Lipton, A. DiMascio, and K. Kiliam, pp. 1437-1450. New York: Raven Press.

Loney, J., Whaley-Klahn, M., Ponto, L., and Adney, K. 1982. Predictors of adolescent height and weight in hyperkinetic boys treated with methylphenidate. Presented at the New Clinical Drug Evaluation Unit (NCDEU) Annual Meeting, May 1982, Key Biscayne, Florida.

Loranger, A. W. Levine, P. M. 1978: Age of onset of bipolar affective illness. *Arch. Gen. Psychiatry,* 35:1345-1348.

Maletzky, B. 1974. Diamphetamine and delinquency, hyperkinesis persisting. *Dis. Nerv. Sys.,* 35:543-547.

Mattes, J., and Gittelman, R. 1983. Growth of hyperactive children on maintenance methylphenidate. *Arch. Gen. Psych.,* 40:317-324.

Medical Letter. 1979. Tardive dyskinesia. *Med. Letter,* 21(529):34-35.

Minde, K. 1980. Some thoughts on the social ecology of present day psychopharmacology. *Can. J. Psych.,* 3:210-212.

Perry, P., Alexander, B., and Liskow, B. 1981. *Psychotrophic drug handbook.* Cincinnati: Harvey Whitney Books.

Pfefferbaum-Levine, B., Kumor, K., Cangir, A., Choroszy, E., and Roseberry, E. 1983. Tricyclic antidepressants for children with cancer. *Am. J. Psych.,* 140:1074-1078.

Platt, J., Campbell, M., Green, W., Perry, R., and Cohen, I. 1981. Effects of lithium carbonate and haloperidol on cognition in aggressive hospitalized school-age children. *J. Clin. Psychopharm.,* 1:8-13.

Pope, H., Hudson, J., Jonas, J., and Yurgelun-Todd, D. 1983. Bulimia treated with imipramine: A placebo-controlled, double-blind study. *Am. J. Psych.,* 140:554-558.

Porrino, L., Rapoport, J., Behar, D., Ismond, D., and Bunney, W. 1983. A naturalistic assessment of the motor activity of hyperactive boys. I. Comparison with normal controls. II. Stimulant drug effects. *Arch. Gen. Psych.,* 40:681-696.

Puig-Antich, J. 1982. Major depression and conduct disorder in prepuberty. *J. Am. Acad. Child Psych.,* 21:118-128.

Puig-Antich, J., and Chambers, W. 1978. The schedule for affective disorders and schizophrenia for school-age children (6-12 years): Kiddie-SADS (K-SADS). For copies of this instrument, contact Drs. Puig-Antich and Chambers at the Department of Child and Adolescent Psychiatry, New York State Psychiatric Institute, 722 West 168 Street, New York, New York 10032.

Puig-Antich, J., Cooper, T., Ambrossini, P., Rabinovitch, H., Ryan, N., Torres, D., and Fried, J. 1983. Plasma level/clinical response in major depressive disorder in adolescents. Presented at the 30th Annual Meeting of the American Academy of Child Psychiatry, October 27, San Francisco, California.

Puig-Antich, J., Greenhill, L., Sassin, J., and Sachar, E. 1978. Growth hormone, prolactin, and cortisol responses and growth patterns in hyperkinetic children treated with dextro-amphetamine: Preliminary findings. *J. Am. Acad. Child Psych.,* 17:457-475.

Puig-Antich, J., Perel, J., Lupatkin, W., Chambers, W., Shea, C., Tabrizi, M., and Stiller, R. 1979. Plasma levels of imipramine and desmethylimipramine and clinical response in prepubertal major depressive disorder: A preliminary report. *J. Am. Acad. Child Psych.,* 18:616-627.

Quitkin, F., Harrison, W., Liebowitz, M., McGrath, P., Rabkin, J.G., Steward, J., and Markowitz, J. Defining the boundaries of atypical depression. *Am. J. Psych.* (in press).

Ranzani, J., White, K., White, L., Simpson, G., Sloane, R., Rebel, R., and Palmer, R. 1983. The safety and efficacy of combined amitriptyline and tranylcypromine antidepressant treatment. *Arch. Gen. Psych.,* 40:657-664.

Rapoport, J., Buchsbaum, M., Zahn, T., Weingartner, H., Ludlow, C., and Mikkelsen, E. 1978. Dextroamphetamine: Cognitive and behavioral effects in normal prepubertal boys. *Science,* 199:560-562.

Rapoport, J., Mikkelsen, E., Zavadi, A., Nee, L., Gruenau, C., Mendelson, W., and Gillin, C. 1980. Childhood enuresis II. Psychopathology, tricyclic concentrations in plasma, and antienuretic effect. *Arch. Gen. Psych.,* 37:1146-1152.

Rapoport, J., Quinn, P., Bradbard, G., Riddle, K., and Bracks, E. 1974. Imipramine and methylphenidate treatment of hyperactive boys. *Arch. Gen. Psych.,* 30:789-793.

Riddle, K., and Rapoport, J. 1976. A two-year follow-up study of seventy-two hyperactive boys. *J. Nerv. Men. Dis.*, 162:126-130.

Rifkin, A., Quitkin, F., Carillo, C., Blumberg, A., and Klein, D. 1972. Lithium carbonate in emotional unstable character disorder. *Arch. Gen. Psych.*, 27:519-523.

Roche, A., Lipman, R., Overall, J., and Hung, W. 1979. The effects of stimulant medication on the growth of hyperkinetic children. *Ped.*, 63:847-849.

Rutter, M., Tizard, J., and Whitmore, K. 1970. *Education, health, and behavior.* London: Longman.

Sachar, E. 1978. Neuroendocrine response to psychotropic drugs. In *Psychopharmacology: A generation of progress,* ed. M. Lipton, A. DiMascio, and K. Killiam, pp. 499-507. New York: Raven Press.

Safer, D., Allen, R., and Barr, E. 1972. Depression of growth in hyperactive children on stimulant drugs. *N. Eng. J. Med.*, 287:217-220.

Saraf, K., Klein, D., Gittelman-Klein, R., and Groff, S. 1974. Imipramine side effects in children. *Psychopharm.*, 37:265-274.

Satterfield, J., Satterfield, B., and Cantwell, D. 1980. Multimodality treatment: A two year evaluation of 61 hyperactive boys. *Arch. Gen. Psych.*, 37:915-919.

Scheel-Kruger, J. 1972. Behavioral and biochemical comparison of amphetamine derivatives, cocaine, benztropine, and tricyclic antidepressant drugs. *Eur. J. Pharmacol.*, 18:63-75.

Schleifer, N., Weiss, G., Cohen, N., Elman, M., Cvejic, H., and Kruger, E. 1975. Hyperactivity in preschoolers and the effect of methylphenidate. *Am. J. Orthopsych.*, 45:38-50.

Schrag, P., and Divoky, D. 1975. *The myth of the hyperactive child.* New York: Pantheon Books.

Schreier, H. 1979. Use of propranolol in the treatment of post-encephalitic psychosis. *Am. J. Psych.*, 136:840-841.

Shabry, F., and Wolk, J. 1980. Granulocytopenia in children after phenothiazine therapy. *Am. J. Psych.*, 137:374-375.

Shaffer, D., and Fisher, P. 1981. The epidemiology of suicide in children and young adolescents. *J. Acad. Am. Child Psych.*, 20:545-565.

Shaffer, D., and Greenhill, L. 1979. A critical note on the predictive validity of "the hyperactive syndrome." *J. Child Psychol. Psych.*, 20:61-72.

Shaffer, D., McNamara, N., and Pincus, J. 1974. Controlled observations on patterns of activity, attention, and impulsivity in brain-damaged and psychiatrically disturbed boys. *J. Psychol. Med.*, 4:14-18.

Shand, D. 1979. Biological determinants of drug disposition in aging. Presentation at the conference on influence of age on the pharmacology of psychoactive drugs, April 16-17, Washington, D.C.

Sheard, M. 1971. Effect of lithium on human aggression. *Nature,* 230:113.

Sjoquist, F. 1979. Overview and future directions of psychopharmacology. Presentation at the conference on influence of age on the pharmacology of psychoactive drugs, April 16-17, Washington, D.C.

Skolnick, P., Paul, S., Hulihan-Giblin, B., and Hauger, R. 1984. The stimulant properties of ritalinic acid esters are highly correlated with their displacement of [^{3}H] methylphenidate binding in striatum. *Nature,* in press.

Sostek, A. J., Buchsbaum, M.S., and Rapoport, J. L. 1980. Effects of amphetamine on vigilance performance in normal and hyperactive children. *J. Abnorm. Child Psychol.*, 8:491-500.

Spitzer, R., and Endicott, J. 1978. Schedule for affective disorders and schizophrenia (SADS). NIMH Clinical Research Branch, Collaborative Program on the Psychology of Depression. Washington, D.C.: U.S. Government Printing Office.

Spitzer, R., and Robins, E. 1978. Research Diagnostic Criteria. *Arch. Gen. Psych.*, 35:773-782.

Sprague, R., and Sleator, E. 1975. What is the proper dose of stimulant drugs in children? *Int. J. Men. Health,* 4:75-104.

Sprague, R., and Sleator, E. 1977. Methylphenidate in hyperkinetic children: Differences in dose effects on learning and social behavior. *Science,* 198:1274-1276.

Swanson, J., and Kinsbourne, M. 1976. Stimulant related state-dependent learning in hyperactive children. *Science,* 192:1354-1357.

Swanson, J., Kinsbourne, M., and Zucker, M. 1977. Time-response analysis of the effect of stimulant medication on the learning ability of children referred for hyperactivity. *Ped.,* 61:21-29.

Trites, R., Dugas, E., Lynch, G., and Ferguson, H. 1979. Prevalence of hyperactivity. *J. Ped. Psychol.,* 4:179-188.

Tupin, J. 1978. Usefulness of lithium for aggressiveness. *Am. J. Psych.,* 135:1118.

Varly, C. 1983. Effects of methylphenidate in adolescents with attention deficit disorder. *J. Am. Acad. Child Psych.,* 22:351-354.

Weingartner, H., Murphy, D., and Stillman, R. 1978. Mood state dependent learning. In *Stimulus properties of drugs: Ten years of progress,* ed. F. Colpaert, and J. Roecrans, pp. 445-453. Janssen Research Foundation. Amsterdam: Elsevier/North-Holland Biomedical Press.

Weiss, B., and Laites, V. 1962. Enhancement of human performance by caffeine and the amphetamines. *Pharmacol. Rev.,* 14:1-36.

Weiss, G., Hechtman, I., Perlman, T., Hopkins, J., and Werner, A. 1979. Hyperactives as young adults: A controlled prospective ten-year follow-up of 75 children. *Arch. Gen. Psych.,* 36:675-681.

Weiss, G., Kruger, E., Danielson, V., and Elman, M. 1975. Effect of long-term treatment of hyperactive children with methylphenidate. *Can. Med. Assoc. J.,* 112:159-165.

Weiss, G., Minde, K., Douglas, V., Werry, J., and Sykes, D. 1971. Comparison of the effects of chlorpromazine, dextroamphetamine, and methylphenidate on the behavior and intellectual functioning of hyperactive children. *Can. Med. Assoc. J.,* 104:20-25.

Weissman, M., and Myers, J. 1978. Affective disorders in a U.S. urban community: The use of Research Diagnostic Criteria in an epidemiological survey. *Arch. Gen. Psych.,* 35:1304-1311.

Weller, E., Preskorn, S., Weller, R., and Croskell, M. 1983. Childhood depression: Imipramine levels and response. *Psychopharm. Bull.,* 19:59-62.

Weller, E., and Weller, R. 1983. Case report of conversion symptom associated with major depressive disorder in a child. *Am. J. Psych.,* 140:1079-1080.

Wender, P. 1971. *Minimal brain dysfunction in children.* New York: Wiley.

Wender, P. 1975. Speculations concerning a possible biochemical basis of minimal brain dysfunction. In *Recent advances in child psychopharmacology,* ed. R. Gittelman-Klein, pp. 14-30. New York: Human Sciences Press.

Werry, J. 1982. An overview of pediatric psychopharmacology. *J. Am. Acad. Child Psych.,* 21:3-9.

Werry, J., and Aman, M. 1975. Methylphenidate and haloperidol in children. *Arch. Gen. Psych.,* 32:790-795.

Whalen, C., Collins, B., Henker, B., Alkus, S., Adams, D., and Stapp, J. 1978. Behavior observations of hyperactive children in systematically structured classroom environments: Now you see them, now you don't. *J. Ped. Psychol.,* 3:177-187.

Whitehouse, D., Shah, U., and Palmer, F. 1980. Comparison of sustained-release and standard methylphenidate in the treatment of minimal brain dysfunction. *J. Clin. Psych.,* 41:282-285.

Williams, D., Mehl, R., Yudofsky, S., Adams, D., and Roseman, B. 1982. The effect of propranolol on uncontrolled rage outbursts in children and adolescents with organic brain dysfunction. *J. Am. Acad. Child Psych.,* 21:129-135.

Winsberg, B., Kupietz, S., Sverd, J., and Hungund, B. 1982. Methylphenidate oral dose, plasma concentrations, and behavioral response in children. *Psychopharmacology* (Berlin), 76:329-332.

Yudofsky, S., Williams, D., and Gorman, J. 1981. Propranolol in the treatment of rage and violent behavior in patients with chronic brain syndrome. *Am. J. Psych.,* 138:218-226.

27

The Behavior Therapies

TOMMIE G. CAYTON / DENNIS C. RUSSO

OVER THE YEARS, the label *behavior therapies* has been applied to an increasingly broader range of techniques and applications. As a result, there has been much disagreement, confusion, and misunderstanding regarding what constitutes a "behavioral therapy." This debate has occasionally resulted in misapplications of the name to poorly conceived and inappropriate treatments, causing behavior therapy to receive undeserved bad press. The area is even further complicated by the existence of similar approaches which are all included under the broad umbrella of the behavior therapies—behavior modification, behavioral medicine, behavioral pediatrics, behavioral health, behaviorism, and the experimental analysis of behavior. Some clinicians have used these terms interchangeably and have applied them to such diverse techniques as psychosurgery, token economies, incarceration, reward system, etc., while others have attempted to differentiate a particular approach from all others. It is therefore not surprising that many newcomers to the area and health providers collaborating with behavior therapists through consults and liaison relationships are sometimes discouraged by the frequent contradictory information they may read and receive.

Ideally, the present chapter would clarify all the discrepancies and thoroughly present all crucial issues such that any reader could become a successful and effective behavior therapist upon completion of this essay. Unfortunately (or fortunately), human behavior is of sufficient complexity to preclude such a simple analysis. The basic tenets of the behavioral approach emphasize the uniqueness of each person's experience and require a separate behavioral analysis for each behavior to be changed. Simplistic "cookbook" recommendations therefore have no validity. The range of potential consequences and complications after implementing an individual program are so diverse that one can no more read about a behavioral technique and successfully implement it across several patients than one could read about an appendectomy and subsequently perform one. In each case it is likely that attempts might be successful with an uncomplicated patient. However, the potential for complexity requires that considerably more training be applied before reaching an acceptable level of proficiency.

As eminent authors have devoted entire volumes to single applications of individual behavioral-therapy techniques, it would be quite presumptuous of the present authors to attempt to present in the space provided the information and skills necessary to become effective behavior therapists. Clinical effectiveness in behavior therapy is determined by many of the same factors that influence the outcomes of any therapy: a therapist who is competent in his or her craft; a thorough understanding of the patient or client under treatment; a prescriptive match between problem presentation and therapeutic process; and, importantly, the development of a positive relationship between therapists and patient. This last point is particularly noteworthy, since popular conceptions of behavioral therapies support the idea of a forceful or coercive therapeutic process. This is quite simply not the case. Behavioral therapies are not so powerful as to be able to produce such changes nor are such programs ethically appropriate. Well-designed behavioral treatments work because they are tailored to fit current circumstances and, often in conjunction with other therapies, because they produce a more adaptive outcome than pretreatment situations.

The intent of the present chapter, then, is to present a brief history and definition of behavior therapy, to give descriptions of the various therapeutic techniques and their application to the problems of children, and to describe variables that influence the effective application of these techniques. Our goal is to provide an information base sufficient for effective interactions between other disciplines and behavior therapists and for entry into training programs specifically designed for the behavior therapies.

Over the past ten years, behavior therapy has assumed an important, complementary role in the psychotherapies. As a methodology for the management and improvement of patient behaviors, it not only provides a potential alternative to traditional theoretical speculation but also provides a productive interface with practitioners in medicine and education, two exceedingly important arenas for psychological practice. Discussion as to the appropriateness of behavior therapy as a therapeutic technique will therefore be set aside. Behavior therapy is a legitimate technique, not only due to its own empirical documentation but additionally to its acceptance in other fields of child therapeutics.

HISTORICAL DEVELOPMENTS

Although an in-depth discussion of the development of behavior therapies with children is beyond the scope of this chapter, a review of some of the major contributing factors in its history will allow the reader to put the behavior therapies in current perspective. Those desiring a more complete historical review are referred to Kazdin (1978).

In ancient times, abnormal behavior was predominantly seen as a result of the effects of demons or evil spirits. Treatments therefore consisted of activities aimed at driving the demons out of the afflicted individual. Since that time there have been multiple retreats and resurgences of the demonic theory of maladaptive behavior. Hippocrates and other eminent Greeks and Romans were perhaps the first to reject the demonic notion of abnormality and attribute the disturbances in behavior to biological causes such as body fluid imbalance. Treatment was therefore removed from the purview of the priests and placed under the realm of physicians. Treatments became more humane and included such things as alterations in diet and exercise. The Middle Ages brought a recurrence of the demonic view of abnormality, a return to treatment by priests, and a resurgence of inhumane treatments intended to drive out evil spirits or to punish sinful behavior.

Advances in medical science and a return to the emphasis on the biological basis of behavior occurred again during the sixteenth and seventeenth centuries. Discoveries of the contribution of microorganisms to disease understandably led to the application of similar theories of etiology for abnormal or maladaptive behavior. Until early in the twentieth century, however, and the discovery of syphilis as the cause of general paresis, no evidence clearly established organic pathology as the source of abnormal or maladaptive behavior. Because of this lack of evidence and the ability of mesmerism and hypnosis to dramatically cure such illnesses as hysterical paralysis, practitioners began to search for psychological and nonbiological causes of abnormality.

Freud was perhaps the first to provide a systematic and comprehensive theory of abnormal behavior that attributed the cause of abnormality to psychological instead of biological pathology. Drawing extensively from the biological (or disease) model, Freud proposed a series of hypotheses on the determinants of behavior, such as conservation of psychic energy, unconscious processes, psychic impulses and conflicts, etc. In spite of the attribution of abnormality to psychological factors, psychodynamic theory is still a "disease model," i.e., instead of an underlying biological process such as the growth of bacteria, maladaptive behavior is assumed to indicate an underlying pathological psychodynamic process. Diagnosis and treatment, therefore, involve the identification and amelioration of the underlying pathological process.

Several factors, however, led to the questioning of Freudian or psychoanalytic theory as a comprehensive theory of human behavior. As a scientific theory, it is difficult to substantiate in that the same behavior may have multiple explanations and the same pathological process may result in different maladaptive behaviors. In addition, the relation between psychodynamic process and behavior and between psychodynamic process and therapy are not always clear, except in retrospect. The applicability of Freudian theory to non-European and non-American cultures has also been questioned. Finally, it is very difficult to conduct traditional psychodynamic therapy with psychotic patients.

Dissatisfacton with psychodynamic theory, or more appropriately, with the subjective method of introspective inquiry in general, led others to investigate more objective measures of behavior and the variables that influence behavior. Although many have influenced the rise of behaviorism (Kazdin, 1978), the three men generally given most credit for its development are Ivan P. Pavlov (1849-1936), John B. Watson (1878-1958), and B. F. Skinner (1904-   ). Their basic theoretical stances and research findings are an appropriate base from which to consider contemporary practices.

While attempting to investigate Sechenov's neurological hypothesis of digestion, Pavlov discovered "psychical secretions." After abandoning subjective approaches to their analysis, he labeled them "conditioned reflexes." In his words:

> At first, in our psychical experiments with the salivary glands (for the time being we will use the term 'psychical'), we conscientiously endeavoured to explain our results by imagining the subjective state of the animal. But nothing came of this except sterile controversy and individual views that could not be reconciled. And so we could do nothing but conduct the research on a purely objective basis; our first and especially important task was completely to abandon the very natural tendency to transfer our own subjective state to the mechanism of the reaction of the animal undergoing the experiment and to concentrate instead on studying the correlation between the external phenomena and the reaction of the organism, i.e., the activity of the salivary glands (Kazdin, 1978, p. 55).

Pavlov's research investigated the salivary reflex in dogs. By repeatedly pairing a stimulus that did not initially elicit salivation (a neutral stimulus such as a tone) with a stimulus that did elicit salivation (the unconditioned response—UCS), the formally neutral stimulus would come to elicit the salivation (the conditioned response—CS). Pavlov's unique contribution was not in the discovery of this reflex, but in the meticulous manner in which he objectively established the lawful nature of the development and elimination of these conditioned reflexes: the temporal relationships required; techniques by which stimuli similar to, but different from, the training stimulus would (stimulus generalization) or would not (stimulus discrimination) elicit the conditioned response; and methods of eliminating the response, i.e., continued presentation of the formally neutral stimulus without pairing it with food (extinction).

John B. Watson is credited with crystalizing the trend toward objectivism in American psychology (Kazdin, 1978). Through many lectures and publications (e.g., Watson, 1913, 1914, 1916, 1919, 1924), he emphasized several methodological points. First, because the study of consciousness led to unresolvable discussions about the nature of "mental events," Watson believed psychology should no longer include consciousness as its domain of study. Second, because introspection did not allow objective assessment, he felt it should no longer be included in the methodology of psychological observation. Third, he believed that inquiry should be focused on the behavior of the organism as a whole. Finally, Watson emphasized the influence of the environment on the development of behavior. The extent of his belief in environmental influences on behavior is demonstrated by one of his more renowned remarks:

> Give me a dozen healthy infants, well-formed, and my own specified world to bring them up in and I'll guarantee to take any one at random and train him to become any type of specialist I might select—doctor, lawyer, artist, merchant—chief, and, yes, even beggar-man and thief, regardless of his talents, penchants, tendencies, abilities, vocations, and race of his ancestors. I am going beyond my facts and I admit it, but so have the advocates of the contrary and they have been doing it for many thousands of years (Watson, 1924, p. 104).

B. F. Skinner has had more impact than any other learning theorist on the development of behavior modification (Kazdin, 1978). Skinner's contributions are seen strongly in explicating the philosophy of behavioral science, in the development of a database, and in envisioning applications to human problems. In addition to further emphasizing the concept of investigating the behavior of the organism as a whole, Skinner developed the use of frequency, or rate, as the appropriate datum for behavioral research. With this concept, Skinner approached all behavior as lawful and attempted to identify those factors that contributed to variation in behavior. Failure of behavior to change in the expected direction was taken to imply lack of control or incomplete understanding of the factors influencing the behavior under study, not individual differences or random uncontrollable factors, as is usually hypothesized in statistical studies. As he continued to study the laws of behavior, Skinner became convinced that reflexes, or respondent conditioning, accounted for only a small part of the complexities of human behavior. As a result, he developed the concept of operant behavior, i.e., most behavior was predominately controlled by the consequences of behavior. While respondent conditioning represented the establishment of a relationship between two stimuli (i.e., the conditioned and the unconditioned stimuli), operant conditioning represented a relationship between a behavior and a stimulus (i.e., future occurrences of the behavior and the consequences of the behavior). Skinner proposed that reinforcement produced an increased probability of occurrence of a class of behaviors and that the best measure of this increased probability was the rate of occurrence of the target behavior.

Skinner also developed many principles and much of the database areound which current research and treatment have evolved. He investigated the effect of "schedules" of reinforcement (the rules by which consequences are applied) and found that different schedules resulted in different rates of behavior. These findings did much to unravel the complexities of behavior. In his writings, Skinner (1948, 1953) also attempted to demonstrate the potential benefits of the application of behavioral technology to human problems, and thereby brought much attention to the behavioral field and its practical applications.

These three individuals provided important conceptual and empirical bases for current practices in behavior therapy. Their insistence on empirical outcome, the lawfulness and predictability of behavior, and the preeminence of assessment over theory form the basis of behavioral practice. Each individual provided concepts and methods that have merged into the variety of approaches encompassing current practice.

Definition of Behavior Therapy

In attempting to define a field of study, what is popularly accepted must be contrasted with what actually represents current practice. Behavior therapy is no exception. Much misconception in both the lay and professional communities still exists regarding the nature, practice, and scope of behavior therapies. Several characteristics of the early behavioral studies, however, differentiated this approach from others and have resulted in steady progress in developing a science of human behavior and a technology of behavior change. As behavior therapy has demonstrated efficacy and received acceptance, more and more diverse techniques have received this label. Some have described this broadening as progress and have stated that the old methods of investigating only observable and measurable events are outdated (e.g., Meichenbaum, 1977). Others herald these developments as diversions from the methodology that brought the science to where it is today (e.g., Rachlin, 1977; Brigham, 1980). Whether or not new explanations are needed to support the current literature on behavior is still the subject of much speculation. The conclusive answer to such speculation will be produced by data derived from experimentation, not from theoretical discussion. A recent assessment of the field attempted to develop an acceptable description of the characteristics unique to behavior therapy (Kazdin and Hersen, as quoted by Calhoun and Turner, 1981, p. 7):

1. A strong commitment to empirical evaluation of treatment and intervention techniques.
2. A general belief that therapeutic experiences must provide opportunities to learn adaptive or prosocial behavior.
3. Specification of treatment in operational and, hence, replicable terms.
4. Evaluation of treatment effects through multiple-response modalities, with particular emphasis on overt behavior.

In one respect, this is an appropriate definition in that it is representative of the kind of research that is taking place in the field as a whole. Therefore, many diverse therapeutic techniques will be discussed in the present chapter. A more conservative stance would add that the patient's behavior should be evaluated frequently as an individual. It is our contention that it is the methodology of behaviorism that has resulted in an effective technology of behavior change. Our future progress will more likely be a function of our assessment methodology than the derived techniques themselves. It is therefore appropriate that those characteristics that have been so successful in the past be maintained as the defining characteristics of behavior therapy.

CURRENT DIMENSIONS OF BEHAVIOR THERAPY

To summarize differences from other psychological approaches, behavior therapy emphasizes the importance of obtaining frequent objective assessments of measurable changes in the patient's behavior, maximizes the importance of present environmental influences on the occurrence of both adaptive and maladaptive patient behaviors, and targets objective, measurable behavior of the patient as an individual. As stated by Russo and Varni (1982), unless data suggest the contrary, the patient/client is considered to be an individual with lawful behavior in a situation that maintains that behavior. Therefore, the most therapeutic changes are those that alter factors of the environment that are influencing the occurrence of the targeted behaviors. No underlying pathological, psychodynamic, or biological processes are automatically assumed. Similarly, events of early childhood or those long past are considered to have little influence on present behavior unless their consequences are being maintained by the present environment. Because it is assumed that every patient is biologically normal until proven otherwise (neurological pathology such as brain tumors, aneurysms, etc., are of course ruled out when appropriate), psychotropics or other behavior control drugs are not considered a part of a behavior-therapy regimen.

These issues begin to differentiate behavior therapy from traditional therapeutic techniques and theories but do not clarify the relationship among techniques within the domain of behavior therapy. It would be useful to understand how these different areas (i.e., behavior modification, behavioral medicine, behavioral pediatrics, and behavioral health) are related. For example, some definitions have limited behavior therapy to the use of techniques derived from the classical or respondent, conditioning paradigm, and behavior modification to techniques developed from the operant paradigm. Others have attempted to classify the two techniques on the types of behaviors that were changed or the settings in which the methods were applied. These differentiations between the two labels are being made less and less. In fact, a comprehensive review of the field (Kazdin, 1978) used the terms interchangeably. These distinctions are apparently not generally drawn by the majority of those in the area, so they will be used interchangeably here as well.

For the purposes of this chapter, we shall use behavior therapy as a superordinate term to encompass the others. Within the area of behavior therapy, four general categories will be reviewed: (1) respondent paradigms, (2) operant paradigms, (3) biofeedback paradigms, and (4) behavioral pediatrics. These areas are differentiated on their theoretical foundations, their sites of conduct, and their utilization of particular methods or apparatus. This breakdown represents one schema of presenting an overview of current practices.

APPLICATIONS OF BEHAVIOR-THERAPY TECHNIQUES TO CHILDREN

In implementing behavioral techniques with children, several factors should be considered. Foremost are ethical considerations (Stolz et al., 1978). Many of the factors that make behavioral treatment with children easier to implement increase the potential for violation of the child's human rights and for violation of accepted ethical principles. Children are generally not capable of nor are they allowed to determine what is in their best interests. This results in a problem of giving informed consent for treatment. As a result it is easy for a parent, teacher, or societal agent to request that a child's behavior be changed such that conditions are easier for the adult caretakers, but may or may not improve the overall functioning of the child (Winnett and Winkler, 1972; Davison and Stuart, 1975; Martin, 1975; Winkler, 1977). Such issues are especially salient when children are institutionalized. Reports of the use of restrictive procedures to produce compliance in institutional settings are often highlighted in this regard.

It is clear that the responsibilities for treatment design exist with the treatment designer; the appropriateness or inappropriateness is not housed within the techniques themselves. Principles of behavior therapy relate to relationships between behavior and events, not to the choice of specific techniques. Practice in an appropriate fashion requires consideration of short- and long-term outcomes, rehabilitative intent, consideration of alternative techniques, and documentation of previous treatment effectiveness. Such treatment selections should be public, that is, subject to the informed scrutiny of peers and others from the community. Implicit in the design of therapeutic programs is the responsiblity to consider within the context of socially accepted practices and current professional standards the goals of therapy, the appropriateness of behavior-change strategies, and the effects on the client or family. Such responsibilities are not limited to behavior therapy, however; they exist for all therapeutic modalities and must concern all providers.

In reviewing the application of behavior therapies to children, we will present a description of the therapeutic technique with a brief statement of its rationale when appropriate. We will then describe the areas of children's problems on which the technique has been applied with comments on critical aspects of their implementation. Our intent is to present a general review and not to give a critical analysis of the literature. Those interested in a critical review of specific areas are referred to table 27–1, which lists significant topic reviews. These reviews summarize the empirical evidence on therapeutic effectiveness in the areas indicated. In general, most articles suggest that the behavioral therapies have demonstrated positive outcomes in most areas but that further and well-controlled clinical trials are still needed.

In order to discuss the different methods, we have divided them into four primary content areas: (a) *the general behavior therapies group*, which will include those techniques not included in the other groups but especially those patterned on respondent conditioning (also known as classical and as Pavlovian conditioning), social learning theory techniques, the cognitive therapies, and self-management or self-control methods; (b) *an operant-conditioning group*, which will contain those applications in which behavior of the child is changed by changing the consequences of that behavior; (c) *a biofeedback group*, in which electronic instruments provide children with information about their physiological status in order to improve their ability to control that physiological behavior; and (d) *a behavioral-pediatrics group*, which will include applications of behavioral techniques in which the goal is improved physical health of the child or which seeks to prevent the occurrence of future health problems. These divisions are admittedly artificial and should be taken as such. Many methods could be considered in several of the areas as defined. Their placement was predominantly determined by convenience in presentation. In all cases, therapies are designed as brief, problem-oriented approaches that allow for the objective assessment of outcome. They view the child as an active learner in an environment that supports current behavior.

TABLE 27-1.
Major Content Area Reviews in Behavior Therapy with Children

Topic	Authors
Cognitive behavior therapy with children	Abikoff (1979)
Classroom behavior	Copeland & Hall (1976)
Cognitive behavior therapy	Craighead et al. (1978)
Enuresis and encopresis	Doleys (1978)
Counterconditioning	Eysenck & Beech (1971)
Noncompliance	Forehand (1977)
Parents as therapists	Forehand & Atkeson (1977)
Methodology	Furman & Drabman (1981)
Review of child behavior therapy	Gelfand & Hartmann (1968)
Treatment of children's fears	Graziano, DeGiovanni, & Garcia (1979)
Cognitive behavior therapy with children	Hobbs et al. (1980)
Childhood obesity	Israel & Stolmaker (1980)
Self-management in children	Karoly (1977)
General behavior therapy review	Kazdin & Wilson (1978)
Asthma	King (1980)
General review of operant techniques	Krasner (1971)
Learning disabilities	Lahey (1976)
Self-control techniques	O'Leary & Dubey (1979)
Treatment of fear in children	Ollendick (1979)
Behavior therapy with children	Phillips & Ray (1980)
Parents as change agents	Reisinger, Ora, & Frangia (1976)
General review of behavior therapy	Rimm & Masters (1974)
Self-control training in the classroom	Rosenbaum & Drabman (1979)
Modeling	Rosenthal & Bandura (1978)
Review of child behavior therapy	Ross (1978)
Self-injurious behavior	Russo, Carr, & Lovaas (1981)
Childhood psychosis	Russo & Newsome (1982)
Behavioral pediatrics	Russo & Varni (1982)
Operant techniques	Sherman & Baer (1969)
Ethics	Stolz et al. (1978)
Children's social withdrawal	Strain & Kerr (1981)

General Behavioral Therapies

SYSTEMATIC DESENSITIZATION. One of the most widely researched behavior-therapy techniques is systematic desensitization (Wolpe, 1958). The rationale for this technique is that the patient's difficulties are a learned maladaptive response to certain stimuli or situations. Therapy therefore consists of unlearning or "counterconditioning" the inappropriate response and replacing it with a more adaptive reaction. This technique consists of developing a hierarchy of situations that are anxiety provoking. The patient is then taught a method of relaxation such as progressive muscle relaxation training (Jacobson, 1938; Wolpe, 1974). Having learned this procedure, the patient is asked to imagine or participate in the least anxious scene or situation until he or she can do so without feeling tense or anxious. As this is accomplished, progressively more anxiety-provoking scenes are similarly presented while the patient remains relaxed. The procedure is continued until the patient has reached the desired level of coping with the formerly anxiety-provoking situation. Variants of this technique include (a) *in vivo* exposure to the anxious situation, and (b) using behaviors other than relaxation that are incompatible with anxiety, such as eating, playing, and listening to music. These techniques have been used very successfully in children ranging in ages from one year to late adolescence for such fears as dogs (Lazarus, 1960: Lazarus and Abramovitz, 1962; Kissel, 1972), separation (Montenegro, 1968; Miller et al., 1972), loud noises (Tasto, 1969; Wish et al., 1973), and many others. Desensitization has also been used to treat problems related to physical health, but this will be discussed in the behavioral-pediatrics section.

IMPLOSIVE THERAPY AND FLOODING. Implosive therapy (Stampfl, 1973) and flooding are other techniques used frequently to treat fears. They are similar in that both involve the patient or client imagining fearful situations. In flooding, the scenes relate to the fearful or phobic situations. In implosive therapy, the scenes involve the phobic situation but are developed according to psychodynamic theory regarding the hypothesized etiology of the fear. Whereas desensitization attempts to decrease the fear response by teaching an incompatible one, implosive therapy and flooding attempt to decrease the response by "putting the avoidance response on extinction," i.e., not allowing the patient to escape from the fearful or phobic situation. By not permitting the patient to leave, the fear responses are not reinforced by termination of the feared stimulation. In this manner their strength is decreased and they are finally eliminated. In contrast to Wolpe's desensitization, which attempts to minimize the anxiety the patient experiences during treatment, flooding and implosive therapy call for deliberate attempts by the therapist to elicit high levels of anxiety. Not surprisingly this approach does not appear to have been used as frequently with children as it has with adults, although one reference was found for a treatment of a school phobia (Smith and Sharpe, 1970). There is some disagreement in the literature regarding the effectiveness of these two techniques (flooding and implosive therapy). They are presented here for completeness and not for recommended use. In fact, when the concept of the child's right to the least restrictive or least aversive treatment is considered with the fact that no study has found implosive therapy to be superior to systematic desensitization, one would appear to be ethically bound to use systematic desensitization prior to using either implosive therapy or flooding.

SOCIAL-LEARNING THEORY. Social-learning theory (Bandura, 1977), in contrast, emphasizes the contribution of vicarious, symbolic, and self-regulatory processes to the maintenance of behavior pattens. Much of the early research investigated the effects of modeling, i.e., how one person's behavior is influenced by watching another. Children were found to increase their rate of nonfear behaviors after observing others behave bravely, especially if their model was similar to them and if the nonfear behavior of the model was reinforced (Bandura, 1965; Bandura and Menlove, 1968; Kornhaber and Schroeder, 1975).

COGNITIVE BEHAVIOR THERAPIES. The cognitive behavior therapies emphasize the mediational effect of a person's cognitions (thoughts, internal or subvocal speech, and images) on his or her behavior. Meichenbaum (1977) has presented the major rationale in the application of cognitive techniques to children. Maladaptive behavior and performance are seen as representing a child's use of inappropriate or poorly organized cognitions. There are several variations in therapeutic approaches (Ellis, 1962; D'Zurilla and Goldfried, 1971; Mahoney, 1974; Beck, 1976; Meichenbaum, 1977), which according to Meichenbaum differ on "the relative emphasis placed on formal logical analysis, the directness with which the therapeutic rationale and procedures are presented to the patient, and the relative reliance on adjunctive behavior therapy procedures" (Meichenbaum, 1977, p. 197). In the application to children, there appear to be three kinds of interventions.

First, there is "problem solving." With this approach the child is either presented with a specific statement (such as, "When I work slower, I do better") or with a series of problem-solving statements (such as, "What is the problem? What are two different ways I can solve it? Which of these ways is the best? I'll try it out and see how well it works. Did it turn out the way I wanted it to?). The child is then taught to vocalize these statements in situations where they are needed. After these statements occur appropriately, the child is taught to make them subvocally.

The second technique is called "self-instruction." In this approach children are taught to vocalize a rule or series of rules to direct their behavior. A child who responds impulsively might be taught the following set of statements for performance situations: "First, I begin at the top and on the left. Next, I make sure that I look at all of the answers. Then I can make my choice. Then I go to the next one. I look at all the answers. . . ."

The third method is called "cognitive modeling." This technique consists of having the child observe another person in real life or on film dealing with the kind of problem facing the child. In addition to modeling the adaptive overt behavior, however, the model also models the verbalizations that the therapist would like the child to use to direct his or her behavior. These statements might be either a problem-solving or self-instruction sequence.

These techniques have been used in attempts to change impulsivity (Kagan et al., 1966; Meichenbaum and Goodman, 1971), hyperactivity (Palkes et al., 1972; Douglas et al., 1976), aggression (Giebink et al., 1968; Goodwin and Mahoney, 1975), academic behavior (Robin et al., 1975; Bornstein and Quevillon, 1976), and delay of gratification (Bandura and Mischel, 1965; Kanfer and Zich, 1974). Reviews of the cognitive behavior therapy literature report mixed results of effectiveness of these techniques, although they appear to have potential. Most of the positive findings are on cognitive types of skills or behaviors. Comparatively few have reported sustained behavioral changes.

A problem that has been identified is the lack of correspondence between a child's verbal report of an event or behavior and the actual occurrence of that event or behavior (Lovaas, 1961, 1964; Sherman, 1964). This problem was addressed in terms of verbal behavior by Risley and Hart (1968) and Risley (1977) by selectively reinforcing not only verbal reports of the occurrence of targeted behavior, but also the correspondence between the children's verbal report and their actual behavior. Only then did increases in the children's reports of favoring clean playgrounds or intentions to pick up trash lead to an increase in actual trash picked up (Risley and Hart, 1978). One might hypothesize that cognitive techniques are effective in the initial development of these behaviors, but that if the environmental consequences do not reward the correspondence of the verbal behavior and the occurrence of the targeted overt behavior, it is unlikely that either will be maintained.

SELF-CONTROL TREATMENTS. Self-control is a related area that has a slightly different emphasis. Children taught from a self-control model are instructed in such tasks as self-monitoring, self-recording, self-assessment or self-evaluation, self-reinforcement, self-punishment, and self-determination of contingencies or goals. These terms are basically used in the manner one would expect from their names. In addition, strategies discussed under cognitive behavior therapy might or might not be included. The difference would be that the focus of the intervention is to have the child perform some of the same tasks as a behavior therapist might in setting up a treatment program. The literature suggests that without external reinforcement for occurrences of the targeted behaviors, self-monitoring, -recording, -assessment, and -evaluation do little to initiate new appropriate behaviors (O'Leary and Dubey, 1979; Rosenbaum and Drabman, 1979), but may augment maintenance of behavioral changes that had previously been maintained by external reinforcement.

Operant Techniques

GENERAL DESCRIPTION. The application of operant techniques to the problem of children has been extensive in terms of numbers, settings, and types of maladaptive behaviors. The operant approach is basically a four-step process: (1) define the problem to be changed in terms of observable, measurable behavior; (2) record the rate of occurrence of the target behavior; (3) apply consequences or treatment interventions; and (4) continue recording to evaluate if the intervention has been effective. Without each of these four steps, a therapeutic method could not be considered as using an operant approach, despite the fact that the intervention itself was describable in operant terms. In addition to the methodology of evaluation, operant techniques are usually derived from the assumption that behavior is a result of its consequences. As a result both "normal" and maladaptive behaviors are considered to follow the same laws and are therefore subject to modification through learning. The classification of abnormal behavior is therefore a function of the behavior of the person being labeled, the situation in which the behavior occurs, the person applying the label, and the societal morals in which the labeling occurs (Ullmann and Krasner, 1969). Thus maladaptive behavior tends to be categorized according to whether it is a behavioral excess (i.e., the problem behavior is occurring too frequently for the situation) or whether it is a behavioral deficit (i.e., not occurring with sufficient frequency in a particular situation). Interventions are directed at increasing or decreasing the rate of occurrence of the target behaviors. Specific technologies have developed to both increase and decrease behaviors. Increasing the rate of occurrence of a behavior involves a one- or two-step intervention process, depending on whether the goal behavior is presently occurring or not. If it is already occurring but at an unacceptably low level, a reinforcement program is developed. If the behavior is not presently occurring, procedures are developed to teach the child how to emit the desired behavior. This can include modeling, verbal instructions, physical guidance through the desired behavioral sequence, "shaping," or some combination of two or more of these techniques.

SHAPING. Shaping is a procedure by which the therapist determines where the child is on the hierarchy of behaviors required to achieve the goal behavior. The child is then rewarded for the occurrence of any behavior that is a closer approximation to the goal behavior. As a level of behavior in the hierarchy is established and begins to occur regularly, less appropriate behaviors are no longer rewarded. The requirements (contingencies) for reward are gradually increased according to the child's performance until the target behavior is reached. The shaping procedure and the reinforcement procedure are implemented simultaneously, as reinforcement is an integral part of the shaping technique. Although logical analyses of what are effective reinforcers are frequently accurate, whether or not a child will increase the rate of a behavior in order to obtain the "reward" cannot be determined except by placing that contingency on the goal behavior. Not everyone likes M&M's® nor will every child work to be told "good job!" Reinforcement procedures may be either of two types.

Positive reinforcement involves the presentation of a desirable (from the view of the child) consequence or event contingent upon the occurrence of the target behavior. Negative reinforcement consists of the termination or removal of an undesirable or unpleasant situation contingent upon the occurrence of the goal behavior. For example, a parent's giving in to a whining child is "negatively reinforced" by the termination of the whining. If the events are effective reinforcers, both procedures result in an increase of the target behavior.

When reinforcement programs are first implemented, they are most effective if the occurrence of the target behavior is put on a "schedule of continuous reinforcement," i.e., each occurrence of the desired behavior is immediately followed by a reinforcer. If the programs have not begun to work within two weeks, different reinforcers might be used and a careful analysis of how the program is being implemented should be conducted. When the program has been successful in increasing the rate of occurrence to the desired level, the reinforcement schedule is gradually "leaned out," i.e., two occurrences of the goal behavior, then four, then eight, then twelve, etc., are required for reinforcement, until the schedule of reinforcement approaches what the child would receive in the normal environment.

TREATING BEHAVIORAL EXCESSES. There are four methods for dealing with behavioral excesses. Positive punishment consists of the presentation of an unpleasant or aversive event or stimulus upon the occurrence of the behavior to be reduced and negative punishment involves the removal or termination of a pleasant situation or stimulus on the occurrence of the targeted behavior. The third technique is extinction. This involves preventing the reinforcing consequences from following the occurrence of the undesirable behavior. Sometimes, however, that which is reinforcing the inappropriate behavior is not always apparent. Another issue to be considered in the use of extinction is that when the reinforcement for a behavior is first removed, the rate of occurrence of that behavior initially increases before it begins to diminish. The reaction of parents to the increase in inappropriate crying that occurs after a therapist has told them to "put it on extinction, or ignore it" is to say "this isn't working" and stop ignoring. This results in inadvertently rewarding the child for crying louder and longer. The fourth method, however, is the treatment of choice whenever possible. It consists of developing a program for increasing the rate of occurrence of the behavior that one would like to have take the place of the undesirable behavior. In this fashion, not only is the undesirable behavior eliminated, but it is replaced with the acceptable responses.

There are additional reasons why this reinforcement paradigm is preferable. When behavior is predominantly controlled by negative consequences, this control is lost whenever the controlling agent is not around (one of the best examples of this phenomena is our speeding when there are no police around). Another problem with the use of punishment programs is the frequent side effects or unintended results of these programs. Children tend to avoid interactions with those who have punished them. This can be very detrimental to families having relational problems. Perhaps the most important factor, however, is that the punishment can result in escalation. The child acts out aggressively when punished which leads to more punishment which leads to more acting out which leads to more punishment and so on until the punishment approaches or is appropriately labeled child abuse. Finally, children who have been disciplined primarily with the punishment paradigm also appear to have less self-confidence.

TIME OUT. The aforementioned techniques have been used on virtually every kind of child behavior problem. Special applications of these paradigms have been developed and have received individual attention as separate techniques. Time out is one example of negative punishment. When a child engages in an undesirable behavior, he or she is "timed out" from positive reinforcement, i.e., removed from the pleasant situation for a set duration of time. During time out each occurrence of inappropriate behavior resets the clock. Time out periods are recommended never to exceed five minutes (although it may take fifteen to twenty minutes before a child has acted appropriately for five consecutive minutes). Because of the difficulties with implementing punishment programs and because of the need to retain a child in the time-out area, time out is not usually the treatment of choice unless staff or parents administering it are well trained. Even then, reinforcement programs should be attempted before resorting to time out.

OVERCORRECTION AND RESTITUTION. Two other techniques also fit the punishment paradigm—overcorrection and restitution. The emphasis is slightly different, but they are similar in their sequence of events. In each the occurrence of an inappropriate behavior is followed by the child being required, with the minimum physical guidance necessary, either to practice the appropriate behavior five to ten times (overcorrection) or to undo or correct the consequences of his or her inappropriate behavior (restitution). An example of overcorrection is a child being required to walk down the hall (that he or she just ran through) five times before being allowed to proceed. If a child had thrown a drink on the floor, a restitution treatment could include having the child mop up the mess. (Although these two techniques are presented as punishment paradigms, they are actually more complex than this in that they include practicing the appropriate or corrective responses as well.

TOKEN ECONOMIES. We will complete the discussion of the operant topics with a technique that has received much use in the child area. Token economies have been used in nearly every setting imaginable (Ayllon and Azrin, 1968; Kazdin, 1977). In a token economy, a child meeting the criteria for reinforcement is given a "token" instead of a primary reinforcer (something for which the child would work that could be given immediately and consumed or enjoyed). The token can be virtually anything that is durable and can be traded in later from a "reinforcement menu." This procedure solves several problems that occur in the regular distribution of reinforcers. The use of tokens makes the distribution of reinforcers easier, in that they are nonperishable, portable, and allow for the cumulative earning of parts of things (it is difficult to give a child a part of a bicycle). In addition, they can be used to teach the child to wait for delayed reinforcers and can be used to instruct the child about money concepts and management. Token economies are best utilized, however, when the distribution of the tokens is preceded by social priase. This procedure helps develop praise as a reinforcer in children who would not normally respond to it.

Biofeedback

Biofeedback is a procedure that attempts to teach the patient improved control over a physiological process by enhancing the patient's ability to perceive changes in the status of that physiological process. This improved sensitivity is most frequently accomplished with the assistance of electronic equipment. Research has indicated that upon receiving such "feedback" of their biological status, many people can learn to predictably alter physiological functioning. The predominant type of feedback used with children has been with the electromyograph (EMG) which translates the minute neuromuscular activity near the surface of the skin into auditory or visual signals. Electrode sensors are attached to the desired site after the area has been cleaned of oils and old skin to insure a good contact. The site depends on the goals of treatment. (For children with cerebral palsy, electrodes may be placed over muscles controlling head position, limb movement, or facial expression, or on opposing muscles where spasticity is involved. For children with headaches, electrodes are connected to frontal muscles of the forehead). The children are then asked to change the muscle activity in the desired direction, increased activity for muscles to be strengthened or activated and decreased activity for muscles to be relaxed.

Several studies have shown EMG feedback to be effective for children with cerebral palsy (Halpern et al., 1970; Harris et al., 1974; Ball et al., 1975; Cataldo et al., 1978). EMG training is also used as a means of training or assessing overall arousal and activity level and is being used as treatment of pediatric headaches as well as hyperactivity (Braud, 1978; Blanchard, 1979). In many situations, however, seeing the needles or lights change or hearing the tones change are not sufficient motivators to get children to work successfully at the tasks. In several studies, token or reward systems have been required to bring about the desired changes in performance on the biofeedback tasks and on the related assessment of functioning in the natural environment.

Another area that has received attention is the use of biofeedback in the control of seizure activity. Electroencephalography (EEG) feedback has been attempted, and several studies have reported success in increasing mu rhythm (which is the human analogue to the sensorimotor rhythm, the increase of which has been associated with increased seizure threshold in cats) and possibly reducing seizures, but in each of the studies these results are potentially attributable to other factors as well. Thus, the clinical usefulness of EEG training has yet to be established (Kuhlman and Kaplan, 1979).

Biofeedback has also been successfully applied to bowel continence training of children with spina bifida or other neurological deficits. For these children the feedback sensors were inflatable balloons which were positioned at each of the anal sphincters and into the large bowel. Children are thereby taught to perceive fullness and to differentially control the sphincter muscles resulting in an improved continence and undoubtedly an increased confidence in their ability to function in social situations (Parker and Whitehead, 1982).

Behavioral Pediatrics

Operant and respondent techniques have most often been applied in home, school, and institutional settings. These environments have been viewed as primary sites for the learning of maladaptive behavior and its maintenance. Much of the literature has therefore concentrated on the modification of specific disciplinary, academic, or social behaviors.

Over the past forty years, it has become increasingly apparent that the epidemiology of disease and the caseload of the practicing pediatrician has rather dramatically changed (Russo and Varni, 1982). While childhood illness and infection are still present, much of the focus of pediatric office practice involves the problems of living, learning, education, and behavior. Similarly, for the hospital-based pediatrician, acute, infectious, and organism-based disease has been replaced by disorders of a chronic nature such as cancer, diabetes, renal disease, and cystic fibrosis.

Accompanying these changes in disease presentation has been a change in the conceptualization of the child with disease and the nature of intervention. For the hospitalized child with serious chronic disease, medical management of symptoms and assisting the child to cope with fear, anxiety, and maladaptive learning around symptoms become primary issues of care.

Clearly, models of personality or behavior focusing on aberrant psychological processes or on history as primary points of intervention do not adequately account for the difficulties faced by children who must undergo years of painful or intrusive treatment, repeated hospitalizations, and the disruption of normal patterns of growth or social maturation, nor do they provide viable treatment strategies for teaching the child to deal with these unusual circumstances. Behavioral pediatrics (Varni and Dietrich, 1981) represents an area of inquiry that merges the methods and assessment base of behavior therapy with the methods and assessment base of pediatric medicine. Within this context, the goal of behavioral pediatrics is seen as the development of procedures to assist patients and their families in coping with and reducing behavioral difficulties that occur as the result of treatment or rehabilitation, and to prevent difficulties that may expose the child to the future development or exacerbation of disease.

As such, behavioral pediatrics utilizes its methods to develop programs aimed at (a) symptom reduction, (b) stress-related disorders, (c) nonadherence to prescribed medical treatments, (d) development of appropriate health-related behaviors in at-risk populations, and (e) assessment of the hospital environment as it affects behavior. Each of these areas represents a productive interface for behavioral techniques and medicine.

Notably, over the past several years, systematic study has demonstrated the applicability of behavioral techniques to disorders such as asthma (Creer et al., 1982), seizures (Cataldo et al., 1980), bowel dysfunction (Parker and Whitehead, 1982), headache (Blanchard et al., 1979), and neuromuscular diseases (Bird, 1982). These studies have demonstrated symptomatic reduction or improved functional outcome in joint behavioral-medical treatment efforts. In addition, general issues of fear and anxiety generated by hospitalization (Melamed et al., 1982) and the productive alteration of hospital environments such as the pediatric intensive-care units (Cataldo et al., 1982) have been modified to the benefit of the child patient. Such changes go hand in hand with the emerging notion of pediatrics, and medicine in general, as being most effective when conceptualized and practiced as a biopsychosocial endeavor (Engel, 1977). What has prompted acceptance by the medical community is the methodological focus and science base of the behavior therapies. The ability to provide brief therapies targeted at the improved function of immediate problems has likewise been a major source of rapid growth. While more data are needed, work at a number of centers is ongoing to assess the initial compatibility seen in early collaborations.

Summary

Behavior therapy has had widespread application to the problems of children and has been demonstrated to be of value in the amelioration of childhood problems. As presented here a behavioral approach is perhaps more a methodology of evaluation than a set of specific techniques. Human behavior is obviously complex and multiply determined. Without an adequate methodology it is unlikely that we will be able to unravel these complexities and bring about predictable behavior changes in the children we treat. The behavioral methodology provides the therapist continual feedback on the progress the child is making, eases the identification of variables influencing the child's behavior by providing continual monitoring of certain behavior, and reemphasizes essential points covered in the therapy sessions through the prompting of the record-keeping process. With this information, insights can be gained regarding which therapeutic procedures are successful and which are not, thus shaping the behavior of the therapist and leading to more effective treatment.

It is clear that within the context of psychological care, behavior therapy has become one of a number of techniques available to the practicing clinician. It must be underscored, however, that these techniques require the same level of careful clinical training and academic study as others. It is impossible to do "a little behavior therapy." A course of treatment is either well designed or it is not. Unless all factors confronting the clinician are considered, successful behavior change will not occur or will not be maintained after therapy is discontinued.

Finally, we should like to raise an important point for consideration. Other theoretical approaches suggest that lasting change is produced by in-depth understanding of life history. It is important to recognize that this is theoretical speculation. It is simply not the case that all patients suffer significant past trauma or that when this is accessed, positive change occurs. For most of us, our life course is predominantly steered by the logic of the present. Our relationships, places of work or sleep, and activities generally present a logical engram to be decoded and modified. Under such circumstances, referral problems when treated are likely to abate; importantly, rather pervasive changes are often seen in child behavior and family interactions. The magnitude and replicability of such changes, in our opinion, is determined by the competency of the behavior therapist and by strict adherence to the methods and tenets of the field.

REFERENCES

Abikoff, H. 1979. Cognitive training interventions in children: Review of a new approach. *J. Learn. Disabil.,* 12:123–135.

Ayllon, T., and Azrin, N. H. 1968. *The token economy: A motivational system for therapy and rehabilitation.* New York: Appleton-Century-Crofts.

Azrin, N. H., and Holz, W. C. 1966. Punishment. In *Operant behavior: Areas of research and application,* ed. W. K. Honig. New York: Appleton-Century-Crofts.

Ball, T. S., McCrady, R. E., and Hart, A. D. 1975. Automated reinforcement of head posture in two cerebral palsied retarded children. *Percep. Motor Skills,* 40:619–622.

Bandura, A. 1965. Influence of model's reinforcement contingencies on the acquisition of imitative responses. *J. Pers. Soc. Psychol.,* 1:589–595.

Bandura, A. 1977. *Social learning theory.* Englewood Cliffs, N.J.: Prentice-Hall.

Bandura, A., and Menlove, F. L. 1968. Factors determining vicarious extinction of avoidance behavior through symbolic modeling. *J. Pers. Soc. Psychol.,* 8:99–108.

Bandura, A., and Mischel, W. 1965. Modification of self-imposed delay of reward through exposure to live and symbolic models. *J. Pers.,* 2:698–705.

Beck, A. 1976. *Cognitive therapy and emotional disorders.* New York: International Universities Press.

Bijou, S. W. 1976. Meeting of the American Psychological Association Commission on Behavior Modification. American Psychological Association, Washington, D.C.

Bird, B. L. 1982. Behavioral interventions in pediatric neurology. In *Behavioral pediatrics: Research and Practice,* ed. D. C. Russo, and J. W. Varni, pp. 101–141. New York: Plenum Press.

Blanchard, E. B., Ahles, T. A., and Shaw, E. R. 1979. Behavioral treatment of headaches. In *Progress in behavior modification,* vol. 8, ed. M. Hersen, R. Eiles, and P. Miller, pp. 207–248. New York: Academic Press.

Bornstein, P., and Quevillon, T. 1976. The effects of a self-instructional package on overactive preschool boys. *J. Appl. Beh. Anal.,* 9:179–188.

Braud, L. W. 1978. The effects of frontal EMG biofeedback and progressive relaxation upon hyperactivity and its behavioral concomitants. *Biofeedback and Self-Regulation,* 3:(1):69–89.

Brigham, T. A. 1980. Self-control revisited: Or why doesn't anyone actually read Skinner (1953). *Beh. Anal.,* 3:25–33.

Calhoun, K. S., and Turner, S. M. 1981. Historical perspectives and current issues in behavior therapy. In *Handbook of clinical behavior therapy,* ed. S. M. Turner, K. S. Calhoun, and H. E. Adams. New York: Wiley.

Cataldo, M. F., Bird, B. L., and Cunningham, C. 1978. Experimental analysis of EMG feedback in treating cerebral palsy. *J. Beh. Med.,* 1:311-322.

Cataldo, M. F., Jacobs, H. E., and Rogers, M. C. 1982. Behavioral/environmental considerations in pediatric inpatient care. In *Behavioral pediatrics research and practice,* ed. D. C. Russo and J. W. Varni, pp. 271-298. New York: Plenum Press.

Cataldo, M. F., Russo, D. C., and Freeman, J. W. 1980. Behavior modification of a 4½ year old child with myoclonic and grand mal seizures, *J. Aut. Dev. Disor.,* 9:413-427.

Copeland, R., and Hall, R. V. 1976. Behavior modification in the classroom. In *Progress in behavior modification,* vol. 4, ed. M. Hersen, R. Eiles, and P. Miller, pp. 45-78. New York: Academic Press.

Craighead, W. E., Wilcoxen-Craighead, L., and Meyers, A. W. 1978. New directions in behavior modification of children. In *Progress in behavior modification,* vol. 6, ed. M. Hersen, R. Eiles, and P. Miller. New York: Academic Press.

Creer, T. L., and Renne, C. M., and Chai, H. 1982. The application of behavioral techniques to childhood asthma. In *Behavioral pediatrics: Research and practice,* ed. D. C. Russo, and J. W. Varni, pp. 27-66. New York: Plenum Press.

Davison, G. C., and Stuart, R. B. 1975. Behavior therapy and civil liberties. *Am. Psychologist,* 30:755-763.

Doleys, D. M. 1978. Assessment and treatment of enuresis and encopresis in children. In *Progress in behavior modification,* vol. 6, ed. M. Hersen, R. Eiles, and P. Miller, pp. 85-123. New York: Academic Press.

Douglas, V., Parry, P., Marton, P., and Garson, C. 1976. Assessment of a cognitive training program for hyperactive children. *J. Abnorm. Child Psychol.,* 4:389-410.

D'Zurilla, T., and Goldfried, M. 1971. Problem solving and behavior modification. *J. Abnorm. Pschol.,*78:107-126.

Ellis, A. 1962. *Reason and emotion in psychotherapy.* New York: Lyle Stuart Press.

Engel, G. L. 1977. The care of the patient: Art or science? *Johns Hop. Med. J.,* 140:222-232.

Eysenck, H. J., and Beech, R. 1971. Counterconditioning and related methods. In *Handbook of psychotherapy and behavior change,* ed. A. E. Bergin, and S. L. Garfield, pp. 543-611. New York: Wiley.

Forehand, R. 1977. Child noncompliance to parental requests: Behavioral analysis and treatment. In *Progress in behavior modification,* vol. 5, ed. M. Hersen, R. Eiles, and P. Miller, pp. 111-148. New York: Academic Press.

Forehand, R., and Atkeson, B. M. 1977. Generality of treatment effects with parents as therapists: A review of assessment and implementation procedures. *Beh. Ther.,* 8:575-593.

Furman, W., and Drabman, R. S. 1981. Methodological issues in child behavior therapy. In *Progress in behavior modification,* vol. 11, ed. M. Hersen, R. Eiles, and P. Miller, pp. 31-65. New York: Academic Press.

Gelfand, D. M., and Hartmann, D. P. 1968. Behavior therapy with children: A review and evaluation of research methodology. *Psychol. Bull.,* 69:204-215.

Giebink, J. W., Stover, D. O., and Fahl, M. A. 1968. Teaching adaptive responses to frustration to emotionally disturbed boys. *J. Counsel. Clin. Psychol.,* 32:366-368.

Goodwin, S. E., and Mahoney, M. J. 1975. Modification of aggression through modeling: An experimental probe. *J. Beh. Ther. Exp. Psych.,* 6:200-202.

Graziano, A. M., DeGiovanni, I. S., and Garcia, K. A. 1979. Behavioral treatment of children's fears: A review. *Psychol. Bull.* 86:804-830.

Halpern, D., Kottke, F. J., and Burrill, C. 1970. Training of control of head posture in children with cerebral palsy. *Dev. Med. Child Neurol.,* 12:290-305.

Harris, F. A., Spelmen, F. A., and Hymer, J. W. 1974. Electronic sensory aids as treatment for cerebral palsied children. *Phys. Ther.,* 54:354-365.

Hobbs, S. A., and Moguin, L. E. 1980. Cognitive behavior therapy with children: Has clinical utility been demonstrated? *Psychol. Bull.,* 87:147-165.

Israel, A. C., and Stolmaker, L. 1980. Behavioral treatment of obesity in children and adolescents. In *Progress in behavior modification,* vol. 10, ed. M. Hersen, R. Eiles, and P. Miller, pp. 81-110. New York: Academic Press.

Jacobson, E. 1938. *Progressive relaxation.* Chicago: University of Chicago Press.

Kagan, J., Pearson, L., and Welch, L. 1966. Modifiability of an impulsive tempo. *J. Ed. Psychol.,* 57:359-365.

Kanfer, F. H., and Zich, J. 1974. Self-control training: The effects of external control on children's resistance to temptation. *Dev. Psychol.,* 10:108-115.

Karoly, P. 1977. Behavioral self-management in children: Concepts, methods, issues, and directions. In *Progress in behavior modification,* vol. 5, ed. M. Hersen, R. Eiles, and P. Miller, pp. 197-263. New York: Academic Press.

Kazdin, A. E. 1977. *The token economy: A review and evaluation.* New York: Plenum Press.

Kazdin, A. E. 1978. *History of behavior modification: Experimental foundations of contempory research.* Baltimore: University Park Press,

Kazdin, A. E., and Wilson, G. T. 1978. *Evaluation of behavior therapy: Issues, evidence, and research strategies.* Cambridge, Mass.: Ballinger Publishing Co.

King, N. J. 1980. The behavioral management of asthma and asthma-related problems in children: A critical review of the literature. *J. Beh. Med.,* 3:169-189.

Kissel, S. 1972. Systematic desensitization therapy with children: A case study and some suggested modifications. *Prof. Psychol.,* 3:164-169.

Klein, R. D. 1979. Modifying academic performance in the grade school classroom. In *Progress in behavior modification,* vol. 8, ed. M. Hersen, R. Eiles, and P. Miller, pp. 293-322. New York: Academic Press.

Kornhaber, R. C., and Schroeder, H. E. 1975. Importance of model similarity on extinction of avoidance behavior in children. *J. Consult. Clin. Psychol.,* 43:601-607.

Krasner, L. 1971. The operant approach in behavior therapy. In *Handbook of psychotherapy and behavior change,* ed. A. E. Bergin, and S. L. Garfied, pp. 612-652. New York: Wiley.

Kuhlman, W. N., and Kaplan, B. J. 1979. Clinical applications of EEG feedback training. In *Clinical applications of biofeedback: Appraisal and status,* ed. R. Gatchel, and K. Price. New York: Pergamon Press.

Lahey, B. B. 1976. Behavior modification with learning disabilities and related problems. In *Progress in behavior modification,* vol. 3, ed. M. Hersen, R. Eiles, and P. Miller, pp. 173-205. New York: Academic Press.

Lazarus, A. A. 1960. The elimination of children's phobias by deconditioning. In *Behavior therapy and the neuroses,* ed. H. J. Eysenck, pp. 114-122. New York: Pergamon Press.

Lazarus, A. A., and Abramovitz, A. 1962. The use of 'emotive imagery' in the treatment of children's phobias. *J. Men. Science,* 108:191-195.

Levitt, E. E. 1963. Psychotherapy with children: A further evaluation. *Bev. Res. Ther.,* 1:45-51.

Lovaas, O. I. 1961. Interaction between verbal and non-verbal behavior. *Child Dev.,* 32:329-336.

Lovaas, O. I. 1964. Control of food intake in children by reinforcement of relevant verbal behavior. *J. Abnorm. Soc. Psychol.,* 68:672-678.

Mahoney, M. 1974. *Cognition and behavior modification.* Cambridge, Mass.: Ballinger Publishing Co.

Martin, R. 1975. *Legal challenges to behavior modification.* Champaign, Ill.: Research Press.

Matarazzo, J. D. 1980. Behavioral health and behavioral medicine: Frontiers for a new health psychology. *Am. Psychologist,* 35:807-817.

Meichenbaum, D. 1977. *Cognitive behavior modification.* New York: Plenum Press.

Meichenbaum, D., and Goodman, J. 1971. Training impulsive children to talk to themselves: A means of developing self-control. *J. Abnorm. Psychol.,* 115-126.

Melamed, B., Robbins, R. L., and Graves, S. 1982. Preparation for surgery and medical procedures. In *Behavioral pediatrics: Research and practice,* ed. D. C. Russo, and J. W. Varni, pp. 225-267. New York: Plenum Press.

Melamed, B., and Siegel, J. 1975. Reduction of anxiety in children facing hospitalization and surgery by use of filmed modeling. *J. Consult. Clin. Psychol.,* 43:511-521.

Miller, L. C., Barett, C. L., Hampe, E., and Noble, H. 1972. Comparison of reciprocal inhibition, psychotherapy, and waiting list control for phobic children. *J. Abnorm. Psychol.,* 79:269-279.

Montenegro, H. 1968. Severe separation anxiety in two preschool children: Successfully treated by reciprocal inhibition. *J. Child Psychol. Psych.,* 9:93-103.

O'Leary, S. G., and Dubey, D. R. 1979. Applications of self-control procedures by children: A review. *J. Appl. Beh. Anal.,* 12:449-465.

Ollendick, T. H. 1979. Fear reduction techniques with children. In *Progress in behavior modification,* vol. 8, ed. M. Hersen, R. Eiles, and P. Miller, pp. 129-168. New York: Academic Press.

Palkes, H., Stewart, M. S., and Freedman, J. 1972. Improvement in maze performance of hyperactive boys as a function of verbal training procedures. *J. Spec. Ed.,* 5:337-342.

Parker, L. H., and Whitehead, W. E. 1982. Treatment of urinary and fecal incontinence in children. In *Behavioral pediatrics: Research and practice,* ed. D. C. Russo, and J. W. Varni, pp. 143-174. New York: Plenum Press.

Phillips, J. S., and Ray, R. S. 1980. Behavioral approaches to childhood disorders. *Beh. Modif.,* 4:3-34.

Pomerleau, O. F., and Brady, J. P. 1979. *Behavioral medicine: Theory and practice.* Baltimore: Williams and Wilkens.

Rachlin, H. A. 1977. Survey of M. J. Mahoney's cognition and behavior modification. *J. Appl. Beh. Anal.,* 10:369-374.

Reisinger, J. J., Ora, J. P., and Frangia, G. W. 1976. Parents as change agents for their children: A review. *J. Community Psychol.,* 4:103-123.

Rimm, D. C., and Masters, J. C. 1974. *Behavior therapy: Techniques and empirical findings.* New York: Academic Press.

Risley, T. R. 1977. The social context of self-control. In *Behavioral self-management,* ed. R. Stuart, pp. 71-81. New York: Brunner/Mazel.

Risley, T. R., and Hart, B. 1968. Developing correspondence between the non-verbal and verbal behavior of preschool children. *J. Appl. Beh. Anal.,* 1:267-281.

Robin, A. L., Armel, S., and O'Leary, K. D. 1975. The effects of self-instruction on writing deficiencies. *Beh. Ther.,* 6:178-187.

Rosen, A. C., Rekers, G. A., and Bentler, P. M. 1978. Ethical issues in the treatment of children. *J. Soc. Issues,* 34:122-136.

Rosenbaum, M. S., and Drabman, R. S. 1979. Self-control training in the classroom: A review and critique. *J. Appl. Beh. Anal.,* 12:467-485.

Rosenthal, T., and Bandura, A. 1978. Psychological modeling: Theory and practice. In *Handbook of psychotherapy and behavior change, 2nd ed.,* ed. S. Garfield, and A. E. Bergin, pp. 621-658. New York: Wiley.

Ross, A. O. (ed.) 1978. *Handbook of treatment of mental disorders in childhood and adolescence.* Englewood, N.J.: Prentice-Hall.

Ross, A. O., and Nelson, R. O. 1979. Behavior therapy, In *Psychopathological disorders of childhood,* ed. H. Quay, and J. Werry, pp. 301-336. New York: Wiley.

Russo, D. C., Carr, E. G., and Lovaas, O. I. 1981. Self-injury in pediatric populations. In *The comprehensive handbook of behavioral medicine,* vol. 3, ed. J. Ferguson, and C. B. Taylor, pp. 23-42. New York: S. P. Medical and Scientific Books.

Russo, D. C., and Newsome, C. D. 1982. Psychotic disorders of childhood. In *Psychopathology in childhood,* ed. J. Lachenmeyer, and M. Gibbs, pp. 120-154. New York: Gardner Press.

Russo, D. C., and Varni, J. W., eds. 1982. *Behavioral pediatrics: Research and practice.* New York: Plenum Press.

Sherman, J. A. 1964. Modification of nonverbal behavior through reinforcement of related verbal behavior. *Child Dev.,* 35:717-723.

Sherman, J. A., and Baer, D. M. 1969. Appraisal of operant therapy techniques with children and adults. In *Behavior therapy: Appraisal and status,* ed. C. M. Franks, pp. 192-219. New York: McGraw-Hill.

Skinner, B. F. 1948. *Walden Two.* New York: Macmillan Co.

Skinner, B. F. 1953. *Science and human behavior.* New York: Free Press.

Smith, R. E., and Sharpe, T. M. 1970. Treatment of a school phobia with implosive therapy. *J. Consult. Clin. Psychol.,* 35:239-243.

Stampfl, T. B. 1973. *Implosive therapy: Theory and techniques.* Morristown, N.J.: General Press.

Stolz, S. B. 1978. *Ethical issues in behavior modification.* San Francisco: Jossey-Bass.

Strain, P. S., and Kerr, M. M. 1981. Modifying children's social withdrawal: Issues in assessment and clinical intervention. In *Progress in behavior modification,* vol. 11, ed. M. Hersen, R. Eiles, and P. Miller, pp. 203-249. New York: Academic Press.

Tasto, D. L. 1969. Systematic desensitization, muscle relaxation, and visual imagery in the counterconditioning of a four-year-old phobic child. *Beh. Res. Ther.,* 7:409-411.

Ullmann, L. P., and Krasner, L. A. 1969. *Psychological approach to abnormal behavior.* Englewood Cliffs, N.J.: Prentice-Hall. p. 21.

Varni, J. W., and Dietrich, S. L. 1981. Behavioral pediatrics: Towards a reconceptualization. *Beh. Med. Update,* 3:13-18.

Watson, J. B. 1913. Psychology as the behaviorist views it. *Psychol. Rev.,* 20:158-177.

Watson, J. B. 1914. *Behavior: An introduction to comparative psychology.* New York: Holt.

Watson, J. B. 1916. The place of the conditioned-reflex in psychology. *Psychol. Rev.,* 23:89-116.

Watson, J. B. 1919. *Psychology, from the standpoint of a behaviorist.* Philadelphia: Lippincott.

Watson, J. B. 1924. *Behaviorism.* Chicago: People's Institute.

Winett, R. A., and Winkler, R. C. 1972. Behavior modification: Be still, be quiet, be docile. *J. Appl. Beh. Anal.,* 5:499-504.

Winkler, R. C. 1977. What types of sex-role behavior should behavior modifiers promote? *J. Appl. Beh. Anal.,* 10:549-552.

Wish, P. A., Hasazi, J. E., and Jurgela, A. R. 1973. Automated direct deconditioning of a childhood phobia. *J. Beh. Ther. Exp. Psych.,* 4:279-283.

Wolpe, J. 1958. *Psychotherapy by reciprocal inhibition.* Stanford: Stanford University Press.

Wolpe, J. 1974. *The practice of behavior therapy.* Elmsford, N.Y.: Pergamon Press.

28

Family Therapy

VIRGINIA GOLDNER

FAMILY THERAPISTS APPROACH pediatric psychiatry from a unique perspective. Their conceptual categories are distinct from both the psychoanalytic and medical models, deriving instead from communications theory and systems theory (Hoffman, 1981). While a thorough exegesis of systemic thinking lies beyond the scope of this chapter, an understanding of certain basic concepts is essential to an application of the family paradigm to child psychiatry.

LOCUS OF PATHOLOGY

From a family systems perspective, psychiatric problems in children are seen as manifestations of a dysfunctional pattern of relationships within a family. It is this *pattern* that constitutes the "presenting problem" for the family therapist, not the child's symptoms in isolation. A childhood disturbance, therefore, is not understood in terms of traditional nosological categories (like those of *DSM-III*) but in terms of its location as part of a transactional sequence between that child and the adults (usually parents) with whom the child is intensely involved. Every symptom is conceptualized as a problem involving two, and usually three, people in the family.

The family therapist, therefore, does not think in terms of "pathology" located within the child, but in terms of "dysfunction" located within the family system which includes that child. This distinction leads to a very different approach to the treatment of childhood disorders. In the individually oriented framework, the main therapeutic input would be with the child alone, and secondary therapeutic efforts (often by different professionals) would be directed at the parents, who might themselves be referred for treatment (either individual or couple). It is also not unusual for the parents to be left out of the process entirely, except for being kept informed about the child's progress.

In the family-oriented framework, the therapeutic intervention *always* includes the parents, since it is believed that the child's problems cannot be considered apart from the context in which they occur and the functions they serve. While therapy might sometimes include sessions for the child alone, the parents are never considered as merely adjuncts to the child's treatment, since they are viewed as *part of the problem to be treated.*

Diagnosis

From a family perspective, a child's symptomatology is seen as embedded in the nexus of family relationships. The family organization is thought to maintain the child as symptomatic, and the symptomatic child is thought to maintain the family organization. Operationalizing this circular relationship in each case is the task of a family diagnosis.

When a family comes for treatment with a symptomatic child, the clinical problem for the therapist is different from the problem the family presents. For the family, the problem is the child's symptoms. For the therapist, the problem is the family's *response* to the child's symptoms. This is because the family seeks professional help when they have been unsuccessful in handling the presenting problem on their own. Thus, the therapist must deal not only with the child's difficulties, but with the family's attempted solutions to those difficulties.

The distinction here is between the factors responsible for the genesis of disturbed behavior, and the factors that determine its maintenance. A child's original difficulties, for example, may arise from biological dysfunction, from problematic family relationships, from problems with peers or teachers, or from a combination of these factors. How the child's distress is handled, however, is a key element in the child's prognosis (Minuchin and Minuchin, 1975). The family, which is a child's primary reference group, can organize itself around the troubled child in such a way as to alleviate, maintain, or exacerbate the child's symptoms. Thus, when a child's psychological problems remain intractable, the family therapist hypothesizes that the structure of family relationships is, in some way, keeping the child symptomatic.

In order to determine how the family's attempts at coping with the problem may be serving to maintain the disturbance, the therapist needs to establish how each member of the family responds to the situation, and whether those responses are part of a repetitive behavioral sequence. For example, a child who is a "slow learner," despite test scores to the contrary, may be participating in a dysfunctional behavioral pattern with his or her parents. A common scenario is one in which the mother, involved in an intense relationship with the child, attempts to help her son with his homework. The more she hovers, the more helpless and agitated the boy becomes. Eventually, this impasse activates the father, who intervenes punitively. Mother then reacts against father, insisting he "does not understand," the father withdraws, and the cycle starts again.

In such a sequence, there is no starting or ending point; there is only endless circular repetition. It is no more accurate, for example, to say that the mother's overinvolvement "causes" the child's incompetence than to say that the father's overcontrol "causes" the mother's overinvolvement, and so on. Each person's behavior is simultaneously "caused" and "causative," and no one can behave differently until the whole sequence changes.

This emphasis on repeating sequences rather than on a linear unfolding of events, and thus on a circular rather than a linear conception of causality, leads the family therapist to think in terms of a symptom's function rather than a symptom's cause. The idea is that if a child's symptom remains intractable, it may be serving a stabilizing function for the family in general, and for the marriage in particular.

This formulation derives, in part, from the concept of *triangulation*. Most family therapists consider the triangle to be the basic building block of the family system. When tension between members of a two-person system becomes too high, there is a tendency to bring in a third person to stabilize the situation. When the tension is in the marital system, the third person can be another adult, such as a lover or grandparent, or it can be a child. Thus, in the example cited earlier, the family therapist can hypothesize that the child's school problems may be serving to perpetuate the overclose relationship between mother and son, which in turn perpetuates the emotional distance between the parents and therefore protects the couple from having to face the problems between them.

This kind of thinking is best illustrated by speculating about the consequences to the marriage if the child were to improve. In this case, the child's improved school functioning would mean that he would be spending less time at home working with his mother and more time outside playing with friends. This would leave the mother free to move closer to the father, which would increase the level of emotional intensity betweem them and therefore increase the potential for conflict. Now, instead of fighting over the handling of the boy's homework, they would be fighting over their relationship, which is much more threatening to family stability.

To the individually oriented therapist, a formulation of this type will appear highly improbable. This is partially a function of perspective. If the child is seen as "figure" and the family as "ground," the speculations about potential marital discord will seem far too removed from the immediacy of the child's experience and dilemma regarding school. But in a family paradigm, the child and parents are seen as parts of a larger whole—the family—which has its own rules of organization. Thus, in order to make sense of the child's symptoms, the therapist must locate them in the context of family relations.

From a systemic perspective, therefore, a family assessment is essential to understanding a child's symptomatology. Thus, whether or not family therapy becomes the treatment of choice in a particular case, family assessment is absolutely crucial to the formulation of a treatment plan. Family assessment is indicated no matter what the nature of the presenting problem, developmental level of the child, or socioeconomic status of the family.

Assessing the Family System

Families can be described along two dimensions: space and time. The spatial dimension refers to the organization of the family system. Assessment along this parameter involves determining the rules that structure relationships in a family. These rules function like social norms, regulating what kind of interactions are permissible among family members and what kind are not; once they have been established, they have the power of unwritten laws that must not be broken. Family rules function to insure the stability and continuity of the family system. Assessment along the spatial or organizational dimension, therefore, highlights the mechanisms the family has developed to resist change and disorganization. These mechanisms are sometimes called *homeostatic regulators*.

The time dimension refers to the developmental process within families. It posits four main developmental stages: couple formation, families with young children, families with school-age or adolescent children, and families with grown children. These stages comprise what is called the "family life cycle." As the family moves through these transitional periods, it must change its internal organization in order to adapt to the changing or maturational needs of its members. Assessment along the time, or life-cycle, dimension involves evaluating the capacity for adaptational change within the family system.

These two parameters, time and space, highlight reciprocal functions in the family. While the spatial dimension evaluates mechanisms for maintaining stability, the time dimension evaluates mechanisms for achieving internal transformation.

The Spatial Dimension: Family Structure

To assess the rule-governed aspects of family transactions, the therapist looks for patterns of behavior that repeat themselves in sequence. For example, in observing a mother, father, and seven-year-old child who came for treatment because the child would become excessively anxious when separated from her parents, the therapist noted a particular transactional sequence, which recurred throughout the session.

Whenever the parents began to talk to one another, they took opposing positions, which created tension between them. Whenever the tension reached a certain level, the child began to clamor for the mother's attention, who would then abandon the conflict with her husband to deal with the child. While mother and child were interacting, the father would become distant and distracted, so that when the child eventually drifted away from her mother, the parents would be too emotionally distant to pick up the threads of the argument. As soon as another conflictual exchange between the parents would begin to develop, the child would once again begin to display helplessness or irritability, pulling the mother toward her.

The repetitive aspects of this sequence suggest that a "rule of the system" has been operating. In this instance, all the parties were behaving as if there were a rule prohibiting the expression of sharp conflict between the parents. Another "rule" required the child to regulate the level of parental conflict by diffusing its intensity through deflection.

Transactional rules govern all aspects of family life, positive as well as negative. These rules organize family members into a unique relational pattern or structure. By watching the sequence of transactions in a family, the therapist can map family structure. Along the vertical axis, the therapist can map hierarchies within a family. This establishes who is in charge of whom. Along the horizontal axis, the therapist can map the degree of closeness and distance between family members. This establishes who is close to whom. These two parameters are interdependent, since people of unequal status and power in any social organization are necessarily more distant from one another than people at the same level. This reciprocal relationship between hierarchy and proximity determines the basic organization of the family system. Adequate family functioning has been positively associated with certain patterns of family organization and negatively associated with others.

GENERATIONAL HIERARCHY AND SUBSYSTEMS. In every family there is a basic family hierarchy which involves the separate generations: grandparents, parents, and children. In a well-functioning family system, the generational hierarchy is clearly defined and conforms to prevailing cultural norms. In the American middle-class family, for example, parents are expected to be in charge of children, while grandparents serve as advisers and assistants to the parents. In traditional Asian societies, the greatest status and power resides with the grandparents, while among poor American blacks, parents and grandparents often share executive responsibilities (Haley, 1976).

When the status positions in a family hierarchy are confused or unclear, family functioning is compromised. For instance, an unclear hierarchy can be inferred when a child has temper tantrums, refusing to obey his mother, who is reciprocally unable to control her son. In such a case, the mother may be indicating that she is in charge, while simultaneously treating her child as a peer (Haley, 1976). This ambiguity can be easily detected in the familiar ineffective injunction, "Johnny, stop yelling! Okay?"

Another kind of confusing hierarchy results when a family member at one level of the generational hierarchy consistently forms a coalition with a member at another level of the hierarchy against a peer of one of them. This arrangement is called a "cross-generational coalition" and it is consistently associated with individual and family dysfunction. The most common example of this pattern occurs when one spouse unites with a child against the other spouse. A variant of this has one parent-child dyad siding against another parent-child dyad. Clearly, if a child has been drawn so close to one of the parents that he or she functions as a peer in the adult conflict, the generational hierarchy has been compromised, hampering the ability of either parent to take charge of the child.

Malfunctioning hierarchies not only interfere with family functioning across the generations but within the generations as well. Every family system differentiates itself into smaller intragenerational subsystems, each with particular social functions. These include, the marital subsystem, the parental subsystem, and the sibling subsystem. If these subsystems are to work effectively, they must be free to operate without interference from participants of other subsystems. For example, the capacity for interdependence and collaboration between spouses requires freedom from interference by in-laws and children. Similarly, the development of skills for negotiating with peers, learned among siblings, requires noninterference from parents (Minuchin, 1974).

For adequate family functioning, each of these subsystems must be demarcated by a clear boundary—a rule governing who participates in a transactional operation, and how (Minuchin, 1974). The following list illustrates a variety of circumstances in which subsystem boundary violations can occur:

1. The marital subsystem boundary can be violated by (a) *members of the sibling subsystem* when a child is co-opted into an alliance with one spouse against the other; or by (b) *members of the parental subsystem* when the couple relates only through their roles as mother and father, and cannot relate as husband and wife.
2. The parental subsystem boundary can be violated by (a) *members of the sibling subsystem* when a child assumes responsibilities for his or her siblings that properly belong to the parents; or by (b) *members of the marital subsystem* when conflicts between the husband and wife are played out as parental conflicts regarding the children.
3. The sibling subsystem boundary can be violated by (a) *members of the parental subsystem* when parents intervene, rather than allowing children to resolve their own conflicts; or by (b) *members of the marital subsystem* when the conflicts between husband and wife are played out between the children, each of whom is allied with one of the parents.

In all of these examples, family functioning is impaired because the tasks appropriate to the various family subsystems cannot be accomplished when there is interference from members of other subsystems.

BOUNDARY DIFFUSION OR RIGIDITY. The clarity of boundaries within a family can vary along a continuum from rigid to permeable. At the extremes of boundary functioning are two family types whose boundaries are either overly permeable, the *enmeshed family,* or overly rigid, the *disengaged family.* Individual and family dysfunction are associated with both of these extremes (Minuchin, 1974).

Enmeshed families operate with a high degree of emotional proximity, causing the boundaries between all subsystems to become blurred. This results in a heightened sense of belonging, but it also discourages autonomous functioning because family members respond to one another with excessive speed and intensity. Disengaged families develop overly rigid boundaries, making communication across subsystems difficult. This results in a heightened sense of autonomy, but the supportive functions of the family are curtailed and members lack feelings of belonging since the family tends not to respond when a response is necessary (Minuchin, 1974).

Minuchin, in his classic textbook, *Families and Family Therapy,* captures the distinction between the two family types:

> The parents in an enmeshed family may become tremendously upset because a child does not eat his dessert. The parents in a disengaged family may feel unconcerned about a child's hatred of school.

In treating enmeshed families, the therapeutic goal is to facilitate differentiation of subsystems by blocking boundary violations between family members. In treating disengaged families, the therapeutic goal is to increase the flow across subsystem boundaries by increasing the emotional proximity between family members.

FAMILY TYPOLOGIES. Research into the relationship between particular patterns of family organization and particular symptom constellations has been inconclusive. One notable exception has been Minuchin's clinical research on the families of children with disorders such as brittle diabetes, intractable asthma, and anorexia nervosa. The characteristics of such "psychosomatic families" typically include overprotectiveness, enmeshment, inability to resolve conflicts, a "peace-at-all-costs" attitude, and extreme rigidity (Minuchin, et al., 1978).

For the most part, however, dysfunctional family structures are not specific to symptoms. In other words, a particular type of family does not produce a particular type of patient. Rather, unclear hierarchies, cross-generational coalitions, subsystem boundary violations, and subsystem boundary rigidities can be considered aspects of "universal pathogenic situations" from which a variety of symptom pictures can emerge.

Instead of typologies of family organization, family therapists take a developmental view of symptom formation. From this perspective, psychiatric symptoms are a consequence of a "lack of fit" between the family organization and the developmental tasks the family must accomplish.

The Time Dimension: Family Life Cycle

As family members age over time, they must change to adapt to their changing bodies and to the changing demands that society places upon them, and they must realign themselves within the family. Family life-cycle passages are concerned with shifting family membership over time and with changing the status of family members in relation to one another. Every stage in the life cycle changes the relative position of all family members. As new members are born into a family, and as other members begin age-appropriate departures, everyone in the family must reorganize his or her position in relation to everybody else.

Adolescents, for example, begin to challenge the hierarchical organization of the family and to distance themselves from it emotionally as well. An accommodation to these age-appropriate demands and needs requires a change in the rules that organize the behavior of a three-person subsystem within the family, the two parents and the adolescent. Changing the structure of this subsystem will necessarily affect other subsystems in the family, such as the other siblings. This in turn will necessitate additional realignments between family members, and so on.

Demands for change in the structure of family relationships also result from unexpected circumstances (as opposed to predictable maturational crises). A father loses his job, an important relative dies, the family moves, a mother goes back to school, someone gets sick. Each of these events reverberate throughout the family system, changing the relative positions of all family members and therefore necessitating a change in the transactional patterns between them.

When a father loses his job, for example, he will necessarily be spending more time at home, which will inevitably alter the rhythms (and therefore the organization) of his relationships with his wife and children. Everyone will then have to accommodate to changes in the degree of emotional distance between dad and the rest of the family, and most likely, to a change in the power hierarchy of the family as well.

If the rules organizing a family's transactional patterns (the homeostatic regulators) are too rigid, the family will be unable to change its internal organization in order to adapt to demands for change originating from within (maturational changes) or from without (changes in the social environment). Not surprisingly, research findings suggest that symptom onset in one family member can be correlated with family life-cycle transitions (Carter and McGoldrick, 1980).

From a clinical perspective, this leads the family therapist to view a child's symptomatology as not only a disturbance pertaining to the child, but as a sign that the family is having trouble negotiating a life transition. Neither the child nor the family is labeled "pathological." Rather, the family is considered to be a normal family in a transitional situation suffering the pains of accommodating to new circumstances.

An important corollary to this developmental formulation is that not only does the child's symptomatology reflect dysfunctional rigidity in the family system, but it serves a function for the family at a developmental impasse. Thus, the adolescent who becomes incapacitated at the point of leaving home can be understood as taking care of his parents who depend upon him to stabilize their troubled marriage. Similarly, the young child who becomes school phobic can be seen as caring for a depressed mother who needs companionship that her husband does not give her.

A Family Systems Diagnosis of a Childhood Disorder

To conceptualize a childhood disorder in a family systems theoretical framework, the therapist operationalizes the symptom-maintaining aspects of the family system, and the system-maintaining aspects of the child's symptomatology. In order to establish how this circular relationship functions in a particular case, the therapist must first: (a) map the family structure (spatial dimension); (b) determine the developmental stage of the family (time, or family life-cycle, dimension); (c) establish whether there have been any recent changes in the family's circumstances (death, divorce, moves, job changes, etc.); (d) get a history of the presenting problem and a description of how the family is currently responding to the problem.

By utilizing information gleaned from the initial phone contact with the family, or from a clinic intake sheet, the therapist can formulate a tentative systemic hypothesis regarding the family structure, the family life cycle, and the presenting problem before the first session. The following guidelines, adapted from Minuchin and Fishman (1981), can facilitate the development of this initial hypothesis.

The therapist can frame a rudimentary hypothesis about family structure from information regarding the number of people living in the home. For example, a single-parent, single-child household is likely to have a different emotional organization than a large, three-generation family or a two-parent nuclear family. Moreover, since family organization will affect how a family functions, each of these family types can be expected to respond to stress in different ways, and therefore to have probable areas of strength and weakness. Knowing the typical problem areas associated with different family types can help the therapist formulate an initial hypothesis about why a child would become symptomatic in this particular family at this particular stage in its development. Some common examples will serve to illustrate this way of thinking.

The most important feature of life in the two-person family is that the parent and child must rely on one another a great deal. This engenders an intense style of relating which fosters mutual dependence and mutual resentment at the same time. Not surprisingly, these families tend to function at the enmeshed end of the boundary continuum, which means that issues of autonomy and separation are likely to be problematic.

From this framework, the therapist can then establish the developmental level of the family (from the age of the child) in order to determine whether the family is facing a life-cycle transition in which separation is demanded. Some common stress points might occur when the child starts school or enters adolescence, or when the single parent finds a suitor. Given any of these situations, the therapist can formulate a tentative hypothesis that this is an enmeshed parent-child dyad having difficulty functioning in new circumstances that demand more distance between them. The child's symptom can then be seen as both a reflection of that difficulty and as a dysfunctional solution to the threat of separation by serving to keep the two together. For instance, a child manifesting symptoms of childhood depression may be reacting to mother's developing a love interest. The depression syndrome both expresses feelings of loss and functions to pull mother and child back together. The assumption here is that mom is clinging to the child, just as the child is clinging to mom.

There are many forms of three-generation families, ranging from the single parent, grandparent, and child combination to a complex network of extended kin who may not live under one roof but who functionally operate as one household with several addresses. In these complex families, there are no explicit cultural norms dictating how authority and responsibility are to be divided. For example, in a household of grandmother, mother, and child, the grandmother can be "head of the house" with mother and child subordinate, or the mother can be in charge with grandmother acting as her assistant, or both adults can share the parenting equally.

Any of these arrangements can be workable if both adults uderstand the organizational schema and agree with it. If, however, they are struggling for positions of primacy, either overtly or covertly, family functioning will be impeded. When presented with this kind of family, therefore, the therapist should question the hierarchical organization of the executive subsystem, being particularly alert for cross-generational coalitions between the symptomatic child and one of the adults. For instance, a child with a conduct disorder may be responding to contradictory injunctions from two competing parental figures. Or, put another way, the child's misbehavior may be the expression of loyalty toward one parental figure who is in a struggle with another.

In a large family, authority must be delegated, since the parent(s) cannot manage all the family responsibilities alone. With many children in the home, usually one and sometimes several older children are given parental responsibilities as representatives of the parent(s). This arrangement can be effective as long as the "parental child's" responsibilities are clearly defined and within his or her developmental capacities. When such children are given responsibilities beyond their years, or are not given the authority to carry out those responsibilities, they can become symptomatic. Similarly, other siblings can develop problems around issues of control since the hierarchy of power in the family is unclear.

Another common presenting problem in this type of family is attention deficit disorder. Insofar as such children do best in a structured, predictable environment, it is not surprising that the often poorly organized large family creates special problems for children with this type of vulnerability. Thus, when presented with a large family, the therapist can speculate that the child's difficulties may be related to a dysfunctional arrangement regarding the delegation of parental authority between the parental and sibling subsystems.

There are many other common family types, e.g., the divorced family, the step family, the foster family, and the intact nuclear family. If the therapist has a basic model of family structure and function, it is possible to extrapolate what would be the likely weak spots in each of these family types and to generate a tentative hypothesis about the relationship of the child's symptom to any particular family constellation.

FAMILY THERAPY TECHNIQUES

Family therapy techniques are directed at changing the structure of the family relationships that are perpetuating the symptomatology of the patient. Since the patient's symptoms are considered to be embedded in an ongoing, repetitive transactional sequence among family members, clinical interventions are focused on present transactions rather than on past memories, and on relationship patterns rather than on separate individuals.

In this section basic techniques for identifying and changing dysfunctional family patterns will be described. These techniques are common to the systems theory, or communications, school of family therapy. These approaches have been selected to illustrate basic family treatment techniques because they most clearly exemplify the clinical application of a family paradigm and because they hold primacy in the field, both in terms of theoretical rigor and clinical innovation.

The systemic approach has been most closely identified with two schools of family therapy: structural family therapy, associated with Salvador Minuchin and the Philadelphia Child Guidance Clinic, and strategic family therapy, associated with a number of prominent family therapists, including Jay Haley and Cloé Madanes of the Family Therapy Institute of Washington, D.C., John Weakland and Paul Watzlawick of the Mental Research Institute of Palo Alto, Mara Selvini-Palazoli and her associates at the Milan Family Studies Center, and Peggy Papp, Lynn Hoffman, and their associates at the Ackerman Institute of Family Therapy in New York City.

There are two basic differences between structural and strategic approaches to family therapy. In structural family therapy there is more emphasis on clinical technique and on structural problems in the family than on the presenting problem, and interventions are geared to create structural change within the therapy session. This means that the structural therapist is not interested in descriptions of the presenting problem or in what goes on at home, but in enactments, within the session, of the problematic transactions. Moreover, it means that the therapist must intervene actively and directively to change dysfunctional transactions as they emerge during the interview.

In strategic family therapy the primary focus is on the presenting problem and on the repetitive interaction cycles that maintain it. The clinical emphasis is on change-producing tasks and directives to be carried out at home, rather than on interventions to create change within the session. This means the strategic therapist is particularly interested in a history of the presenting problem and how the family has dealt with it in the past. It also means that the strategic therapist does not comment on or intervene to change interaction patterns observed in the session. Rather, these observations, together with information the family provides about life at home, are used to plan change-producing directives that the family is to carry out between therapy sessions.

These distinctions are not absolute, however. Since proponents of both approaches hold similar views on theory and treatment, they tend to incorporate one another's techniques when appropriate. Thus, structural therapists will often prescribe tasks between sessions, and strategic therapists can be quite challenging (although in a more covert fashion) during an interview.

In order to convey the therapeutic context which determines when and how systemic interventions of both types are used, the following section will describe the format of an initial interview. Parts of this material have been adapted from Minuchin (1974) and Haley (1976).

Stages of the Initial Interview

The initial interview is divided into four stages. These are (1) a social stage, in which the family is greeted and put at ease, (2) a problem stage, in which the therapist elicits information regarding the presenting problem, (3) an interaction stage, in which family members are instructed to talk to one another while the therapist observes, and (4) a goal-setting stage, in which the therapist reformulates the presenting problem in a way that can involve the whole family, and if desired, proposes a task for the family to carry out at home.

In structural family therapy, these content-oriented stages are roughly paralleled by a sequence of process-oriented goals. These include transforming the family system into a therapeutic system, formulating a systemic hypothesis, providing family members with an alternative experience of one another, and of the problem, so that they can begin to change their habitual patterns of organization.

SOCIAL STAGE. The tone of the social stage is the etiquette of a host-guest relationship. The therapist acts as a host, putting the family at ease and establishing the rules by which they are to conduct themselves. She or he makes contact with each family member, getting introduced to everyone and chatting informally with each person for a few minutes. Children should be contacted in age-appropriate ways. An infant or toddler can be touched, an elementary-school child addressed in short sentences, an adolescent treated in an adult fashion. It is best to begin with the parents, since this conveys the message that they are "in charge" of the family.

Because the tone of this phase of the interview is informal, it provides the therapist with a chance to observe the family before they begin to behave in "official" ways. For example, the therapist should have the family seat themselves, and should remain standing until everyone else is seated. This is because the seating arrangement often reflects patterns of closeness and distance among family members, and the process by which seats are taken can illustrate aspects of the family hierarchy.

Do the children clamor for seats, scuffling with one another, ignoring the mother who attempts to guide them, and being ignored by the father, who takes a seat off to the side? Do the children wait anxiously for the parents to instruct them on where to sit? Or do they compete for a seat next to mom? Special notice should be taken of the problem child. Is she or he seated alone, while the parents and another sibling are seated together, suggesting a position of isolation? Or is the problem child seated between the parents, suggesting that the child's problem serves a function in the marriage? Inferences at this stage should be very tentative, and should be utilized as hypotheses to be tested as the session proceeds.

PROBLEM STAGE. The therapist shifts to the problem stage when the family seems to be feeling more comfortable, or when they appear to be getting impatient with the informalities. Since the family has come to an expert for help with a problem that has defeated them, the therapist should not delay too long in shifting to a professional tone.

In asking about the problem, it is best to begin with the parents in order to convey an appreciation of the family hierarchy. Once both spouses have spoken, the therapist moves on to other family members. If there is more than one child present, it is best to delay contacting the problem child until other siblings have spoken. This is because if the parents have focused on the symptomatic child, she or he will be feeling increasingly overwhelmed or defensive. By asking the child to respond immediately, the therapist conveys the appearance of agreeing with the parents. Contacting another sibling first gives the message that the therapist is not necessarily accepting the parents' view, and it also allows the child time to prepare a response.

The therapist should hear from everyone in the family. What is said about the problem, how it is said, and how other family members react to what is said, provide a great deal of data about the family system. As various people speak, patterns of agreement and disagreement and of interruption or facilitation will emerge. These reveal family coalition patterns and power hierarchies that almost certainly operate with regard to the presenting problem. For example, in a three-generation family the therapist may observe that the grandmother and mother disagree about the child's problem, and that the grandmother consistently interrupts mother while encouraging the child to speak. Such a pattern suggests that the two adults are in conflict over the family hierarchy and that the grandmother and child are in a coalition against the mother.

Similarly, the way family members describe the presenting problem and how they have attempted to manage it, tells the therapist how the family has organized itself around the symptomatic child. This organizational pattern probably mirrors the family structure. In a family with a child manifesting chronic enuresis, for example, the therapist may discover a repetitive behavioral cycle around the symptom in which mother hears the child whimpering, goes into his room, comforts him, changes the sheets, and stays in bed with him until he falls back to sleep. Returning to her husband, the two fight over her "babying" the child. Such a cycle points to the structure of family relations. The way mother, father, and child transact around the symptom suggests that mother and son are overly involved, that husband and wife are distant, and that father is peripheral to the parent-child interactions. The therapist can also hypothesize that the child's symptom may be serving to maintain this structure. By keeping mother and child together at night, husband and wife are kept apart.

During the social and problem stages, the therapist attempts to form a *therapeutic system* with the family. This is a difficult and subtle task because, unlike individual therapy, family therapy is an arrangement between a natural group, with its strong bonds and complex organization, and a lone professional. If the therapist cannot gain entry into this natural group and establish a therapeutic system, the therapy will fail.

Strategies designed to facilitate the therapist's entry into the family system are called *joining techniques*. All of them can be likened to the task of an anthropologist who must both join a culture and observe it at the same time. If therapists do not experience the idiosyncratic demands and prohibitions of the family system, their formulations will be sterile; if therapists cannot disengage from the family's powerful norms, their interventions will be ineffective.

Joining techniques include system maintenance, tracking, and mimesis. System maintenance refers to an accommodation technique in which the therapist conforms to the rules of the family system, even if they are clearly dysfunctional. The rationale here is that a premature challenge will mobilize the family's resistance and highlight the therapist as "different" and therefore an outsider. Thus, the therapist temporarily accepts the family's characterization of the patient as "bad" or "sick." Similarly, in a family where the mother speaks for everyone, the therapist does not contact family members directly, but rather asks the mother, "Can I speak to your son now?"

In tracking, the therapist follows the content and the sequencing of communication among family members. This involves asking clarifying questions, eliciting additional information, and conveying understanding. It explicitly excludes challenge.

Mimesis involves accommodating to the cultural style of the family, which includes responding to nonverbal cues. The therapist tries to match the family's tempo of communication, its level of loudness, and its affective tone. The goal here is to increase the sense of kinship and familiarity between therapist and family so that the family can more easily reveal itself.

INTERACTION STAGE. In the social and problem stages, the therapist has operated from a position of centrality, directing the flow of communication and responding to what every person says. During the *interaction stage,* the therapist moves from a position of centrality to a position of disengagement, from that of an actor in the session to that of a director of the session. The goal at this stage of the interview is to get family members to talk together so that the therapist can observe how they function when there is no intermediary. Arranging these interaction scenarios is called creating an *enactment*.

The therapist can begin by listening for a natural transition point, such as when a child says, "My father doesn't like it when I cry." The therapist can then say, "Talk with your father about that. I bet he can help you understand what he really means." At first, the therapist might meet with resistance, but if she or he persists, the family will eventually accept the rule of talking to one another.

Once the resistance to the enactment has been overcome, the transaction develops a life of its own. Without an intermediary, the usual rules that control these interchanges will operate, creating an affective intensity similar to that which occurs at home. This provides compelling data about the family system. Family members cannot actually tell a therapist about the structure of their relationships and their patterns of behavior, because they don't really know what they are. But if encouraged to interact, the family can enact these patterns for the therapist to observe.

For example, in the three-generation family described earlier, the mother may complain that she cannot get the child to "mind her." The therapist can then wait for a moment in the

The pioneer work in the field of play psychotherapy is attributed to Anna Freud and Melanie Klein. The theoretical assumption was that children could use play as a means of expressing unconscious conflict and fantasy, much in the same way as the adult patient in psychoanalytic treatment uses free association. Others have modified the theory over the years, most notably Otto Rank, Frederick Allen, Carl Rogers, Margaret Lowenfeld, Virginia Axline, and David Levy.

The child-guidance clinic movement which started in the United States in the 1920s incorporated the thinking of these theorists and adapted it to clinical work with children. Initially, the main thrust for the development of psychotherapeutic theory and technique came from psychoanalysis. However, as the field of psychotherapy expanded its scope, modifications of the methodology occurred both within and outside of the psychoanalytic movement.

Studies on the effectiveness of individual psychotherapy as a treatment modality helpful to children have been few and equivocal (Levitt, 1957). Attempted comparisons with other treatment modalities have suffered from serious methodological flaws, from lack of proper controls both in patient populations and in psychotherapists, and from the difficulties inherent in longitudinal studies where a large number of uncontrollable variables intrude over the course of time.

RATIONALE FOR DYADIC PSYCHOTHERAPY

Dyadic psychotherapy, or one-to-one psychotherapy, is a process by which one person who is trained in the fields of social and biological development, psychopathology, and psychotherapeutic techniques assists another person through psychological measures, with regard to mental processes and adaptation to life. Its purpose is to bring about the patient's readjustment and to promote more comfort in emotions, mental life, attitudes, and behavior so that social relationships, a sense of well-being, and functional adaptation will be improved. Such improvement can take place by means of various features inherent to the psychotherapeutic process. These psychological elements can be summarized as follows:

1. Relationship—The patient-therapist interaction promotes the development of a relationship that is mostly accepting and nonjudgmental. The patient forms this alliance with someone who can understand and empathize with his or her suffering, guilt, anger, and other feelings.
2. Emotional release—The psychotherapeutic encounter provides a situation in which the expression, the understanding, and the proper channeling of feelings, both acceptable and unacceptable, supersede judgments about right or wrong or whether logic or justification exists in regard to these feelings. In this parameter the psychotherapeutic relationship differs from any other relationship in the patient's life.
3. Insight—Through the therapist's knowledge and understanding of human psychological processes, he or she attempts to make the patient aware of the forces within himself and in his environment which generate symptoms or difficulties and which interfere with successful adaptation. This is not limited to an emotional understanding of possible unconscious elements, but also involves an increased awareness of the interrelationships between a broad variety of conscious elements.

It includes the processes of uncovering or gaining insight, of emotional reconciliation, and of redirecting.
4. Reeducation and suggestion—The therapist can provide alternative points of view and alternative modes of adjusting. He or she personifies a benevolent authority figure and an alternative role model for identification.
5. Support—The therapist leads the patient toward the establishment or the strengthening of adaptive capabilities. Together patient and therapist elaborate new and better mechanisms of dealing with stressful situations and with feelings.

Emphasis on any of these psychotherapeutic elements with a particular patient, or at a given phase of treatment, is determined by the therapist's clinical judgment after thorough assessment of the child's strengths, cognitive functions, developmental profile and psychopathology, environmental situation, and social support systems. The focus of treatment is the patient's presenting symptomatology within the context of the patient's total picture as a social being.

The ideal therapist is one who is warm, empathic, and open, and who can reflect accurately and sensitively the feelings and experiences of the patient (Truax and Charkhuff, 1967). He or she should be knowledgeable and thoroughly immersed in various theoretical views about child development, child psychopathology, and psychotherapeutic treatment process. The therapist should be tolerant and receptive without being weak or passive, as well as authoritative without being rigid or dogmatic, and should be relatively free of serious psychopathology or character disturbance.

Indications for Dyadic Psychotherapy

Dyadic psychotherapy is the treatment method traditionally associated with psychiatry as well as with child psychiatry. The descriptive and phenomenologic nature of current psychiatric nosology precludes the utilization of diagnosis as the sole criterion upon which to base one's decision of assigning a child for individual psychotherapy or any other therapy as the treatment of choice. Any one, or several, of the elements of psychotherapy previously outlined could be justified as potentially useful in the management of most childhood disorders, whether used exclusively or in combination with other measures. Because the therapeutic intervention provides such a broad spectrum of potentially beneficial effects, one must view dyadic psychotherapy as a treatment that lacks specificity. Additionally, one cannot utilize the child's experience of subjective distress as the criterion. Most children come to clinical attention because they are presenting problems to their parents, their teachers, or important others, rather than because of any personal awareness of difficulties.

Generalizing, one could say that this method of treatment is most applicable to the child whose condition and whose state of well-being is likely to be improved by all of the components of psychotherapy previously outlined, i.e., the relationship with the therapist, emotional release and rechanneling of feelings, insight, reeducation and suggestion, and support. This would apply mostly to children who are cognitively unimpaired, who are not compromised in their capacity to establish an affective bond, and who are suffering from emotional disorders that seem to be sufficiently severe so that healthy maturation and development are being impeded. Rutter (1975) suggests that "individual psychotherapy...is most likely to be required when the child's problems stem from some form of emotional disturbance concerned either with internal conflicts and stresses or with the way he feels about some unalterable stress in the past or present" (p. 306). We might add that the interest, flexibility, and willingness to cooperate of at least one, if not both, of the child's parents is of utmost importance.

Though these criteria define the child most likely to benefit from individual psychotherapy, they by no means preclude the application of this treatment modality to other children manifesting various forms of psychopathology. However, the goals of treatment as well as the statement of a favorable prognosis would be lessened with certain children. For instance, a child of below average intelligence might benefit from an accepting relationship or from the emotional release available in the psychotherapeutic setting, and yet be cognitively unable to arrive at meaningful insights or to integrate and apply any alternative point of view provided by the therapist. Similarly, a child with an organic mental syndrome who would also profit from the relationship and from the supportive strengthening of his adaptive capabilities, might be unable to restrict emotional release to the psychotherapeutic hour. The inappropriate carry-over to other situations would make it appear as if treatment were aggravating rather than helping the child's condition.

The child psychotherapist must be first and foremost a competent diagnostician. It is necessary to reiterate the importance of a comprehensive assessment by clinicians, who will take into account all aspects of the child's life—psychologic, constitutional, personal, interpersonal, and environmental. Such an assessment will determine whether individual psychotherapy will be useful, which of the elements of individual psychotherapy need to be emphasized and which are contraindicated, and whether it is to be utilized as the sole form of treatment or as an adjunct to other measures—psychopharmacologic, environmental, family counseling—that might be of equal or even greater clinical value.

Approaches to Treatment

Over the past several decades a broad variety of psychotherapeutic measures have been proposed. Ultimately, the theoretical aim of any technique or strategy is to enhance the communication between the patient and the therapist, so as to promote one or more of the psychotherapeutic features previously outlined. Whether this communication takes the form of verbal dialogue or a combination of verbalization and expression through play and/or fantasy will be dictated by the particular child's capabilities as well as by the therapist's dexterity in utilizing certain techniques. It is hoped that the child in psychotherapy will eventually acquire the ability to communicate with words rather than through actions. This is a goal in the development of any person, since language is the most precise of our communicative tools.

Nonetheless, we assume that in the schema of cognitive development, true deftness with the use of language as a means of communication is not fully achieved until the stage of formal operations when the adolescent can deal effectively with the abstractions inherent in language (Inhelder and Piaget, 1958). The importance of play in the development of any child is common knowledge. In general, fantasy can be seen as having a fundamental role in human psychological functioning. The human organism at any stage of development has the capacity to resolve conflict and to pattern future behavior by first "playacting" it in his mind. Even as adults we "toy around" with ideas before deciding upon a course of action. In the child, play is a powerful instrument in attaining mastery over various forms of emotional conflict. Erikson (1964) has concluded that playacting is probably the most natural self-therapy method in childhood.

Psychotherapy with children, whether verbal or otherwise, can be classified in different ways based on various features of the process. Thus one can speak of the aim or type of treatment and refer to it as supportive, suppressive, directive or nondirective, exploratory or "insight oriented," or expressive and abreactive. If one should focus on the influence that the therapist is attempting to exert on the patient, psychotherapy could be classified as interpretative, suggestive, or educative. Emphasis on the theory behind the strategy leads to labeling the psychotherapy as Freudian, Kleinian, Rogerian, Rankian, and so forth.

The more strictly psychoanalytic approach places a great deal of emphasis on the content of the child's play during the therapeutic session. The child analyst systematically interprets the unconscious elements in the sequence of affect-defense-impulse, focusing on the unconscious and on transference reactions. The therapist's interpretations of what the child brings forth, whether verbally or during play, are expected to provide the child with emotional insight into his or her conflicts. This interpretative process can take place in a very direct verbal manner or through less direct means of communication, whereby the same elements of play or fantasy that the child has provided are utilized to speak back to the child.

The child, for example, might draw a series of pictures depicting a small person being attacked and destroyed by monsters and giants. The therapist could infer that the patient is troubled by a sense of weakness or helplessness for whatever reasons and might point this out to the child, proceeding then to explore that feeling. The therapist could also provide the child with an alternative series of drawings, utilizing the same characters but providing other outcomes; the small person might befriend the monsters or possibly postpone the conflict with the reassurance that the small person will eventually grow up, thus the therapist is dealing with the affect without necessarily bringing the interpretation too close to the child's own world. This approach has also been used with children's fantasies and stories and has been elaborated into the mutual storytelling technique (Gardner, 1971).

In either case the interpretative approach is heavily laden with inferences that the therapist makes about the significance of the symbolic communication provided by the child in his or her play or fantasy projections. The inferences are generally made within the context of a particular psychological theory of human development. Assuming that the hypothetical constructs of psychoanalytic theory represent true facts, these inferences lend themselves to varying degrees of inaccuracy or accuracy and potential therapeutic usefulness, depending on the therapist's clinical skills, basic knowledge, sensitivity, and scientific discipline.

Different approaches to play psychotherapy advocate the use of play activities as a medium on which to base other aspects of the intervention. The Rogerian approach, elaborated most extensively by Axline (1969) for the purposes of child treatment, emphasizes the use of play to foster the therapeutic relationship and to create within the therapeutic situation a climate of acceptance and trust. This approach is nondirective and allows the child freedom of emotional expression with a minimum of intervention on the therapist's part. In theory, at least, the therapist is completely accepting and permissive, merely reflecting back the emotions that the child is manifesting through play. Axline has proposed eight basic principles of nondirective psychotherapy. These include:

1. the development of a warm friendly relationship with the child;
2. acceptance of the child as he or she is;
3. establishment of a feeling of permissiveness in the relationship;
4. reflecting back to the child the feelings he or she is expressing;
5. respect for the child's ability to solve his or her own problems;
6. allowing the child to lead the way;

7. recognition of the therapy as a gradual process so that no push for change is made;
8. imposing a minimum of limitations—only those needed to anchor the therapy to reality.

The hypothesis is that by playing out their feelings, children will be able to face these emotions and will learn to control them or abandon them. Thus, the emphasis of this method is on abreaction and on providing a corrective emotional experience in the therapeutic relationship. Although there is limited clinical applicability to the exclusive use of this approach, it has the distinct advantage of keeping inference and interpretation at a minimum.

Levy (1939) proposed a more structured and directive use of the abreactive method, in which the therapist structures the play materials in a way that focuses on a particular conflictual feeling, so as to provide the child with means of ventilating and working out emotional conflicts. This is again done with a minimum of interpretation, but there is little emphasis on fostering the relationship with the therapist. Levy's series of reported cases showed positive therapeutic results in a selected clinical sample. When applicable, this method has the added advantage of providing a relatively brief, goal-oriented treatment approach.

Other approaches to the utilization of play place greater emphasis on its usefulness as a means of setting limits or for the establishment of enforceable rules regarding the child's behavior. One expects that learned principles of fair play and competition will carry over from the therapeutic setting to other areas of the child's life. Behaviorists emphasize this aspect of treatment, utilizing play as a way of implementing principles of learning, such as positive reinforcement, to help the child abandon maladaptive behaviors and learn other more adaptive modes.

In general terms, research evidence is lacking as to whether one approach is better than any other approach. A competent therapist should have the knowledge and skills to apply a broad variety of psychotherapeutic strategies as determined by clinical judgment. Children with underlying emotional or neurotic conflicts may profit most from a psychoanalytic, interpretative approach. Those children who are inhibited in their emotional expression, or who need a situation that will allow emotional abreaction about traumatic events in their lives, are more likely to benefit from a release approach. A conscious effort toward fostering a positive and accepting patient-therapist relationship is probably important in any psychotherapeutic endeavor, but is a *sine qua non* with an insecure child who needs to gain self-confidence or trust in others. Impulsive children require an emphasis on limit setting, whereas those with habit or conduct disorders may show a better response to a behavioral repatterning approach. These are, however, only points of emphasis. The complexities of human beings and of psychopathology will evidently require that a variety of strategies be utilized in the treatment of any child. Any approach or approaches to be utilized must be based on a sound clinical rationale. Sitting in an office and talking or playing a game with a child may be enjoyable for both patient and therapist, but is not necessarily to be considered psychotherapeutic.

Children in treatment are generally integral components of a family. The parents exercise the ultimate authority over them, dictating and regulating their vital activities. It is usually parental motivation that keeps a child in treatment. More so than with adult patients, some level of involvement of the child's family in the treatment effort is necessary. This involvement can range from occasional encounters to obtain information and to provide feedback as to the progress of treatment, through actual family counseling or family therapy sessions, to possible referral of one or both parents for their own psychotherapy with a collaborator. Thus the child psychotherapist must also be a family diagnostician and must always be conscious of the possible effects of his or her individual intervention with the child on the family system as a whole. The therapeutic alliance must exist not only with the child, but with the family as well. In a broad sense all of child psychotherapy is family therapy, even when the bulk of the therapeutic intervention focuses on the child, since it must take into account the shifts in balance between the family and individual systems.

Case Examples

There are obvious limitations in attempting to describe the course of a psychotherapeutic intervention in summary fashion. The following two case examples have been considerably abridged for the sake of conciseness, pointing out the highlights of assessment and treatment. Doubtlessly, much more goes on in psychotherapy than actually meets the eye or that could be delineated in even a lengthier exposition.

Case 1

> John was a nine year old brought to clinical attention by his mother because of "stealing." On one occasion he had taken a pair of roller skates from the school gym, had used them in the park that afternoon, and left them behind some bushes with the alleged intention of picking them up the following day to return them. However, the next day the roller skates had disappeared from their hiding place and another child who had seen John removing them from the gym reported it to the school principal. John's parents were informed and asked to pay for the roller skates, much to their embarrassment and consternation. On another occasion his mother had asked John to buy some milk at the corner grocery store. He purchased the milk but took the change from the twenty-dollar bill his mother had given him and spent it on a set of model airplanes at a toy store.
>
> John was the second of four boys. An older sibling aged eleven was described by the mother as a model child. The younger siblings were two preschoolers aged two and three. John's father was a successful executive whose involvement with his family was minimal. Two years prior to the consultation John's mother had enrolled in a doctoral program which occupied much of her time. The care of the children was mostly in the hands of house servants.
>
> The family was highly religious and of strict moral standards. The mother described herself as an undemonstrative person who, even though she loved all her children dearly, felt uncomfortable with open manifestations of her affection. John's physical resemblance to his mother was striking, a fact that both recognized and that set him apart from his siblings, all of whom were said to resemble his father.
>
> John was an attractive boy, well developed for his age. In the initial encounters he was shy and reserved. After the first few visits, he was allowed to come to the therapist's office on his own, since his home was within walking distance. He was always punctual and his face lit up on meeting the therapist. The assessment made it clear that he had better-than-average cognitive functioning. He reiterated his mother's opinion that he was a terrible child and a thief, and he admitted to the

therapist that there had been other incidents of petty stealing, mostly money at home, of which his parents were unaware. He also expressed a profound dislike for females, a fact that was corroborated by his female teachers with whom he was negativistic and defiant in the classroom. He was also known to play pranks on the girls in school, such as spilling water over their sandwiches at lunchtime or cracking raw eggs inside their bookbags. His teachers saw him as an underachiever in school, obtaining only average grades when all of them felt he had the potential to excel.

John was much relieved when the therapist told him that he did not share the opinion that he was a terrible child or a crook. Instead, he was reassured that he was basically a good boy who had done some stealing and who was angry inside for reasons that had to be found out and understood. Subsequent to this he became much more open and verbal.

In exploring his feelings about his family and his perception of his family's feelings toward him, John was always adamant about his professed love for his parents and siblings as well as of their love for him. In spite of his mother's low opinion of him, he was extremely defensive of her and explained that everything she did, including an incident where she punished his defiance by biting his arm, was all done "for his own good."

It was clearly evident to the therapist that John's treatment could not be carried out in isolation from his mother. John was seen initially twice weekly for a period of four months and subsequently weekly for another six months. Additional sessions for both John and his mother were scheduled on alternate weeks during the entire treatment period.

John felt that playing with doll figures was "sissy stuff." However, he was rather talented in drawing and selected this medium as his favorite way of expressing fantasy. He was asked to draw pictures of anything he liked, but told that each picture should have some kind of story behind it. His drawings of human figures were rather suggestive. Females would be consistently extremely large in size as compared to any other human figure he drew. They had open, gaping mouths with innumerable sharp teeth and frowning faces. They were often described as witches. In the stories they would always be angry, screaming, and harshly punitive. By contrast, all male figures, whether adults or children, would be small in size, dejected, often without hands or with arms behind their backs. John was always asked about what these figures were saying, or thinking, and feeling. The monstrous females were consistently described as cursing, reprimanding, threatening, and angry, whereas the men were generally said to be frightened, would speak very little, and thought of ways of avoiding the situation. Eventually, after several weeks of repetition of these leitmotifs, John was able to relate these perceptions to his mother, his family, and himself with a minimum of suggestion on the therapist's part.

The sessions with John's mother did not always include John. On several occasions she was seen individually. Initially, John's perception of her as an angry and punitive figure was pointed out to her. John's "stealing" was explained to her as his way of obtaining something at a concrete level that he felt was missing in his life at an emotional level. Her immediate reaction was one of sadness and guilt. She felt she should abandon her professional aspirations and devote all her time to her children. The therapist strongly advised her against doing this and instead suggested that she set aside a specified amount of time each day to devote individually to each of her children in mutually enjoyable activities. She faithfully executed this prescription, which much to her surprise was pleasurable to her and resulted in much more compliance on John's part and in less rivalry among the siblings.

A significant event, which occurred during a joint session, was that John at one point got up and sat on the therapist's lap. This was followed by an immediate reprimand from his mother for "acting like a baby." The therapist intervened by giving John an affectionate hug and pointing out that perhaps John was trying to tell them something with this gesture, since it was uncharacteristic of his behavior with the therapist during his individual sessions. His mother asked him to come and sit by her instead, gave him a kiss, and kept her arm around his shoulder during the remainder of the session.

In a subsequent individual meeting, she proudly reported how she had been making a conscious effort to be more openly affectionate with her children. She elaborated on her own strict upbringing which had followed a predominantly disciplinarian pattern, and how she had grown up with the mistaken notion that open expressions of affection were a sign of weakness and would result in spoiled children.

Attempts at bringing the father directly into the treatment effort were met with much resistance. However, there were several long telephone conversations in which the therapist stressed the crucial importance of his becoming more involved with his son. This was also pointed out to John's mother. The family joined an equestrian club and started to spend Sundays together, picnicking and horseback riding. John proudly reported that his father was much better at the sport than his mother.

The quality of John's drawings and his fantasies changed dramatically over the course of treatment. Comparisons with the earlier drawings were made and it became clear to him how his perceptions of himself and of his family were changing. It was then easier to bring out how sad and rejected he had felt and how deep down inside he had really thought his parents didn't love him. He could see the connection between these feelings and his urge to steal, as well as between his defiance toward his teachers and his feelings for his mother. He felt this had all changed, and indeed his behavior in school markedly improved; he finished the school year with excellent grades. At that point, regular sessions were terminated, but open contact was maintained with John and his family. He was seen for a yearly visit for the next five years. On one occasion he invited the therapist to a school musical performance which the therapist attended. It may not have been pure coincidence that John's role in the show was that of Hansel in *Hansel and Gretel*. At fourteen John continued to excel in school and brought a picture of his girlfriend for the therapist's comments and approval.

Case 2

Billy was just six and beginning the first grade when brought to clinical attention. On his second day at school he was one of four boys who had been reprimanded by the teacher for getting out of their seats during class. For the following two days he had absolutely refused to attend school and his mother's attempt to bring him to school on the second of those days was accompanied by a violent temper tantrum and a state of panic which moved her to bring him home.

Billy had attended the same school during the previous two years in the pre-kindergarten and kindergarten classes. Except for a few new children in the first-grade class, he was essentially in the company of familiar friends. His mother had observed a change in Billy's behavior during the previous summer vacation. He had become extremely clinging and wanted to be with her all the time. She had discussed with him the possibility of attending a summer day camp, but he had preferred to stay home. He had a younger sister aged two years. His mother's physical health had been relatively good except for a two-year history of back pains which had been finally diagnosed as a herniated lumbar disk. In recent months the periods of back pain had been more frequent and more severe, often requiring her to stay in bed for most of the day. Billy's father was a technical supervisor in a factory somewhat distant from home. He would leave home early in the morning and would return at around the time when Billy was going to bed. However, weekends were family days and he would devote his spare time to his children. He also noted that during the summer Billy had been recalcitrant about going places with him unless his mother came along. During the previous months Billy had expressed fears of remaining in his room alone, and his mother would sit by his bedside until he fell asleep.

Billy's family was initially seen on a Friday. They were instructed to take Billy to school as usual on Monday, and the mother was told to ask permission to remain in Billy's classroom if necessary. There were two favorite television programs that Billy watched every evening. The parents were also instructed to tell Billy that only children who attended school were allowed to watch television, and to curtail his viewing of these programs unless he attended school.

When Billy was seen on Monday, his mother reported that the morning experience had been a fiasco. Her entry into the classroom was begrudgingly accepted by the teacher, but Billy became so disruptive that the teacher asked her to leave. On her departure Billy had again panicked and she felt obligated to take him home.

Billy agreed to stay in the therapist's office without his mother as long as the door to the waiting room was left ajar. During the session he went to the door three times to say hello to his mother. He was quite eager to play with the mini-dolls and puppets. The therapist first created a family situation consisting of a mother, a father, a boy, and a baby. The dolls were all placed in their respective beds in the dollhouse. Billy was told that it was early in the morning and asked to show the therapist what happened in that family. He immediately got the father doll out of bed and sent him off to work. Then the boy doll was brought from his room to lie down next to the mother where the father had been. The boy doll started nudging the mother doll to wake her up, and upon awakening she started complaining of a terrible headache and saying she couldn't move. Billy was asked how the boy felt, to which he replied that the boy was hungry and there was no one who could fix his breakfast. He subsequently added that perhaps the mother doll was going to die. The therapist told Billy that this reminded him of something that sometimes happened in Billy's home. His mother was asked to come into the office and was told in his presence that apparently Billy didn't understand her back pain problems and might be afraid she would die. At this point the mother laughed and told Billy that this was a silly notion, that there was something pinched in the bones of her back which made it hurt sometimes, but that her life was not in any danger. Billy then asked some questions about the anatomical aspects of the problem which were answered in a straightforward fashion by both the therapist and the mother.

During the same session Billy was shown a calendar of the month and was told that for each day he attended school, a gold star would be placed over the calendar date. The mother added that when he had ten stars in a row, there would be a special surprise. On leaving the office, Billy asked if he could watch his television programs that evening. He was again told that television was for children who went to school so that he could watch his programs the following evening if he stayed in school that day.

That night the therapist had a long conversation with Billy's schoolteacher, stressing her crucial role in helping Billy, explaining some of the elements involved in the problem, and suggesting some ways in which she might be of assistance. The following day Billy went to school with some hesitancy and got as far as the classroom door before he started whimpering and saying he wouldn't stay. At this point the teacher intervened and said "Welcome back, Billy. Children, Billy is back." She started to applaud and the entire class broke into a loud round of applause. Billy smiled and took his seat. Although the teacher had agreed to allow Billy's mother to remain in the classroom that day, Billy himself went over and asked his mother to go home and to come back for him at dismissal time. He was allowed to watch television that evening and he attended school regularly until his next session three days later. The therapist spoke with the family on the telephone every evening to ascertain that the progress was sustained and to offer advice and encouragement. Billy was very proud on his second session when the therapist pasted the four gold stars on his calendar. Visits were stopped at that point and an appointment was given for the following month. His mother was given the calendar and the stars, and instructed to continue using them over the next few weeks. At the follow-up visit the child was reported to be attending school regularly, and he proudly showed the therapist his star-studded calendar and the surprise present that he had selected—a set of mini-dolls.

Discussion and Summary

The foregoing cases exemplify what could be considered two success stories in child psychotherapy. Evidently not every intervention will yield such favorable results. The interventions also illustrate an eclectic approach toward the management of childhood problems where a broad variety of theoretical strategies were applied. These were dictated by the therapist's clinical knowledge, intuition, acquired skills, and personal style. What was utilized at any given time followed a rationale, but was modified to take into account unplanned, fortuitous circumstances.

In John's case a concerted effort was made to establish an accepting relationship which would foster a positive self-image. His symptoms were set up, in John's mind as well as in his mother's as elements outside of his true self which became issues to be dealt with, rather than as integral components of his personality. Straightforward advice was provided to both parents in order to achieve some level of modification in the child's environment. Some of the mother's conflicts were addressed in order to alter her rejecting stance. John's individual therapeutic sessions allowed the abreaction of his feelings and his perceptions. This was facilitated through the utilization of play materials chosen by the child. Through interpretative work John was made aware of his feelings of rejection, his perceptions, and of the transference of his feelings toward his mother onto his teachers and other females. He was also able to grasp the meaning of his symptoms.

In the case of Billy the intervention was not sufficiently extensive to foster the establishment of a warm, trusting relationship. Play techniques were utilized to arrive at unverbalized misperceptions that had psychological meaning. This information was employed to clarify a distortion and the clarification was provided by the mother herself, with the therapist's prompting. This was followed by further elaboration of the child's misconceptions and reeducation. Measures were taken to manipulate the environment through specific instructions to both parents and teachers. Of crucial importance was the emphasis placed on repatterning and positive reinforcement, including visible rewards as well as praise and acceptance by teachers and peers.

In each instance of child psychotherapy, the therapeutic elements of a positive relationship, insight, abreaction, support, and reeducation and suggestion enter into the picture to one extent or another. The data obtained and the therapeutic gains made during the course of individual treatment must be enhanced, when common sense and clinical judgment so dictate, through properly timed family interventions, clinically guided environmental manipulation, and other known therapeutic measures. No one has determined conclusively which of the elements of psychotherapy prove to be most therapeutic in a given case, though one might provide reasonably sound hypotheses for any intervention. A different therapist, utilizing other strategies and having a different style might obtain similar results. A child might improve even without psychotherapy due to changing circumstances in the patient's life.

In the present state of knowledge about this art, one must view individual child psychotherapy, if not as a curative treatment modality by itself, certainly as a potentially useful facilitator in fostering the normative development and personal well-being of disturbed children.

References

Axline, V.M. 1969. *Play therapy.* New York: Ballantine Books.

Erikson, E.H. 1964. Toys and reasons. In *Child psychotherapy,* ed. M.R. Haworth, pp. 3-11. New York: Basic Books.

Freud, S. 1955. *Analysis of a phobia in a five year old boy. Standard edition,* vol. 10, pp. 5-149.

Gardner, R.A. 1971. *Therapeutic communication with children: The Mutual storytelling technique.* New York: Science House.

Inhelder, B., and Piaget, J. 1958. *The growth of logical thinking.* New York: Basic Books.

Levitt, E.F. 1957. The results of psychotherapy with children. An evaluation. *J. Consult. Psychol.,* 21: 189-196.

Levy, D.M. 1939. Trends in therapy: Release therapy. *Am. J. Orthopsych.,* 9:713-736.

Rutter, M. 1975. *Helping troubled children.* New York: Plenum Press.

Truax, C.B., and Carkhuff, R.R. 1976. *Toward effective counseling and psychotherapy: Training and practice.* Chicago: Aldine Press.

30

Focused Short-term Treatment in Clinical Social Work

BOBBA JEAN MOODY / REGGIE SWENSON / ANNA WELTON / PENNY GOLDBERG

DEFINITION OF MODEL

Focused short-term treatment as defined and used in this chapter emphasizes the resolution of immediate reality problems, or "problems of living." In this model the patient or client and the social worker enter into a contractual agreement, working together to solve the individual's or family's difficulty. In contrast to long-term psychoanalytically oriented treatments—which aim for reparative or reconstructive goals—focused short-term work has as its goal the resolution of one or two problems related to current social and emotional functioning.

This form of treatment is particularly applicable in child mental-health care where services must be provided to both the child and the family. For this reason, the social worker's patient in child psychiatry and child mental-health settings is just as likely to be the family as the child. In this model the practitioner and the patient agree to work collaboratively to resolve or ameliorate specific problems within a limited period of time or a predetermined number of sessions. Planned short-term treatment by social workers draws upon traditional casework principles and uses techniques based primarily on psychodynamic and learning theory with some incorporation of role theory. The model is indebted conceptually and operationally to Helen Harris Perlman's "problem solving approach" (Perlman, 1957), to Parad's and Rapoport's work on "crisis intervention" (Parad and Parad, 1968; Parad, 1971; Rapoport, 1965, 1967), and to Reid, Shyne, and Epstein's "task centered" casework (Reid and Shyne, 1969; Reid, 1970; Reid and Epstein, 1972; Reid and Epstein, 1977).

Problem solving for Perlman is a systematically organized process, making use of a rational, directive approach focusing on the person's reality situation. It requires that the caseworker "understand the structure and function of the personality" and use the professional relationship to mobilize the patient's adaptive mechanisms for resolving his problem

(Perlman, 1957, pp. 16–17). As this occurs, integration takes place and further growth is experienced as the problem is mastered.

Crisis theory provides the conceptual frame of reference for a large part of the practice in family agencies, public welfare offices, medical facilities, mental-health clinics, and school social services (Golan, 1974). The worker intervenes at a point of psychosocial stress and disorganization with the aim of shifting the balance in the individual's disrupted equilibrium toward the forces of health. It is theorized that during the crisis situation the person's customary coping and defense mechanisms have become weakened and he is more susceptible to outside influences for change. "A little help, rationally directed and purposefully focused at a strategic time, is more effective than more extensive help given at a period of less emotional accessibility" (Rapoport, 1965, p. 30). Parad (1971) believes that the stressful event typically reactivates old problems as well, providing an opportunity—"a second chance"—to rework unresolved problems (p. 198). If there is no intervention, the individual may move toward a more maladaptive style of coping. For a child, the crisis may interfere with the normal course of psychological growth, resulting in regression and fixation. Intervention therefore becomes crucial in preventing developmental arrest.

Planned short-term models of treatment began to receive more attention after publication in 1969 of the Reid and Shyne Community Service Society Study. This rigorously controlled study challenged the long-accepted hypothesis that continuous open-ended casework treatment would produce better results. The data consistently showed that adults receiving planned, brief service were able to achieve more positive change than those who received open-ended, continuous casework service (Reid and Shyne, 1969). A year earlier, the publication of a national survey of family services and psychiatric clinics for children, conducted in 1965–66, had brought to the profession's attention the relative effectiveness and wide use of short-term crisis-oriented programs (Parad and Parad, 1968).

The problem-solving approach presented here represents basic casework treatment practiced within the specific framework of delimited goals and number of sessions. Reid comments that "the main issue concerns the *degree* of focus or delimitation in defining the major problems and goals in a case—for example, whether a practitioner should strive to help a child improve his impulse-control generally or to help him stay in school" (Reid and Epstein, 1977, p. 8).

BRIEF MODEL VS. OPEN-ENDED TREATMENT METHODS

Focused treatment attempts to support and reinforce areas of intact functioning rather than opening them up to exploration for the purposes of reparation or reconstruction—as would intensive psychotherapy or child analysis. One of the primary aims in short-term focused treatment is to restore the individual to his previous level of functioning and, hopefully, enable him to strengthen his coping mechanisms and learn new patterns of adaptation. If the individual has never functioned well, the goal would be to maximize his ability to function socially and emotionally up to his fullest capacity. For example, an eight year old with a diagnosis of schizophrenia and a history of hyperactivity who has never been able to be maintained in a classroom setting would be helped to function in a special class.

Short-term counseling *bolsters whatever is healthy,* while *closing off* options for the patient. Providing closure serves to lower the individual's anxiety by focusing more keenly upon the nature of the immediate difficulty. This is in contrast to long-term psychoanalytic psychotherapy and psychoanalysis—treatments in which the goal encompasses changes in many more areas of functioning and personality. These longer-term, less-structured treatments also assume that the individual has a high degree of anxiety tolerance and is capable of considerable self-analysis, which may not be the case with the short-term focused-treatment patient. The social worker's saying, for example, "Tell me how I can be of help to you" is much more limiting than "Tell me about yourself." Or again, "What is the problem?" closes off, while "How did you come to be here?" opens up many more areas for exploration. Another example can be shown by the adolescent patient who has listed a number of solutions to a problem. In open-ended treatment the caseworker might say, "What comes to mind about the solutions you have just enumerated?" while in brief focused intervention the worker might say, "Well, you yourself have suggested one solution that you have already given a lot of thought to. Why don't we take a look at that together and see how that might work out for you?" The worker focuses on one of the solutions, thereby closing off options and refraining from opening up the whole issue for lengthy and time-consuming exploration. The work is also carried out at a conscious level of awareness with no attempt being made to elicit unconscious material (dreams, free associations, and interpretation of the transference relationship). Limiting the treatment to problems and symptoms in the present, to the here and now, helps to meet the individual's need for answers to pressing reality questions. Short-term casework also avoids the development of a regressive transference.

When unconscious material is brought into treatment, which often happens in the case of young children, the therapist helps the child differentiate between reality and fantasy or dreams. One boy dreamed that snakes had invaded his bookbag and consequently was afraid to take his books out when he arrived at school. Short-term treatment would aim at reducing the child's fears in school by helping him to understand that the snakes represent his own internal fears and fantasies, that they are symbolic, and do not really exist as snakes in his bookbag (explained in whatever language the child is capable of understanding). This reassures him that the snakes do not exist in reality and that the therapist understands his situation, feelings, thoughts, and fears.

APPLICATIONS IN TREATMENT OF CHILDREN AND PARENTS

In the field of child psychiatry, the focused short-term model is a valuable addition to the clinician's treatment armamentarium, as it is responsive to a variety of child and family needs. The model is ideal for resolving crisis situations brought to the mental-health practitioner. It also is useful for ameliorating specific reality problems associated with chronic conditions, which cannot themselves be resolved by the short-term method. This treatment approach would not be appropriate for children with serious personality disorders or multiple personality problems, such as obsessive-compulsive disorder, conduct disorder (undersocialized, aggressive type), Tourette's syndrome, or anorexia nervosa. Though even in these situations the family and child can be helped with associated living problems such as family fighting, child-management and limit-setting difficulties, need for medication compliance, and excessive parental guilt and anxiety.

If child neglect results from chronic depression on the part of the mother, she will respond better to long-term treatment than to focused short-term intervention. While the mother may do well caring for her children during the period of short-term treatment, the situation typically deteriorates when the worker terminates counseling. Teenage or adult alcoholism or drug addiction by themselves also are not suitable for the short-term treatment approach. However, problems of living (either an outgrowth of the substance abuse or unrelated to it) can be addressed in brief treatment, and include resolving living arrangements, getting medical treatment, entering a special treatment program related to chemical abuse, or reestablishing relationships with family members. Reid and Epstein (1972) have suggested that in such situations short-term work should be offered in conjunction with other forms of treatment that address the major illness. This has been borne out by the experience of the authors as well.

The short-term focused approach is well-suited to working with multiproblem families where one specific area is identified for focused work. The other problem areas are not treated, thus making it possible to resolve or ameliorate the one most compelling reality problem for which the family has come for help. By identifying and limiting focus to one area, the "bottomless-pit" syndrome (for both client and worker) is avoided with its attendant hopelessness and therapeutic drift.

Crises require rapid and active intervention by the child psychiatrist or social worker. The crisis may be precipitated by an environmental or developmental stress—a major breach can occur between appropriate developmental stages. A variety of examples may be cited: pregnancy in an eleven year old; a family thrown into crisis by a fire-setting child or a knifing incident; a child becoming panicky over a real or perceived trauma (surgery, incest, sexual attack, rape); a family becoming exhausted and overwhelmed in dealing with an angry schizophrenic adolescent son living at home. Assertive, active intervention using the focused model can rapidly engage the child and family, limiting focus and identifying and working directively on targeted problems. Anxiety of the child and family will decrease, so they can use their adaptive and coping skills to best advantage. As such, the model can diminish excessive guilt and anxiety of parents in crisis over a hospitalized child, helping them to continue functioning at home or at work. Assistance can take the form of providing individual or joint parent counseling, involving parents in a support group, and establishing supervised visits with the disturbed child.

With chronic conditions such as childhood schizophrenia or severe developmental disabilities, the short-term model has particular relevance. The therapist may focus on the child's chronic regressed condition and its impact on the day-to-day life functioning of the family. The therapist and parent can then select segments of the problems that are most amenable to short-term intervention. For example, if the patient has a diagnosis of mild mental retardation, the parents can work to enhance their child's travel skills. If the child can learn to take the subway to school, the therapist might help by breaking down this activity into simple tasks: "How do you buy a token? How do you go through a turnstile? How do you know which train goes where (learning to read the subway map)? How do you recognize the station where you get off, and how do you exit from the station?"

The short-term model can be adapted to groups as well as to individual and family approaches. For example, the parents of depressed children might utilize a task-centered group to learn behavior-management skills. A ten-session contract, one and a half hours each, can focus on the child's behavior and the effectiveness of the parent's reaction to the child. This can be done through behavioral rehearsal and role playing, so the parents can practice their new management skills.

One parent spent a considerable amount of time rehearsing her reaction to her eight-year-old daughter's temper tantrums in front of the group. She learned to stop and think before reacting. After several weeks the child's temper tantrums decreased markedly. The group helped another mother to establish a goal of getting her son to work on his homework for one hour each day. She planned to reach this goal by rewarding him with something desirable each time he did his homework. She began with ten minutes a day, gradually working toward her target goal of sixty minutes. As her son progressed in accomplishing his task, she provided enough positive reinforcement to motivate him to go on. This type of group raises parental self-esteem and ability to cope with a situation formerly experienced as overwhelming. As they begin to share their difficulties and feelings with other parents in the same situation, parents realize that they are not so "odd" and "different" as they had imagined. The experience of mutuality with those similarly affected reduces parental blame and feelings of incompetence and failure. The parents' sense of self-esteem is additionally enhanced by seeing their children do more for themselves.

Several issues arise perennially: whether the child or the parent should be treated; whether separately or together; by one or two therapists. Whatever decisions are made concerning these questions, the parent must be counseled if short-term focused treatment is to be successful A chaotic home environment or pathologic parental attitude can have a major impact on the child's functioning. With a very young child with anxiety disorders, counseling with the mother alone is frequently the most economic and effective method of treatment. In cases of severe "disturbance of the vital functions of the child, such as food intake, sleep, excretion and respiration," Melitta Sperling (1974) believes that "interpretations exposing the unconscious motivations and conflicts of the mother" are necessary in resolving the disorder and finds that this "can often be accomplished even in brief contacts with the mother." (p. 3). She observes that indirect treatment of the parent is the only method by which infants and preverbal children can be successfully treated.

Sperling considers simultaneous treatment of mother and child by the same therapist the preferred treatment for children suffering from psychosomatic disorders. An alternate method is the technique of treating the mother first for a period of time before beginning the treatment of the child, particularly in cases of younger children up to the age of eight or nine (Sperling, 1974). Sperling's observations on simultaneous treatment and preparatory treatment of the mother are based on long-term psychoanalytic treatment of mothers and children, but her basic concepts of joint and separate treatment of parent and child—depending on the child's developmental stage and diagnosis—are applicable to the short-term model as well. Particularly in short-term treatment of adolescents, two therapists may need to be assigned when patients are unable to fully trust their secrets to a therapist who is also treating the mother or father.

The short-term focused model is often used on child inpatient psychiatric units. Tasks or behavioral goals are set up that combine treatment of the individual child and the family with total milieu treatment, utilizing group, occupational, and recreational therapy. The duality of this treatment approach greatly enhances the chances that short-term intervention will be successful. Token-economy reward systems are often used in conjunction with this approach as a way of reinforcing positive behavior change in the child patient.

Work with children on an outpatient basis must take into account the lack of the continuous reinforcement available in the inpatient setting. In such treatment settings, the patient can be asked to complete certain tasks as part of a direct problem-solving approach. The task selected must be appropriate to the child's level of affective and cognitive development (Ziegler, 1980). The therapist may invoke other techniques, such as role playing, to rehearse the child for carrying out feared or difficult assignments in his environment. The patient's self-esteem is increased when he is able to make specific behavioral changes or accomplish agreed upon tasks, promoting better functioning.

Ziegler has attempted to apply Reid's task-centered treatment to short-term work with children and their families by using tasks to help the parents and child focus on one central problem. If the child's main problem is low self-esteem, for example, the parental task could be to give the child praise and support whenever he is in a difficult situation at home. To the child, Ziegler might assign the task of selecting a competitive game, playing it with the therapist in the treatment session, and talking about his feelings of not being good enough while competing. Similarly, symptom relief is often possible when there is agreement between the child or parent and the practitioner on what needs to be changed.

For example, an eleven-year-old boy was brought for treatment following the birth of a sibling because he began to take money from his mother's purse. The therapist helped the child to identify that the stealing occurs at a point where he feels his mother is not paying sufficient attention to him. He was given the task of learning to translate his previously unrecognized feelings into a verbal communication such as, "I need to talk with you now, Mom," or, "I need your help now to . . . " In other words, the nonverbal, angry acting-out of feelings of deprivation and rejection can be converted into constructive behavior. At the same time, the work with the mother focuses on increasing her understanding of her child's motivation—that his feelings of being unloved are being acted out by stealing material objects from her. She can then be counseled to respond to her son when he verbally communicates a need for her time and attention and involve him in the care of the newborn so that he no longer feels excluded. Specific time could be set aside for him. In addition, the parents could spend time reading to their son before bedtime or take him on a special outing alone.

IMPLEMENTATION OF MODEL

The emphasis when targeting goals for the short-term treatment process should be on defining problems that have specific behavioral manifestations or are connected to specific circumstances (Reid and Epstein, 1972). Some examples of such reality problems in the current life situation are divorce, out-of-wedlock pregnancy, birth of a handicapped child, admission of a child to a psychiatric hospital or to foster care, terminal illness, rape, death of a parent or sibling. All of these situations involve separation and loss which may precipitate the individual or family into a crisis state.

Once selected as the treatment modality, focused short-term treatment requires that certain sequential steps be taken if it is to be effective. These include: (a) exploration, definition, and clarification of the problem, (b) selection of target problems, (c) selection of target goals (Reid and Epstein, 1977), (d) contracting with the client, (e) structuring interviews, (f) termination.

Exploration, Definition, and Clarification of Problem

"Problem definition is perhaps the most significant element in the helping process. All else that is done hinges on the way problems and needs are defined" (Germain, 1980, p. 5).

The social worker's nonjudgmental attitude, respect for the adult's or child's autonomy and wishes, warmth, and empathic understanding are communicated through a detailed and specific eliciting of the facts surrounding the patient's situation. The process of information gathering is in itself narcissistically gratifying to the individual and is a building block in the relationship between patient and worker. With a child, the therapist's physical approach and friendly attitude is of particular importance for the development of rapport. During the first session, the therapist explores the presenting problem(s), elicits relevant history, and assesses motivation, developmental level of the child, and capacity for change. This will include the collection of demographic data and information about family constellation, support network, medical and psychiatric history, and functioning in major areas. The initial focus is on the patient's perception of the problem. In the practitioner's mind are the questions: What is the problem? Why is the individual patient or family coming now (precipitating event)? How can the worker and agency be of help?

This process applies as well to those situations where the patient does not initiate the request for help. This frequently is the case in acute general-hospital settings where the patient or family may not know that social work services exist or may not have conceptualized a need for help. Here, the worker or therapist must "reach out" to the patient and family to provide information about the service available. For example, on a pediatric oncology service, a worker may not see every child admitted but will select those children and families considered to be at high social-emotional risk according to a predetermined set of criteria. The worker will go to the child and family, explaining that he or she is from the Social Work Department and meets with all families whose children have this illness. The practitioner may try to engage them by universalizing the experience of coming into a hospital and undergoing all the tests, describing it as a difficult and often anxiety-provoking time. What has it been like for them? Could they describe it?

Our experience has shown that it is difficult for some individuals to maintain focus after the initial information-gathering session due either to the overwhelming and immobilizing nature of the stressful reality situation or to internal disorganization and difficulty with thought processes. In such instances the therapist may need to repeatedly refocus and bring the individual back to the task at hand. With a parent, the worker might say, "I would be interested in hearing more about..." "Can we go back to your description of..." or "I wonder if you could talk more about the feelings you experienced when..." With the child, the worker might say, "Tell me more about what happens to you inside when your teacher asks you to read in front of the class," or "Your story about how your puppy died sounded very upsetting. Could you tell me more about what did happen that day?" Refocusing can also affirm interest in the adult or child.

Families who have difficulty acknowledging their problems present a particular challenge to the short-term case method. For example, parents may have been told that their eight-year-old daughter disrupts her class by repeatedly lifting her skirt in front of the boys. The parents see their child as "bad," plan to punish her, and blame the teacher for not providing proper supervision. They reluctantly come for treatment to appease the school principal who has insisted that the child and parents need psychological counseling. During the initial interview they refuse to see their daughter's behavior as signifying emotional problems and believe that the school exaggerated.

In such a case, the clinician moves from the presenting problem to "join" the parents' resistance, empathizing with the parents and dealing with the issue as understood by them. The parents are asked to explain how they perceive the child's skirt-lifting behavior and why she might be doing this at school. By saying, "Tell me how she is bad" and asking questions like "Is this the only bad thing she does?" or "Do you have any other worries or concerns about her?" the parents can begin to discuss other behavior demonstrated at home that is upsetting to them. In joining the resistance, the worker turns the situation around, directing empathy and understanding toward the parents' needs and toward helping them with their concerns. This technique is useful for example, in working with impulse-ridden mothers. A woman who wants to free her newborn child for adoption is offended by what she perceives as rude and insulting behavior on the part of the city child welfare worker. She refuses to sign the necessary papers and threatens to throw the city worker out of her apartment when she visits the next day bringing the forms. The hospital social worker empathizes with the mother's feelings of vulnerability but points out that by refusing to sign the voluntary placement papers, she is hurting herself and preventing her baby from having the good home she wants for him. The mother recognizes the priority of the child's welfare over her own impulses and is able to follow through on signing the appropriate forms so that the adoption process can begin. It has become increasingly recognized that arousing motivation and diminishing resistance may be one of the essential tasks of the initial period of treatment (Hollis, 1971).

As in other treatment modalities, there are some parents who are never really able to come to terms with the fact that their child has problems. It often takes a serious crisis before the parents recognize any need for help. It has been the experience of the authors, however, that these parents often leave treatment once the critical phase of the crisis is over or when the child begins to improve. It may not be possible to engage such clients in even short-term focused treatment, no matter how skilled the worker.

Selection of Target Problems

During the phase of exploration and clarification, a large number and variety of problems may be presented. In addition, the therapist is likely to identify several other problems the patient may not have recognized as contributing to the difficulty. However, the practitioner and patient must select one or two core issues that will become the focus of their work together. This is critical, since the individual or family may want help with many serious problems which may not be resolvable within the context of time-limited treatment. It is the worker's responsibility at this juncture to help narrow the field of focus, selecting problems that are specific and have the highest priority in the individual's or the family's current life situation. This will prevent "overload."

Selection of Target Goals

Once the target problems have been delineated, appropriate treatment goals must be selected. These include both broad goals for the treatment process and more narrow or subgoals. The aim is to develop specific, realistic, and manageable goals, thereby maximizing the potential for success. This selection process is crucial, as reaching one small goal successfully can provide incentive for future problem solving and goal accomplishment. The following examples of some broad and narrow treatment goals illustrate the application of this concept:

    1. The target goal with an out-of-wedlock pregnant teenager is to help her make a realistic plan for her baby. This overall goal can, however, be broken down into subgoals which might include: obtaining prenatal care, telling her parents of the pregnancy, making a decision about adoption versus keeping the baby, contacting the baby's father, and making future plans for herself following delivery.

    2. A couple has come for marital guidance. It is easier to work on one aspect of poor communication rather than to work on the global concept of "poor communication." A first step would be to teach them to stop interrupting each other while talking.

Contracting with the Child and Family

In focused short-term work the practitioner must be prepared to give a clear and direct statement about what he or she can offer, and the patient must agree that there are indeed problems to be worked on. This defines the purpose for them to meet and helps the patient and worker gain clarity and focus about their joint task. This step is generally referred to as the development of a contract. In discussing this issue, Reid notes:

> The major function of the contract is to ensure that the practitioner and client have a shared understanding of the purposes and content of treatment. The contract is formed at the beginning of service and, unless both parties agree to changing it, serves to guide the course of service. A contract may be oral or written; the understanding reached may be fairly general or quite detailed. Use of contracts helps avoid certain perennial problems in social work practice: misunderstandings between worker and client as to the nature of the former's intentions and the latter's difficulty . . . , lack of clarity on the part of both as to what they are to do together; drift and scatter in the focus of treatment" (Reid and Epstein, 1977, p. 9).

Contracting is the core of mutuality in the professional relationship. It ensures that the patient will not be "treated behind his back" for conditions of which he is unaware (Reid and Epstein, 1977) and reduces the chance of there being hidden agendas. It forces the worker to conceptualize and crystallize his or her role. If an individual cannot be involved in contracting (such as with a young child, or a legally incompetent adult), then the goals of service are determined which meet the client's best interests (Berkman and Rehr, 1978). With a child, especially a very young child, who does not have adult verbal capabilities and has not developed the ability to think abstractly, the contract has to be translated into the child's language and understanding—e.g., "I think I can help you with those worries you are having about being in school," or ". . . worries you are having about what is happening to your mother while you are at school." Proskauer (1971) believes:

> It is unnecessary in most cases, and especially so with younger children, to confront the child with a verbal statement of the focus (of treatment). The focal issue serves best as a guiding and organizing idea in the therapist's mind, enabling him to intervene selectively through therapy. With adolescents, however, both the time limit and the focal issue are best negotiated explicitly from the start, with the patient having some say about how many months and how often to meet. Thereby resistance related to the normal adolescent ambivalence toward external authority can be minimized (p. 622).

Structuring the Interviews

ROLE OF THE THERAPIST. Treatment begins with the first contact—whether by phone or in person. In the initial stage of treatment, emphasis is on establishing and building a relationship of trust between the worker and the child or family which will mobilize the patient's efforts and energy to solve his or her problems. The therapist must assume an active, assertive role in order for short-term treatment to be successful. A positive alliance with the client must be formed rapidly, as only a strong positive partnership will allow the therapist to structure the process of treatment without undue resistance.

Rather than waiting for the treatment to unfold, the worker directs and focuses the content and flow of the sessions. Within the session itself the amount of structuring will vary somewhat with the client, the targeted problem and goals, and the style and training of the practitioner. However, within the interview certain specific material related to the target problem and goals should be covered, if not by the client, then by the worker. In a highly structured approach the worker may begin the session by asking specific questions, e.g., "What happened when you and your wife went to see your son's teacher on Monday?"

The therapist serves as a positive identification and role model for the patient. Throughout their interactions the worker who is psychodynamically trained seeks to diminish the patient's anxiety and guilt and to increase self-esteem, capacity for pleasure, and sense of competence through the use of techniques familiar to clinical social workers. The worker's goal here is to restore and enhance the patient's functioning as rapidly as possible. The counselor offers recognition of and support in whatever areas of success and competence can be found in the individual's life situation—at work, at school, in sports, or in parenting. In the worker-patient contact the problem is repeatedly clarified, reformulated, and restated, and the worker helps the child or parent understand and identify feelings related to the situation. The therapist also has a responsibility to increase the individual's reality testing by helping him or her to sort out and differentiate what is going on in the world from the patient's own distorted perceptions. Making order out of a seemingly chaotic situation—breaking it into parts small enough to be dealt with and clarifying what is going on internally and externally—is in itself stabilizing and ego-supportive for the individual.

The worker must also be able to convey a sense of hope that the treatment will be effective. The aspect of hope is conveyed through the "worker's authority based on professional competence and expertise" (Golan, 1974, p. 434). The demonstration of empathic understanding is necessary for encouraging patient's self-expression and helping them to feel accepted and understood, and is an important factor in the outcome of any psychotherapeutic treatment.

ROLE OF THE PATIENT. The patient is not a passive recipient in focused short-term treatment, but must be mobilized by the clinician to assume an active role in the work. The worker may assign certain tasks to be carried out during the treatment, or the patient may be required to make certain decisions within a specified period of time. This may include doing homework between sessions—going to a medical clinic, going to the Welfare Department, keeping a diary of thoughts, fantasies, symptoms, or behavior. It will be easier to activate patients' own problem-solving capacities, whether children or adults, if the target problems and goals are ones they feel are most important to them.

ROLE OF ADVICE GIVING. In the opinion of the authors there is an important place for advice giving in short-term treatment. It can provide the patient with the stimulation necessary for task accomplishment and can convey that the worker is fully participating with the client in problem-solving work. Reid and Epstein (1972) feel that the only limitation on direction in task-centered casework is that it must be aimed at furthering the client's progress on the task. Advice should not be offered indiscriminately or gratuitously but in the context of the patient's own desire to solve the targeted problems.

There are situations where workers would be abdicating their professional responsibilities if they did not give advice. In an emergency situation, firm and emphatic (even authoritarian) advice and direction must be given and may even be lifesaving. Acting-out patients and those who are suicidal risks often require explicit instructions as to which actions they are to take and which they should avoid. Agreement to abide by the worker's instructions may be made a condition of continuing the treatment relationship.

In all situations great care should be given to the subtleties of advice giving and what is communicated to the patient. Advice may be offered in many "face-saving" ways attuned to the individual's narcissism (which is more apt to be injured in a direct "thou shalt not" edict). This avoids increasing the patient's resistance to further exploration of feelings and behavior by creating a power struggle in which the treatment itself is likely to be the loser. It is usually best in nonemergency situations to couch advice as a question: "I wonder if you have thought of . . . . ?" or "I wonder if you have considered . . . ?" Prohibitions on potentially self-injurious actions can be combined with other techniques. For example, with a parent: "We both know that you are furious and are planning to go into the principal's office and make a scene. I wonder if that is really in your best interest? Why don't we look together at how that might work out." Here the worker increases the individual's reality testing by clarification of the planned behavior, identification of the feelings involved (rage), and a suggested prohibition, while making an appeal to the patient's healthy, adaptive functioning. One may need to let any patient know that "this is not a criticism," that "I am on your side."

Some patients will experience advice as criticism, especially those who have had very critical, hard-to-please parents (in particular, overly critical and obsessive mothers). It is therefore especially important to provide recognition of and to appeal to the client's healthy functioning and healthy sense of values—"I know you want the best for your child. That is why I want you to think about what will happen if . . . " This softens the advice giving so that the worker is not experienced as issuing emphatic directives and nurtures the patient's better functioning. Empathy and commitment to the patient's best interests are the *sine qua non* of treatment. Generally, if the practitioner has a high regard and respect for the patient and is sensitively attuned to his or her needs, feelings, and functional capacities, the worker is not likely to act in a way that would communicate a "holier-than-thou" attitude to the patient.

Termination

In short-term focused treatment, termination is addressed explicitly from the beginning (Small, 1971). It arises as an issue during formulation of the therapeutic contract by the fact of setting a time limit on the treatment. There are a variety of ways that termination may be effected by the therapist: (1) the agreed upon contract is met and services are completed (e.g., when the disturbed child is transferred from an acute hospital to a residential treatment center, or when the contracted number of outpatient interviews are completed); (2) the patient is told that he or she can return in case of future problems; (3) referral is made for another type of treatment or to another agency.

It is common practice to leave an "open door" where patients are made to feel welcome to return if they wish. Some individuals may continue to call or write from time to time for several years to let the worker know how they are doing and to keep in touch. Not totally breaking the tie to the worker serves the function of allowing the patient to maintain a relationship with a positive, interested, and benign powerful "parental" figure, which in itself can greatly increase the individual's coping and adaptive capacities.

One of the major findings from the Reid and Shyne (1969) study was that termination modes and problems were dramatically different in time-limited than in open-ended treatments. It was found that clients in brief treatments were more apt to like the caseworker's personality and attitude and to view their caseworkers as having "moderately" or "very positive" feelings toward them. Only a minority of the clients who received continuous open-ended services thought their caseworkers had "clearly positive" feelings toward them, and about one-third left treatment feeling less positive toward the caseworker than they had at the beginning of treatment. The clients in short-term treatment were also more likely to see termination in neutral terms at the completion of a service contract. On the other hand, the continuous-service clients more often saw termination in negative terms and as having occurred because of lack of progress. Reid and Shyne hypothesized that the time limitation in the brief model may have enabled the client to lower expectations for change, so that he or she could end treatment with a feeling of having made some progress within the given period of time with feelings of mastery and accomplishment. In contrast, the structure of open-ended treatment permitted the client to determine the point of termination in most cases, leaving open the possibility of clients blaming themselves for lack of progress. Some clients, Reid and Shyne felt, may have experienced termination as a rejection of them by the caseworker, especially if the caseworker had encouraged the client to leave. Reid and Shyne concluded that a predetermined point of termination "may lessen feelings of inadequacy and rejection" (pp. 162–163).

It was also found that fewer families dropped out of treatment after the first interview when the brief treatment approach was used as compared to the continuous open-ended service model. Reid and Shyne felt that the presentation to clients of a plan for limited services, as was done in the first interview of the brief treatment program, may have provided an incentive necessary for clients to return that had not been offered in continuous service. They hypothesized that the potential or actual length of the open-ended service may have had negative effects that precipitated early withdrawals. Clients may be more willing to complete a service they know to be short in duration than to start a therapy of undetermined length.

Case Example

The following vignette demonstrates how the model works in actual practice. In particular, this case example highlights the importance of selection of target problems for work. The target problem here was narrowly defined, and important family issues were set aside even though they affected the child. The sequential steps essential in utilizing focused short-term treatment are illustrated.

Presurgical Counseling of a Pubertal Child

(*DSM-III* Diagnosis: 309.28 Adjustment Disorder with Mixed Emotional Features)
Anne was a twelve-year-old, intellectually gifted, pretty blond child with cerebral palsy who had undergone two surgical procedures (at the ages of four and ten). Both operations were successful medically, but following her second hospitalization (which was uneventful), she developed increasing resistance to follow-up care. She refused to attend her regular clinic appointments and carried out her prescribed program of physical therapy only sporadically. She became strongly invested in her schoolwork and involved herself in after-school activities with her friends, none of whom was disabled. Though outreach attempts had been made, Anne was resistant to preventive social-work services.

A crisis situation occurred for Anne when, on her latest visit to the clinic, she was informed by the orthopedist that another surgical procedure (on her feet) was indicated. She became extremely upset, crying, screaming, and cursing that she would never return to the clinic, that she would never undergo surgery again. Her mother,

Mrs. M., was completely unprepared for the recommendation of surgery and felt helpless and frustrated by her inability to allay her daughter's fears. She was caught between intellectually recognizing the need for surgery and emotionally wishing to shield her daughter from any further suffering and fear.

The social worker met with Mrs. M. alone following the mother's discussion with the physician. Mrs. M. confided that she was burdened by feelings of guilt about Anne's last surgery, as she and her husband had not visited regularly during the hospitalization. They had been experiencing considerable financial and marital strains as well over the last few years. Unbeknownst to Anne, Mrs. M. and her husband had recently been talking about a separation. She was aware that her daughter's feet were becoming increasingly deformed but did not feel committed to influencing Anne to agree to surgery. As she was in the throes of facing her own marital conflicts and needed to reserve her emotional energies for this "battleground," Mrs. M. felt overburdened and emotionally overloaded. She stated that she could not force the child to undergo surgery, that Anne was too old to be left out of the decision-making process. Mrs. M. welcomed the worker's suggestion of meeting with Anne for the purpose of engaging her in a problem-solving endeavor around the issue of surgery.

Anne entered the worker's office truculently, announcing that she was not going to be convinced by her to have surgery. The worker shared with Anne that she had no intention of doing this but was concerned about Anne and her mother being so upset following the orthopedic examination. Could Anne tell the worker what had happened? Reluctantly, Anne began to share some experiences of what had occurred earlier that day. The more the worker probed, empathized, and joined her in her misery and anger, the freer Anne felt to expose her own vulnerabilities, expressing considerable ambivalence about future surgery. When this conflict was pointed out to her, she recognized that surgical repair of her feet would probably benefit her. However, it was clear to the worker that Anne's fears (based on past experiences) prevented her from moving beyond an impulse level. Anne and the worker agreed to meet again to further explore her feelings about surgery, with the ultimate goal of helping her make a rational decision about this procedure. A time limit of two months was settled on, since Anne indicated that, should she agree to have the surgery, she wanted both the operation and recuperation period completed before the beginning of the fall school term.

Due to her discomfort in the clinic setting, Anne asked the worker to come to her home. This healthy manipulative ploy was responded to positively—fostering a sense of mastery and control for the child while capitalizing on her willingness to participate in problem-solving work. During the home visit the worker met with Anne and her mother (at Anne's request) to more fully understand and develop the subjective significance surgery held for her.

Anne crystallized her fantasies and fears regarding the recommended surgery, confiding that she was afraid to have another operation for fear of disturbing her relationship with her friends. She felt she "belonged" even though she had difficulty walking. She felt that her absence from her friends (two in particular) during the hospitalization of a few weeks would breach her ties with them. As the worker explored further and searched for details, Anne was able to admit to feelings of anger and hurt toward her parents for not visiting often during her last hospitalization. Anne thought she had caused them to be angry at her because she needed surgery, had special needs, and had imposed financial burdens on them. Mrs. M. was helpful in clarifying that this was not the case, that the problems she and her husband were having were not related to Anne's cerebral palsy or to her need for surgery. They talked together for a long time and Mrs. M. was able to move toward Anne, holding her in her arms and expressing feelings of love and compassion. Anne began to cry, saying, "I'm afraid of surgery. I don't want to be cut anymore, I'm afraid I'll get worse." When this was explored, Anne said that after her second operation people had told her she was "lucky" that the operation went well and that "other kids who had surgery didn't always get better." She was scared to risk it again. She did not really understand what the surgery entailed and she had blocked out whatever the doctor had told her. Anne admitted she did not know if the other kids—the ones who did not improve—had undergone the same surgery.

Once these objective and subjective facts were culled, Anne was able to recognize and act on the evident gaps in her knowledge—particularly the specific aspects of the surgery itself and her parents' thoughts and feelings about her as an individual. Four more sessions were arranged with Anne during the next seven weeks. The first session was with Anne, her mother, and the surgeon to explain in detail the proposed surgery, the risk, and expectations for improvement; the second was with Anne alone to rethink and rework the information gathered and the feelings of abandonment. During these interviews the primary goal was to sharpen, reclarify, rethink, and reorganize the facts, feelings, and thoughts as they emerged, in order to mobilize Anne to act in consonance with her understanding of what was best for her. The worker's role was active and hopeful, encouraging Anne's growth by linking her good emotional and intellectual capacities with her ability to translate her fears and thoughts into words where they could be examined one by one.

The third and fourth sessions were spent with Anne alone and focused on role playing, task identification, and anticipatory guidance. Anne was able to bring her dilemma under conscious management and agreed to the surgery. The following practical plan, developed to maintain Anne's sense of equilibrium, was crucial in helping her make a favorable decision: (1) parents' visiting hours were planned to assuage Anne's fears of being abandoned (mother to visit each afternoon within certain hours, and father at night at least three times during the week); (2) a presurgical visit to the pediatric unit where Anne would be hospitalized was conducted where she had an opportunity to meet the chief resident, the nursing coordinator, and the play therapist; (3) special passes were to be arranged for her two closest friends to visit once each during the course of the hospitalization to reinforce Anne's fragile sense of belonging. In addition, Anne and the worker agreed to meet regularly at least three times a week during Anne's hospitalization and to maintain contact once a week for two weeks during her planned outpatient rehabilitation. Anne felt her most acute need for support would be just before surgery and at the time of her first session in physical therapy. The availability of the worker was essential during these two periods. Phone contact was maintained with the family during Anne's hospitalization on a once-per-week basis to reinforce the positive effects of the active involvement of Anne's parents.

Anne's surgery and early rehabilitation were very encouraging. Her feet were markedly improved, allowing better anatomical alignment and correction of her poor posture. Just as important, however, was Anne's pleasure with the results.

She felt she had made the right decision. In the last planned session Anne thanked the worker for helping her deal with a "scary" problem. She felt she could now handle the rest of the rehabilitative process without the worker's direct involvement but asked, "Can I show you my new shoes when I get them?" Anne was assured that the worker's door would always be open to her.

During the concluding meeting with Anne's parents, they recognized how much their participation had contributed to Anne's consistent progress. Their marital and financial problems, not directly dealt with in the short-term intervention, still remained. They were encouraged to consider marital treatment at a family agency in their community.

This case example illustrates how planned short-term treatment was used to facilitate resolution of a reality conflict which had crucial implications for the whole of this child's future development. The worker did not try to deal with all of the social and emotional issues (marital conflict, financial burdens, parental guilt related to Anne's impairment) but separated out those issues most imperative to solution of the overall problem (surgery). Through the technique of targeting problems and goals, practical aspects of Anne's situation were selected, allowing for facts and feelings to be looked at objectively. Helping Anne to work through her feelings and fantasies on a conscious level enabled her to make a decision that furthered her healthy development. The successful outcome of surgery and rehabilitation served to bolster this child's positive sense of self and increased her coping and adaptive capacities. At termination, Anne and her family expressed a sense of accomplishment and pride at having overcome a difficult problem in their lives.

Suitability of Model

Focused short-term treatment is an economic and efficient way of helping individuals and families solve problems of living. The time limit in this treatment model can serve as an incentive for both worker and patient to focus on the problems and utilize the interviews in a more productive way. By selecting problems limited in scope, patients can take satisfaction in knowing that their problems have a chance of being resolved in a short period of time. This can motivate them to work harder and increase confidence and self-esteem so that more difficult problems can be addressed in the future.

This treatment model can be used effectively with a wide range of patients to help them solve immediate reality problems. The essential components are the ability on the part of the patient to engage cognitively in a problem-solving process and the patient's motivation to do something about his or her life situation. This would rule out actively psychotic or severely retarded individuals and individuals who are too depressed to mobilize themselves. Also ruled out would be individuals who do not wish to change their life situations, although it may be viewed by the social worker as maladaptive.

It is often thought that more progress can be made in short-term focused treatment with patients who are capable of higher levels of intellectual and emotional functioning. However, this may not always be true; some patients who seem to have very limited intellectual or emotional resources are able to utilize the process maximally, whereas others who initially appear to have much greater capacity for change may not make progress. The authors have been impressed by the fact that the degree of pathology does not necessarily correlate with the child's or the family's ability to benefit from this kind of social-psychological counseling. Benefiting from treatment seems to be related to motivation, the amount of distress experienced, the ability to trust and make attachments, and to the specific type of impairment. Highly motivated patients are usually able to engage actively in the problem-solving process, which promotes more rapid and effective change.

In summary, this model can be applied to a wide range of biopsychosocial problems and patient needs. It is suitable for the resolution of specific immediate reality problems and crises. These involve situations where: (1) the problem requires immediate resolution and decision making, and neither worker nor patient has the luxury of using a long-term treatment process (a child expelled from school, fire setting); and (2) the problem is not suitable for an uncovering, anxiety-provoking type of treatment. In a case of rape or terminal illness, the goal is to help the person deal with the immediate and overwhelming anxiety, to allay rather than stimulate anxiety.

Focused short-term treatment is an ideal model for clinical social workers whose master's level training prepares them specifically to deal with reality problems. Individual, group, and family treatment modalities, requiring basic social-work skills, are an integral part of this treatment method. The practice of developing a contract is a social-work concept which promotes the client's right to self-determination and validates social work's concern with basic human rights.

The short-term approach can play a legitimate and useful role in the social worker's repertoire of treatment interventions. Its applicability to a wide range of clients is suitable for the wide variety of social-work practice settings. The social worker often is the only mental-health professional working to intervene between individuals and interacting agencies (child welfare, courts, schools, general hospitals). Since the bulk of mental-health counseling and psychotherapy in the United States is performed by social workers, short-term treatment is an important model, making it possible to extend services more broadly with available resources.

REFERENCES

Berkman, B., and Rehr, H. 1978. Social work undertakes its own audit. *Soc. Work Health Care,* 3(3):273-286.

Germain, C. B. 1980. Social work identity, competence, and autonomy: The ecological perspective. *Soc. Work Health Care,* 6(1):1-10.

Golan, N. 1974. Crisis theory. In *Social work treatment: Interlocking theoretical approaches,* ed. F. J. Turner, pp. 420-455. New York: Free Press.

Hollis, F. 1971. Social casework: The psychosocial approach. In *Encyclopedia of social work,* vol. 16, ed. R. Morris, pp. 1217-1226. New York: National Association of Social Workers.

Parad, H. J., and Parad, L. 1968. A study of crisis-oriented short-term treatment. *Soc. Casework.,* 49:346-355, 418-426.

Parad, H. J. 1971. Crisis intervention. In *Encyclopedia of social work,* vol. 16, ed. R. Morris, pp. 196-202. New York: National Association of Social Workers.

Perlman, H. H. 1957. *Social casework: A problem-solving process.* Chicago: University of Chicago Press.

Proskauer, S. 1971. Focused time-limited psychotherapy with children. *J. Am. Child Psych.,* 10(1): 614-639.

Rapoport, L 1965. Crisis: Some theoretical considerations. In *Crisis intervention: Selected readings,* ed. H. J. Parad, pp. 22-31. New York: Family Service Association of America.

Rapoport, L. 1967. Crisis-oriented short-term casework. *Soc. Serv. Rev.,* 41(1):31–42.

Reid, W. J., and Shyne, A. W. 1969. *Brief and extended casework.* New York: Columbia University Press.

Reid, W. J. 1970. Implications of research for the goals of casework. *Smith Coll. Studies Soc. Work,* 40:140–154.

Reid, W. J., and Epstein, L. 1972. *Task-centered casework.* New York: Columbia University Press.

Reid, W. J., and Epstein, L. 1977. *Task-centered practice.* New York: Columbia University Press.

Small, L. 1971. *The briefer psychotherapies.* New York: Brunner/Mazel.

Sperling, M. 1974. *The major neuroses and behavior disorders in children.* New York: Jason Aronson.

Ziegler, R. G. 1980. Task-focused therapy with children and families. *Am. J. Psychother.,* 34(1):107–111.

31

Establishment of Accessible and Relevant Services for Adolescents

Lorraine E. Henricks

History of Services to the Adolescent Population

In the late 1960s the problems of adolescents reached crisis proportions in this country. Teenage pregnancy, inadequate parenting and child neglect among adolescent mothers, death and disability due to illegal abortion, venereal disease, prostitution, and sexual exploitation of the young, drug and alcohol abuse, suicides, homicides, accidents, delinquency, emotional problems, and the "runaway phenomenon" were among the most outstanding problems. The need for services and the lack of housing and basic survival resources, especially in the inner cities, demonstrated the lack of adequate mental-health, health and social services. Poor attendance figures at school and high unemployment among youth demonstrated the need for more relevant educational and vocational programs for adolescents.

Services that did exist were accessible to only a few adolescents—those who had parental approval for their choice of help and those compelled to services by the schools or courts. The services were fragmented and contributed to the already poorly integrated identity of the adolescent.

Few professionals knew this population or how to reach them. These glaring problems, the high mortality rate among fifteen to twenty-four year olds, and the lack of services and expertise finally forced society and helping professionals to recognize this population as a population at very high risk and with a need for new and innovative service-delivery approaches.

In response to the crises of adolescent needs and the paucity of relevant services, professionals and youth leaders from a variety of backgrounds began to meet in various settings with the purpose of developing a meaningful response to this problem. The unique characteristics and needs of this age population were taken into account, i.e., identity formation, emancipation, need to develop mastery over drives, need to develop a sense of competency, and need to develop one's own value system. Societies of adolescent medicine and adolescent psychiatry emerged, and specialized training in adolescent health and mental health began to evolve.

In 1972 a critical conference was held in Breckenridge, Colorado, entitled "Youth, Health, and Social Systems." It was sponsored by the National Institute of Mental Health. It brought together professionals from a variety of disciplines interested in youth, as well as youth leaders, to study the problem and make recommendations to the Department of Health, Education, and Welfare. Several models that seemed to have been effectively reaching this population, ranging from the free-clinic models established in several cities to school-based programs and to the multiservice concept represented by the Jeanne Mance Clinic in Montreal and The Door—A Center of Alternatives in New York City, were presented and examined. From these a variety of models were recommended in a report to the Department of Health, Education, and Welfare, but more importantly, a network of concerned youth-serving professionals began and continued to experiment with these approaches in different parts of the country.

The Population

In a paper presented by Henricks (1978), characteristics of the adolescent target population were identified as having to be considered in program development. One must take time to think about what a program is ideally aiming to accomplish, who the target population is, and how to develop a health service-delivery system to meet their specific needs. Some important considerations follow:

1. Adolescence is a time of extremely rapid change, second only to the first two years of life. Therefore it is a time of great vulnerability as well as extreme resilience, i.e., a time of great therapeutic advantage and an opportunity for prevention and early intervention.
2. Specific dramatic changes are occurring in several areas of the young person's life:
   - physical, physiological, and sexual changes
   - emotional changes; shift of bonding from parents to peers and other adults
   - intellectual changes; moving from concrete to abstract thought
   - social changes; move to junior high school and to high school, with shift in peer pressure.
   - spiritual changes; beginning of ability to examine belief system, meaning of life and death, value system, etc.
3. Specific developmental tasks must be accomplished during this time. A service-delivery program must support these normal tasks just as an early child development center must take into consideration the developmental tasks of the "toddler," e.g., large blocks to develop gross motor skills. To summarize these tasks:
   - The adolescent must move away from the family toward autonomy or independence.
   - The adolescent must establish a sense of personal identity without crystallization, i.e., in Eric Erikson's terms identity diffusion vs. integration. This includes sexual identity, body image, work identity, and personal identity.
   - The adolescent must develop the capacity for intimacy and commitment.
   - The adolescent must develop a sense of mastery over basic drives, i.e., sexual, aggressive, self-actualization drives.

- The adolescent must develop his or her own value system, i.e., the integration of the ego and the superego (Kohlberg, 1964).
- The adolescent must develop a sense of competency, or competent ego function, e.g., ability to read, work, and be creative.
- The adolescent must accomplish ego maturation (see Loevinger ego-development scales for adolescents—Loevinger and Wessler, 1970).

4. There are specific needs and problems in this particular population which are as follows:
    - Health-Related Problems—pregnancy, birth control, venereal disease, prenatal care, abortion, parenting, and child care; chronic illnesses such as asthma and physically handicapping conditions; dental and dermatology problems; immunization; physical examination for work.
    - Mental-Health Problems—suicide, homicide, accidents; substance abuse; depression; acute psychosis, schizophrenia; family problems, adolescent abuse, and incest; antisocial behavior and delinquency.
    - Educational/Vocational Problems—learning problems, either organic or social/cultural; unemployment and lack of vocational training.
    - Social Needs—housing; financial support; Medicaid; welfare.

Adolescents are the only age group in which the mortality rates are rising. The three leading causes of death are accidents, suicide, and homicide. All three of these causes of death may be seen as behaviorally related or mental-health problems.

IMPLICATIONS FOR PROGRAM PLANNING

Henricks (1978) identified certain principles of service delivery as having to be considered in developing a program for adolescents.

Availability and Accessibility

A service center should be highly visible and freely accessible to young people. The program should be a community-based rather than an institution-based program. A youth center environment is ideal, i.e., open space, colorful, spaces for group activities and gatherings.

The program should have multiple points of entrance or access; e.g., a young person may come for a dance workshop and eventually go for needed family-planning services or drug-treatment services. Young people avoid situations in which they are labeled, because of their own struggles with their emerging identities. In a Service Utilization Study conducted at The Door—A Center of Alternatives (1980) in New York City where all services are equally accessible, only 9% entered through the general counseling service. Thirty-eight percent entered seeking reproductive-health, general-health, nutrition, and food services; 25% entered seeking recreation or creative and performing arts activities; only 5% initially came seeking psychiatric counseling and substance-abuse services (see table 31-1).

When the same five hundred clients, all of whom had been in the program at least three months, were questioned as to which services they had ever used, 35% declared they had used psychiatric counseling and substance-abuse-treatment counseling services, a majority declared they had used reproductive-health and general-health services, and about two-

TABLE 31-1.
Distribution of Reasons for First Visit to The Door—1980

REASON	PERCENTAGE*
Family Planning and Sex Counseling	21
Medical Services	13
Nutrition	2
Food Services	1
Perinatal Counseling	1
"To Check It Out"	13
Creative Workshops	12
Gym	7
Yoga and Martial Arts	4
Learning Center	10
Career Counseling	2
Psychiatric Counseling	4
General Counseling	9
Drug and Alcohol Counseling	1
Social Services	2
To Get Involved	6
To Socialize	2
To Work at The Door	1

*Some young people gave more than one reason for coming to The Door. Thus, percentages do not add to 100.

thirds declared they had used creative workshops, gymnastics, or martial arts programs (see table 31–2).

CONFIDENTIALITY. Parental consent cannot be required at first contact, especially if a program wishes to meet the needs of adolescents with sensitive health issues such as substance abuse, incest, or contraceptive services. The adolescent must be seen as the primary client and the family as the secondary client, in keeping with the task of the adolescent moving toward independence. In the Urban and Rural Systems Associates (U.R.S.A.) study (1976), "Improving Family Planning Services for Teenagers," in which teenagers and providers in forty clinic sites across the country were interviewed, it was found that before large numbers of teenagers would utilize a program they had to feel it was available and confidential.

A program was believed to be available if it was open to their participation without eligibility restrictions such as minimum age levels or parental consent. To be considered confidential, the teenagers stated they must feel that their decision to seek contraceptive services would not be made known to their parents, other influential adults in their lives, or to their peers. The single most important deterrent to clinic use mentioned by teenagers was "fear of parents finding out." Teens perceived a program as assuring confidentiality based on two factors: clinic location (they perferred teen clinics that are not highly visible) and clinic procedures, i.e., appreciation was voiced for special precautions that clinics took to protect confidentiality and to let young people know, up front, that services were confidential. Interestingly, confidentiality was valued both by teenagers who did not have parental consent and teenagers whose parents were aware that they were sexually active.

COST. Affordable services must be offered. In the same U.R.S.A. study teenagers felt that clinic services should either be free or that the cost of the service be very reason-

TABLE 31-2.
Distribution of Services Ever Used

Services Ever Used	Percentage*
Medical Services/General Health	70
Family Planning/Sex Counseling	45
Health Awareness	8
Perinatal Counseling	6
Nutrition	30
Food Services/Meal Program	53
Creative Workshops	44
Gym	31
Yoga/Martial Arts	17
Psychiatric Counseling	29
Drug/Alcohol Counseling	6
Rap Group	21
Community Meeting	12
Learning Center	41
Career Counseling	17
Social Services	15
Legal Counseling	17
Orientation Tour	43
Other Door Activity	7

*Since a young person could have used more than one service, these percentages do not add to 100. In addition, Medical Services and Family Planning may be excessively high because of misinterpretation of the difference between them.

able. In an unpublished Fee for Service Study done at The Door in 1979 by Henricks, L., Kunkes, C., and Rothenberg, P., the subjects were 112 male and female young people waiting for their visit in the health center. An analysis of the data was conducted and the results are as follows.

The distribution of the ages of the participants is presented in table 31-3.

The majority of the young people who responded to questions indicated that their families earned under $10,000 per year. Differences emerged, as expected, in the levels of personal weekly income. A substantial proportion of adolescents in each age group had no personal income. The majority of the younger teens (groups I and II) earned nothing or only a minimal amount and were dependent on their families or other external sources for money. In contrast, a majority of the older teens (groups III and IV) had some source of personal income and were, therefore, more financially independent.

A presentation of the subjects' responses to questions asking about their ability to pay and the degree to which such a policy would affect their involvement at The Door is provided in table 31-4.

Generally, the majority of subjects in each age group could pay up to $1 per visit with no concomitant reduction in their use of the health center's services. On an intragroup comparative basis, far fewer adolescents in all groups could afford to use the services to the same degree if $1.50 or more was charged per visit. It is of importance to note that the youngest teens (group I: 14-15) would experience the greatest hardship with a "fee for service" policy. Generalizations from these data should be made in conjunction with the fact that this group has the smallest number of subjects but is also at the highest risk.

It is also of interest to note that many teens in group III (18-19) indicated that they

TABLE 31-3.
Ages of the Subjects

Group	Age Range	Number
I	14–15	12
II	16–17	25
III	18–19	42
IV	20–21	28

TABLE 31-4.
Reactions to "Fee for Service" System on a Per Visit Basis

Group	$.50/visit Y	Y/N	N	$1/visit Y	Y/N	N	$1.50/visit Y	Y/N	N	$2/visit Y	Y/N	N
I	67	25	8	58	25	17	42	25	33	42	25	33
II	92	8	0	92	8	0	68	25	7	52	32	16
III	84	14	2	70	28	2	50	44	6	48	38	14
IV	93	7	0	90	10	0	65	25	10	61	25	14

NOTES: The numbers represent the percentage of subjects within each group who responded to the questions.

Y = *Yes,* I would still come to The Door as often as I do now.
Y/N = *Yes,* but I would *not* come to The Door as often as I do now.
N = *No,* I would not come to The Door anymore.

would not utilize the health center's services to the same extent if the higher fees were instituted. Since these teens were usually earning more money than those in group II (16–17), these findings are curious. An analysis of their reactions provides some clarification. Basically, the 18–19 year olds felt that this was a moral issue, and the implementation of a "fee for service" system would run counter to the philosophical premise of The Door and their concept of health care.

ORGANIZATION. Location and availability of clinic services are critical if one wishes to reach young people who are unlikely to go to traditional settings. Programs must make it explicit that they are "teen" programs. It is not sufficient that the program just be there buried amidst pediatric and adult services. Access and utilization can be increased by the way services are organized and administered. The U.R.S.A. study showed a number of key features in this regard:

Convenient Hours. It seems important for services to be available for teenagers at a time that does not conflict with school hours or parental demands. Teenagers' preference in this regard seems to relate to the maintenance of confidentiality as much as to convenience. According to questionnaire responses and patient interviews, the best times for teenagers to attend clinics seem to be during the after-school hours and early evening hours. A client questionnaire distributed at The Door indicated that the hours between 5:00 P.M. and 9:00 P.M. were the most desirable to clients.

Convenient Location. The U.R.S.A study indicated to the extent possible clinics should be located in a place that is not highly visible (i.e., teens did not want their parents or other familiar adults to know they were seeking help). On the other hand, transportation was a problem for many teens and these two factors must be balanced.

Simplified Admission Procedures. The U.R.S.A. study observed that complicated admission procedures acted to deter patients from receiving initial services. Procedures that were time-consuming or that required patients to come for admission processing first and then to return for clinic services on another day were not highly utilzed by teenagers.

Youth Participation in Program Design and Implementation. Peer counseling, youth work, and youth consumer advisory boards make it easier for teenagers to enter the peer environment of the youth program and to experience a sense of ownership or empowerment.

Visibility Must Be in the Youth Community Not the Adult Community. This could be attained by outreach in schools, courts, residences, parks, and hospitals. At The Door—A Center of Alternatives, 65% of young people were referred by a friend or another Door member.

Comprehensiveness

The program must consist of a comprehensive, integrated multiservice center that will attempt to deal with the multiple problems of adolescents in a holistic manner, dealing with the causes of the problems as well as the symptoms. All services relevant to youth should be included under one roof if possible in order to avoid fragmentation and to facilitate integration. If this is not possible given the resources of the community, these services should be clustered and linked as closely as possible.

This implies a total person approach which would include the young person's physical, emotional, intellectual, interpersonal, creative, and developmental dynamics and his or her family, legal, educational, vocational, and other life needs. It is well-known that adolescents do very poorly with referrals, thus the more services that can be incorporated and consolidated under one roof the better.

Therapeutic Milieu

This service system must be developed within a therapeutic milieu which can offer growth opportunities and opportunities for creative expression as well as educational and vocational opportunities, thus dealing with the developmental needs for identity formation, ego competency, value formation, and independence. It is necessary within this milieu with its multiple points of access to develop ongoing more intensive supportive and treatment programs, e.g., a psychiatric treatment program, a substance-abuse treatment program, a perinatal program, an educational and vocational training program, a creative and performing arts program for those adolescents with greater therapeutic or growth-oriented needs, but who may have an initial difficulty acknowledging their problems or making a commitment to intensive treatment.

Linkage

This service center, having all of the services relevant to youth within a single unit, should provide multiple points of linkage with the existing service systems in the community. These linkages to encourage interagency treatment planning will more effectively utilize the existing resources of the city as well as provide daily feedback mechanisms for communication of experiences learned and modalities tried. In addition, they will provide a continuum of services ranging from the community-based ambulatory setting to institution-based or residential services, i.e., consolidation of services.

Youth Participation

Vehicles and mechanisms for input and involvement of the consumer—youth work program, community meetings, consumer advisory board, youth leadership program—are a necessity. Youth participation in program development and program responsibility can lead to a sense of empowerment among young people.

A Program Model: The Door—A Center of Alternatives

The Program

The Door—A Center of Alternatives is a comprehensive community-based multiservice center for adolescents between the ages of twelve and twenty-one in New York City. It was modeled on a pilot project developed in Montreal, Canada, in 1967—the Jeanne Mance Clinic. The Door is an after-school and evening program; services are free or low cost and provided without the requirement of parental consent. It offers medical and gynecological services, family planning, pregnancy diagnosis, prenatal and postpartum care, nutrition counseling services, psychiatric counseling and therapy, and social and legal services.

The Door also includes educational and vocational counseling, has a learning center, and a variety of prevocational and vocational training opportunities. It offers creative and rehabilitative workshops in art, crafts, poetry, music, dance, and theater as well as offering gymnastic, recreational, and martial arts programs. In addition, The Door has several ongoing, structured treatment programs within this multiservice and creative activity center for youth. These include a prenatal, young parents, and child health program, a drug- and alcohol-abuse treatment program, a psychiatric treatment program, an educational and prevocational training program, and a youth leadership and youth empowerment program.

The Door serves approximately 350 teenagers daily. The center utilizes an approach aimed at dealing with the whole person: with his or her physical, emotional, intellectual, and interpersonal dynamics and with family, education, and life problems rather than with one or two problems or symptoms. Within The Door, issues of sex education, counseling, family-planning and contraceptive services, prenatal care, early child care, postnatal services, treatment for venereal disease, substance-abuse issues, psychological problems, and family problems are dealt with in the context of total life needs. The program has attempted to integrate services within the therapeutic milieu concepts of Maxwell Jones (1953).

The program also works actively on a preventive and early intervention level. If offers opportunities for exploring issues around roles including sex roles, and behavior, parenting issues, health-awareness issues, values clarification, and decision making. Through its educational, vocational, and creative activities The Door offers alternatives to premature sexual behavior, pregnancy or abortion, substance abuse, delinquency, antisocial and suicidal behavior.

The program has also been actively engaged in outreach and health-education programs in local junior high and high schools as well as in providing training and consultation to other youth service agencies.

The Door came into being at a time when drug abuse, delinquency, dropping out of school, venereal disease, and other problems among New York's youth had reached crisis proportions. The immediate challenge to be met at that time was to develop a full spectrum of innovative services, programs, and resources for dealing with the acute problems and needs of adolescents.

In the summer of 1970 an interdisciplinary group of professionals, who shared an interest in youth problems, met to discuss the acute crisis that was affecting the lives of the urban adolescent population of New York City. They were convinced that the life needs of these young people could only be met by new approaches to the delivery of youth services. The pilot project in Montreal, Canada, had demonstrated that the multiservice center was effective. Out of these meetings came the concepts that formed the basic underlying principles of the The Door—A Center of Alternatives. After several months of initial planning, this group invited colleagues and friends to join them in developing an integrated youth service center. People with commitment, training, and experience in human service delivery to adolescents and a capacity for creative treamwork began to join the initial group. They set about establishing a demonstration project that would provide relevant services and meaningful life alternatives to young people in an effective and nonalienating way.

By March 1971 the development group had grown considerably and detailing of program elements began. Task forces were developed to address issues around health, mental health, drug and alcohol abuse, sexual health and family planning, nutrition, social services, runaway and homeless youth, education, vocation, and legal problems, as well as recreation and the creative arts. Each task force met once a week on a volunteer basis to plan and develop the service programs. During this period the task forces met individually and with other task forces in order to gather and share information regarding existing services, to develop information and resource files, and to conceptualize new ways to deliver services.

The basic philosophic outlook underlying The Door's program has always been the total person approach influenced by Kurt Lewin, Maxwell Jones, Abraham Maslow, and the Gestalt therapists. The use of this integrative method enabled The Door to address a client's whole life situation.

Functioning as a comprehensive service-delivery system, The Door developed all of its services for young people within a single facility which made it possible to avoid the traditional fragmentation that occurs between separate service systems. This system facilitated continuity of care and integration of services.

The Door put an emphasis on the creation of a therapeutic milieu, focusing on the causes of problems as well as their symptoms. This also made it possible to go beyond a young person's immediate needs to explore his or her special growth dimensions and potentials. This kind of milieu encouraged the development of new therapeutic modalities, where staff could experiment with promising new treatment methods which seemed to be more appropriate to the life realities and health needs of young people. It has been a setting which allowed relevant methods of treatment, rehabilitation, and education to be integrated into a total therapeutic process. The Door also focused on the development of primary health-care services involved in the restoration and maintenance of the physical and mental well-being of adolescents.

The Door intentionally sought to become highly visible and easily accessible to the youth population. Community based rather than institution based, with multiple points of entry, free to low-cost services, and no parental consent required, it provided easy access to services for those who would otherwise be unlikely to seek or receive help or guidance.

Over fourteen years have passed since The Door initiated its operations, providing a broad range of services and programs to three to four hundred young people each day. It has served as a model for many agencies and institutions concerned with serving the critical needs of the urban adolescent population both nationally and internationally. Several thousand private and governmental agency administrators and others involved in youth service delivery have come to The Door to explore and learn from the program. Through this process The Door has served to stimulate new program designs for adolescents.

Clientele

The Door has been able to attract large numbers of young people who generally are not reached by traditional agencies and institutions. It has been particularly important for minority populations (greater than 67% have been black, Hispanic, and Oriental youth), disadvantaged young people from areas in which there are no youth services available. Most young people have heard about The Door by word of mouth from friends and other Door members (67%); others are referred by families, schools, hospitals, drug programs, police, courts, or other agencies whose staff have learned about The Door through its outreach activities.

There are various reasons why young people turn to The Door. Many of its clients seek help because of emotional, sexual, family, or peer relationship problems or health problems. Many are drug and/or alcohol abusers. Pregnancy, trouble with the law, difficulty with finding and keeping a job, dropping out of school, running away from home—these, too, are crisis situations that bring young people to The Door.

Attracted initially by a spectrum of services, programs, and activities that adolescents are not likely to find elsewhere, young people can find opportunities for new forms of self-expression and personal growth within a supportive environment. They may wish to explore the creative or martial arts or become interested in job or educational possibilities or simply establish a stronger sense of personal identity with the guidance of sympathetic adult staff and the support of their peers.

The Door is open to all young people, whether or not they have identified problems, whether they are in need of help or just want to engage in creative interaction with other young people or adults. Young people come to The Door on their own initiative and identify the problem that is most important to them. They are not labeled with diagnostic terms which would only add further stigma to an already confused identity.

In the Service Utilization Study (1980) referred to earlier, at the time of entry into the program, 49% of the young people claimed to be financially supported by parents or relatives, many of whom were welfare recipients; 23% supported themselves, largely through unskilled jobs; 11% were on welfare; and 17% had no regular source of support. Thirteen percent of these young people had completed primary-school education or less; 48% had completed a junior-high-school education; 39% had completed a high-school education, including 10% enrolled in college. A total of 62% of these youth were enrolled in elementary school, junior high school, high school, high-school equivalency programs, or college. Twenty-seven percent had dropped out before completing high school and lacked the necessary skills or experience to gain meaningful employment or qualify for job training programs.

When they entered the program, 48% of the youth were living with one or both parents (23% with only one parent), 14% with friends, 13% in agency residences, 9% with relatives, 8% alone, and 8% were undomiciled.

The Door's clients ranged in age from twelve to twenty-one years, with 29% seventeen years or younger. At the time of this study 66% were female and 34% were male.

Although many of these young people were in urgent need of psychiatric, medical, and other kinds of help, they were often too distrustful to utilize existing professional services and institutions. It is these interrelated social and developmental crises that lead many young people to The Door. These young people needed a nonthreatening place where they could feel free to come for help.

Client Flow within the Program

As a human service system in the broadest sense, The Door has developed an integrative approach combining the best features of a free medical youth clinic, an education center, a social-services center, a community mental-health center, a community youth center, a cultural center, and a therapeutic drug, alcohol, and delinquency prevention and rehabilitative center. Initially, new clients of The Door have tended to utilize only those services that are relevant to the specific problems they see as important—and usually their initial involvement is on an as-needed, short-term, or crisis-intervention basis. For example, some young people might come for the medical or vocational services if they are experiencing difficulties in these areas. As they begin to deal realistically with their identified problems and needs, however, many have begun to identify other problems and eventually make a commitment to participate in long-term structured programs.

The Door has developed intensive, ongoing programs to serve the entire range of its client population, from young people with serious psychological problems, drug and alcohol abuse, legal, educational, and vocational problems, to youth who are generally functioning well but who are struggling with the psychological dynamics of adolescence, such as peer relationships, parental authority, sexual and human identity, and the search for authentic means of self-expression. Through involvement in these programs, young people have been able to participate in an intensive, ongoing process of therapy and rehabilitation, change of negative and destructive patterns of behavior, resolution of personal and interpersonal problems, learning and self-actualization.

Ongoing participation in these structured programs has helped young people to develop a sense of common interest, respect, and concern. They have been able to come to see themselves as a community of people who share a willingness to help each other, to relate and communicate, and to work together toward common goals. They have been able to lose a sense of impotence and develop a sense of empowerment.

Through The Door's crisis-intervention and short-term treatment programs, young people who are not yet ready to become involved in more intensive therapy have received needed counseling and treatment in a broad spectrum of specific problem areas. As they deepen their involvement, they are able to decide to join the creative and rehabilitative workshops, take part in orientation and rap groups, and participate in youth awareness seminars. Within the supportive environment of The Door, these individuals become involved in alternative activities before destructive behavior patterns develop into a lifestyle and have a major impact on their lives and on society.

Some young people whose immediate needs are met by the crisis-intervention program terminate their involvement with an option to return at a later date for additional help. Other clients—those with serious drug, alcohol, and other mental-health problems such as severe anxiety, depressive reactions, suicidal behavior, acute or chronic psychotic disorders, long-standing aggressive, self-destructive, delinquent, or other dysfunctional behavior patterns, crises of premature and unplanned pregnancy, and the debilitation of being unemployable—have chosen to become involved in the structured long-term programs. Many of these young people have grown up in institutions, foster homes, or families devoid of love or stability and have become bitter, distrustful, and unable to function or to maintain long-term constructive relationships.

Following entry into the program a team of staff members who have had relevant contact with the client jointly evaluate the young person with regard to life and family situation, educational, vocational, and economic status, as well as his or her potential and life goals. The evaluation also serves to identify medical, emotional, and other problem areas, the client's ability to use existing services and support systems, and his or her motivation for dealing with problems and for becoming involved in structured, task-oriented therapy.

Following this evaluation a primary counselor acts to coordinate and supervise the client's overall treatment program. This counselor—together with the interdisciplinary team who plan the client's therapy—is responsible for the continuity of the client's care throughout his or her involvement in the program.

An individualized treatment plan, with specific goals, is designed for each client. It deals with the strengths as well as the problem areas of the young person's life, including family dynamics, in an effort to provide challenge as well as support and to involve him or her in a process of change that deals with behavior patterns and with related psychosocial problems.

Young people involved in the intensive programs are treated in a socially constructive therapeutic milieu where they can be part of a more varied peer group with a wider range of social experiences and thus have an opportunity to experiment with alternative viewpoints and more constructive lifestyles. The use of group modalities allows individuals to explore their lives and behavior and has made the therapeutic approach concrete, pragmatic, and reality oriented. This exposure to a new, growth-oriented peer environment and social setting can help the young person to develop new ways of relating to others, to learn about the advantages as well as responsibilities of being a member of a larger human community, and to establish a positive self-image. The therapeutic environment also can provide a sense of warmth and belonging which is often absent in the lives of many of these youth.

Within the context of real life situations at The Door, educational and vocational counselors can help the client develop academic and basic skills required for meaningful work. In order to develop a sense of responsibility, participants have been able to take on tasks on a regular basis, such as assisting in workshops, peer counseling, peer tutoring, and helping new participants at The Door.

On a structural level The Door has used a growth phase process to measure change. On a quarterly basis the primary counselor and client assess twelve major life areas, ranging from family relations to substance use to emotional status and health status, and grade them according to five phases (see fig. 31-1):

1. Denial of problem, i.e., the young person does not feel there is a problem, when there is a very definite problem.
2. Recognition of the problem without action, i.e., the young person begins to recognize that there is a problem, but is unable to take any action to change the situation.
3. Directed action on the problem, i.e., the young person begins to take some action toward resolution of the problem, but only with much support from the counselor.
4. Self-initiated action on the problem, i.e., the young person takes initiative in changing behavior.
5. Autonomy, i.e., the young person is able to perceive his or her situation and is able to make changes on his or her own.

In short-term goal-oriented individual counseling, with the help, support, and challenge

NAME _____ PROGRAM _____ CHART # _____

PRIMARY PERSON _____ TEAM _____ DATE OF REVIEW _____

I. LIFE AREAS* (check)   PHASE**   PROGRESS**   I. LIFE AREAS* (check)   PHASE**   PROGRESS**
                                                          (continued)
         DATE: DATE:
              (prior) (current)   (prior) (current)
                                        ***   ***
                                        | W | S | I | | W | S | I |
                                        |---|---|---| |---|---|---|
( ) 1. Psychological   ( )   ( ) | | | | ( ) 7. Health, Nutrition ( )   ( ) | | | |
       Functioning | | | | ( ) 8. Family Planning,   ( )   ( ) | | | |
( ) 2. Family Situation/ ( )   ( ) | | | | Perinatal | | | |
       Relationships | | | | ( ) 9. Leisure, Recreation ( )   ( )
( ) 3. Peer Relations   ( )   ( )   ( ) 10. Social Responsi- ( )   ( )
( ) 4. Substance Use   ( )   ( )   bility/Leadership
( ) 5. Work, Self-Support ( ) ( )   ( ) 11. Legal   ( )   ( )
( ) 6. Career, Education ( )   ( )   ( ) 12. Other   ( )   ( )

* Check areas of current concern only.   ** Evaluate ALL areas of functioning.
                                                   W = worsened; S = same; I = improved
                                                *** R = Resolved; U = Unresolved; A = Attained; N = Unattained

II. PROBLEM IDENTIFICATION AND TREATMENT PLAN   (R = Resolved; U = Unresolved; A = Attained; N = Unattained)

LIFE AR.#	NEEDS/PROBLEMS		SHORT-TERM GOALS	ACTION PLAN/ TARGET DATE		LONG-TERM GOALS
1.		R U			A N	
2.		R U			A N	
3.		R U			A N	
4.		R U			A N	
5.		R U			A N	

OTHER COMMENTS _____

COUNSELOR _____ SUPERVISOR _____

DATE FOLLOW-UP COMPLETED _____ COUNSELOR _____

Fig. 31-1. PROGRESS REVIEW

of the therapist, the young person is able to explore and deal with anxieties, negative self-images, destructive behavior patterns, and distorted perceptions of reality. Through the ongoing therapeutic process, more constructive ways of functioning and relating, a healthier self-image, and better reality testing can be established. Young people have been able to move from a state of confusion, isolation, withdrawal, or destructive acting out toward a more resolved and active life.

Group therapy brings young people into a peer environment where, under the guidance of the therapist, they can learn skills in communication, establishment of trust, mutual care, and concern. Exploration of common themes and problems offers opportunities to share experiences, inhibitions, and fears, to explore common defense patterns, and to find new, workable alternatives to old patterns.

The use of relevant services provides concrete opportunities to resolve long-standing housing, education, job- or career-related, legal, medical, nutritional, and other problem areas and to develop new and better mechanisms to deal with the functional realities of life.

The creative and vocational training workshops provide young people with opportunities to explore their own potentials for creative expression, to develop work-related skills, and to gain a sense of confidence and self-esteem. In the workshops young people have learned to relate to peers and adults in a constructive atmosphere of respect and trust, while learning skills and developing problem-solving capabilities which could help them to achieve their full human potential.

Some young people especially have been initially attracted to The Door by creative activities that are of particular interest to them. At a later time they may make use of the services to resolve problems that they had not felt comfortable in revealing earlier. The workshops and other special activities have been individually structured to augment the psychotherapeutic, educational, or vocational program in which a young person has been involved. Through this process of creative self-expression, participants have been able to experience a growing sense of respect for themselves and for their individual worth,

In the workshops young people have been able to test out a wide range of possible career choices and creative expressions, to learn to work cooperatively with others, and to develop pride in the quality of their skills. The workshops therefore have served as a valuable vocational and life training modality. Arrangements were made for young people to receive credit in New York City high schools for participation in various workshops and learning center programs.

The recreation and physical-education program offers the opportunity to engage in constructive physical activities and to establish positive peer relationships. As part of The Door's program of exploring alternative lifestyles and providing positive group support and identification, the martial arts program also has exposed young people to a variety of Eastern cultures, philosophies, and disciplines, many of which are in sharp contrast to their current lifestyles. The aim of these programs has been to help individuals improve their general physical condition and self-images, and become more aware of and responsible for their bodily health as well as to deal with issues of aggression and respect for others.

The youth work and youth leadership program provides paraprofessional training and education for youth who are concerned with problems and issues relevant to young people, who are seeking opportunities to be of service to others, and who are ready to assume leadership among their peers at The Door and in their schools and communities. Youth workers have been assigned to various service components of The Door and receive ongoing in-service training from supervisory staff members. The youth workers assist staff through peer counseling and tutoring, provide introductory information about specific programs, and orient new young people to the services, activities, and programs at The Door.

Youth workers participate in outreach activities outside The Door and assist with follow-up and home visits. They participate in weekly youth awareness seminars and ongoing group supervision to review questions and dynamics encountered in their work with other youth and staff, and take part in weekly in-service education meetings with the supervisory staff who have coordinated their activities and training within a particular service.

Other young people who are interested in developing leadership skills and acting as liaison persons between The Door and their schools and communities have been involved in youth leadership and advocacy workshops and youth awareness seminars and have participated in an in-depth, service-by-service orientation to The Door. Where possible, these youth also have taken part in the development and planning of projects at The Door and in their own schools and communities in order to express the interests and concerns of youth and mobilize the energies of young people in constructive ways.

Community, Youth, and Agency Outreach

The Door developed an extensive community and youth outreach program from the beginning in order to contact and involve young people in need of services and to develop referral arrangements with professionals, paraprofessionals, agencies, and institutions which work with adolescents throughout New York City.

Youth-oriented outreach activities have focused on contacting young people such as school dropouts, members of youth gangs, and youth who come from deprived and troubled inner-city families. Outreach workers have attempted to reach those who are bored, lonely, and alienated, who are into drugs and drug-oriented lifestyles, who are prematurely sexually active, and who are reluctant to seek help for their problems from traditional agencies or institutions or who are unaware of the existence of services and resources relevant to their needs. Outreach workers have visited local hangouts, schools, hospitals, parks, and recreation areas and have engaged young people in music sessions and informal rap sessions about The Door and issues relevant to youth. Youth have been encouraged to return to The Door with the outreach staff or to visit it at a later time at their convenience.

Other youth-oriented outreach activities in the community have included contact with youth in agencies and institutions that provide direct services to adolescents. Visits have been made to special school programs and student groups, and to teachers, guidance counselors, and street workers from junior high schools, high schools, and alternative education programs. All students have been invited to come to The Door. Similar outreach visits have been made to residential treatment centers, detention programs, psychiatric hospitals, residences, and drug treatment detoxification centers to offer a continuum of care.

Interdisciplinary teams of staff have also conducted agency outreach through speakers and seminar programs which have been directed toward increasing communication and cooperation among agencies and institutions serving youth. Education and training sessions have been provided for a wide range of professionals and paraprofessionals, including drug counselors, social workers, lawyers, teachers, nurses, psychiatrists, and others working with youth. Through agreement with the Board of Education, The Door has conducted seminars for in-service training credit for teachers, drug education specialists, drug coordinators, and guidance counselors in public primary, junior high, and high schools throughout New York City.

Evaluation of Program Effectiveness

The Service Utilization Study is an example of the broad application that can be made of evaluation techniques. Client interviews were done each day over a three-month period in May 1978 and again in June 1981. Staff members interviewed approximately five hundred clients as they were about to leave the center at the end of the evening. The clients had to have been at The Door a minimum of three months. These interviews were conducted to determine the demographic characteristics of clients and their patterns of service utilization. Results showed that the typical client contacted an average of 5.3 services—an extremely important fact in terms of demonstrating the need for integrated service delivery. It also showed that a large percentage of new clients first used the health services and that the most extensively used programs included medical and family-planning services, creative workshops, the gym, and creative workshops. These and other statistics in the Service Utilization Study shed important light on such questions as quantitative patterns of program utilization, major points of entry into service delivery for adolescents, and patterns of referral sources for adolescents.

The results of the Service Utilization Study prompted the service staff to explore such questions as why the family-planning program referred more clients to psychiatric services than to any other activity, why the recreation and creative workshops tend to attract clients who are younger, more often Hispanic, black, and male, and why the medical component attracted a larger number of white, older adolescents than the other services of The Door. Answers to these and other questions yield vital insights into client motivation, attitudes, and life concerns as they relate to the utilization of multiple services and treatment modalities. In the larger sense, such insights can prove to be important guidelines for redefining service goals, planning program changes and new program initiatives, and in improving the integration of activities to better reach and meet the overall needs of its clients. In addition, it provides material for evaluation of program effectiveness.

In addition to investigating what a program is doing and whom it is serving, a key function of a sound evaluation system is to measure, as accurately as possible, how well any given program is accomplishing its goals, and why it is or is not succeeding. When evaluations are conducted throughtfully, they can help staff discover why specific modalities and techniques are effective with certain groups of people, while others may fail with the same age group. Beyond that, they can help identify the variety of reasons why a particular program is or is not achieving its objectives, and may identify some of the barriers to their successful achievement.

The usefulness of conducting carefully conceived and executed research was confirmed by a three-year study of the Learning Laboratory Program. The purpose of this research and evaluation study was to test the validity of a highly individualized, meaningful education program as a form of treatment for drug-abusing youth. Toward this end, three basic variables in the clients' lives were measured: educational progress during the program, i.e., change in reading level and math skills; change in drug use patterns; and involvement in purposeful activities, including employment, training, and continuing education (see table 31-5).

Results showed a significant improvement in all three areas and indicated that the program as a whole was more therapeutically effective than other types of drug-abuse programs. Forty percent of the participants either stopped using drugs or significantly reduced their use. Furthermore, the young people made encouraging educational progress and became increasingly involved in many constructive life activities. In addition, the enlistment

TABLE 31-5.
Composite Success Classification System

	EDUCATION		PURPOSEFUL ACTIVITIES		DRUG USE	
	Code	Description	Code	Description	Code	Description
Top quarter (TQ)	4	No worse than 3 on short- and long-term goals *and* current educational involvement	4	Positive, full-time activity; stable living situation; finances OK	3	From minimal drug use or regular soft drug use to minimal or no drug use
Must receive only those codes indicated on this level	3	*Either*: average of 3 or more on short- and long-term goals and no educational involvement *Or*: pattern of 3, 2 or 2, 3 on short- and long-term goals and educational involvement	3	Positive, full-time activity; stable living situation; in need of money	4	From regular hard drug use to minimal or no drug use
					5	From regular hard drug use to regular soft drug use
					(2)	Regular soft drug use with no significant change—only if combined with a 3.5 code average on education and purposeful activities

(*continued*)

TABLE 31-5. (continued)

	Education		Purposeful activities		Drug use	
	Code	Description	Code	Description	Code	Description
Bottom quarter (BQ) Must receive only those codes indicated on this level	2	*Either:* pattern of 3, 2 or 2, 3 on short- and long-term goals and no educational involvement *Or:* pattern of 1, 2 or 2, 1 on short- and long-term goals and educational involvement	2	Positive, part-time activity; stable or fair living situation; in need of money	2	Regular soft drug use to regular hard drug use or regular soft drug use with no significant change
			1	*Either:* no positive activity and stable or fair living situation *Or:* unstable living situation	6	Regular hard drug use with no significant change
	1	Average of 1.5 or less on short- and long-term goals and no current educational invovement			7	From minimal drug use to regular soft drug use
					(5)	From some hard drug use to regular soft drug use—only if combined with code average of 1.5 or less on education and purposeful activites

of clients in evaluating their own progress helped them to become more realistic in assessing their strengths and weaknesses, and more independent in planning their educational programs.

On the other hand, the evaluation suggested a need for additional psychological counseling services and financial aid for some young people, since these were among the primary reasons why some participants dropped out of the program. On the basis of these findings, it was recommended that professional psychological assessment, stipends for the participants, and vocational skills training be incorporated into future programs of this kind. A monograph on this evaluation study has been published and distributed by the National Institute on Drug Abuse (1980).

Another more recent evaluation was conducted to determine the effectiveness of The Door's family-planning program for young people. Using change in contraceptive behavior over time, pregnancy rate, childbirth rate, and program continuation rate as major criteria, this two-year study found that an overwhelming majority of the clients continued to successfully use contraception and continued in the program longer than in other single-purpose adolescent programs. In accounting for the success of the program, the most important features were found to be: the provision of sexuality counseling and contraceptive services in a confidential, personal, and caring way, and the provision of these services within the context of a comprehensive medical and multiservice center for adolescents that could respond to their other needs which might lead to unintended pregnancy.

A major study of broader implications done by C. Kunkes and I. Hilton (1979), in which The Door collaborated with Yeshiva University, concerns the underlying determinants of teenage pregnancy. This study has compared a group of young people who use contraception with young people who choose early abortion and a group of young people who go to term with their pregnancies. On an age-matched group the young women who go to term score on an ego-maturation scale (Loevinger scale) at a remarkably less mature level than the other two groups, as well as having a more external locus of decision making and lack of future direction vis-à-vis careers.

Together with Columbia University's Center for Population and Family Health, The Door has also conducted a study on decision-making and risk-taking behavior among adolescents in relation to sexuality and contraception utilization assuming controlled access to services. The Lukar (1975) Cost-Benefit Model of Pregnancy Risk Taking was used as the major research instrument. The results of this study are currently being analyzed. These projects will contribute significantly to scientific and applied professional knowledge in the youth service field as well as to program development designs. The collaborating principal investigators in this project were C. Kunkes, S. Phillibes and P. Rothenberg.

The Door is currently in the process of extending its evaluation capacity to carry out studies on a multidimensional scope with regard to its programs and activities. The Door is undertaking a comprehensive evaluation of its overall program, focusing on the different structural and functional levels of program components. The central concern of this large-scale evaluation is to investigate how interrelated and interdisciplinary approaches affect the total program operations, how the benefits of this approach can be maximized, and how shortcomings can be minimized. As part of its objectives, the study includes a more comprehensive evaluation of services, staff, resource utilization, cost effectiveness, and therapeutic milieu than has been possible in the past without funding.

As part of this expanded evaluation effort, follow-up studies are currently being conducted on client "alumni" to determine how their current life situation has been influenced by their involvement in programs at The Door. Follow-up studies aim to determine how successful these previous clients have been in dealing with peer, family, and authority relationships, with community and social activities, and in fulfilling creative, educational, vocational, and other goals. The studies are also seeking to detemine what impact The Door's integrative approach has had on such dysfunctions as serious psychological disturbances, unplanned pregnancy, substance abuse, criminal and other antisocial behavior. This report will shortly be completed and published with the support of the Commonwealth Foundation.

Other Existing Comprehensive Models

Many programs have been developed over the past several years, all with the same underlying concept of dealing with as many problems as possible under one roof and focusing on the growth potential of young people. In Mexico City, CORA, a project that provides comprehensive services and activities to teenagers, inspired by The Door, has been in existence for seven years and operates six satellite programs. In Saskatchewan, Canada, the Youth Services Center has been providing comprehensive services to multiethnic youth for three years. It was initiated by one of the original Jeanne Mance Clinic founders. In Washington, D.C., a program called "The Center for Youth Services" opened a full-service system in 1981 specifically designed to meet the multiple problems and needs related to the adolescent population. In Hartford, Connecticut, the city health department has initiated a comprehensive youth program.

These programs all utilize concepts of the whole-person approach, comprehensiveness, complete services, multiple activities under one roof, and extensive links with other service systems in the community. Other examples include: the Eden Youth Center in Alameda County, California; El Cameno in Guatemala City; the Adolescent Center in Panama City, Panama; The Rainbow Youth Center in Regina, Saskatchewan, Canada; Task Force in Melbourne, Australia; Young Detroit in Detroit, Michigan, The High Risk Young Peoples Program in Los Angeles, and many others.

Twenty programs across the country have just been funded by The Robert Wood Johnson Foundation with the mandate to provide comprehensive, consolidated services. Different programs take on slightly different forms but the underlying principles are the same.

A great deal has been accomplished during the past few years through family-planning services, prenatal services, drug and alcohol treatment services, runaway services, and sex and drug education and counseling programs for teenagers. The mandate now is to look creatively at the integration and consolidation of these services and programs within settings that are truly youth oriented.

A possible treatment flow chart (fig. 31–2) which includes intake sources, multiple points of access to service delivery, and intensive treatment programs follows.

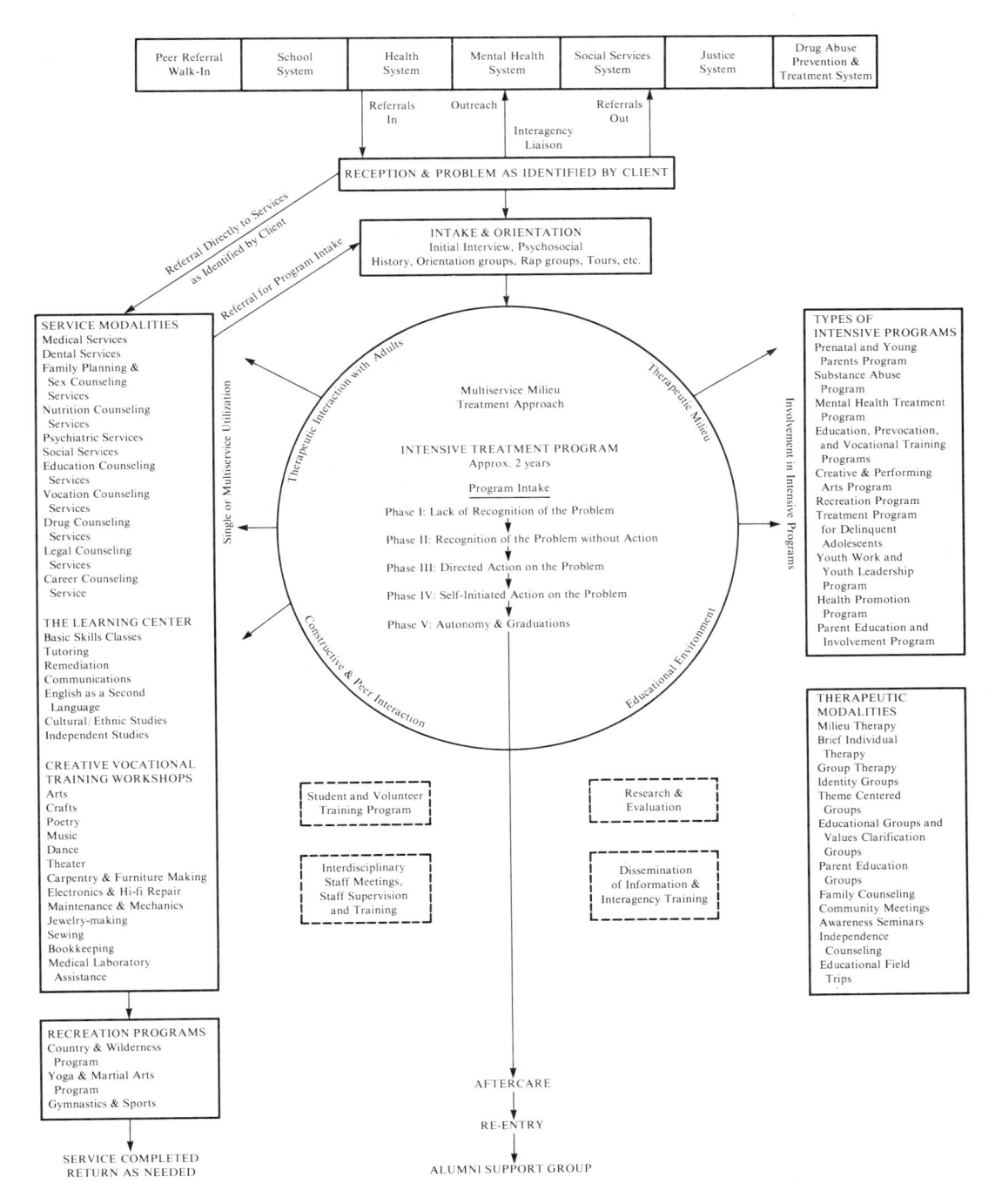

Fig. 31-2. TREATMENT PROGRAM FLOW CHART

REFERENCES

Erikson, E. H. 1959. *Identity and the life cycle: Selected papers.* Psychological Issues, Monograph I. New York: International Universities Press, Inc.

Henricks, L. 1978. Sexual health in adolescents: The mandate for an integrated service delivery response. Paper presented at the meeting of the American Public Health Association. Los Angeles, California.

Henricks, L., and Kunkes, C. 1979. Fee for service study. New York: The Door—A Center of Alternatives.

Henricks, L., Kunkes, C., and Rothenberg, P. 1980. Service utilization study. New York: The Door—A Center of Alternatives.

Dept. of Health, Education, and Welfare. 1972. *Youth, health, and social systems: An integrated service delivery approach.* Monograph Series.

Henricks, L., Lecker, S., and Turanski, J. 1973. New dimensions in adolescent psychotherapy: A therapeutic system approach. *Psychiat. Clin. North Am.,* 20:4.

Jones, M. 1953. *The therapeutic community.* New York: Basic Books.

Kohlberg, L. 1964. Development of moral character and moral ideology. In *Review of child development research,* eds. M. L. Hoffman and L. W. Hoffman. New York: Russell Sage Foundation.

Kunkes, C., and Hilton, I. 1979. Predictors of teenage pregnancy: Psychological and demographic factors. Paper presented at the meeting of the Society for Adolescent Medicine. Los Angeles, California.

Loevinger, J., and Wessler, R. 1970. *Ego development measuring.* Vols. 1 and 2. San Francisco: Jossey-Bass.

Lukar, K. 1975. *Taking chances: Abortion and the decision not to contracept.* Los Angeles: University of California Press.

National Institute on Drug Abuse. 1980. The Learning Laboratory. The Door—A Center of Alternatives. Service Research Monograph Series, OHHS Pub. No. (ADM) 80-928.

National Institute on Drug Abuse. 1981. Monograph ser. The Door: A model youth center. Treatment Program Monograph Series, OHHS Pub. No. (ADM) 81-1132.

Urban and Rural Systems Associates. 1976. Improving family planning services for teenagers. Dept. of Health, Education, and Welfare, Office of the Assistant Secretary for Planning and Evaluation/Health.

Index

Abdominal examination, 428
Abnormal puberty: see Puberty, abnormal
Abstraction ability, 420
Academic skills: see School performance
Accidental injuries vs. child abuse, 317
Achenbach Teacher's Report Form, 261
Acting-out behavior, sexual abuse and, 341
Activity of daily living (ADL) assessment, 417
Adenoma sebaceum, 63
Adolescent services, 583–603
   history of, 583–584
   implications for program planning, 585–590
   population, 584–585
   program models, 590–603
Advice-giving in short-term treatment, 575–576
Aggressive behavior, 229–247
   assessment of, 235–240
   common characteristics of, 231
   differential diagnosis and, 230–231
   epidemiology of, 231–232
   etiology of, 233–235
   history taking and, 235–237
   hyperkinetic syndrome and, 255
   psychopharmacology and, 509–511
   in school, 294, 295
   treatment of, 237–247
Airflow, controlled, 104

Ambrosini, Paul J., 182–190
American Speech, Language, and Hearing Association, The (ASHA), 81, 92, 93
Amitriptyline
   anorexia nervosa and, 226
   nocturnal enuresis and, 38
Amphetamines, 37, 502–504
Androgren insensitivity syndrome, 157
Androgen therapy, 159
Anger, sexual abuse and, 347
Anorexia nervosa, 218–227
   assessment of, 221–223
   clinical features of, 218–219
   demographic features of, 219–220
   differential diagnosis and, 220–221
   major depressive disorder and, 184
   obsessive-compulsive disorder and, 209
   treatment of, 223–227
   Turner's syndrome and, 161
Antiandrogenic drugs, 156–157
Anticholinergic drugs, 37
Antidepressants: see Tricyclic antidepressants (TCAs)
Anti-Parkinsonian agents, 21
Antipsychotic medications, 268–269
Antisocial behavior: see Aggressive behavior
Anxiety, in school children, 294, 297, 453
Aphasia
   vs. autism, 65–66
   defined, 83

605

Arithmetic tests, 468
Art therapy, 348
Articulation disorders, 80, 99, 102
Asocial behavior in school, 294, 299
Assertiveness training, 303-304
Attention deficit disorder (ADD)
  with hyperactivity: see Hyperkinetic syndrome
  Tourette syndrome and, 7, 11-12, 14
Attention dysregulation as core dysfunction, 258
Attitude/stuttering modification approaches, 105
Atypical affective disorders, 185
Audiological tests, 83, 416
Audiologist, 92
Auditory acuity, 427
Auditory impairment, 85, 87, 88, 92
Auditory memory, short term, 419-420
Autism, infantile, 48-74
  assessment of, 51-63
  associated features of, 50
  clinical characteristics of, 48-50
  cognitive development and, 50, 51, 60-62, 64, 65, 67
  course of, 51
  development sequence assessment, 52-54
  differential diagnosis and, 63-68
  epimediology of, 50-51
  history taking and, 51-58
  language and, 49-51, 53-55, 62, 64-69, 86
  medical assessment and, 62-63
  observation/interview and, 58-59
  play behavior and, 49-50, 53-54, 57-58, 60-61, 65
  social interaction and, 53-57, 65, 69-70
  vs. Tourette syndrome, 15
  treatment of, 68-74
Awareness of others' feelings, 303

Battered child syndrome: see Child abuse
Bayley Scales of Infant Development, 460, 473
Becker, Judith V., 336-350
Behavior analysis: see Functional behavior analysis
Behavior checklists, 439
Behavior therapies, 519-534
  aggressive behavior and, 237-247
  anorexia nervosa and, 224-226
  behavioral-pediatrics group of, 525, 533-534
  biofeedback group of, 525, 531-532
  current dimensions of, 524
  defined, 523-524
  fears and, 174-177
  general group of, 526-528
  historical developments in, 520-523
  hyperkinetic syndrome and, 269
  nocturnal enuresis and, 39-43
  obsessive-compulsive disorder and, 214-215
  operant-conditioning group of, 525, 529-531
  sexual abuse and, 348
  somatoform disorders and, 205
  stuttering and, 105-107
Behavioral pediatrics, 525, 532-533
Bell-and-pad conditioning, 39-43
Belladonna, 37
"Belle indifference, la," 202
Bender-Gestalt test, 470, 473
Benton Visual Retention Test, 471, 473
Biofeedback, 525, 531-532
Bird, Hector R., 554-565
Bladder disturbances, nocturnal enuresis and, 32
Bleeding disorders vs. child abuse, 317
Block Design Test, 471
Bone diseases vs. child abuse, 317
Brain damage
  child abuse and, 325-326
  hyperkinetic syndrome and, 255-257
  obsessive-compulsive disorder and, 209, 210
  tests of, 470-471
Bryant Reading Test, 467
Bulimia, 221
Butyrophenones: see Haloperidol

Calculations, simple, 420
Canino, Ian A., 393-407
Cantwell, Dennis P., 475-489
Carbamazepine, 511
Catecholamine hypothesis of hyperkinesis, 256
Categorical approach to classification, 477-479
Cayton, Tommie G., 519-534
Central auditory processing disorder, 83
Central nervous system impairment
  brain damage: see Brain damage
  child abuse and, 325-326
Cerebral dwarfism, 113

Chamberlain, P., 229-247
Change, managing family resistance to, 552-553
Chemotherapy: see Psychopharmacology
Chest examination, 427
Child abuse, 282, 315-332
    assessment of, 316-317
    characteristics of children, 321-322
    characteristics of parents, 318-319
    defined, 315-316
    epidemiology of, 317-318
    etiology of, 320-328
    parent-child interaction and, 319-320
    treatment of, 328-332
Child neglect, 315-316
Childhood language disorders: see Language disorders
Children's Apperception Test (CAT), 456, 473
Children's Embedded Figures Test, 470, 473
Chlorpromazine, 226
Chronic multiple tics (CMT), 3
Chronic tics, 3
Clarification of problem situation, 435
Classification principles, 477-479
Clonidine, 17, 21-23, 511
Clorgyline, 214
Cluttering, 99
Cognitive behavior therapies, 527-528
Cognitive development, 557
    abnormal puberty and, 148, 152, 161
    assessment of, 459-471
    autism and, 50, 51, 60-62, 64, 65, 67
    child abuse and, 322
    hyperkinetic syndrome and, 254
    language disorders and, 81-82
    short stature and, 112-113
    Tourette syndrome, 16
Cognitive modeling, 528
Cohen, Donald J., 3-28
Complex motor tics, 4, 5
Complex phonic tics, 5-7
Compliant behavior, sexual abuse and, 341
Conditioning, 525, 529-531
    fears and, 175-177
    nocturnal enuresis and, 39-43
Conduct disorders, 185, 230, 244-245; see also Juvenile delinquency; School disturbances
Conners Parent Questionnaire, 266-267
Conners Teacher Questionnaire, 261, 496
Consequence cards, 302

Constitutional growth delay, 111-113, 125
Contracting, 574
Control, sexual abuse and, 348
Conversion disorders, 192-193, 497; see also Somatoform disorders
Coprolalia, 6-7
Coproxaxia, 6
CORA (Mexico City), 602
Cortical arousal, hyperkinetic syndrome and, 258
Corticosteroid therapy, 156
Cortisol, 183
Counseling; see also Focused short-term treatment in social work
    child abuse and, 329
    divorcing family and, 364-365
    sexual abuse and, 345-346
    Turner's syndrome and, 163
Counterconditioning, fears and, 174-175
Coverage of classification systems, 479
Crisis intervention, child abuse and, 330
Crisis theory, 567
Cyclothymia, 185
Cylert, 268
Cyproheptadine, 226
Cyproterone acetate, 157

"Damaged goods" syndrome, 346-347
Data collection methods, 436-444; see also Interviews; Observation
Deanol, 268
Decision-tree approach to diagnosis, 485-486
Deep-tendon reflexes, 415
Defense mechanisms, child abuse and, 324
Delayed adolescence, 154-155
Delinquency: see Juvenile delinquency
Denial, 377
Depression
    abnormal puberty and, 148
    vs. anorexia nervosa, 220
    major: see Major depressive disorder
    obsessive-compulsive disorder and, 209
    psychopharmacology and, 506-507
    in school children, 294, 296-298
    sexual abuse and, 340, 347
    Tourette syndrome and, 11
Desensitization, 526-527
    obsessive-compulsive disorder and, 214, 215
    stuttering and, 105-107
Desmethylimipramine, 38
Developmental analysis, 435

608 / INDEX

Developmental aphasia, 83
Developmental framework of classification systems, 479
Developmental history, 397-400, 411-412
 autism and, 52-54, 64
 language disorders and, 87-91
Developmental lag, psychological testing and, 453
Developmental stuttering, 98
Developmental tasks, sexual abuse and, 348
Deviant language, 82-83
Dextroamphetamine, 13
Dextroamphetamine sulfate, 267
Diabetes insipidus, 209
Diagnostic approaches, 371-512
 to abnormal puberty, 152-159, 163
 to aggressive behavior, 230-231, 235-237
 to anorexia nervosa, 220-223
 to autism, 51-68
 to child abuse, 316-317
 to divorcing family, 356-362
 DSM-III and: see *Diagnostic and Statistical Manual of Mental Disorders*
 family therapy and, 540-547
 to fears (and phobias), 171-174
 functional behavior analysis: see Functional behavior analysis
 to hyperkinetic syndrome, 259-267, 412, 418, 419
 initial clinical evaluation: see Initial clinical evaluation
 intensive evaluation: see Intensive clinical evaluation
 to juvenile delinquency, 281-288
 to language disorders, 84-93
 to major depressive disorders, 186-187
 mental status evaluation: see Mental status evaluation
 to nocturnal enuresis, 33-35
 to obsessive-compulsive disorders, 211-213
 physical examination: see Physical examination
 psychological tests: see Psychological tests
 to school disturbances, 299-301, 306-311
 to sexual abuse, 340-344
 to short stature, 115-118
 to somatoform disorders, 199-202
 to stuttering, 101-103
 to Tourette syndrome, 13-19
Diagnostic and Statistical Manual of Mental Disorders (DSM-III), 475-489
 advantages and disadvantages of, 486-489
 basic features of, 480-483
 classification principles and, 477-479
 decision-tree approach to diagnosis in, 485-486
 infancy, childhood, and adolescence section of, 483-484
 necessity of using, 476-477
 questions in diagnostic process, 475-476
 use of, 484-485
Differentiation in classification systems, 479
Dimensional approach to classification, 477
Disengaged families, 544
Disintegrative psychosis, 65, 66
Disruptive behavior, 294-296
Dissociation, 198-199
Divorcing family, 353-367
 assessment of, 356-362
 associated conditions and, 355-356
 clinical features of, 354-355
 epidemiology of, 353-354
 guidelines to decision making and, 362
 joint or shared custody and, 363-364
 treatment of, 364-366
 written psychiatric report and, 366-367
DMI, 189
Door, The,-A Center of Alternatives, 584-602
Dopamine, 12, 256, 508
Dopamine-deficiency hypothesis, 503
Dose-response studies, 500-501
Draw-A-Person Test, 382-383, 457
Drawing pictures, 379-380, 382-383, 418-419, 457
Drug therapy: see Psychopharmacology
"Dry-bed" procedure, 41
DSM-III: see *Diagnostic and Statistical Manual of Mental Disorders*
Durell Analysis of Reading Difficulty Test, 467, 473
Durrell-Sullivan Reading Capacity and Achievement Tests, 466, 473
Dyad therapy in incest cases, 346
Dysarthrias, 80
Dysfluency, normal, vs. stuttering, 97-98, 102-103, 106
Dysgraphesthesia, 415
Dysmorphic short stature, 111, 112
Dysphasia, 83
Dysthymia, 185

Easier stuttering approach, 105, 107
Echolalia, 7-8

Echopraxia, 7-8
Education for All Handicapped Children Act, 93
Ego functioning impairment, child abuse and, 322-323
Ehrhardt, Anke A., 145-164
Electroencephalography (EEG)
 feedback, 532
 hyperkinetic syndrome and, 266
 juvenile delinquency and, 288
 Tourette syndrome and, 14, 16
Electromyograph (EMG) feedback, 531-532
Emotional release, 555
Endocrine clinics, 127-128
Endocrinologists, 150, 154, 162
Enmeshed families, 544
Enuresis, nocturnal, 29-44
 assessment of, 33-34
 associated conditions and, 30-31
 bladder disturbances and, 32
 clinical features of, 29
 conditioning and, 39-43
 differential diagnosis and, 31
 epidemiology of, 29-30
 etiology of, 31-32
 fluid restriction and, 34, 36
 genetic transmission of, 31
 hypnosis and, 37
 initial observation and, 42
 mental-status evaluation and, 35
 natural history of, 30
 night waking and, 36
 overlearning and, 43, 44
 physical examination and, 35
 psychometric evaluation and, 35
 psychopharmacology and, 37-38, 43-44, 504-505
 psychotherapy for, 37
 reassurance and, 35-36
 retention-control training for, 38-39
 social-learning factors in, 32
 surgery for, 36-37
 treatment of, 35-44
Environmental analysis, 435-436
Epilepsy
 autism and, 51
 juvenile delinquency and, 278, 280
 vs. nocturnal enuresis, 31
 vs. Tourette syndrome, 14
Estrogen, 146
Estorgen therapy, 159, 161
Estrogen-progestin therapy, 156

Exposure treatment, obsessive-compulsive disorder and, 214
Extinction, 530
Eye examination, 427

Face tests, 414
Factitious disorder, 185-186, 196
Familial short stature, 111
Family
 aggressive behavior and, 232-235
 autism and, 72-74
 divorce and: see Divorcing family
 fears and, 173, 179
 hyperkinetic syndrome and, 253
 individual psychotherapy and, 559-560
 language disorders and, 87
 short stature and, 122-123
 Turner's syndrome and, 163-164
Family history, 401-404
Family life cycle, 544-545
Family structure, 542-544
Family therapy, 539-553
 anorexia nervosa and, 226
 child abuse and, 329-330
 diagnosis in, 540-541
 divorce and, 365
 family system assessment, 541-547
 indications and contraindications for, 553
 locus of pathology and, 539-540
 sexual abuse and, 346
 somatoform disorders and, 203-204
 techniques of, 547-553
Fears (and phobias), 169-180
 assessment of, 172-174
 clinical features of, 169
 content of, 169-170
 differential diagnosis and, 171-172
 epidemiology of, 169-170
 etiology of, 170-171
 vs. obsessive-compulsive disorder, 210
 sexual abuse and, 340, 347
 stuttering and, 102, 103
 treatment of, 174-180, 526-527
Feldman, Richard S., 432-444
Fenfluramine, 509
Ferry, P. C., 84, 87, 93
Finger-to-nose test, 414
Flooding, 527
 fears and, 175
 obsessive-compulsive disorder and, 214
Fluency-shaping approaches to stuttering, 104

Fluid restriction, nocturnal enuresis and, 34, 36
Focused short-term treatment in social work, 566-581
　applications of, 568-571
　brief model vs. open-ended treatment methods, 567-568
　case example, 577-580
　definition of model, 566-567
　implementation of model, 571-577
　suitability of model, 580-581
Food additives, hyperkinetic syndrome and, 257-258
Formal test administration, 443-444
Freud, Sigmund, 521, 554
Frustration, stuttering and, 99, 102, 103
Functional behavior analysis, 432-444
　data collection methods, 436-444
　scope of inquiry, 434-436
　target behaviors selection, 444
　unit of analysis, 433-434

Gardner, Richard A., 371-391
Generational hierarchy and subsystems, 542-543
Genetic counseling, 24
Genetic transmission
　aggressive behavior, 233
　autism, 51
　hyperkinetic syndrome, 253, 257
　juvenile delinquency, 279-280
　nocturnal enuresis, 31
　obsessive-compulsive disorder, 210
　stuttering, 100
　Tourette syndrome, 11-12
Genital examination, 428
Gilles de la Tourette syndrome: *see* Tourette syndrome
Gilmore Oral Reading Test, 466, 473
Gittleman, Rachel, 447-474
Goldberg, Penny, 566-581
Goldner, Virginia, 539-553
Goodenough-Harris Drawing Test, 418-419
Gratification of dependency needs, somatoform disorders and, 198
Gray Oral Reading Test, 466, 473
Green, Arthur, 315-332
Greenhill, Laurence L., 251-272, 409-429, 493-512
Group vs. individual testing, 449-450
Group therapy
　child abuse and, 329

　language disorders and, 94
　sexual abuse and, 345
Growing Up Small (Phifer), 127
Growth disorders: *see* Short stature
Growth hormone problems, 111-113, 154
Growth hormone therapy, 115, 125, 159-160, 162
Growth-rate evaluation, 421-424
Guilt, sexual abuse and, 347
Guitar, Barry, 97-108
Gynecomastia, 155

Hallucinations, 420
　depressive, 185
　juvenile delinquency and, 279
Halmi, Katherine A., 218-227
Haloperidol, 507
　autism and, 72
　stuttering and, 104
　Tourette syndrome and, 10, 12, 17, 20-23
Hand tests, 414-415
Head circumference measurement, 424-426
Head tests, 414
Hearing impairment, 85, 87, 88, 92
Heart examination, 427-428
Henricks, Lorraine, 583-603
Heritability: *see* Genetic transmission
Hirschberg test, 416
Hirsutism, 155-157
History taking, 393-407
　abnormal puberty and, 152-153
　aggressive behavior and, 235-237
　autism and, 51-58
　chief complaints and, 397
　child abuse and, 316
　child's psychiatric history and, 397
　clinician variables and, 395
　data and informants identification in, 397
　developmental: *see* Developmental history
　divorcing family and, 356-358
　family: *see* Family history
　fears and phobias and, 172-173
　general suggestions for, 395-396
　hyperkinetic syndrome and, 259-264
　juvenile delinquency and, 282-283
　language disorders and, 84-87
　major depressive disorder and, 186-187
　medical: *see* Medical history
　nocturnal enuresis and, 33-34
　obsessive-compulsive disorder and, 211-212

parents' contribution to, 393-394
patient variables and, 394
present illness and, 397
school, 405-406
sociocultural, 404
somatoform disorders and, 199-200
special problems in, 395
stuttering and, 101-102
Tourette syndrome and, 15, 18
Hoover test, 201
Hopping test, 416
Hormonal control of puberty, 146
Hormone therapy
abnormal puberty and, 159-162
hirsutism and, 156
short stature and, 115, 125
Hostility, sexual abuse and, 347
House-Tree-Person Test, 419, 457
Human Growth Foundation (HGF), 124, 126-127
Hyperkinetic syndrome, 251-272
assessment of, 259-267, 412, 418, 419
associated conditions and, 253-255
clinical features of, 251-252
differential diagnosis and, 259
epidemiology of, 252
etiology of, 255-259
juvenile delinquency and, 278, 280
major depressive disorder and, 184
natural history of, 252-253
psychopharmacology and, 496, 499-505
treatment of, 267-272
Hypnosis
nocturnal enuresis and, 37
somatoform disorders and, 199, 204-205
Hypnotics, autism and, 72
Hypochondriasis, 194
Hypopituitarism, 113, 115, 125

Idiopathic hirsutism, 156
Illinois Test of Psycholinguistic Abilities (ITPA), 469, 473
Imipramine, 498, 506
major depressive disorder and, 187-189
nocturnal enuresis and, 38, 43-44, 504-505
obsessive-compulsive disorder and, 214
somatoform disorders and, 206
Implosion therapy, 527
fears and, 175
obsessive-compulsive disorder and, 214

Impulse control, 304-305, 324, 331
Impulsivity
cognitive behavior therapies and, 527-528
hyperkinetic syndrome and, 251, 252, 261
Inappropriate inattention, 251
Incest, 339, 346, 349
Incongruous pubertal development, 155-157
Individual vs. group testing, 449-450
Infantile autism: see Autism, infantile
Initial clinical evaluation, 371-386, 434-435
decision whether therapy is warranted and, 384-385
interview with child, 377-383
interview with parents, 376-377
interview with parents and child, 373-376
recommendations, 385-386
screening for mild neurological impairment, 384
telephone call, 372
Insight, 555-556
Intellectual ability assessment, 459-471
Intelligence
abnormal puberty and, 146, 148, 152, 161
short stature and, 112-113
Intelligence quotient (IQ) testing, 459-466
autism and, 50, 51, 61, 62, 64, 67
child abuse and, 322
Intensive clinical evaluation, 386-391
final presentation of findings, 390-391
interviews with child, 387-390
interviews with parents, 386-387
interviews with parents and children, 387
Intermittent reinforcement, nocturnal enuresis and, 40
International Classification of Diseases-Ninth Edition, 479, 489
Interviews
aggressive behavior and, 245-247
autism and, 58-60
divorcing family and, 356, 358-360
in family therapy, 548-552
focused short-term treatment and, 574-576
functional behavior analysis and, 437-439
initial, 373-383
intensive, 386-390
juvenile delinquency and, 281-284
major depressive disorder and, 186
school disturbances and, 300, 301
sexual abuse and, 342-344
with siblings, 360-361
stuttering and, 101-102

Iowa, University of, Child Psychiatry Clinic, 300, 306-311
Iowa Silent Reading tests, 467

Johnson, Robert Wood, Foundation, 602
Johnson, Suzanne Bennett, 169-180
Joint custody, 363-364
Juvenile delinquency, 276-290
　assessment of, 281-288
　associated disorders and, 277-281
　concept of, 276-277
　epidemiology of, 277
　treatment of, 288-290

Kiddie-SADS (Schedule for Affective Disorders and Schizophrenia for Schoolage Children), 182, 186, 494

Language acquisition device, 80
Language disorders, 79-95
　assessment of, 84-93
　autism and, 49-51, 53-55, 62, 64-69
　case history, 84, 87-91
　developmental, 82
　developmental milestones for, 87, 89-91
　diagnosis of, 84, 87-93
　epidemiology of, 82
　hearing impairment and, 85, 87, 88, 92
　interdisciplinary teams and, 88, 92-93
　interviews and, 87-88
　language, defined, 81
　learning disorder and, 81-82
　medical advances and, 84
　nature of, 82-84
　neurological orientation to, 83
　psycholinguistic orientation to, 82-83
　stuttering and, 99, 102
　tests of, 469-470
　treatment of, 94-95
　types of, 84-86
Language processing disorder, 83
Language therapy, 94-95
Lead-induced brain damage, 257
Learning disabilities
　autism and, 70-71
　juvenile delinquency and, 279, 287
　language problems and, 81-82
Learning Laboratory Programs, 598-601
Learning theory, somatoform disorders and, 198
Lecithin, 23

Leckman, James F., 3-28
Levy, Alan M., 353-367
Lewis, Dorothy Otnow, 276-290
Leyton Obsessional Inventory, 212-213
Life space interviews, 302
Lithium, 226, 509-510
Little People of America (LPA), 124, 126-127
Lung examination, 427

Magnesium pemoline, 268
Major depressive disorder (MDD), 182-190
　assessment of, 186-187
　associated clinical conditions and, 184
　clincial features of, 182
　differential diagnosis and, 184-186
　epidemiology of, 183
　historical development of, 182-183
　natural history of, 183-184
　psychopharmacology and, 187-190, 497, 505, 511
Make-A-Picture Story test (MAPS), 383, 388
Malingering, 196
Mance, Jeanne, Clinic, 584
Manic depressive disorder, 497-498
Maprotiline, 38
Masochistic behavior, 325
Matching Familiar Figures Test, 470-471, 473
McCarthy Scales of Children's Abilities, 460-461, 474
McKirdy, Laura S., 79-95
Medical examination: see Physical examination
Medical history, 401-411
　autism and, 62
　juvenile delinquency and, 282-283
　nocturnal enuresis and, 33
Medical tests
　audiological, 83, 92
　autism and, 63
　language disorders, 83, 84
　of short stature, 119-121
Medication: see Psychopharmacology
Mellaril, 508
Mental retardation
　autism and, 50, 67
　language disorders and, 98
　major depressive disorder and, 186
　obsessive-compulsive disorder and, 209
　as separate axis, 487-488
　short stature and, 113

vs. Tourette syndrome, 15
    Turner's syndrome and, 162
Mental-status evaluation
    anorexia nervosa and, 223
    hyperkinetic syndrome and, 264–265
    juvenile delinquency and, 284–286
    nocturnal enuresis and, 35
    obsessive-compulsive disorder and, 213
    as part of sequence in general physical examination, 417–421
    somatoform disorders and, 201–202
Methscopolamine, 37
Methylphenidate, 499–501, 503
    hyperkinetic syndrome and, 267–268
    Tourette syndrome and, 13
Meyer-Bahlburg, Heino F. L., 110–128
Minimal brain dysfunction, 255, 265
Mirroring, Tourette syndrome and, 7–8
Moban, 508
Modeling, fears and, 177–178
Molindone hydrochloride, 508
Monoamine oxidase inhibitors, 189, 505, 506
Moody, Bobba Jean, 566–581
Motivational analysis, 435
Motor disturbances, 4–5, 192–193, 201
Mouth-opening finger-spreading phenomenon, 415–416
Multiaxial diagnosis, autism and, 63–65
Muscle strength evaluation, 415
Musculoskeletal system examination, 428
Mutual storytelling technique, 380–382

National Center on Child Abuse and Neglect, 318
National Society for Autistic Children, 74
Natural history, 476
Neck examination, 424
Negative punishment, 530
Neuroleptics, 507–509; see also Haloperidol
Neurological approach to language disorders, 83
Neurological examination
    hyperkinetic syndrome and, 266
    juvenile delinquency and, 287–288
    obsessive-compulsive disorder and, 212
    Tourette syndrome and, 16
Neurological impairment
    autism and, 50
    child abuse and, 325–326
    brain damage: see Brain damage
    screening for, 384
Neurological signs, soft, 412–417

Neurologists, 93
Neurotransmitter systems, Tourette syndrome and, 12
New York State Child Protective Services Act of 1973, 315–316
Night waking, nocturnal enuresis and, 36
Nocturnal enuresis. See Enuresis, nocturnal
Nortriptyline, 189, 507

Object phobias: see Fears
Obscene language (coprolalia), 6–7
Observation
    aggressive behavior and, 238–240
    autism and, 58–60
    functional behavior analysis and, 440–443
    hyperkinetic syndrome and, 264–265
    in physical examination, 412, 417–418
    stuttering and, 101
Obsessive-compulsive disorder, 208–215
    assessment of, 211–213
    associated conditions and, 208–209
    clinical features of, 208
    differential diagnosis and, 209–210
    etiology of, 210–211
    history-taking and, 211–212
    Tourette syndrome and, 11, 12, 14
    treatment of, 213–215
Oedipus complex, somatoform disorders and, 197–198
Onset enuresis, 30
Operant conditioning, 175–177, 525, 529–531
Opposition test, 415
Oppositional behavior, 230, 240–244
Outreach services, 330
Outward Bound, 305
Overactivity, 251, 252, 262
Overcorrection, 531
Overlearning, nocturnal enuresis and, 40–41, 43, 44

Palilalia, 7–8
Paranoid symptomatology, juvenile delinquency and, 285
Parent Daily Report (PDR), 235, 236
Parents; see also Family; Family history; Genetic transmission; Interviews
    abusing: see Child abuse
    focused short-term treatment and, 568–571
    history taking and, 393–396
    -infant speech and language therapy, 94
    psychopathology of, delinquency and, 279–280
    stuttering and, 101

Pathological object relationships, child abuse and, 223-324
Patterson, G. R., 229-247
Pavlov, Ivan P., 521-522
Peabody Individual Achievement Test (PIAT), 254, 467, 468, 474
Peabody Picture Vocabulary Test, 62, 463, 474
Peabody Picture Vocabulary Test-Revised (PPVT-R), 378
Peer relations
  hyperkinetic syndrome and, 254
  short stature and, 114, 123-124
Pemoline, 13, 268
Personality testing, 457-458
Pervasive developmental disorders: see Autism, infantile
Pharmacotherapy: see Psychopharmacology
Phenothiazines, 495
  autism and, 71-72
  Tourette syndrome and, 23
Phifer, Kate G., 127
Phobias: see Fears
Phonation, gentle onset of, 104
Phonic tics, 4-7
Physical approaches to school disturbances, 305
Physical examination, 409-429
  of abdomen, 428
  anorexia nervosa and, 222-223
  approach to the patient, 410
  of auditory acuity, 427
  autism and, 62-63
  of chest, heart, and lungs, 427-428
  child abuse and, 316-317
  of eyes, 427
  of genitals and rectum, 428
  of growth-rate, 421-424
  of head circumference, 424-426
  history taking and: see Medical history
  major depressive disorder and, 187
  mental status: see Mental status evaluation
  of musculoskeletal system, 428
  nocturnal enuresis and, 35
  observation and, 412
  obsessive-compulsive disorder and, 212
  sexual abuse and, 342
  short stature and, 115-116, 119
  of skull and neck, 424
  for soft neurological signs, 412-417
  somatoform disorders and, 200-201
  Tourette syndrome and, 16
  of vital signs, 424

Physical illness
  symptoms complicating, 193
  symptoms simulating, 193
  undiagnosed, 195-196
Physical symptoms of sexual abuse, 342
Physical therapy, somatoform disorders and, 205
Physostigmine, 23
Picture drawing, 379-380, 382-383, 418-419, 457
Pimozinde, 22-23
Placebos, 203, 496
Playacting, 557
Play behavior
  autism and, 49-50, 53-54, 57-58, 60-61, 65
  psychotherapy and, 558-559
Play therapy, sexual abuse and, 348
Point contract, 240-242, 246, 247
Polyuria vs. nocturnal enuresis, 31
Porteus Maze Test, 470, 474
Positive punishment, 530
Positive reinforcement, 529-530
Precocious puberty, 149-154
Premarin, 159
Problem exploration, definition and clarification, 571-573
Problem solving, 304, 527-528; see also Focused short-term treatment in social work
Progesterone, 146, 159
Projective tests, 455-459
Propantheline, 37
Propranolol, 510-511
Provera, 159
Proverbs, 420
Pseudo-maturity, sexual abuse and, 341, 348
Psychiatric reports, divorcing families and, 366-367
Psychoactive medication. see Psychopharmacology
Psychoanalytic theory, somatoform disorders and, 197-198, 204
Psychogenic pain disorder, 193; see also Somatoform disorders
Psycholinguistic approach to language disorders, 82-83
Psychological tests, 447-474
  anorexia nervosa and, 222-223
  autism and, 58-62
  fears and phobias and, 173
  functional behavior analysis and, 443-444
  general issues in, 447-452

hyperkinetic syndrome and, 265-266
initial, 378-383, 387-390
intellectual ability assessment, 459-471
juvenile delinquency and, 286-287
language disorders and, 93
list of, 473-474
nocturnal enuresis and, 35
obsessive-compulsive disorder and, 212
practical issues in, 453-455
projective, 455-459
short stature and, 118
somatoform disorders and, 202
Psychopharmacology, 493-512
abnormal puberty and, 153-154, 156-157, 159-161
ages-associated differences in, 496-498
aggressive, 509-511
anorexia nervosa and, 226
autism and, 71-72
disturbed adolescents and, 498
drug management issues, 494-496
fears and, 178
history of, 493-494
hyperkinetic syndrome and, 267-271, 496, 499-505
major depressive disorder and, 187-190, 497, 505, 511
nocturnal enuresis and, 37-38, 43-44, 504-505
obsessive-compulsive disorder and, 213-214
review of, 499-511
somatoform disorders and, 206
stuttering and, 104
Tourette syndrome and, 10, 12-13, 20-23, 511
Psychosexual development
abnormal puberty and, 147, 150-155, 160
short stature and, 124-125
Psychosocial schedule (PSS), 186-187
Psychosocial short stature, 111, 112
Psychotherapy, 554-565
abnormal puberty and, 153
aggressive behavior and, 237
anorexia nervosa and, 224, 226-227
approaches to treatment, 557-560
case examples, 560-565
child abuse and, 329, 331
divorcing family and, 364-365
hyperkinetic syndrome and, 269
indications for, 555-557
juvenile delinquency and, 289

major depressive disorder and, 189
nocturnal enuresis and, 37
obsessive-compulsive disorder and, 213
rationale for, 555-556
sexual abuse and, 345-346, 348
somatoform disorders and, 203-204
stuttering and, 105, 106
Pubertal failure, 157-164
Puberty, abnormal, 145-164
behavior changes and disturbances, 147-148
behavior problems associated with, 148-164
delayed adolescence, 154-155
epidemiology of, 147-148
gynecomastia, 155
hirsutism, 155-157
incongruous pubertal development, 155-157
mental functioning and, 148
vs. normal puberty, 145-146
precocious puberty, 149-154
psychopathology and, 147-148, 151-152
psychosexual development and, 147, 150-151, 154
pubertal failure, 157-164
Turner's syndrome, 158-164
Puig-Antich, Joaquim, 182-190
Punishment for aversive behavior, 243-244, 246-247
Purdue Pegboard, 470, 474

Race
IQ testing and, 465-466
juvenile delinquency and, 280-281
Rape crisis centers, 350
Rapid Automatized Naming Test, 469, 474
Rapoport, Judith L., 208-215
Rating scales, 439
Raven's Progressive Matrices, 61-62
Reading tests, 466-468
Reassurance
anorexia nervosa and, 223-224
child abuse and, 331
fears and, 174
nocturnal enuresis and, 35-36
somatoform disorders and, 203
Tourette syndrome and, 19
Receptive-Expressive Emergent Language Scale, 87
Recommendation, initial, 385-386
Rectal examination, 428

Reeducation, 556
Regressive behavior, sexual abuse and, 340
Reinforcement, 529–531
  nocturnal enuresis and, 40
  of prosocial behavior, 240–242, 246
Reinforcement contingency, 433–434
Reinforcement menus, 440, 531
Relationship, 555
Reliability
  of diagnostic categories, 478
  of tests, 448–449
Research Diagnostic Criteria (RDC), 183, 185, 494
Resistant children, enticement of, 378–379
Respiration, controlled, 104
Restitution, 531
Restless behavior in school, 294–296
Retardation: see Mental retardation
Retention-control training, 38–39
Rhythm disorders, 80
Rhythmic speech, 104
Right-left orientation, 413–414
Ritalin, 267–271
Role confusion, sexual abuse and, 347–348
Role reversal, child abuse and, 320–321
Romberg examination, modified, 415
Rorschach test, 286, 456, 458, 474
Rostra-caudal progression of motor tics, 10
Roswell-Chall tests, 467, 474
Running test, 416
Russo, Dennis C., 519–534
Rutter, Michael, 48–74

Scapegoating, 321
Schizophrenia
  vs. anorexia nervosa, 221
  vs. autism, 66
  juvenile delinquency and, 278, 280
  language disorders and, 86
  obsessive-compulsive disorder and, 209
  psychopharmacology and, 507–508
School
  autistic children and, 73–74
  language disorders and, 93, 94
  short stature and, 117–118, 121, 123, 125–126, 136–138
  Tourette syndrome and, 23–24
School disturbances, 293–311
  assessment of, 299–301, 306–311
  child abuse and, 325, 331
  epidemiology of, 293–294

psychological testing and, 453
treatment of, 302–305
types of problems, 294–299
School history, 405–406
School performance; see also School disturbances
  hyperkinetic syndrome and, 254
  psychological testing and, 453, 466–468
  sexual abuse and, 341
  Tourette syndrome and, 16
School phobia, 497, 507
Secondary enuresis, 30
Self-awareness, school disturbances and, 302–303
Self-concept, child abuse and, 324
Self-control analysis, 435
Self-control treatments, 178, 528
Self-destructive behavior, Tourette syndrome and, 5
Self-esteem
  school disturbances and, 294, 298–299, 301
  sexual abuse and, 347
Self-instruction, 528
Sensitivity cards, 302
Sensitivity values, 450–452
Sensory-discharge cycle in Tourette syndrome, 8–9
Sensory disturbances, 193, 200–201
Serotonergic mechanisms, Tourette syndrome and, 12
Serotonin, 256
Service Utilization Study, 585
Services for adolescents: see Adolescent services
Sex chromosome abnormalities, 157–164
Sex hormones
  abnormal puberty and, 158, 159, 161
  normal puberty and, 146
  short stature and, 125
Sexual abuse, 336–350
  assessment of, 340–344
  defining characteristics of, 336
  epidemiology of, 338–340
  myths about, 337–338
  prevalence of, 336–337
  prevention of, 349–350
  treatment of, 344–348
Shaffer, David, 29–44
Shame, stuttering and, 102, 103
Shaping, 529–530
Shared custody, 363–364
Shaywitz, Bennett A., 3–28

Short stature, 110-144
  assessment of, 115-118
  assessment guide for, 130-135
  behavioral development and, 112-113
  classification of, 111-112
  literature on, 127
  management team and, 127-128
  medical education and, 119-121
  medical treatment of, 119
  physical environment and, 110, 116, 121, 137-144
  physical examination and, 115-116, 119
  psychiatric sequelae and, 113-117, 122-125
  psychometric examination and, 118
  psychosocial management of, 118-128
  school and, 117-118, 121, 123, 125-126, 136-138
  self-help organizations and, 126-127
Short-term treatment: see Focused short-term treatment in social work
Shy school children, 294, 296-299
Siblings
  abuse committed by, 317
  aggressive behavior and, 233
  fears and, 173
  history taking and, 394
  hyperkinetic syndrome and, 260
  incest and, 339
  joint interviews in divorcing families and, 360-361
  Turner's syndrome and, 163-164
Similarities, 420
Simple motor tics, 4, 5
Simple phonic tics, 5
Situational fears: see Fears
Skeletal dysplasias, 111-113, 122, 125
Skinner, B. F., 521-523
Skinner, Linda J., 336-350
Skull examination, 424
Slow speech, 104, 107
Social factors
  in hyperkinetic syndrome, 256
  in juvenile delinquency, 280
Social interaction
  aggressive children and, 233-235
  autism and, 55-57
  short stature and, 110, 113-115, 122-124
Social learning
  aggressive behavior and, 237-247
  nocturnal enuresis and, 32
Social-learning theory, 527
Social relationships analysis, 435

Social work, focused short-term treatment in: see Focused short-term treatment in social work
Socialized conduct disorder, 294, 296
Sociocultural history, 404
Sodium amobarbital, 203
Soft neurological signs, 412-417
Somatoform disorders, 192-206
  vs. anorexia nervosa, 221
  assessment of, 199-202
  clinical features of, 192-194
  differential diagnosis of, 195-197
  epidemiology of, 195
  etiology of, 197-199
  treatment of, 202-206
S-O-R-K-C model, 434-436
Specific language deficit, 83
Specificity values, 450-452
Speech disorders, 79-80
  autism and, 49, 51, 55, 69
  developmental milestones and, 87, 88
  incidence of, 82
  stuttering: see Stuttering
Speech evaluation, 416
Speech Foundation of America, 100
Speech and language pathologist, 92
Speech therapy, 94-95
Spelling tests, 468
Spreen-Benton Memory for Sentences Test, 469
Squeeze-clip test, 415
SRA Achievement Series, 467, 474
Stammering: see Stuttering
Standard Reading Test, 467, 474
Standardization of tests, 447-448
Stanford Achievement Tests, 467, 474
Stanford-Binet Intelligence Scale, 460-462, 474
Stanford-Binet Memory Test for Sentences, 469
Star chart, 36
Stereognosis, 414-415
Stewart, Mark A., 293-311
Stigmatization, short stature and, 110, 114
Stimulants
  hyperkinetic syndrome and, 267-268, 270-271, 499-504
  Tourette syndrome and, 12-13
Stimulus feeding, fears and, 176-177
Stimulus prepotency, 171
Storytelling, mutual, 380-382
Strabismus test, 416

618 / INDEX

Strategic family therapy, 547
Structural abnormalities, speech and, 80
Structural family therapy, 547
Stuttering, 97-108
   assessment of, 101-103
   associated conditions and, 99-100
   attitude/stuttering modification approaches to, 105
   developmental, 98
   etiology of, 100-101
   fluency-shaping approaches to, 104
   vs. normal childhood dysfluency, 97-98, 102-103, 106
   treatment of, 103-108
Subacute sclerosing panencephalitis (SSPE), 15
Suggestion, 203, 556
Suicidal ideation, 420-421
Suicide, 497
Support, 556
Surgical treatment
   nocturnal enuresis and, 36-37
   obsessive-compulsive disorder and, 215
Swenson, Reggie, 556-581
Syndenham's chorea vs. Tourette syndrome, 15
Systematic desensitization, 526-527

Talking, Feeling, and Doing Game, The, 389
Tandem gait, 416
Tardive dyskinesia (TD), 20, 22, 509
Task Force on Nomenclature and Statistics of American Psychiatric Association, 479-480
Telephone call, initial, 372
Testosterone, 154, 156
Tests: see Medical tests; Psychological tests
Thematic Apperception Test (TAT), 383, 456, 457, 474
Thioridazine, 508
Tic disorders
   chronic, 3
   Tourette syndrome: see Tourette syndrome
   transient, 31, 13-14
Time-out procedure, 243-244, 530-531
Timing errors, pubertal, 148-155
Tiptoe walking, 416
Token economies, 531
Token Test, 469
Total Aversive Behavior, 229
Tourette syndrome (TS), 3-28, 418
   academic intervention and, 23-24
   assessment of, 15-19
   associated disorders, 7
   behavioral symptoms of, 4, 7-9
   clinical expression of, 4-7
   coprolalia and, 6-7
   differential diagnosis of, 13-15
   epidemiology of, 11
   etiology of, 12-13
   genetic counseling and, 24
   genetic transmission of, 11-12
   monitoring of, 19
   motor symptoms of, 4-5
   multiply handicapped patients, 24-25
   natural history of, 10-11
   obsessive-compulsive disorder and, 209
   phenomenology of, 7-9
   phonic symptoms of, 4-7
   psychopharmacology and, 10, 20-23, 511
   reassurance and, 19
   research on, 26
   treatment of, 19-25
   Yale Tourette Syndrome Sympton List, 27-28
Tranquilizers, major, 71-72, 507-509
Transactional analysis, 302
Transient tics, 3, 13-14
Traumatic reaction to child abuse, 323
Treatment approaches
   to aggressive behavior, 237-247
   to anorexia nervosa, 223-227
   to autism, 68-74
   behavior therapies: see Behavior therapies
   to child abuse victims, 328-332
   to child molestation victims, 344-348
   decision about need for, 384-385
   to divorcing family, 364-367
   family therapy: see Family therapy
   to fears, 174-180
   focused short-term: see Focused short-term treatment in social work
   to hyperkinetic syndrome, 267-272
   to juvenile delinquency, 288-390
   to language disorders, 94-95
   to major depressive disorders, 187-190
   to nocturnal enuresis, 35-44
   to obsessive-compulsive disorder, 213-215
   psychopharmacology: see Psychopharmacology
   psychotherapy: see Psychotherapy
   to school disturbances, 302-305
   to short stature, 119, 125, 127
   to somatoform disorders, 202-206

to stuttering, 103–108
to Tourette syndrome, 19–25
to Turner's syndrome, 159–160, 163, 164
Tricyclic antidepressants (TCAs): *see also* Imipramine
anorexia nervosa and, 226
conversion disorders and, 497
hyperkinetic syndrome and, 505
major depressive disorder and, 187–189, 505
mood disorder and, 506–507
nocturnal enuresis and, 38, 43–44, 504–505
toxicity of, 498
Trust, sexual abuse and, 340, 347
Turner, Henry, 158
Turner's syndrome, 113, 116, 118, 125, 157–164

Undiagnosed physical illness, 195–196
Urinary tract infection, nocturnal enuresis and, 31
Utility of classification systems, 479

Validity of diagnostic categories, 478–479
Verbal apraxias, 80
Verbal Language Development Scale, 87
Vineland Social Maturity Scale, 60, 122
Vital-sign measures, 424

Vitamin therapy, autism and, 72
Voice disorders, 80

Watson, John B., 521, 522
Wechsler Intelligence Scale for Children (WISC), 61, 286
Wechsler Intelligence Scale for Children-Revised (WISC-R), 266, 462–463, 468, 471, 474
Wechsler Intelligence Scale for Preschool Children, 61
Wechsler Preschool and Primary Scales of Intelligence (WPPSI), 461, 474
Welton, Anna, 566–581
Wide Range Achievement Test (WRAT), 254, 466, 468, 474
Williams, Daniel T., 192–206
Wilson's disease vs. Tourette syndrome, 15
Winnicott's Squiggle Technique, 389
Withdrawal, short stature and, 114
Withdrawn school children, 294, 296–299
Woodcock Reading Mastery Test, 167, 474

Yale Child Study Center Tourette Syndrome research group, 3*n*
Yale Tourette Syndrome Symptom List, 27–28
Youth Services Center (Canada), 602